Communication Sciences and Disorders

An Introduction

Communication Sciences and Disorders

An Introduction

Laura M. Justice

University of Virginia

PEARSON
Merrill
Prentice Hall

Upper Saddle River, New Jersey
Columbus, Ohio

Library of Congress Cataloging-in-Publication Data

Justice, Laura M.
Communication sciences and disorders : an introduction / Laura M. Justice.—1st ed.
p. cm.
Includes bibliographical references and index.
ISBN 0-13-113518-X (paper)
1. Communicative disorders. 2. Speech disorders. 3. Language disorders. I. Title.

RC523.J87 2006
616.85′5—dc22

2005046950

Vice President and Executive Publisher: Jeffery W. Johnston
Acquisitions Editor: Allyson P. Sharp
Development Editor: Heather Doyle Fraser
Editorial Assistant: Kathleen S. Burk
Production Editor: Sheryl Glicker Langner
Photo Coordinator: Valerie Schultz
Design Coordinator: Diane C. Lorenzo
Cover Design: Ali Mohrman
Cover Image: Corbis
Production Manager: Laura Messerly
Director of Marketing: Ann Castel Davis
Marketing Manager: Autumn Purdy
Marketing Coordinator: Brian Mounts

This book was set in Berkeley Book by TechBooks/GTS York, PA. It was printed and bound by Courier/Kendallville. The cover was printed by The Lehigh Press, Inc.

Photo Credits: Patrick White/Merrill, p. 2; Trish Gant © Dorling Kindersley, pp. 7, 325; Tracy Morgan © Dorling Kindersley, p. 10; Scott Cunningham/Merrill, pp. 18, 75, 111, 117, 120, 147, 190, 357, 428, 432; Anne Vega/Merrill, pp. 23, 113, 142, 182, 204, 225, 246, 396; Todd Yarrington/Merrill, pp. 38, 284, 286; Shirley Zeiberg/PH College, p. 43; Eddie Lawrence © Dorling Kindersley, pp. 48, 290, 406; David Mager/Pearson Learning Photo Studio, p. 69; Anthony Magnacca/Merrill, pp. 78, 212, 228, 348, 358, 405, 510; Dan Floss/Merrill, pp. 84, 443; Silver Burdett Ginn, pp. 85, 93; Simon Brown © Dorling Kindersley, courtesy of Simon Brown, p. 101; Laura Dwight/Peter Arnold, Inc., p. 106; Barbara Schwartz/Merrill, pp. 155, 436, 442; Michael Newman/PhotoEdit, p. 162; Larissa Siebicke/Das Fotoarchiv/Peter Arnold, Inc., p. 164; Tom Watson/Merrill, p. 168; Susanna Price © Dorling Kindersley, p. 180; Tom Wilcox/Merrill, pp. 198, 322; EMG Education Management Group, pp. 216, 484; Spencer Grant/PhotoEdit, pp. 254, 266; Bill Aron/PhotoEdit, p. 258; EyeWire Collection/Getty Images—Photodisc, pp. 259, 260; Dave King © Dorling Kindersley, p. 301; Vanessa Davies © Dorling Kindersley, p. 303; David Young-Wolff/PhotoEdit, p. 324; Ed Young/Photo Researchers, Inc., p. 332; Ken Glaser/Index Stock Imagery, Inc., p. 337; AP/Wide World Photos, p. 351; William Philpott/Getty Images/Time Life Pictures, p. 354; Photolibrary.com, p. 386; Robin Sachs/PhotoEdit, p. 393; Mike Peters/Silver Burdett Ginn, p. 468; Tessa Codrington/Getty Images, Inc.—Stone Allstock, p. 474; Francesca Yorke © Dorling Kindersley, p. 478; Tony Freeman/PhotoEdit, p. 492; Richard Lord/PhotoEdit, p. 500; Eric Fowke/PhotoEdit, p. 504; Ariel Skelley/Corbis/Bettmann, p. 519; p. 522 Courtesy of DynaVox Systems LLC, Pittsburgh, PA (1-866-DYNAVOX).

Pearson Education Ltd.
Pearson Education Singapore Pte. Ltd.
Pearson Education Canada, Ltd.
Pearson Education—Japan
Pearson Education Australia Pty. Limited
Pearson Education North Asia Ltd.
Pearson Educación de Mexico, S.A. de C.V.
Pearson Education Malaysia Pte. Ltd.

PEARSON
Merrill
Prentice Hall

10 9 8 7 6 5 4 3 2 1
ISBN: 0-13-113518-X

I dedicate this book to Ian and Addie Mykel.
Ian, I thank you for your
unwavering support, kindness,
and humor; Addie, I thank you for being an
amazing and delightful inspiration every day of my life.

Preface

Developing the Text: A New Approach

The summer of 2002 found me at home on maternity leave, learning how to be a mother to a new daughter. I used this time not only to learn how to be a mom but also to think, from a distance, about my discipline of communication sciences and disorders and to consider where we have come from as a field and where we are going in this new century. I thought about how rapidly our field seems to change to keep pace with innovations in technology, new educational policies, the shifting demographics of the population, the emerging scientific literature on disease and disability, and the like.

I conceived this book that summer as I considered the communication sciences and disorders disciplines and examined how well they are assimilating the changes affecting our knowledge base and our practices. As a university professor, I was familiar with the available texts that both provided a survey of the field and introduced promising scholars to the study and practice of human communication disorders. As a practicing clinician, I realized that these books did not contain enough authentic, real-life examples to engage my students' interest in or understanding of the field. I wanted an innovative and contemporary textbook that would not only be up-to-date in its substantive content, including theory and research, but would also bring the field to life for the introductory student. Such a text would have to provide students with a foundation in communication sciences and expose them to the primary types of communication disorders, while also presenting this core information in a new light.

Communication Sciences and Disorders: An Introduction introduces students to the field in a clear and succinct manner that allows access to the most current theories, research, and practices through rich examples and anecdotes. It employs a clinical case-based, lifespan approach with special attention given to certain areas:

- The application of knowledge, skills, and concepts through comprehensive case studies, which include evaluation and treatment plans and multimedia samples
- The ecological impact of communication disorders at home, at school, at work, and in the community, with an emphasis on functional assessment and outcomes
- Multicultural issues, emphasizing the interactions among culture, communication ability, and communication disability
- Research-based practices in assessment and intervention
- Pediatric impairments in feeding and swallowing
- Contemporary hot topics associated with the ongoing evolution of the speech, language, and hearing disciplines

Organization of the Text: A Unique Perspective

The organization of this textbook provides a useful framework to ensure students' understanding of basic concepts and principles in part I. Then, in part II students can apply these concepts and principles to each disorder presented. Within part II each disorder appears in a self-contained chapter. Thus, instructors can follow the suggested order of presentation or adopt an order based on their own preferences.

Part I includes four chapters that introduce the key principles and theories in communication sciences and disorders that are needed to understand disordered communication. Chapter 1 defines communication, provides an overview of different types of communication disorders, and identifies those professionals who work most closely with persons with communication disorders. Chapter 2 describes communication development across the lifespan, including major milestones from birth through adolescence. Chapter 3 describes the anatomical and physiological bases of communication and communication disorders, including key terms and concepts required to understand the structures and functions of the human body involved with speech, hearing, language, and swallowing. Chapter 4 discusses general principles and practices of communication assessment and intervention, laying a foundation for concepts such as psychometric terminology, categories of common tests and measures, and prevalent intervention approaches.

Part II includes eleven chapters, each surveying a particular disorder of communication and following a similar organization to provide coherence to the discussion. Each chapter addresses a set of key questions concerning the definition, classification, defining characteristics, identification, and treatment of a disorder. Chapters 5 and 6 describe disorders of speech-sound production, with chapter 5 devoted to phonological disorders and chapter 6 to motor speech disorders. Chapters 7 and 8 describe disorders of language, with chapter 7 focusing on disorders affecting children and adolescents and chapter 8 addressing acquired disorders and other cognitive-based dysfunctions in adults. Chapters 9 and 10 both describe disorders of swallowing, or dysphagia. Chapter 9 examines swallowing and feeding disorders in pediatric populations, whereas chapter 10 describes dysphagia in adults. Chapter 11 describes voice disorders as they affect the young through the elderly, and chapter 12 describes fluency disorders, or stuttering. Chapters 13 and 14 examine hearing loss, with chapter 13 focusing on pediatric populations and chapter 14 focusing on the adult population. Chapter 15 describes a special population of individuals, those whose communication needs are significant enough to require an augmentative and alternative system for communicating.

Key Features of the Text: Bringing the Field to Life

Throughout all of the chapters in the text, students receive ample opportunities to build and extend their knowledge. Each feature is designed not only to facilitate students' comprehension of key topics, but also to entice their interest in the field through clinical case-based connections, a lifespan perspective, and active learning.

Clinical, Case-Based Connections

- *Clinical problem-solving:* Each of the 11 disorders chapters features an authentic case providing assessment and/or treatment reports for students to study and discuss. For instance, in chapter 9, students read a clinical report for Joshua Harvey, 32 months, who is being enrolled in an outpatient feeding program for young children. In this way students receive authentic examples from the field to contextualize information in the chapter and to extend their learning.
- *Case examples:* Each of the 11 disorders chapters also features three case examples at the opening of the chapter. These vignettes provide examples of how disorders of communication affect children and adults in various ways, enabling students to draw connections among research, theory, and practice through discussion and reflection.
- *Multicultural considerations:* Each chapter features a special boxed insert that introduces a topic related to multicultural influences on the field of communication sciences and disorders. For instance, one of the inserts (Box 8-2, page 270) discusses the issue of

bilingualism in adult language disorders and the ways an acquired disorder of language affects bilingual individuals.

- *Ecological contexts:* Each of the 11 disorders chapters features a special boxed insert that considers how a specific disorder of communication affects an individual's life at home, school, and work and in the community. This boxed insert focuses on the *functional impact* of different communicative impairments and asks students to reflect on various ways communicative difficulties affect a person's life in different contexts. In chapter 13, for instance, the ecological contexts insert considers how hearing loss in children affects their access to educational programs.
- *Research and practice spotlights:* Each chapter features two special boxed inserts that spotlight individuals currently working as researchers and practitioners in the field of communication sciences and disorders. These special inserts introduce students to the wealth of possibilities available in both research and clinical practice. Chapter 2, for instance, spotlights Jennifer Anderson, a program manager at Microsoft who works to develop speech recognition software; chapter 7 spotlights Claudia Dunaway, a lead speech-language pathologist in San Diego Public Schools. Speaking in their own words, 30 researchers and practitioners tell what they are currently doing in the field.

A Lifespan Perspective

This book carefully considers the impact of communication disorders across the lifespan. In part I a foundation is laid for students to consider communication development and its disorders across the human lifespan; students then apply this foundation throughout part II as they study disorders affecting communication processes in infants, young children, adolescents, adults, and the elderly. Departing from other introductory textbooks, I include both a hearing loss chapter and a chapter on feeding and swallowing disorders focused exclusively on children, with companion chapters addressing these topics in the adult population.

Active Learning

This book is unique among introductory texts in communication sciences and disorders in its emphasis on active learning by students. Active learning occurs when students engage with the material through reflection and discussion. To promote students' active engagement, this text includes a variety of special features:

- *Focus questions:* Each chapter opens with a series of focus questions to orient the learner to the content of the chapter and the way the content is organized.
- *Discussion points:* Each chapter is peppered with discussion points as margin notes, which ask students to pause and consider various provocative topics associated with the content.
- *Boxed features:* The special boxed features focused on multicultural issues and ecological contexts also include discussion and reflection questions that will help to extend students' learning.

Supplementary Materials: A Wealth of Resources for Students and Professors

The text itself is designed to support learning and facilitate better understanding of chapter concepts through the features discussed here. In addition, both students and professors can benefit from a wealth of supplementary materials.

Companion Website

Located at **http://www.prenhall.com/justice**, the Companion Website for this text includes a wealth of resources for both professors and students. The Syllabus Manager™ enables professors to create and maintain the class syllabus online, while also allowing the student access to the syllabus at any time from any computer on the Internet. The student portion of the Companion Website helps students gauge their understanding of chapter content through the use of online chapter overviews, reflection questions, suggested readings and other resources, and interactive self-assessments (multiple choice, true/false, and short-answer quizzes).

Communication Sciences and Disorders: An Interactive Multimedia Introduction CD-ROM

The CD-ROM that accompanies the text provides immediate access to clinical case examples of the communication disorders presented in the text. Each of the five cases on the CD contains nine video clips, which give students an opportunity to hear directly from individuals experiencing communicative impairments and to observe authentic assessment and treatment activities. These video snapshots provide a means for the instructor to bring the field to life for students—through observation, discussion, and reflection.

Instructor's Manual with Test Items and TestGen Software

Instructors will find a wealth of resources to support their introductory course within the text itself. Each chapter contains focus questions, key terms, chapter summaries, and numerous discussion questions to be infused throughout lectures and to engage students' interest. Beyond the text, instructors receive a manual (also available online at the Instructor Resource Center, described here, at **www.prenhall.com**), which includes chapter overviews, chapter outlines and instructional guides, key terms, discussion questions, suggested readings and resources, and a list of PowerPoint slides and transparency masters. Test items include multiple choice, true/false, short answer, and essay (40–45 questions per chapter). The computerized version of these test items (TestGen) is available in both Windows and Macintosh format, along with assessment software allowing professors to create and customize exams and track student progress.

Overhead Transparencies/PowerPoints

The transparencies—available in PowerPoint slide format by going to the Instructor Resource Center, described next, at **www.prenhall.com**—highlight key concepts and summarize content from the text.

Instructor Resource Center

The Instructor Resource Center at **www.prenhall.com** has a variety of print and media resources available in downloadable, digital format—all in one location. As a registered faculty member, you can access and download pass-code protected resource files, course management content, and other premium online content directly to your computer.

Digital resources available for *Communication Sciences and Disorders: An Introduction* include:

- Text-specific PowerPoint lectures
- An online version of the Instructor's Manual

To access these items online, go to **www.prenhall.com** and click on the Instructor Support button; then go to the Download Supplements section. Here you will be able to log in or complete a one-time registration for a user name and password. If you have any questions regarding this process or the materials available online, please contact your local Prentice Hall sales representative.

Acknowledgments

This book has moved from a glimmer of an idea to an actuality because of the support of two persons. My husband, Ian Mykel, deserves more gratitude than I can ever express for calmly pushing me onward when I most needed it. Heather Doyle Fraser, development editor at Merrill/Prentice Hall, also deserves a special and sincere thank you for her behind-the-scenes confidence in this book and for sharing her knowledge about and experience with projects of this magnitude.

I also want to acknowledge several colleagues at the University of Virginia for their support and generosity in recent years, which enabled me to take the time needed to write this book: Alice Wiggins and Khara Pence, colleagues in the Preschool Language & Literacy Lab; Laura Smolkin and Marcia Invernizzi, colleagues in the McGuffey Reading Center; Dan Hallahan, chair of the Department of Curriculum, Instruction, and Special Education; Sara Rimm-Kaufman and Robert Pianta, colleagues in the Curry School of Education's Interdisciplinary Doctoral Training Program in Risk and Prevention; and students Lori Skibbe, Angela Beckman, Jessica Kingsley, Sarah Greene, Tamika Lucas, Ryan Bowles, Caroline Streppa, Darcy Crocker, and Maurie Sutton.

I am also grateful to have several close colleagues in the communication disorders discipline who continually motivate me by their own contributions to research and practice, including Joan Kaderavek, Melanie Schuele, Gail Gillon, Claudia Dunaway, Hugh Catts, Wayne Secord, Teresa Ukrainetz, Ilsa Schwarz, Gary Pillow, and my mentor, Helen Ezell.

At Merrill/Prentice Hall, Allyson Sharp and Jeffery Johnston require a special note of gratitude for supporting this project from inception to completion. The opportunity to work with Merrill/Prentice Hall is an honor.

Finally, a number of experts served as reviewers of this manuscript in its various stages of development. I am very grateful for their constructive input. The reviewers included Eileen P. Abrahamsen, Old Dominion University; Tracy Acevedo, formerly of the University of Mississippi; Linda C. Badon, University of Louisiana at Lafayette; Stephanie H. Beebe, Pontotoc City Schools; Sandra R. Ciocci, Bridgewater State College; Rebecca A. Gavin, Indiana University; Carole J. Hardiman, Florida State University; Judith B. King, Northern Arizona University; Sara Elizabeth Runyan, James Madison University; Rosalind R. Scudder, Wichita State University; Elnita Stanley, Stephen F. Austin State University; and Louise Van Vliet, Miami University.

Brief Contents

Contents

Note: Every effort has been made to provide accurate and current Internet information in this book. However, the Internet and information posted on it are constantly changing, so it is inevitable that some of the Internet addresses listed in this textbook will change.

Communication Sciences and Disorders

An Introduction

Companion CD-ROM

Communication Sciences and Disorders: An Interactive Multimedia Introduction CD-ROM presents five studies of individuals with communication impairments or a history of communication difficulties, and provides a unique opportunity to bring the field to life for the introductory student. The following discussion provides a summary of the five individuals featured on the CD-ROM as well as topics for exploration and questions for discussion. Each of the five studies contains nine video clips designed to feature:

- *Personal story:* Several clips feature the personal background story of the individual as told by him/herself, close family members (parent, spouse), and professionals with whom they work. For instance, in our first study, Diana's mother tells us about her daughter Diana and how she was adopted at age two from Ukraine.
- *Communication assessment:* Several clips in each study demonstrate various assessment tasks characteristically used by professionals in the communication sciences and disorders disciplines. For instance, in our second study, Mr. Lamm's speech-language pathologist examines his abilities to coordinate precise oral-motor movements, like pursing his lips and moving his tongue laterally. In our third study, Ashley's audiologist evaluates her hearing using audiometry.
- *Communication intervention.* Several clips in each study demonstrate various intervention tasks characteristically used by professionals in the communication sciences and disorders disciplines. For instance, in our fourth study, Mr. Johnson receives counseling on his hearing aids from his audiologist, Dr. Pillow, which is an important aspect of aural rehabilitation. In the fifth study, Dr. Justice engages La'Kori in completing an alphabet puzzle and naming letters of the alphabet, an activity which is important for building early literacy abilities for typical children and those with communication impairments.

STUDY 1: DIANA

The video study of Diana provides a useful supplement to the following chapters:

Chapter 1: Fundamentals of Communication Sciences and Disorders

Chapter 4: Communication Assessment and Intervention: Principles and Practices

Chapter 5: Phonological Disorders

Chapter 7: Language Disorders in Early and Later Childhood

Diana is a 5-year-old girl with Down syndrome who was adopted at 2½ years from an orphanage near Kiev, Ukraine. Diana was adopted into a family residing in central Virginia; her mother is a teacher and her father is a school administrator. She has a sister similar in age who also has Down syndrome. Diana has received speech-language therapy since her arrival to the United States. Since coming to the United States, Diana has progressed from using few if any words (in Ukrainian) to communicating well in the English language for a variety of purposes and to using her language base for literacy activities, such as reading and writing. She attends kindergarten in the regular education program at her elementary school, and receives some special education services specifically for reading and speech/language therapy.

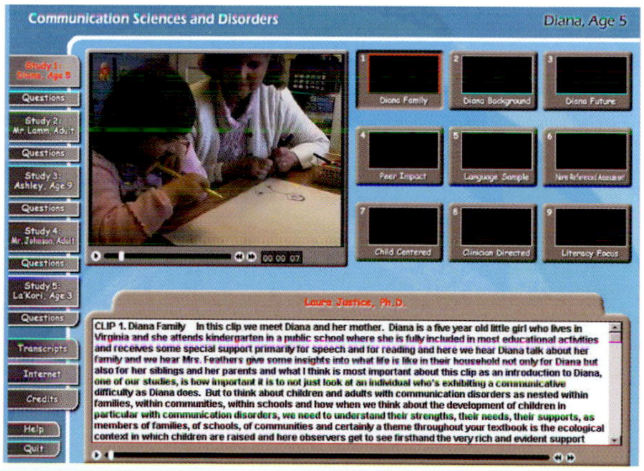

View Diana's video study on the CD-ROM and use the clips to explore the following topics:

- The impact of family support systems on communication development in young children
- The critical period of language development
- The impact of Down syndrome on speech, language, and communication
- The inclusion of children with communication disabilities in regular education

Use Diana's video study to answer the following questions:

1. Diana has a unique developmental history. In what ways might her early experiences in an orphanage affect her present level of skills in communication?
2. Describe Diana's abilities in language, speech, and communication. What are her strengths in each area? What are her needs?
3. Diana communicates for many different reasons. What are some communication intentions or functions observed in the videos of Diana?
4. Discuss Diana's family and educational support systems. What are some aspects of Diana's life at home and school that support her communication development?

STUDY 2: MR. LAMM

The video study of Mr. Lamm provides a useful supplement to the following chapters:

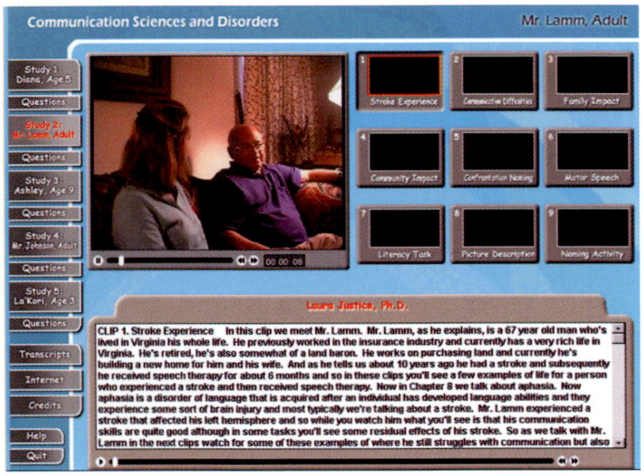

Chapter 1: Fundamentals of Communication Sciences and Disorders

Chapter 4: Communication Assessment and Intervention: Principles and Practices

Chapter 8: Adult Aphasia and Other Cognitive-Based Dysfunctions

Mr. Lamm is a 68-year-old man who experienced a stroke approximately ten years ago. Mr. Lamm is retired from his career in the insurance industry, but has an active real estate portfolio and is in the process of designing and contracting a new home for his wife and himself. Mr. Lamm's stroke affected the left hemisphere of his brain and significantly affected his language and speech immediately after the injury. His reading and writing abilities were also seriously affected. Mr. Lamm received speech-language therapy for about six months, during which his communication improved to result in mild word-finding difficulties.

View Mr. Lamm's video study on the CD-ROM and use the clips to explore the following topics:

- The impact of family support systems on helping an individual cope with communicative disabilities after stroke
- The effectiveness of speech-language therapy
- The impact of stroke on speech, language, and communication
- The impact of acquired disorders of communication on an individual's community participation.

Use Mr. Lamm's video study to answer the following questions:

1. Mr. Lamm experienced a stroke approximately ten years ago, yet currently shows few physical or cognitive difficulties related to his stroke. What aspects of his personality do you believe contributed to his successful outcomes?
2. Describe Mr. Lamm's current abilities in language, speech, and communication. What are his strengths in each area? What are his needs?
3. Mr. Lamm communicates for many different reasons. What are some communication intentions or functions observed in the videos of Mr. Lamm?
4. Discuss Mr. Lamm's support systems available at home and in the community and how these have contributed to his successful communication outcomes.

STUDY 3: ASHLEY

The video study of Ashley provides a useful supplement to the following chapters:

Chapter 1: Fundamentals of Communication Sciences and Disorders

Chapter 4: Communication Assessment and Intervention: Principles and Practices

Chapter 7: Language Disorders in Early and Later Childhood

Chapter 13: Pediatric Hearing Loss

Ashley is a 9-year-old girl who has a severe bilateral sensorineural hearing loss. The cause of her hearing loss is unknown. Ashley also has experienced recurrent otitis media and has had five sets of pressure-equalizing tubes for treatment. Ashley is fully included in regular education, is an above average student, and is gifted in math. Ashley wears bilateral hearing aids, and receives support from a deaf/hard of hearing teacher twice weekly in her school. She is interested in animals, has two horses of her own, and hopes to be an animal control agent when she gets older. Ashley lives in a small rural community in West Virginia with her mother.

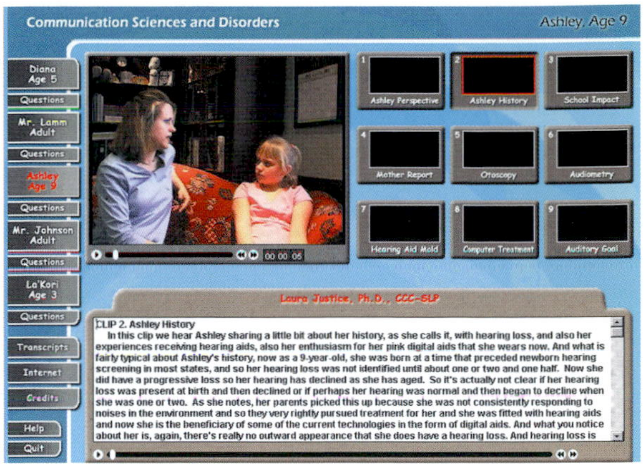

View Ashley's video study on the CD-ROM and use the clips to explore the following topics:

- The importance of early identification of hearing loss
- The role of parental advocacy in supporting children with hearing loss
- The impact of hearing loss on speech, language, and communication
- The impact of hearing loss on a child's educational achievement

Use Ashley's video study to answer the following questions:

1. Ashley has a severe bilateral hearing loss. Describe the extent to which her hearing loss has had a handicapping influence on her life and the extent to which her hearing loss will affect her future ambitions.
2. Describe Ashley's current abilities in language, speech, and communication. What are her strengths in each area? What are her needs?
3. Ashley communicates for many different reasons. What are some communication intentions or functions observed in the videos of Ashley?
4. Discuss Ashley's support systems available at home, at school, and in the community, and how these have contributed to her successful communication outcomes.

STUDY 4: MR. JOHNSON

The video study of Mr. Johnson provides a useful supplement to the following chapters:

Chapter 1: Fundamentals of Communication Sciences and Disorders

Chapter 4: Communication Assessment and Intervention: Principles and Practices

Chapter 14: Hearing Loss in Adults

Mr. Johnson is a 70-year-old male who has an acquired sensorineural hearing loss, most likely due to noise exposure. Mr. Johnson is retired from the construction industry. Mr. Johnson was referred to a hearing specialist due to the persistent requests of his wife, who noticed a decline in his hearing. Mr. Johnson is extremely pleased with his hearing ability when using his aids. Mr. Johnson currently wears hearing aids and sees an audiologist for their maintenance and for counseling on their use.

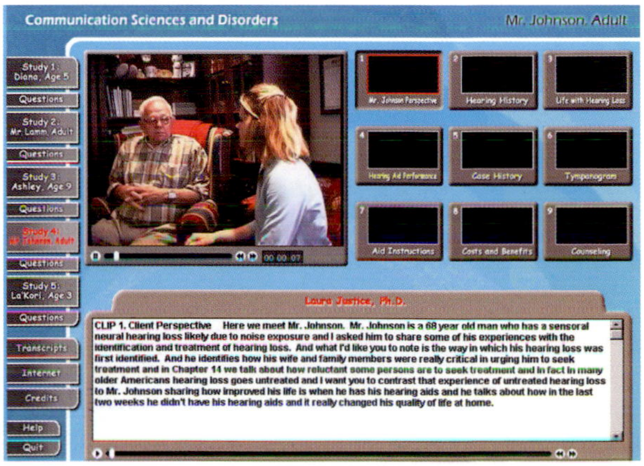

View Mr. Johnson's video study on the CD-ROM and use the clips to explore the following topics:

- The impact of environmental noise exposure on hearing
- The ways in which hearing loss may be identified
- The impact of hearing loss on speech, language, and communication
- The impact of hearing loss on an individual's quality of life

Use Mr. Johnson's video study to answer the following questions:

1. Mr. Johnson has a significant bilateral hearing loss yet communicates quite well. What aspects of his personality do you believe contributed to his successful outcomes?

2. Describe Mr. Johnson's current abilities in hearing and communication. What are his strengths in each area? What are his needs?
3. Discuss Mr. Johnson's support systems available at home and in the community and how these may have contributed to his successful communication outcomes.
4. Discuss the counseling provided to Mr. Johnson, and consider how the information provided may improve Mr. Johnson's aural outcomes.

STUDY 5: LA'KORI

The video study of La'Kori provides a useful supplement to the following chapters:

Chapter 1: Fundamentals of Communication Sciences and Disorders
Chapter 2: An Overview of Communication Development
Chapter 4: Communication Assessment and Intervention: Principles and Practices
Chapter 7: Language Disorders in Early and Later Childhood

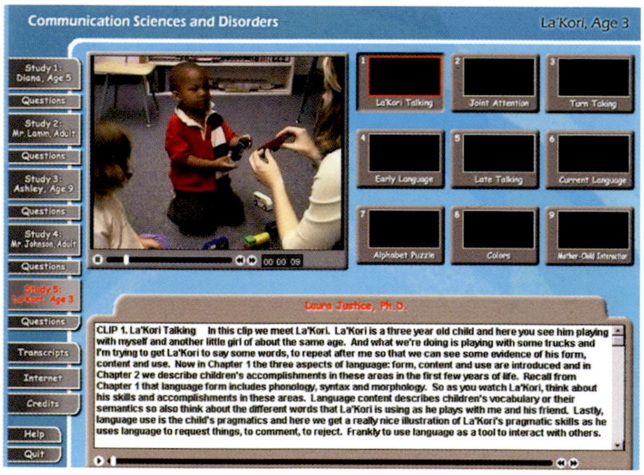

La'Kori is a 3-year-old who was slow to talk. Although La'Kori currently appears to be progressing well in his speech and language, his mother was concerned about his communication development when he failed to use words during the second year of life. Currently, La'Kori uses a variety of words and sentences to express himself for a variety of purposes, and is able to meet his needs through effective communication. La'Kori's mother notes that he sometimes surprises her with the words he uses, like "delicious." La'Kori attends a daycare center in which his mother is a teacher, and plays well with the other children.

View La'Kori's video study on the CD-ROM and use the clips to explore the following topics:

- The role of caregivers in identifying communicative delays in children
- Individual differences among children in rate of communicative achievements
- The reasons for which young children communicate with others
- Factors that influence the rate of language acquisition among children

Use La'Kori's video study to answer the following questions:

1. La'Kori is a typically developing 3-year-old. Describe his current abilities in speech, language, and communication.
2. La'Kori's mother had some concerns about La'Kori's early communication development. Based on her description of his development, to what extent were her concerns warranted?
3. La'Kori communicates for many different reasons. What are some communication intentions or functions observed in the videos of La'Kori?
4. Discuss the support systems available to La'Kori at home and at school. How do these systems support his communication development?

Companion Website

To answer these questions online, go to the CD-ROM Activities link on the home page of the Companion Website at http://www.prenhall.com/justice.

PART I

Foundations of Communication Sciences and Disorders

Fundamentals of Communication Sciences and Disorders

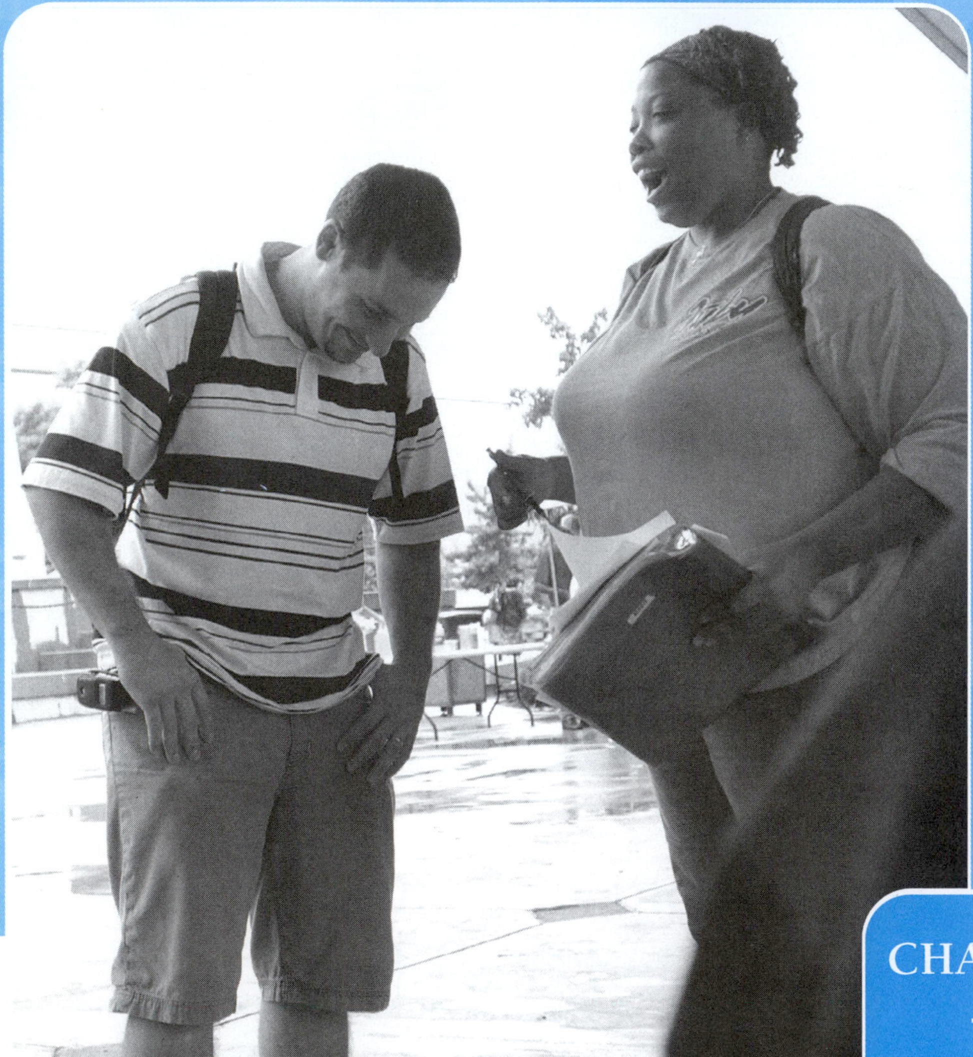

CHAPTER 1

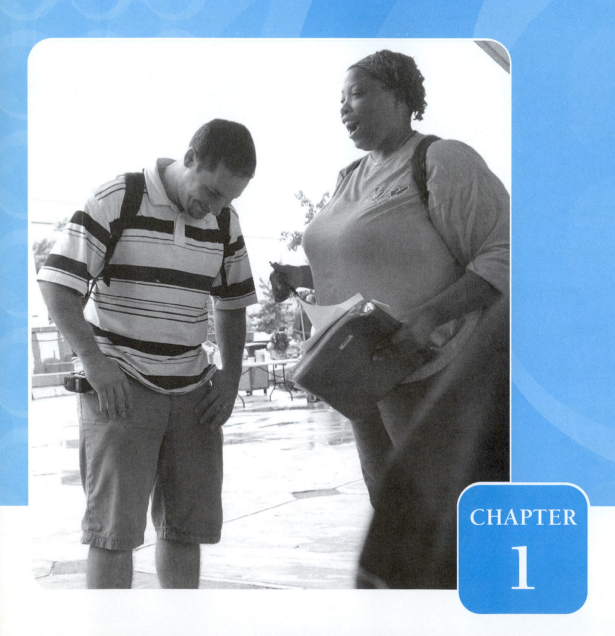

FOCUS QUESTIONS

This chapter answers the following questions:

1. What is communication?
2. How does communication relate to language, speech, and hearing?
3. What is a communication disorder?
4. What careers are available in the field of communication sciences and disorders?

INTRODUCTION

How important is communication to you? If you give this question serious consideration, you will likely realize that your ability to communicate is essential to who you are and is something you would never want to do without. Your understanding of the importance of communication is likely what drew you to this textbook. All of us have at some time been in a situation in which we had difficulty communicating. Perhaps you were visiting another country and did not know the language. Perhaps you were at the dentist, mouth numb from anesthesia, and you could not articulate well. Perhaps you had a panic attack and were too nervous to talk. Or perhaps you had laryngitis and temporarily lost your voice. It is usually times like these that remind us how important our ability to communicate is to us and how unpleasant and challenging it is to lose this ability.

While experiences like losing your voice or having your mouth numbed from anesthesia are inconvenient, they are temporary. Many other types of communication difficulties are more long lasting, such as those resulting from vocal nodules (calluses on the vocal cords), aphasia (loss of language skill following a brain injury), dysarthria (imprecise speech due to nervous system dysfunction), or noise-induced hearing loss (hearing loss from noise exposure). People experiencing these significant communication challenges need medical or therapeutic interventions, or both, to improve their experiences of and increase their enjoyment of life at home, at work, in school, and in the community. These people do not take their communication skills for granted. Indeed, they realize that communication is "the heart of life's experience" (American Speech-Language-Hearing Association [ASHA], 2003b).

Discussion Point: *Can you think of someone in the popular media who has a communication disorder? Or a movie or book that featured a communication disorder? One example is* Rainman, *the 1988 film drama that told the story of a man with autism, a developmental disorder discussed in chapter 7. Autism is typically accompanied by significant communication difficulties.*

Communication disorders are relatively common. The National Institutes of Health estimate that 42 million Americans, or one out of every six persons, have a communication disorder (National Institute on Deafness and Other Communication Disorders [NIDCD], 1995). It is likely that everyone reading this book knows someone who has a disorder of communication or has experienced a significant communication disorder himself or herself.

This chapter defines communication, provides an overview of different types of communication disorders, and identifies those professionals who work most closely with people with communication disorders. As you read this chapter, think about the role of communication in your life and the importance of communication in our society. Let me

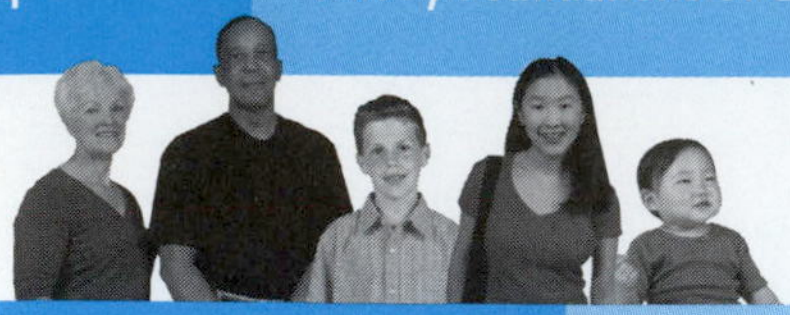

BOX 1-1 **Communication Disorders Across the Lifespan: Case Examples**

Ten weeks premature and weighing 2 pounds, 1 ounce, **Anika** was born on August 14, 2003, to single parent Lina Roster. Her prematurity and low birth weight were attributed to lack of prenatal care and prenatal exposure to high carbon monoxide levels—Anika's mother smoked two packs of cigarettes daily throughout her pregnancy. The neonatal intensive care unit attempted to feed Anika orally using maternal breast milk for one week, at which time Anika was diagnosed by her neonatal specialist as severely undernourished and too weak to be fed orally. Anika was then placed on a nasogastric tube (NG tube), fed through her nose to her stomach. NG tube feedings were supplemented three times daily with oral feeding of breast milk by her mother. A neonatal intensive-care nurse trained Ms. Roster to give Anika the tube feedings and to replace the tube each week. At 4 weeks of age, Anika is consistently gaining weight but is no longer interested in breastfeeding or in any type of oral activity. A speech-language pathologist has been called in to consult with Ms. Roster and the medical team on ways to promote Anika's oral interest and oral intake.

Internet research

1. What is the general developmental prognosis for infants born at very low birth weights?
2. How common are feeding problems in infants?
3. What supports are available for families when babies are born prematurely or with significant medical concerns?

Brainstorm and discussion

1. What are some strategies that the speech-language pathologist might use to promote Anika's interest in oral exploration?
2. What types of supports should be provided to Ms. Roster to help her cope with the challenges of giving birth to a medically fragile infant?

....

Jan Shen is a 62-year-old man who has worked in a print shop at a local community college for the last 35 years. His hearing has been steadily decreasing, and during the last several years Mr. Shen has been unable to actively participate in most conversations. He recently was in a car accident that his wife believes was caused by his inability to hear what was happening around him. In the weeks since the accident, Mr. Shen has been very depressed, refusing to participate in many activities that previously gave him pleasure (e.g., walking each morning, talking on the phone to his daughter). At his wife's request, Mr. Shen received a comprehensive audiological evaluation last week, which showed a severe hearing loss, likely due to ongoing exposure to noise. The audiologist recommended use of a hearing aid, but also indicated that because of the type and the nature of the hearing loss, the hearing aid would not fully restore Mr. Shen's hearing to the level Mr. Shen would like. The audiologist also asked Mr. Shen to participate in a hearing-loss support group, and has recommended he receive auditory rehabilitation therapy to help him best use his residual hearing and hearing aid. Mr. Shen has told his wife that he will not be returning to the audiologist and he does not think that the hearing aid, support group, or therapies are needed.

also encourage you to use this introduction to the study of communication sciences and disorders as a springboard to a future career helping people with communication disorders—as a teacher, a clinician, a researcher, or a public-policy advocate.

What Is Communication?

Definition

Understanding the meaning of the term *communication* is, of course, critical for the study of human communication sciences and disorders. **Communication** refers to the process of

Internet research

1. How common is noise-induced hearing loss?
2. What is the best way to protect yourself against noise-induced hearing loss if your work exposes you to noise?

Brainstorm and discussion

1. Why did Mr. Shen not seek help for his deteriorating hearing prior to his wife's urging after the car accident?
2. What are some possible reasons for Mr. Shen's refusing to return to the audiologist and follow the prescribed course of action?

Anna Parish is a 52-year-old wife, mother, and grandmother, who lives in a small, rural community in northern Alabama. Mrs. Parish has long served as the coordinator of her church's charity drives. One year ago, Mrs. Parish had a stroke, which left her completely paralyzed on the right side and with significant speech impairment. Although Mrs. Parish seems to understand everything that is said to her, she is unable to produce speech that is intelligible to others. When trying to speak, Mrs. Parish often becomes very frustrated and sometimes cries. Although she received individual and then group therapy for apraxia, a motor speech disorder often associated with stroke, she did not make much progress and her insurance will no longer cover the costs of treatment. Mr. Parish has been pushing Mrs. Parish to become involved in her church's charity activities again, and twice a week he drops her off at the church, where she helps to organize materials for the church's literacy program. Mrs. Parish refuses to take on any of her former fund-raising responsibilities, as she feels that without speech she will be unable to do the job successfully.

Internet research

1. What is the leading cause of stroke?
2. What are the warning signs of stroke?
3. How often are people who have experienced a stroke able to fully resume their previous life responsibilities?

Brainstorm and discussion

1. What are some possible supports that could be put in place to help Mrs. Parish take on more responsibility with her charity work?
2. What are some barriers that may be keeping Mrs. Parish from taking on more responsibility with her charity work?

sharing information between two or more persons, or more specifically, "the transmission of thoughts or feelings from the mind of a speaker to the mind of a listener" (Borden, Harris, & Raphael, 1994, p. 174). People share their thoughts and feelings for many reasons, the three most basic being to request ("I need some coffee."), to reject ("This coffee is awful!"), and to comment ("Ah, that's much better."). Even children as young as 1 year are able to communicate for these three basic purposes ("Milk?" "Milk!" "Milk.").

Communication involves two main players, a sender and a receiver, and four processes: formulation, transmission, reception, and comprehension. The sender formulates and then transmits the information being conveyed, and the receiver receives and then comprehends the information. **Formulation** is the process of pulling together one's thoughts or ideas for sharing with another: What is the thought or feeling I want to share? **Transmission** is the process of conveying those ideas to another person, often by speaking but also by signing, gesturing, or writing. **Reception** is the process of receiving the information from another person, and **comprehension** is the process of making sense of that message.

Although speaking is one of the most frequent modes of communication, communication need not be spoken. A person can reject by turning away, a baby can comment by smiling, and a dog can request by panting at the door. However, what is particularly unique about human communication is the use of language and speech in the communication process. Much of this text, and indeed much of the study of human communication science and disorders, emphasizes the use and breakdown of these uniquely human processes for communication.

Discussion Point: *People who use sign language to communicate sometimes refer to themselves as members of the deaf culture. What does the use of the term* culture *imply regarding people who use sign as a communication modality?*

Modality describes the manner in which information conveyed via communication is transmitted and received. Speech is the most common modality of communication for humans. For people who cannot speak, hear, or both, sign language is a prevalent modality for communication, particularly among members of the deaf and hard of hearing community. In literate cultures, reading and writing are also common means of communication. People who cannot read or write—who are illiterate—cannot participate in this communication modality.

Obviously just being able to speak, hear, read, write, and sign does not ensure effective communication. For instance, if I wrote *¿Qué crees que esto dice aquí?* and you did not know Spanish, our communication would not be successful. Why? Although we are both able to participate in the modality (reading and writing), we do not fully share the symbolic system being used. For communication between two individuals to be effective, they must have an agreement as to the symbol system to be used to communicate, and they must be proficient in that system. Language is one symbol system with many variations (e.g., Spanish, English, Chinese, Swahili, American Sign Language[ASL]); it is also the most sophisticated symbol system used for communication. Other, less sophisticated symbol systems include gestures, pictures, and facial expressions.

A Model of Communication

Figure 1-1 provides a model of communication that includes three essential components: (1) a sender to formulate and transmit a message, (2) a receiver to receive and comprehend the message, and (3) a shared symbolic system. An additional component, feedback, is also included in this model. **Feedback** is information provided by the receiver to the sender. In effective communication, feedback is continually provided by the receiver, and the sender responds to this feedback to maintain the effectiveness of the communication process. This

FIGURE 1-1 Model of communication.

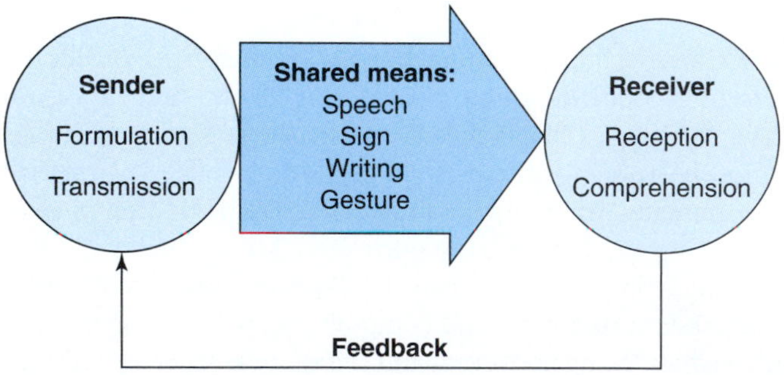

feedback system is what makes communication active and dynamic. Communication is active because both sender and receiver must be fully engaged. It is dynamic because the receiver is constantly sending feedback that is interpreted and used by the sender to modulate the flow of communication.

Feedback is provided in numerous ways by the receiver. **Linguistic feedback** includes speaking, such as saying, "I totally agree," "I hear what you are saying," or "Wait, I don't get it." It also includes vocalizing, such as saying "mm-hmm" or "uh-oh." **Nonlinguistic** or **extralinguistic feedback** refers to the use of eye contact, facial expression, posture, and proximity. This type of feedback may supplement linguistic feedback, or it may stand alone. **Paralinguistic feedback** refers to the use of pitch, loudness, and pausing, all of which are superimposed over linguistic feedback. These linguistic and nonlinguistic forms of feedback keep communication flowing and provide the speaker with valuable information concerning the receiver's comprehension.

Discussion Point: *Our cultural backgrounds influence the type of feedback that we use in communication. What does your feedback package look like?*

You can probably think of a time when you were trying to communicate something and you got the impression the receiver was not getting it. What kind of feedback was the receiver using to give you this message? Perhaps he or she looked away while you were talking or interrupted you frequently for clarification. You can also probably think of a time when you were on the receiving end and your feedback was not being attended to. Perhaps you were having a difficult time understanding what someone was telling you. What kind of feedback did you give to the sender? Perhaps a few linguistic cues ("Well, this is all very interesting, but . . .") and some paralinguistic cues too (e.g., looking at your watch).

For communication to be effective, feedback from the receiver is just as important as the information being provided by the sender. Feedback is used by the sender and receiver to prevent a **communication breakdown** from occurring:

Sender: His whole demeanor is totally insouciant. It drives me crazy.

Receiver furrows her brow in confusion.

Sender: I mean, he is so indifferent! How can he not care about this stuff?

Receiver (nodding): Oh, I totally know what you mean. Like the other day . . .

If you look closely at this snippet of conversation, you should be able to find a communication breakdown. It centered on the word *insouciant*, which the sender used but the receiver did not understand. By giving the speaker prompt feedback (a furrowed brow, which is a type of nonlinguistic feedback), the sender was able to repair the breakdown by indicating that *insouciant* means "indifferent." This is called a conversational repair. Minor communication breakdowns happen in every conversation but are easily recognized and repaired if the receiver is sending ongoing feedback and the sender is closely monitoring that feedback. More serious communication breakdowns occur when receivers do not send appropriate types or amounts of feedback or when senders do not attend

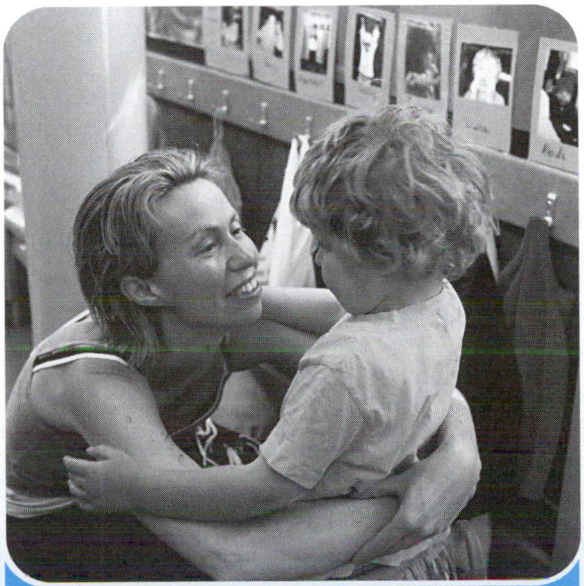

We communicate through linguistic, nonlinguistic, and paralinguistic ways.

to the feedback. In such cases, the communication interaction is ineffective, as it does not meet the purposes of the participants.

The Purpose of Communication

The main purpose of communication is to provide and solicit information. We communicate to provide information about our feelings ("I love you.") and to get information from others ("Do you love me?"). We communicate to share information about trivial ("Ouch! I stubbed my toe.") and exciting events ("Today I won a new car!") and to describe our needs and desires ("Won't you please lend me $5.00 for lunch?"). Halliday (1975) differentiated the purposes of communication into seven categories, or **communication functions:**

1. *Instrumental communication:* used to ask for something ("I would like the shrimp, please.")
2. *Regulatory communication:* used to give directions and to direct others ("You need to take a right here.")
3. *Interactional communication:* used to interact and converse with others in a social way ("What did you think of the game yesterday?")
4. *Personal communication:* used to express a state of mind or feelings about something ("I am just furious about this!")
5. *Heuristic communication:* used to find out information and to inquire ("Do you know when this dam was built?")
6. *Imaginative communication:* used to tell stories and to role-play ("If I had a million dollars, I would . . .")
7. *Informative communication:* used to provide an organized description of an event or object ("What happened was, we got to the game, and then it began to rain . . .")

All of these purposes are vitally important to developing and maintaining social relationships with other people and for meeting our own basic needs and desires. These diverse functions are used by effective communicators every day in various ecological contexts, including home, school, work, and community.

Discussion Point:
Communication helps us maintain our relationships with those in our lives. Consider the case of Mr. Shen, detailed in Box 1-1. How might his difficulties with hearing impact his relationship with his wife?

People who have a restricted range of communication functions face significant challenges and frustrations in these ecological contexts. As will be discussed later in this chapter, a communication disorder is present when a person experiences a substantial impairment in his or her ability to communicate. Often, a restricted range of communication functions is one of the first signs of a communication disorder. This is the case for very young children who develop communication skills more slowly than their peers, as commonly happens with children who have mental retardation. Children who are unable to use communication for diverse purposes feel great frustration, as do their parents. Adults who have experienced neurological injury, such as a stroke, may lose the ability to communicate for diverse purposes, such as asking for a prescription at the pharmacy or telling a friend how much they enjoy their company, and feel similar frustration.

Effective Communication

We can all think of instances when we did not communicate as effectively as we needed to. Effective communication occurs when information is successfully shared between a sender and a receiver; there is no breakdown in formulation, transmission, reception, or comprehension. An effective communicator is one whose communications with others are effective most of the time. Effective communicators communicate through a modality that is shared by important people in their lives and communities, such as speaking and hearing, reading and writing, or signing. Effective communicators avoid communication breakdowns by responding to and giving feedback during conversations. They use communication for diverse purposes: to ask for things, to direct others, to interact with others in a social way, to express their own feelings, to find out information, and to tell stories. Additionally, effective communicators abide by four principles known as **Grice's maxims** (Grice, 1975): (1) quantity, (2) quality, (3) relevance, and (4) manner. These principles refer specifically to the way in which senders formulate and transmit information, as described by Damico (1991):

1. *Principle of quantity:* The sender provides the right amount and type of information needed by the receiver, uses clear and concise vocabulary, and is not redundant. The following breakdown results from the speaker's lack of adherence to this principle:

   Speaker: He is not coming! Can you believe it?
   Receiver: Who is "he"? What are you talking about?

2. *Principle of quality:* The sender shares information that is accurate. The following breakdown results from a speaker ignoring this principle:

   Speaker: I am *not* angry at you.
   Receiver: Why are you shouting at me?

3. *Principle of relevance:* The sender maintains the topic and uses appropriate transitions as needed; the sender communicates in a way that is appropriate to the situation and to his or her relationship with the receiver. The following speaker is not abiding by this principle:

   Speaker: I am so worried about the test tomorrow. This is such crazy weather! What do you think?
   Receiver: It is kind of hot.
   Speaker: I was asking you about the test!

4. *Principle of manner:* The sender speaks fluently without frequent hesitations or revisions, takes appropriate turns, pauses as needed but does not delay responses longer than called for, uses appropriate loudness and pitch, and engages in eye contact as expected by cultural norms. The following communication exchange breaks down by inordinate pauses, going against this principle of manner:

   Speaker: You want to know what time it is? Um, um. Uh (pauses for 10 seconds). I don't have a watch.

How Does Communication Relate to Language, Speech, and Hearing?

Language, speech, and hearing are the essential ingredients of human communication. The sophisticated use of these three processes for communication is what makes the human species unique. This textbook focuses on language, speech, and hearing as key communication tools and on how difficulties in these areas can result in disorders of communication.

Language, speech, and hearing are used for the formulation, transmission, reception, and comprehension of information using spoken channels (see Figure 1-2). Language is used for formulation and comprehension. Speech is used for transmission. Hearing is used for reception. Although the terms *language, speech,* and *communication* are often used synonymously, they describe very different processes.

The term *language* describes the cognitive process by which we formulate ideas and thoughts. Once these ideas and thoughts are formulated, we can orally communicate them

FIGURE 1-2 Key processes in spoken communication.

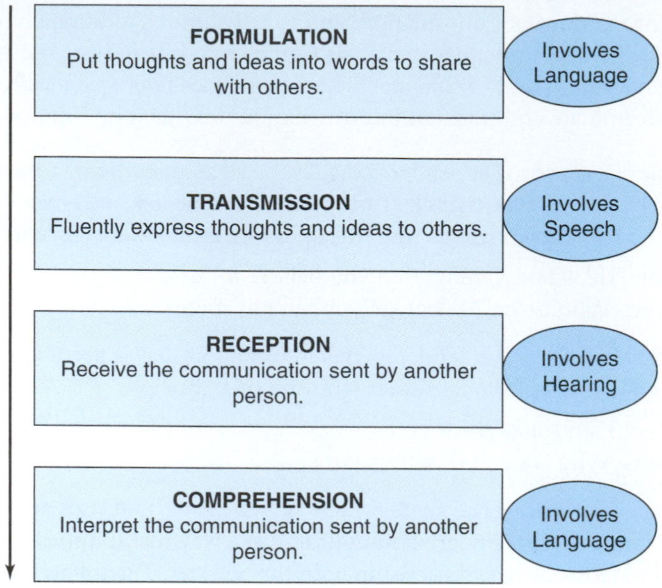
FORMULATION
Put thoughts and ideas into words to share with others.
Involves Language
TRANSMISSION
Fluently express thoughts and ideas to others.
Involves Speech
RECEPTION
Receive the communication sent by another person.
Involves Hearing
COMPREHENSION
Interpret the communication sent by another person.
Involves Language

Source: From "Cultural Competence and Communication Disorders" from C. Tolmeda & K. Bayles (2002, April 2). *Cultivating cultural competence in the workplace, classroom, and clinic.* ASHA Leader Online. [Online]. http://professional.asha.org/news/020402d.cfm

to others through speech. We can also choose to keep these thoughts and ideas to ourselves (inner language) or to write them down (written language).

The term *speech* describes the neuromuscular process by which we turn language into a sound signal that is transmitted through the air (or other medium, like a telephone line) to a receiver. Speech involves using voice and articulators (e.g., tongue, lips, palate) to make the sounds that produce words and sentences.

Why do humans have speech and language? These evolved for only one purpose: to communicate. The information shared through communication

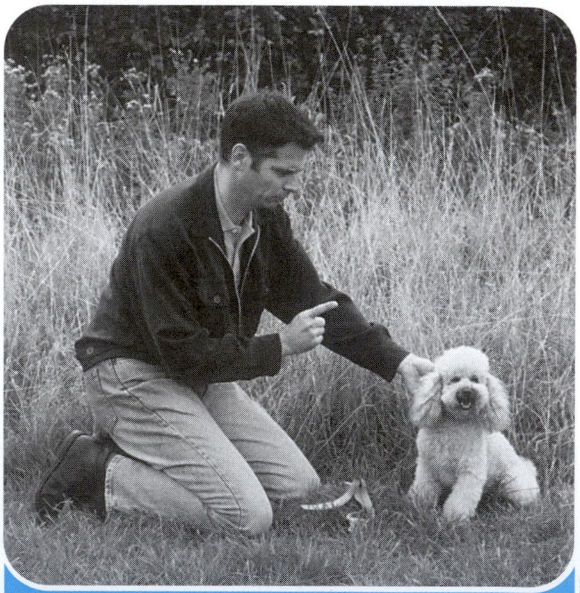

Other species are able to communicate, but only humans have the capacity for speech and language.

is language, and speech is a primary means by which language is transmitted. Although many other species are able to communicate, only humans have speech and language. The capacities for speech and language allow humans to share remarkably complex ideas and thoughts with one another, a feat that is not possible for other species.

Language

Definition

Language, as defined by Nelson (1998, p. 26), is the "socially shared code that uses a conventional system of arbitrary symbols to represent ideas about the world that are meaningful to others who know the same code." The key elements of this definition are:

1. *Language is* socially shared: A community of speakers shares the same system for communicating their ideas. For example, everyone reading this textbook shares the English language as a means for communicating ideas about communication sciences and disorders.

2. *Language is a* code: Ideas about the world are communicated using a set of symbols. The symbols used in language are words, which are made up of sounds that are combined in various ways. The code for what you are holding in your hand right now involves three sounds—b + oo + k—blended together to form a word (*book*). Those of us who speak English and therefore know this particular code are a linguistic community. The word itself (in this case, *book*) is completely arbitrary; the thing in your hand could just as well be called a *trift*, formed by blending five sounds—t + r + i + f + t.

3. *Language is* conventional: Language follows specific, systematic conventions; it is a rule-governed code. Strict rules govern the way a linguistic community organizes words into sentences, the way word units are put together, and the way sounds are combined to make words. The rules of English constrain English speakers from saying things like *Sat cat the the on hat, He drankeding the milk,* and *Thit rinches shug gfmiiikn nink.* Speakers in a linguistic community abide by a strict set of rules when they produce words and sentences and converse with others. When someone in the linguistic community violates those rules, we tend to be aware of it. For instance, if a doctor said to you, "Need prescription store go," you would be cognizant of the fact that some linguistic rules were being violated. If a young child said, "He goed to the store," you would also probably recognize that a rule was being violated, but you would be more accepting, knowing that the child was still learning the rules of language and would shortly figure out that the past tense of *go* is *went*.

4. *Language is a* representational tool: Language allows us to represent our thoughts and ideas to others. Language is a tool for communication, and the only reason humans evolved language was to communicate with one another. In addition to allowing us to represent our ideas to others for communication purposes, language enables our brains to store information and to carry out many cognitive processes, such as reasoning, hypothesizing, and planning (Bickerton, 1995). Although the relationship between thought and language continues to spur controversy (Can we think without using language?), we do know that much of human thought uses the code of language.

Remarkable Features of Language

Language is beyond a doubt one of the most remarkable capacities of the human species. It is what makes humans human, and it is what makes our species uniquely different from other species. Language is studied by more disciplines than any other subject. It commands the interest of psychologists, speech-language pathologists, audiologists, linguists, sociologists, philosophers, biologists, anthropologists, childhood educators, special educators, neuroscientists, nurses, physicians, mathematicians, and musicians, among others. Several of the remarkable features of language that attract scholars include its universality, species specificity, semanticity, productivity, and rate of acquisition.

Universality. Language is ubiquitous. Every human culture has one and sometimes many languages, and all languages are equally complex. The universality of language, as Steven Pinker wrote in *The Language Instinct* (1994, p. 26),

> fills linguists with awe, and is the first reason to suspect that language is not just any cultural invention but the product of a special human instinct. . . . Cultural inventions vary widely in their sophistication from society to society. . . . language, however, ruins this correlation. There are Stone Age societies, but there is no such thing as a Stone Age language.

Species Specificity. Language is a human capacity, and no other animals share this aptitude. Although many nonhuman species are able to communicate, their communication abilities are wholly iconic (Bickerton, 1995). Iconic communication systems are those for which there is a transparent relation between what is being communicated and how it is being communicated. For instance, the purring of a cat is a fairly transparent way to say "I like your petting." If the purring goes up a notch to a veritable roar, it says, "I *really* like your petting. Keep it up." All nonhuman communication systems are more or less iconic, whereas there is little that is iconic about human language.

Semanticity. Human language allows us to represent events that are decontextualized, or removed from the present—what happened before this moment or that may happen after this moment. We need not talk only about what is concrete and in the here and now; rather, language allows us to talk about things that are decidedly not concrete, that are intangible, abstract, hypothetical, complex, and far removed from the present. Semanticity is this unique aspect of language, and it relates to the noniconic aspect of human language. Because the relations between our language and what we are talking about are not tied together, we have an immensely powerful tool for use.

Productivity. Productivity is the principle of combination, specifically, the combination of a small number of discrete units into seemingly infinite novel creations. Productivity is a phenomenon that applies to other human activities—such as mathematics and music—as well as to language. With a relatively small set of rules governing language, humans are capable of producing an endless number of ideas and new constructions. For instance, humans use only a small set of sounds (for speakers of Standard American English, there are about 40 or so), and we can combine these small units on the basis of a set of rules we intuitively know (e.g., /g/ cannot follow /l/) into an infinite number of words and syllables. Similarly, with a relatively small number of words, humans are capable of creating an infinite variety of sentences, the majority of which no one has ever heard before. If you desired, right now, you could produce a sentence that no person has ever uttered before because of the remarkable principle of productivity.

The principle of productivity is inherent to language in its earliest stages of acquisition. Children who are 18 months of age who have about 50 words in their vocabulary begin to combine and recombine this small set of words to produce sentences that express a range of needs. The productivity feature of language is unique to humans, as the units of nonhuman communication systems cannot be recombined to make new meanings. For instance, night monkeys have 16 communication units. These 16 units cannot be recombined to make more than 16 possible ways to communicate, as the principle of productivity is not operating (Bickerton, 1995).

Rate of Acquisition. Hoff-Ginsberg (1997, p. 3) has stated that language development "reveals the genius in all children . . . it is remarkable that 3-year-olds who can't tie their shoes or cross the street alone have vocabularies of thousands of words and can produce sentences with relative clauses." For many of us who are researchers of child language, this is the remarkable feature of language that drew us to the field—the sheer rate of acquisition, the marvelous feat of children in learning so much so fast. Children go from using perhaps 5 words at 12 months, to two-word sentences and about 50 words at 18 months, to thousands of words and complex sentences by 5 years. Spend a few minutes with a 3-year-old child in the next week, and it is likely that you will be amazed by the language you hear. The rate of language acquisition is a key achievement of early childhood, and many scholars view language development as fairly complete by about 5 years of age, although the system is continually refined during middle and later childhood (e.g., new words are added to the vocabulary). Thus the first 5 years of life are a critical period for language development; after this period, the rate of language development slows, and never again will so many linguistic achievements be possible in such a short period of time.

Language Domains

Language consists of three rule-governed domains that together reflect an integrated whole: content, form, and use (Lahey, 1988). **Content** refers to the meaning of language—the words we use and the meaning behind them. Content is conveyed through our vocabulary system, or lexicon, as we select and organize words to express our ideas or to understand what others are saying. **Form** is how words, sentences, and sounds are organized and arranged to convey content. **Use** is how language is used functionally for meeting personal and social needs.

Let's take, for instance, the two-word sentence spoken by 2-year-old Dakota: "Daddy's cup." This sentence can be analyzed for its content, form, and use. The content is the words Dakota selected from her vocabulary and the meaning behind those words; concepts expressed here include Daddy's ownership and an object used to hold liquid and to drink from. Form is how these concepts are conveyed by organizing sounds (eight sounds are used), by manipulating word structure (*'s* is added to *Daddy* to convey possession), and by organizing words in a particular order (*cup* comes after *Daddy's*). Use is how the content and forms function within a social routine. In this case, Dakota says "Daddy's cup" while pointing to a cup sitting on a table. Although there are many possible functions for Dakota's utterance, in this case she appears simply to be commenting, possibly to initiate a conversation with her mother.

Dakota: Daddy's cup.

Mother (looking up): Yes, that is Daddy's cup.

Dakota: Mommy's cup.

Mother: You're right. This is my cup.

Dakota: That Mommy.

Mother: Yep, this one's mine. Where's your cup?

Dakota: My cup.

Content, form, and use thus constitute a three-domain system used to represent and organize the major dimensions of language. A five-domain system is also often used to provide a slightly more refined description of language dimensions (see Figure 1-3). The five domains are semantics, syntax, morphology, phonology, and pragmatics. The domains of semantics and pragmatics are synonymous with the domains of content and use, respectively. The domains of syntax, morphology, and phonology reflect three elements of form.

FIGURE 1-3 The domains of language.

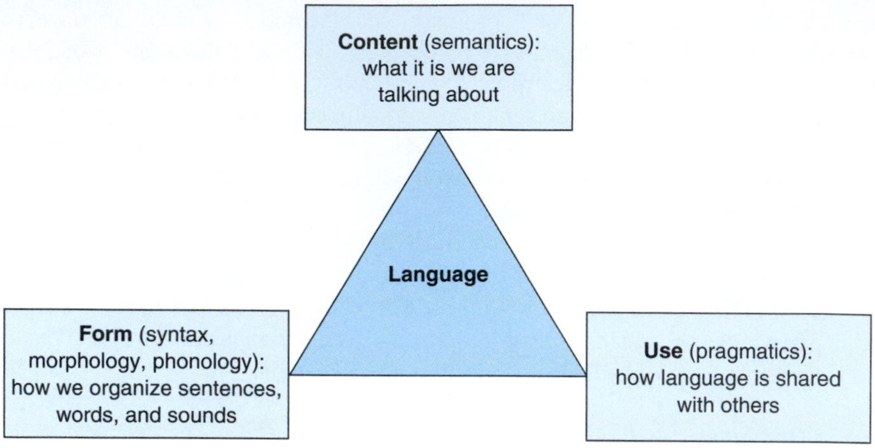

1. **Semantics** (content): The rules of language governing the meaning of individual words and word combinations. For instance, we know that a *culprit* is someone who has done something wrong, and that *green* and *blue* go together meaningfully. Our knowledge of semantics tells us that something is wrong with the sentence *Colorless green ideas sleep furiously,* a sentence produced by the linguist Noam Chomsky to differentiate semantics and syntax (Pinker, 1994).

2. **Syntax** (form): The rules of language governing the internal organization of sentences. The sentence *Colorless green ideas sleeps furiously* abides by conventional rules of syntax: its word order is acceptable despite its lack of meaning.

3. **Morphology** (form): The rules of language governing the internal organization of words. Words can be morphed (manipulated) to change their meanings; for instance, *-ed* can be added to *walk* to show that this activity happened in the past (*walked*), or *-er* can be added to turn the verb *walk* into a noun to describe a person who is walking (*walker*).

4. **Phonology** (form): The rules of language governing the sounds we use to make syllables and words. Every language has a relatively small number of sounds, called phonemes. Standard American English (SAE) uses about 40 phonemes (depending on the dialect), as shown in Figure 1-4. SAE relies on the combination of 15 vowels and 25 consonants to create some 100,000 words. Some languages use more phonemes, and others use less. (For instance, the Lakhota language, a Sioux language, uses 34 phonemes [Rood & Taylor, 1996], many of which would be unfamiliar to speakers of Standard American English.) In addition, each language has rules governing how sounds are organized in words, called phonotactics. In English, for instance, the sound /g/ never follows /s/ or /l/ at the beginning of a word.

Discussion Point: *Can you think of some other phonotactic rules that govern the organization of American English speech sounds?*

5. **Pragmatics** (use): The rules of language governing how language is used for social purposes. Pragmatics governs three important aspects of the social use of language: (1) using language for different purposes (communication functions), (2) organizing language for discourse (conversation) (Lahey, 1988), and (3) knowing what to say and when and how to say it (social conventions). In using language for social purposes, pragmatic rules govern linguistic, extralinguistic, and paralinguistic aspects of communication. The latter two include word choice, turn taking, posture, gestures, eye contact, proximity, pitch, loudness, and pausing.

Metalinguistic Awareness

The ability to deliberately scrutinize language as an object of attention is called **metalinguistic awareness.** Because language is a highly abstract concept, working at a metalinguistic level

FIGURE 1-4 The phonemes of Standard American English.

Consonants						*Vowels*			
/p/	pat	/t/	tip	/g/	go	/i/	feet	/ɪ/	fit
/b/	bat	/d/	dip	/ɳ/	sing	/e/	fate	/ɛ/	fret
/m/	mat	/n/	not	/h/	hop	/u/	food	/u/	foot
/f/	fit	/s/	sun	/?/	uh-oh	/o/	phone	/ɔ/	fought
/v/	vat	/z/	zoo	/l/	lose	/æ/	fan	/a/	hot
/θ/	think	/c/	chew	/r/	rose	/ʌ/	cut	/ə/	bathtub
/ð/	those	/j/	jeep	/j/	young	/aɪ/	fight	/au/	found
/s/	shop	/k/	kiln	/w/	week	/ɔɪ/	toy		
/z/	measure								

can be challenging. For instance, if you were asked to find the first article in this paragraph, you would have to think about the meaning of the linguistic term *article* before doing so. Then, starting at the beginning of the paragraph, you would look at each word and consider whether it was an article. Thinking about the various parts of speech and then analyzing words for their linguistic category (article, noun, etc.) is a metalinguistic act, and a certain degree of metalinguistic awareness is needed to be successful at this task.

Each domain of language can be the object of metalinguistic scrutiny. Semantic awareness is needed to analyze words or concepts explicitly. For example, asking, "What does *shipwreck* mean?" makes the word *shipwreck* an object of scrutiny much as asking, "What is the cat doing?" makes the cat an object of scrutiny. Obviously, the *shipwreck* task is more challenging, as it involves working at an abstract level. When a person says, "I can't come up with the right word," this, too, is a metalinguistic comment. Syntactic awareness is needed to analyze sentence grammar explicitly, as in asking what is wrong with the sentence *Her did it.* Morphological awareness is needed to analyze the structure of words in a deliberate way, as in asking, "What do I add to the word *walk* to show that it already happened?" Phonological awareness involves analyzing the sound structure of language, as in asking, "What is the first sound in the word *bottle?*" Pragmatic awareness involves analyzing language use in social situations, as in asking a child, "How could you phrase that to be more polite?" or "Why do we not talk loudly in libraries?"

Speech

Definition

Speech is the neuromuscular process that allows humans to express language. In spoken communication, after our ideas are formulated (language), they must be transmitted. Speech involves the very precise activation of muscles in three systems to transmit ideas: respiration, phonation, and articulation (Duffy, 1995). These three systems represent the remarkable coordination of a breath of air that begins in the lungs (respiration), travels up

FIGURE 1-5 Systems involved with speech.

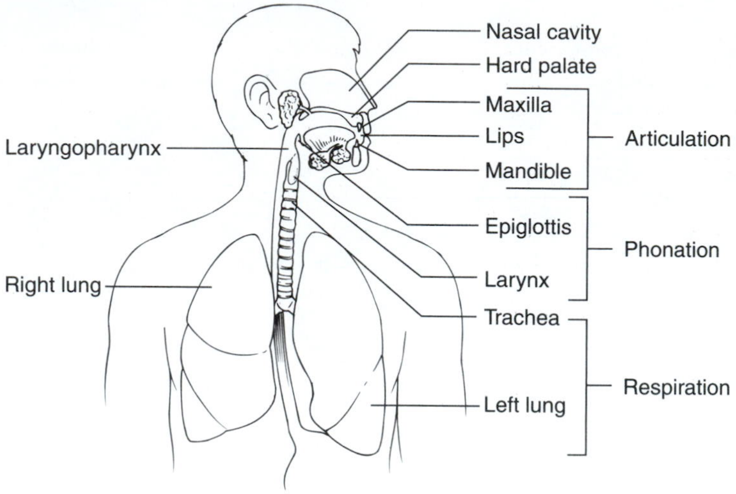

through the trachea or windpipe, over the vocal cords, and into the oral and nasal cavities (phonation), and then is manipulated by the oral articulators—tongue, teeth, and jaw (articulation)—to come out as a series of speech sounds that another person can understand and attribute meaning to (see Figure 1-5).

***Discussion Point:** The concepts of speech and language are often confused and considered synonyms. Why is it important to distinguish between these two concepts? How would you explain the distinction?*

To understand better the processes involved with speech, say the word *eat* slowly and deliberately and think about the process as you do so. You will see that the speech process begins with the intake of a breath of air, which is then exhaled; this is the basic fuel needed for all speech. The exhalation travels up from the lungs through the windpipe (trachea) and over the vocal cords, which begin to vibrate and create the "eeeee" sound. This "eeeee" sound is then sent into the oral cavity, which is open and marked by a big, toothy smile with the lips pulled wide. Notice that the upper and lower jaws are held fairly close together but are not closed; the tongue sits low in the mouth, with the tip tucked behind the lower row of teeth and the middle rounded up on the sides to touch the upper teeth. Once the "eeee" sound is in the oral cavity, a brief "ea" escapes and then the tongue comes quickly up behind the teeth to produce the "t" sound following the "ea."

The complete neuromuscular and neuroanatomical description of this process is provided in later chapters. For now, it is important to recognize that speech is a neuromuscular act involving precise coordination of three systems. It is also important to appreciate how highly complex speech is. As a neuromuscular activity requiring considerable accuracy across a number of biological systems, there are many sites of possible breakdowns. Breakdowns in these systems, if serious enough, can result in a variety of communication disorders. Go ahead and produce the word *eat* again; as you do so, think about each stage of the speech production process and consider where breakdowns might occur.

The systems used by humans for speech—respiration, phonation, and articulation—did not evolve for the purpose of speech. Rather, speech as an evolutionary capacity superimposed itself on systems that were already in place. The structures of the respiratory and phonatory systems allow us to breathe, and the structures of the articulatory system allow us to eat and drink. Although when and how humans first began to use speech is the subject of considerable popular, philosophical, and scientific debate, it is generally accepted that speech became the mode for language expression because of its advantages over other possible modalities. Unlike gestured, signed, or written communication, speech

FIGURE 1-6 Model of speech production.

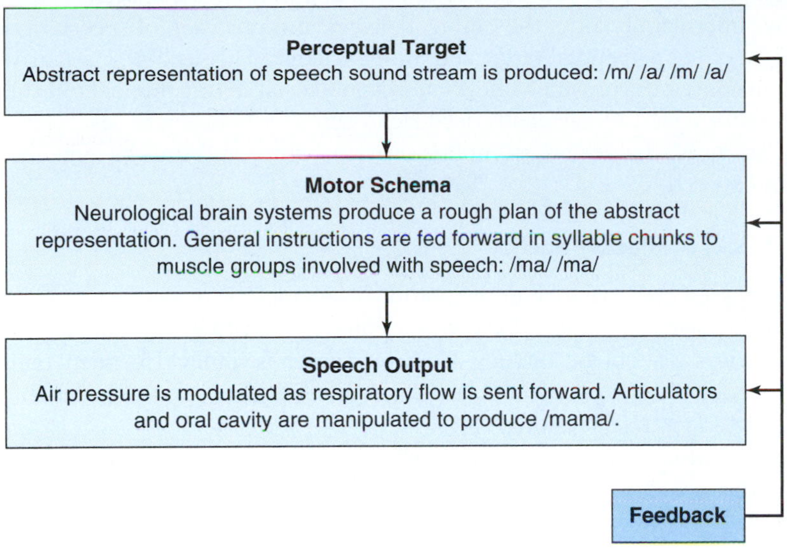
Perceptual Target
Abstract representation of speech sound stream is produced: /m/ /a/ /m/ /a/
Motor Schema
Neurological brain systems produce a rough plan of the abstract representation. General instructions are fed forward in syllable chunks to muscle groups involved with speech: /ma/ /ma/
Speech Output
Air pressure is modulated as respiratory flow is sent forward. Articulators and oral cavity are manipulated to produce /mama/.
Feedback

Source: Adapted from Borden, Harris, & Raphael (1994).

can be used in the dark, around corners, at a distance, and even when a person's hands are occupied (Borden et al., 1994).

Model of Speech Production

How a human being is able to go from an idea ("I am hungry.") to a clearly articulated spoken product ("Let's eat!") is a question that has yet to be fully answered. This question is interesting to scientists in diverse disciplines because speech is one of several critical capacities that make humans human.

Figure 1-6 presents a basic model of speech production. A model is a way to represent an unknown event based on the current best evidence governing that event. This model shows speech production as a three-stage process (Borden et al., 1994) initiated with an abstract mental representation of the speech stream to be produced. This perceptual target is a cognitively based conceptualization of a series of individual sounds, or phonemes. A **phoneme** is the smallest unit of sound. The word *mama,* for instance, is made up of four phonemes strung together. These phonemes are represented in Figure 1-6 as /m/ /a/ /m/ /a/. (Phonemic representations are usually bounded by slashes.) The symbols of the International Phonetic Alphabet (see Figure 1-4) are used to represent individual phonemes.

The next stage is development of a motor schema to represent this sound sequence. The motor schema is a rough motor plan based on the abstract representation of the perceptual target. The rough plan organizes the phonemes into syllable chunks; *mama* is represented as two syllables to be executed—/ma/ /ma/. The rough plan is sent forward to the major muscle groups involved with speech production. These include muscle groups in the respiratory system, which will initiate and modulate the flow of air, the larynx, which contains the voice box, and the muscle groups of the oral cavity, which govern the movement of the tongue and the positioning of the upper and lower jaws and lips.

Sending forward the motor schema stimulates the production of speech, or speech output. The flow of air, use of the voice box, and movements of the oral cavity are all finely manipulated to carry out the motor schema and to create speech. Ongoing feedback relays information about the timing, delivery, and precision of speech output back to the origin of the perceptual target and motor schema. This feedback, occurring in the speaker's unconscious, provides information about what is to come next at the perceptual and motor levels. Occasionally, feedback occurs at a conscious level, for example, when we are aware that we are stumbling over our words and thus become more deliberate in our speech.

Building Blocks of Effective Speech

Speech is a representational tool for the sharing of language. Language is not dependent on speech, as language can be shared via other means (e.g., writing, sign language) or can be kept to ourselves as a tool for thinking. However, speech is wholly dependent on language; speech is a tool for language. Without language, speech is just a series of grunts and groans. Language gives speech its meaning.

Speech is normal when we are able to use it to accurately translate our thoughts as language for other people to hear. We want our speech to be as clear and fluent as it can be to serve this purpose. Speech that is not clear and is dysfluent is a barrier to sharing our language and may signify the presence of a speech disorder. A person can have a speech disorder and still have excellent language and communication skills, as speech is itself a process that is distinct from communication and language.

Discussion Point: *Can you think of another illustration of how speech and language are distinct processes?*

For instance, Stephen Hawking, the famous theoretical physicist at Cambridge University, has a profound speech disorder resulting from amyotrophic lateral sclerosis (ALS), a disease of the motor neurons. Hawking was diagnosed with ALS while completing his doctorate at Oxford University. Over the next decade the disease progressed to the point that Hawking had serious difficulties with any motor task and eventually he was no longer able to speak. As we are well aware, however, Hawking's language and communication skills are as intact as ever. Like many people who have a severe or profound speech disorder, Hawking uses augmentative/alternative communication (AAC) to express himself. Although he is satisfied with the speech synthesizer he uses, Hawking has complained that it gives him an American accent (Hawking, 2003).

There are four essential building blocks of normal speech: (1) breathstream, (2) voice, (3) articulation, and (4) fluency.

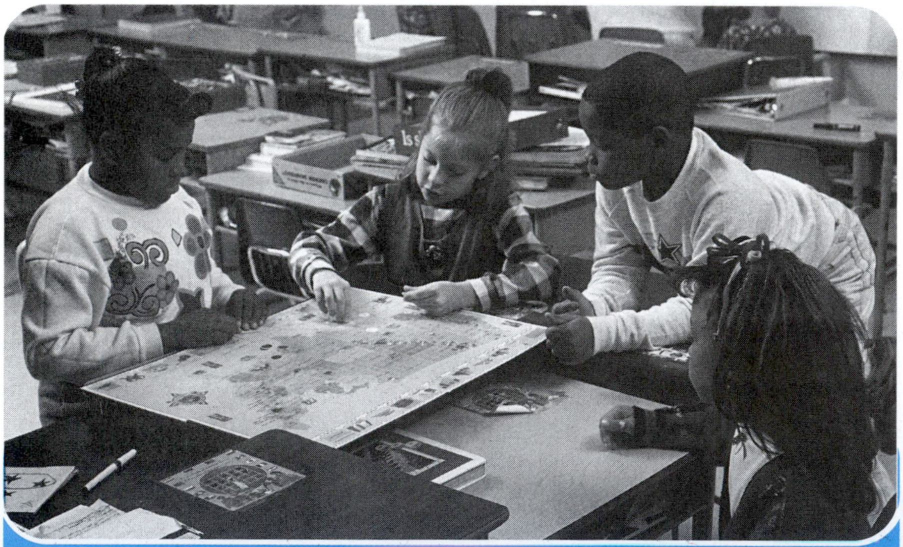

A person who is unable to speak does not necessarily have impaired language abilities.

1. *Breathstream.* Speech begins with the exhalation of breath. A speaker must have an adequate breathstream that is exhaled consistently and evenly for good speech to occur. A speech disorder can result from an inability to produce or maintain a strong breathstream.
2. *Voice.* Speech requires a strong and even voice. Voice quality can affect speech significantly; a breathy, hoarse, broken, or nasal voice can distract a listener and undermine the effectiveness of speech. Likewise, a voice that is too loud, too soft, too high, or too low can also undermine speech quality. Loud and soft describe vocal intensity, whereas high and low describe vocal pitch.
3. *Articulation.* Speech requires precision in phoneme production. In Standard American English, roughly 40 phonemes are used and reused to produce a seemingly endless supply of words. The difference between two words—like *bat* and *pat,* or *pin* and *pen*—may be only one phoneme. Phonemes must be produced accurately and consistently for effective speech. There is room for some minor variation in how particular phonemes in a language are produced, as in dialects, which are the systematic variations of a particular language that arise in social or geographic communities. However, consistent omission (e.g., saying "tee" for *tree*) or distortion (e.g., saying "bark" for *park*) of phonemes can lead to significant problems in using speech to accurately reflect language.
4. *Fluency.* Speech is most effective when it is produced effortlessly and smoothly, with few hesitations, interjections, and circumlocutions. Hesitations are long pauses. Interjections are the use of filler words (*um, er*) and phrases (*I mean, like, you know*). Circumlocution is talking around a word by describing features of it (e.g., "That thing you keep dishes in"), and is accompanied by hesitations and interjections ("I put it on the, on the, uh, you know . . . the thing you keep dishes in."). Speech is fluent when all the elements of good delivery come together.

Hearing

Definition

In the spoken communication process, there is a sender and a receiver. The receiver's job includes reception and comprehension of the information being conveyed, namely, language via speech. Hearing is essential to reception and comprehension. Hearing, or **audition,** is the perception of sound; applied to the communication process, audition involves specifically the perception of speech.

Sound Fundamentals

To understand hearing, it is important to have a general sense of acoustics. **Acoustics** is the study of sound (Borden et al., 1994). To understand acoustics, we'll use a demonstration. Clap your hands. Your clap creates a sound, which is subsequently registered in the auditory portion of your brain. What is the chain of events that gets the clap sound from your hands to your brain, where the sound is processed? There are four essential steps, as shown in Figure 1-7: creation of sound source, vibration of air particles, reception by ear, and comprehension by brain (Champlin, 2000).

FIGURE 1-7 Role of hearing in spoken communication.

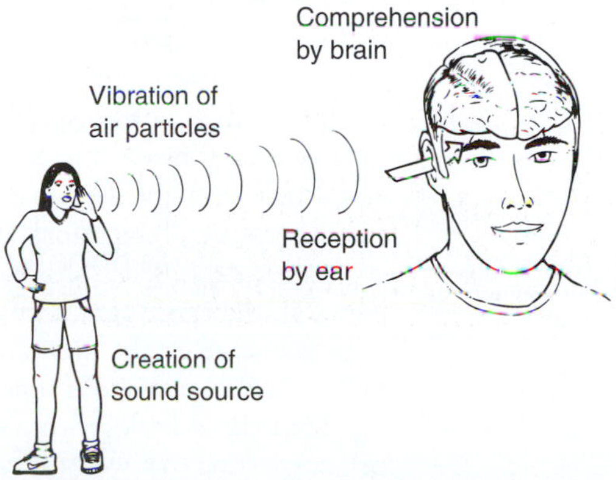

1. *Creation of sound source:* A sound source sets in motion a series of events. The sound source creates a disturbance, a set of vibrations, in the surrounding air particles. When you bring your hands together to clap, this sets the air particles near the sound source into a complex vibratory pattern.
2. *Vibration of air particles.* Sound is, fundamentally, the movement or vibration of air particles. The air particles, set in motion by the sound source, move back and forth through the air (or other medium, such as water). How fast the particles move back and forth is the sound **frequency**, or pitch. How far apart the particles move when going back and forth relates to **intensity**, or the loudness of the sound. When you clap your hands, you set the air particles around the sound source into a vibratory pattern, and how the particles move carries information about frequency (pitch) and intensity (loudness); this information is carried through the air to the ear of the receiver.
3. *Reception by ear.* The ear is specially designed to channel information carried by the air particle vibrations into the human body. The ear is a complex structure with three chambers. The outer chamber (outer ear) captures the sound and channels it to the middle chamber (middle ear). The third chamber then receives the sound information (inner ear); this chamber is connected to a nerve that leads to the brain. Information from the air particle vibrations—and particularly information about frequency and intensity—is sent through these three chambers and then along the auditory nerve to the audition centers of the brain.
4. *Comprehension by brain.* The auditory centers of the brain, located in the left hemisphere, translate frequency and intensity information sent through the ear and along the auditory nerve. If the information that arrives at the brain involves speech sounds, the speech and language centers of the brain help in the comprehension process. If the information that arrives at the brain is not a speech sound—as is the case with a clap—the speech and language centers are not involved. Sound information is differentiated by the human brain as speech or nonspeech. The human ear and brain are designed to be "remarkably responsive" to processing the sounds that humans use for speech (Borden et al., 1994, p. 176).

Speech Perception

Speech perception is the processing of human speech. Speech perception is different from auditory perception, a more general term that describes the brain's processing of any type of auditory information. The processing of a clap or an insect's buzz involves auditory perception, but processing the word *Help!* requires speech perception. As sound information is sent from the ear and auditory nerve to the brain, the brain differentiates between general auditory information and speech sounds. Speech perception involves specialized processors in the brain that have evolved specifically to make sense of human speech.

Figure 1-8 shows a spectrogram of a person saying the word *judge*. A spectrogram provides a three-dimensional depiction of the speech signal that is carried by the movement of air particles into the human ear (Kent, 1997). The spectrogram is included here to provide a general sense of the information that is translated by the human brain in the speech perception process. It also shows how complicated speech information is! The word *judge* depicted in the spectrogram involves three phonemes: /ʤ/ /^/ /ʤ/. To the trained observer, each phoneme can be identified based on its particular sound structure using information in the spectrogram about time, frequency/pitch, and amplitude/loudness.

Sometimes analogies are made between reading a spectrogram and reading the alphabet, suggesting that we can read a sequence of phonemes (e.g., /ʤ/ + /^/ + /ʤ/ = /ʤ ^ ʤ /

FIGURE 1-8 Spectogram for *judge*.

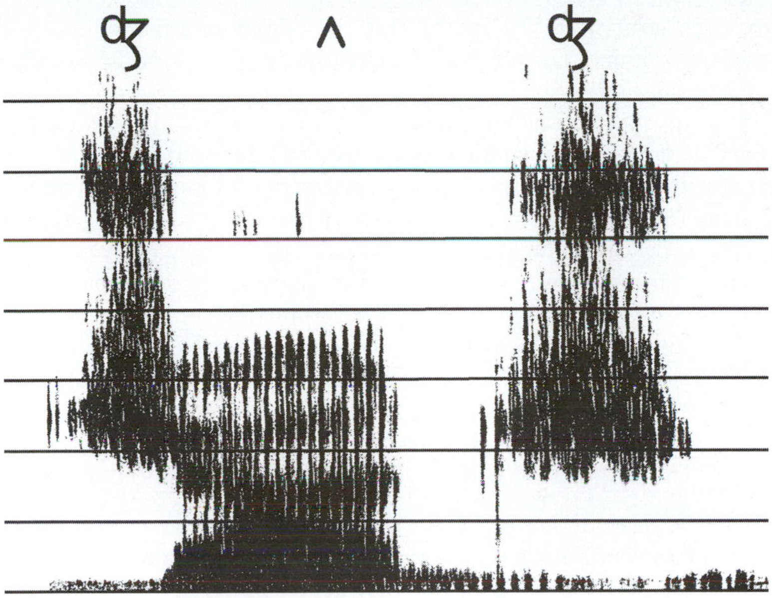

Source: From *The Speech Sciences* 1st edition by KENT. Reprinted with permission of Delmar Learning, a division of Thomson Learning: www.thomsonrights.com. Fax 800 730-2215.

just as we can read a series of letters (e.g., j + u + d + g + e = judge). Scientists have shown that this analogy is incorrect. When humans produce phonemes, the phonemes overlap with one another, a process called co-articulation. For instance, say the word *judge* and think closely about your production of the first /ʤ/ sound. You will realize that it carries information about the next sound—the /^/. Hold the /ʤ/ for a moment or two before releasing to the vowel and notice that your lips are jutting forward in a rounded position, as if you are about to give your pet a kiss. Now note how this initial /ʤ/ in *judge* is quite different from the final /ʤ/, in which the lips are not rounded in anticipation of the vowel. Co-articulation is the term used to describe this "smearing," or overlapping, of phonemes in the production of strings of speech sounds. The articulators (lips, tongue, etc.) co-articulate speech sounds because it is much quicker than producing just one sound at a time, and the brain has evolved to make sense of co-articulated speech sounds. The production and processing of co-articulated phonemes are what allow humans to produce words at incredibly rapid rates and what undermine the notion of speech as a sort of spoken alphabet.

Discussion Point: *In your own words, describe the difference between the terms* communication, speech, language, *and* hearing.

What is a Communication Disorder?

Normal and Disordered Communication

Whether communication occurs via speech and hearing, writing and reading, or sign or other manual means, individuals are normal and effective communicators when they are able to formulate, transmit, receive, and comprehend information from other individuals successfully. A communication disorder or impairment is present when a person has significant difficulty in one or more of these aspects of communication when compared with other people sharing the same language, dialect, and culture. Formulation and comprehension difficulties usually signal a language impairment; problems with transmission usually suggest a speech impairment; and problems with reception usually signal a hearing impairment. The term *significant* means that the communication difficulty is serious enough to adversely impact an individual's ability to participate in the home, school, work, or community environment.

The process of communication is remarkably complex and involves many biological systems. For instance, spoken communication involves the hearing apparatus, the visual system, the articulators, the left and right hemispheres of the brain, the larynx, and the respiratory system. (The way in which these systems are used for communication will be described in chapter 3.) Given the many systems involved, there are many possible points at which a breakdown can occur, resulting in communication impairment. For instance, a stroke can cause damage to the brain regions governing the comprehension of language, which can affect the communication process to the extent that the person might not be able to understand spoken language. Traumatic brain injuries, developmental disabilities, hearing loss, and aging are other factors that can have an adverse influence on communication and can result in significant communication impairment.

There are four key points at which a breakdown in communication may occur (see Figure 1-2):

1. *Formulation:* Difficulty in effectively formulating a message for communication. Aphasia is a type of communication disorder resulting from stroke in which people can have significant problems formulating their thoughts and ideas into words. Aphasia is described in chapter 8.
2. *Transmission:* Difficulty in effectively transmitting a message for communication. Motor speech disorders are a type of communication disorder affecting the neuromuscular systems governing the articulators, such as the tongue, lips, and palate. People with cerebral palsy, for instance, may experience a motor speech disorder resulting in difficulty in effectively transmitting their thoughts and ideas through speech, even if these ideas are formulated well. Motor speech disorders are described in chapter 6.
3. *Reception:* Difficulty in effectively receiving a message being communicated. Noise-induced hearing loss, a type of communication disorder in which significant hearing loss is caused by prolonged exposure to loud noise, can result in a problem with reception. Noise-induced hearing loss is described in chapter 14.
4. *Comprehension:* Difficulty in effectively decoding or comprehending a message being communicated. Mental retardation is a developmental disorder characterized by mild to severe intellectual difficulties. Individuals with moderate to profound levels of mental retardation often have problems comprehending what others are saying, even though their reception is intact. Mental retardation is discussed in chapter 7.

Communication Disorders and Communication Differences

The way an individual communicates with others is highly influenced by the individual's culture. Culture describes a system of knowledge comprising beliefs, behavior, and values that is shared by a particular community (Battle, 2002, p. 3). The community may be defined by many diverse parameters, including language (speakers of African American English), religion (people who are Catholic), geography (inhabitants of Brooklyn), ethnicity (people who are Hispanic), race (people who are Asian), health status (people with diabetes), sexual identity (people who are heterosexual), marital status (unmarried people), and so forth.

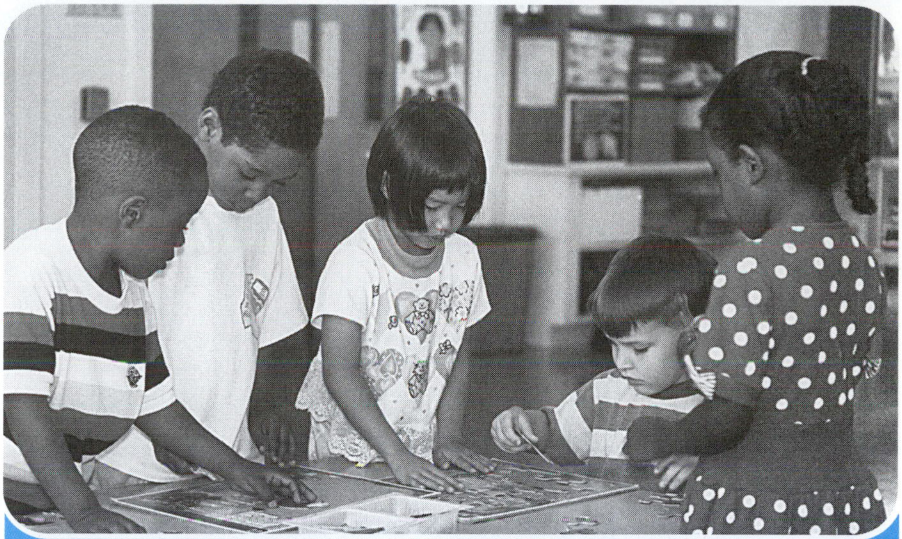

Our cultural identity strongly influences the way we communicate with each other.

Any one person's cultural identity is likely to be influenced by these many dimensions as well as others. Likewise, the way a person communicates is also influenced by these diverse dimensions, and there is no one way to communicate that is better than others. Rather, "speech, language and communication are embedded in culture" (Battle, 2002, p. 3). Accordingly, culture influences communication, and communication influences culture. The two cannot be separated.

Because communication is so heavily influenced by culture, it is important when trying to identify a communication disorder to first rule out the presence of a communication difference. In our increasingly diverse country, communication differences are common. Consider two kindergarten children on a playground in Charlottesville, Virginia. One child, JaJuan, lives in a Latino household in which only Spanish is spoken. The family recently immigrated to the United States from Cuba. JaJuan knows very few words in English and tends to be unresponsive to the communication of adults and children in his classroom. The other child, Gabrielle, has lived in central Virginia her whole life. She is African American, speaks the local dialect of African American English, and is one of the more communicative children in her classroom, often persistently asking questions of her teachers and initiating conversations with her peers. The communication skills of these two children are very different. An observer might view JaJuan as having poor communication skills—on the playground, he doesn't understand what others are saying, he doesn't initiate conversations with his peers, and he has a difficult time getting his needs met.

Could we say that JaJuan has a communication disorder? After all, earlier in this chapter, a communication disorder was defined as significant difficulties in formulation, transmission, reception, and/or comprehension. Clearly JaJuan has difficulties in all four of these areas, at least on this English-speaking playground. However, in identifying communication disorders, an individual's communication skills must be significantly discrepant when compared with those of others who have the same language, dialect, and cultural background. Thus it would be inappropriate to view JaJuan's communication skills as anything more than simply different from those of the children around him. JaJuan's communication difficulties are most appropriately viewed as a communication difference, not a communication disorder.

A communication difference is present when an individual's communication patterns differ substantially from those of the person or persons with whom he or she is communicating. The differences between speakers may be relatively minor, as in the case of people using different dialects of English. Dialects are the variations of a language shared by a particular group of speakers; dialectical variations of a language affect all domains of language, including content, form, and use. In many cases, however, the communication differences among speakers may be significant, particularly when they do not share the same language or when they speak

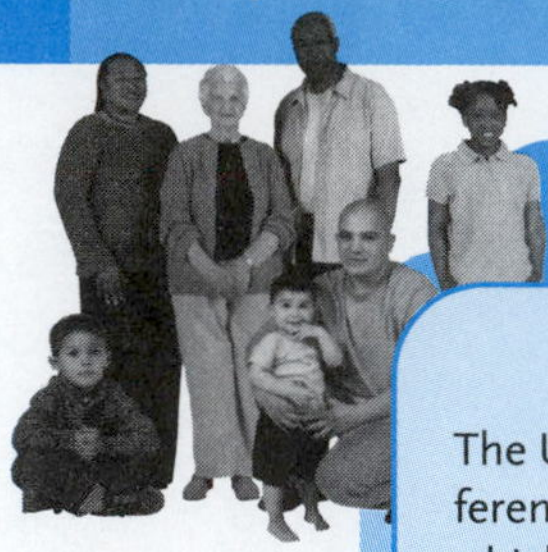

BOX 1-2 Multicultural Focus

Cultural Competence and Communication Disorders

The United States is a culturally rich society, one that not only brings together people of many different cultures, but that also embraces the differences among us. Today, the communities in which we live comprise people from hundreds if not thousands of diverse ancestries. Because the way we communicate is linked to our cultural identity, the study of human communication disorders must be attuned to appreciating and recognizing human diversity. This diversity encompasses race, ethnicity, language, and religion; all these pieces contribute to individual differences and preferences in communication patterns and beliefs.

People who study and treat communication disorders must have a keen awareness of, sensitivity to, and appreciation for human diversity in communication; in short, they require cultural competence. Cultural competence means being sensitive to nine cultural parameters (Tomoeda & Bayles, 2002).

Individualism and Collectivism. Individualistic cultures place great value on individuals and their decisions and accomplishments; collectivist cultures place greater value on group membership.

Views of Time and Space. Individuals in clock-oriented cultures organize their days around clocks, schedules, and daily planners and emphasize punctuality. Individuals in event-oriented cultures emphasize completion of one event (however long that takes) before beginning another.

Roles of Men and Women. The roles of men and women vary substantially across cultures, influencing access to education, ownership, and choice of profession. Some cultures are relatively patriarchal, whereas others are relatively matriarchal, with males or females, respectively, dominating rule and decision making.

Concepts of Class and Status. Cultural communities attribute class and status to their members in diverse ways. In capitalistic cultures, class is hierarchical and derived from income, job prestige, and level of education. Some cultures derive hierarchies from familial lineage and heritance. Other cultures are egalitarian, with all members provided equal status.

Values. Cultures are diverse concerning the relationship of humans to nature, to other human beings, to ancestors, and to the environment.

distinct dialects of one language. Having spent a year in a Chinese-speaking country without speaking Chinese, I can attest to the frustration that can result from communication differences. While it would not be appropriate to say that I had a communication disorder during that year in Taiwan, significant communication differences made some daily living activities challenging indeed.

For professionals working in the fields of communication sciences and disorders, understanding the distinction between a communication disorder and a communication difference is not a light matter. Mistaking a communication difference as a disorder has likely contributed to the overrepresentation of children from minority populations, such as Native Americans, among those receiving special education services in U.S. schools (Battle, 2002). Professionals who diagnose or treat communication disorders must study an individual's communication performance within the context of the indigenous culture or language group. A communication disorder is present only when an individual's communication ability

1. operates outside the minimal norms of acceptability of one's culture or language group

Communication. Cultures vary on a continuum ranging from high to low context, which relates to how much context contributes to communicating meaning. In low-context cultures, the words themselves are crucial, and contextual information is often superfluous. In high-context cultures, contextual information may be more important than the words used during communication.

Rituals. Each culture has its own rituals for commemorating meaningful historical events, life changes, and commitments to shared values, including weddings, births, deaths, and worship.

Significance of Work. Cultures differ in their perceptions of work and recreation. In some cultures, people identify themselves by their work from the earliest of ages (e.g., "What do you want to be when you grow up?"), whereas in other cultures people are defined by the groups to which they belong and by their role in the community.

Beliefs about Health. Cultures differ in the ways disabilities and illnesses are explained. Some cultures may view individuals with disabilities and illnesses as special or as bewitched. In many cultures, people believe that illness occurs when an individual is out of harmony with nature or the universe. Cultural differences also exist in determining the appropriate person to provide health care or restore well-being to one who is ill.

For Discussion

What are some ways to develop cultural competence?

What are some ways in which concepts about status and time might influence communication between two people?

The last decade has seen an increase in Americans' use of Asian healing arts, including acupuncture, shiatsu, and yoga. What other aspects of American culture have seen great changes in recent years as a result of Asian influence?

Adapted from Tomoeda, C., & Bayles, K. (2002, April 2). Cultivating cultural competence in the workplace, classroom, and clinic. *ASHA Leader Online*. Retrieved October, 2, 2004, from http://professional.asha.org/news/020402d.cfm. Reprinted with permission.

Companion Website

To answer these questions online, go to the Multicultural Focus module in chapter 1 of the Companion Website.

2. is considered disordered by one's culture or language group, and
3. interferes with communication or calls attention to itself within one's culture or language group (Taylor, 1986, p. 13).

Classification

Language, speech, and hearing are the fundamental elements of spoken communication. A breakdown in any one of these three areas can result in a communication disorder. Communication disorders are generally differentiated into three broad categories: disorders of language, disorders of speech, and disorders of hearing. An additional category of communication disorder is discussed in this textbook: disorders of feeding and swallowing. Because the feeding and swallowing processes are so intricately tied to the communication system—particularly the areas involved with speech—feeding and swallowing problems are increasingly considered under the communication disorders umbrella. The entire umbrella is presented in Figure 1-9.

FIGURE 1-9 The communication disorders umbrella.

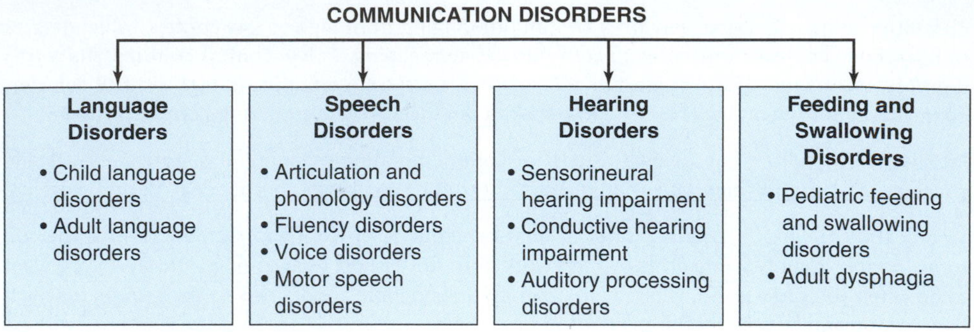

Disorders of Language

A language disorder refers to a breakdown in the linguistic system that has an impact on one or more of the following domains: semantics, syntax, morphology, phonology, or pragmatics. Language disorders are differentiated according to whether they affect children or adults.

Child Language Disorders. Child language disorders are one of the most common disorders of early childhood. Children with language disorders have problems communicating with others because of difficulties in the development of semantics, syntax, morphology, phonology, or pragmatics. Language disorders in children may be developmental or acquired. Developmental disorders are present at or soon after birth, and symptoms are manifested as children develop. Acquired disorders are experienced after birth, usually as a result of an injury. One of the most prevalent types of child language disorders is specific language impairment (SLI), which affects about 7% of children (Tomblin et al., 1997). SLI refers to a significant disorder of language in the absence of any other developmental disability. Language disorders are also common in children who have mental retardation, autism, and traumatic brain injury. Altogether, about 12% of young children exhibit a language disorder (NIDCD, 1995).

Adult Language Disorders. Adult language disorders comprise a diverse range of developmental (present since birth, e.g., adult SLI) and acquired disorders. Aphasia is a prevalent adult language disorder that results from damage to the brain, particularly the language areas of the left hemisphere. Aphasia is a frequent consequence of stroke, but it can also result from traumatic brain injuries, such as would be caused by a gunshot wound or car accident. Aphasia takes different forms, depending on the location and severity of the brain injury. Some people with aphasia have problems only with complex language tasks, such as reading and writing or following complicated directions, whereas others are unable to produce or understand any language at all. Approximately 80,000 people are diagnosed with aphasia each year. While this disorder can affect adults of any age, the majority of people with aphasia are 65 or older (ASHA, 2003a).

Disorders of Speech

A speech disorder refers to a breakdown in one or more of the systems involved with speech production: respiration, phonation, and articulation.

Disorders of Articulation and Phonology. Articulation and phonological disorders are two varieties of speech production impairments characterized by distortions, substitutions, and omissions of speech sounds. Speech production impairments are most common in young children, affecting about 10% of youngsters (Gierut, 1998). An articulation or phonological impairment is present when a child fails to use speech sounds at a level appropriate for his or her age and cultural and linguistic background.

Disorders of articulation occur at the site of speech output, shown in the speech production model in Figure 1-6, and are usually attributed to some sort of structural problem or problem with articulatory placement. Articulation disorders are a common consequence of cleft palate, which is a congenital malformation of the lip and/or palate. Disorders of phonology occur at the site of the perceptual representation of speech sounds (see Figure 1-6), resulting in underdeveloped or faulty representations of speech sounds, which undermines production of those sounds. Although the point of breakdown differs in these two varieties of speech disorders, the manifestation is similar in that the child has difficulties with the production of speech sounds. Technically, phonological disorders are best viewed as disorders of language, but because the disorder is evidenced as a problem with speech sound production, they are typically viewed under the umbrella of speech disorders.

Fluency Disorders. Communication difficulties that are characterized by "an abnormally high frequency or duration of stoppages in the forward flow of speech" are referred to as fluency disorders (Peters & Guitar, 1991, p. 9). Their most common characteristics are repetition and prolongation of sounds and complete blockages of the airflow, usually accompanied by body movements (e.g., head nods, blinking) in an attempt to stop or reduce these disfluencies. As might be expected, many people with disorders of fluency have tense, negative feelings about speaking. Many young children go through a stage of normal dysfluency, which should be differentiated from true fluency disorders. Fluency disorders affect about 1% of the general population (Bloodstein, 1987).

Voice Disorders. Communication difficulties characterized by difficulties with the voice are voice disorders. An underlying difficulty with voice production usually manifests itself as either a complete lack of voice (aphonia) or a hoarse voice (dysphonia). Aphonia and dysphonia affect nearly everyone at some point, as they can result from illness or isolated overuse of the voice (e.g., cheering at a football game). However, chronic aphonia or dysphonia due to ongoing overuse or misuse of the voice or that results from an underlying pathology, such as cancer of the vocal folds, can seriously affect one's life.

Severe voice disorders, including a complete lack of voice, can result from injuries or illnesses to the vocal folds or the surrounding tissues or organs. One of the most common reasons for a complete loss of voice is laryngeal cancer. The larynx is the cartilaginous container that holds the vocal folds. The vocal folds vibrate to produce voice. Cancer of the vocal folds, a risk for smokers, particularly older men, may necessitate surgery to remove vocal fold growths or, in some cases, to remove the larynx. In such cases, a loss of voice is the trade-off for survival.

Motor Speech Disorders. Like the speech production impairments previously described, motor speech disorders are communication disorders characterized by distortions, substitutions, and omissions of speech sounds. However, with motor speech disorders, the pathology is attributed to a dysfunction with the nervous system that controls motor output of the speech stream. Motor speech disorders are also often referred to as *neurogenic speech disorders* to emphasize their neurological underpinnings. There are two major types of motor speech disorders, apraxia and dysarthria, both of which affect children and adults.

Discussion Point: *Mrs. Parish, described in Box 1-1, has a severe motor speech disorder resulting from stroke. How has it affected her life?*

Disorders of Hearing

Hearing disorders occur when there is a breakdown in the reception or transmission of sound along the auditory pathways traveling from the ear to the brain.

Sensorineural Hearing Impairment. Sensorineural hearing loss refers to a breakdown in the hearing system in the inner ear or in the auditory nerve that runs from the inner ear to the brain centers. Sensorineural hearing loss can be congenital (present at birth) or acquired, as in the case of noise-induced hearing loss, in which the hair cells of the inner ear are damaged and become less sensitive to sound. Sensorineural hearing loss can range from mild, requiring no or minimal treatment, to profound. Cochlear implants are a late-twentieth-century cutting-edge treatment used to enhance or restore hearing ability in people with profound sensorineural loss, also referred to as deafness.

Conductive Hearing Impairment. Conductive hearing impairment describes a breakdown in the hearing system in the outer or middle ear. Malformation of the outer ear, a torn eardrum, and the buildup of fluid in the middle ear (associated with middle-ear infections) are common causes of conductive hearing loss, particularly in children. Middle-ear infections, or otitis media, are increasingly common in young children. One recent study conducted with 2,253 infants in Pittsburgh found that 91% of children experienced otitis media between birth and 2 years of age (Paradise et al., 1999). Chronic otitis media during the first few years of life has been linked (although not definitively) to delays in communication development (Friel-Patti & Finitzo, 1990; Roberts, Burchinal, & Zeisel, 2002; Roberts, Wallace, & Henderson, 1997).

Discussion Point: *Middle-ear infections have become much more common in recent decades. Brainstorm some reasons why this might be so.*

Auditory Processing Disorder. An auditory processing disorder (APD) is a breakdown in the processing of speech sounds in the auditory center in the brain. This center is responsible for localizing sounds, discriminating sounds, and recognizing auditory patterns. Auditory processing disorders have been linked to specific nervous system disorders, such as Alzheimer's disease; however, in many cases, no neuropathology can be identified (ASHA, 1996). Symptoms of APD overlap with those of other learning and attentional difficulties, making it difficult to accurately diagnose this disorder. Symptoms include difficulty paying attention, poor listening skills, difficulty following multistep directions, slow processing time, and impaired language and literacy development (NIDCD, 2003).

Disorders of Feeding and Swallowing

Feeding and swallowing problems are considered within the spectrum of communication disorders because of the functional overlap of the neurological systems that control feeding and swallowing functions and those that control communication. The treatment of feeding and swallowing problems has received little attention historically. Traditional treatment for children and adults who could not eat or swallow focused on bypassing the feeding/swallowing systems (e.g., putting the person on a feeding tube) with little attempt to improve or restore feeding and swallowing. The recognition that the ability to eat and drink is a critical aspect of quality of life for people of all ages has brought changes in the last two decades, and there has been significant progress in the design and delivery of treatments focused on improving or restoring feeding and swallowing functions.

Pediatric Feeding and Swallowing Problems. Pediatric feeding and swallowing problems tend to be associated with specific developmental disorders, such as cleft palate or cerebral palsy, and prematurity or low birth weight. In addition to undermining the child's growth and development, feeding and swallowing disorders may bring adverse behavioral reactions to feeding and may compromise the caregiver-child relationship. Children with structural impairments, such as cleft palate, may not be able to feed or to swallow because of lip or palate malformations. Children with neurological impairments, as in the case of cerebral palsy, may not be able to manage the precise motor control needed to feed and to swallow. Children who are born prematurely or are of a low birth weight may not have the neurological maturity to handle the complexities of the feeding/swallowing process. Children with chronic reflux, or regurgitation of stomach acids into the oral cavities, may resist eating altogether. Pediatric feeding and swallowing problems can also result from traumatic events, such as brain injuries, stroke, and infections (Arvedson & Rogers, 1997). When children are unable to feed or swallow, it is critical that their nutritional needs be met in other ways. One common method is tube feeding, as when a nasogastric tube is run through the nose down into the stomach. It is important to provide children who are being tube fed with therapies to promote feeding and swallowing skills so that they can later be transitioned to oral means of nutrition.

Adult Dysphagia. Adult dysphagia refers to a swallowing disorder. Often the result of a nervous system dysfunction, such as that resulting from stroke or a progressive ailment like Alzheimer's disease, dysphagia includes such problems as difficulty with chewing or managing food orally and difficulty with triggering or maintaining a swallow. Symptoms of these difficulties include choking and coughing while eating, repetitive swallows or throat clearing, regurgitation of food after eating, pain while swallowing, loss of weight or energy, and change in appetite (Schulze-Delrieu & Miller, 1997). Swallowing problems should always be treated quickly and aggressively, as people with dysphagia are at risk for choking and for malnourishment, both of which can have fatal consequences.

Discussion Point: *Box 1-1 discusses a case of infant feeding and swallowing problems. Why was a nasogastric tube used?*

What Careers Are Available in the Field of Communication Sciences and Disorders?

As a broad discipline that brings together psychology, education, health, technology, and linguistics, the field of communication science and disorders attracts many people from diverse backgrounds. The disciplines most closely aligned with the study and treatment of communication disorders are speech-language pathology and audiology. Within these disciplines, specialization is available in many areas, among them speech science, hearing science, multicultural issues, geriatrics, child language, phonology, and neurogenics. Increasingly, treatment of communication disorders involves a multidisciplinary, team-based approach involving many educational, medical, and allied health professionals, such as special educators, pediatricians, occupational therapists, physical therapists, and nurses.

Speech-Language Pathology

Speech-language pathologists, or SLPs, are frequently the lead service providers for people with speech and language disorders and are also key members of the treatment team for people with hearing, swallowing, and feeding disorders. The scope of practice for speech-language pathologists is presented in Figure 1-10. As can be seen, these professionals have diverse responsibilities, from evaluating infant feeding and swallowing problems to identifying alternative communication techniques for people who have severe communicative difficulties. Speech-language pathology assistants (SLPAs) are paraprofessionals who work under the supervision of SLPs to conduct speech-language screenings, assist in assessment, and implement treatment plans with clients. The roles and responsibilities of SLPAs, as well as training avenues, are still evolving, and the extent to which SLPAs are involved in speech-language services can vary significantly across states.

Employment Contexts

Speech-language pathologists work in a variety of settings, including public and private schools, hospitals, rehabilitation facilities, home health agencies, community and university clinics, private practices, group homes, state agencies, universities, and corporations (ASHA, 2001). Currently more than 100,000 speech-language pathologists in the United States are certified by the American Speech-Language-Hearing Association (ASHA), yet there remains a

FIGURE 1-10 Scope of practice for speech-language pathology.

The practice of speech-language pathology includes prevention, diagnosis, habilitation, and rehabilitation of communication, swallowing, or other upper aerodigestive disorders; elective modification of communication behaviors; and enhancement of communication. The practice involves the following activities.

1. Providing prevention, screening, consultation, assessment and diagnosis, treatment, intervention, management, counseling, and follow-up services for disorders of (1) speech, including articulation, fluency, resonance, and voice; (2) language, including comprehension and expression in oral, written, graphic, and manual modalities; language-based processing; and preliteracy and language-based literacy skills; (3) swallowing or other upper aerodigestive functions; (4) cognitive aspects of communication; and (5) sensory awareness related to communication, swallowing, or other upper aerodigestive functions.
2. Establishing augmentative and alternative communication techniques and strategies.
3. Providing services, such as speech-reading, to individuals with hearing loss and their families and caregivers and providing hearing screening.
4. Using instrumentation to observe, collect data, and measure parameters of communication and scaffolding.
5. Selecting, fitting, and establishing effective use of prosthetic/adaptive devices for communication and swallowing.
6. Collaborating to assess central auditory processing disorders and providing treatment when speech, language, and other cognitive abilities are affected.
7. Educating and counseling individuals and families about communication and swallowing.
8. Advocating for persons with communication disorders through community awareness, education, and training programs to promote and facilitate access to full participation in communication.
9. Collaborating with other health professionals, including providing referrals as individual needs dictate.
10. Addressing behaviors and environments that affect communication and swallowing functions.
11. Providing services to modify or enhance communication performance, such as accent modification and care and improvement of the professional voice or the transgendered voice.
12. Recognizing the need to provide and appropriately adopt services to individuals from diverse cultural backgrounds.

Source: Adapted from the American Speech-Language-Hearing Association. (2001). *Scope of practice in speech-language pathology.* Rockville, MD: Author. Reprinted with permission.

significant shortage of speech-language pathologists in most regions of North America. The U.S. Department of Labor (Hecker, 2001) named speech-language pathology as one of the top 30 fastest-growing professions of the next decade. Reasons for the shortage—and for the continued growth of this profession—include: (1) an increased awareness of the importance of early intervention, (2) greater success in life-saving measures for children born with significant health impairments, (3) the aging of the U.S. population, (4) an increased awareness of health promotion and disease prevention, (5) a nationwide increase in implementation of newborn hearing-screening measures, and (6) the passage of federal laws focused on improving the rights and addressing the needs of people with disabilities (e.g., Individuals with Disability Education Act, Medicare, and Medicaid) (ASHA, 2003e). In addition, there is great demand for doctoral-level speech-language pathologists to fulfill university research and teaching positions in part because of the overall growth of the profession and in part because of the retirement of baby boomers holding faculty positions.

Employment benefits, including overall job satisfaction as well as compensation, are high for speech-language pathologists. The median annual salary for speech-language pathologists in 2002 was $51,000, with a starting salary of about $43,000 (ASHA, 2002e). In a recent survey of more than 500 speech-language pathologists, the majority reported high satisfaction with their work and low overall job stress levels (Blood, Thomas, Ridenour, Qualls, & Hammer, 2002). On the other hand, like many other professionals in the education and health disciplines, SLPs currently face many challenges in effectively executing their jobs. In education, some SLPs face inappropriately high caseloads, excessive paperwork, isolation from other professionals, lack of support for collaboration, inadequate access to up-to-date materials, and the like. In health care, SLPs face many of the same challenges, compounded by constantly changing federal and state regulations regarding reimbursement for therapies. To address these challenges, speech-language pathologists organize themselves through state-level organizations, such as the Speech and Hearing Association of Virginia (SHAV), and national organizations, such as the American Speech-Language-Hearing Association (ASHA), to lobby for improved working conditions.

Credentials

The entry-level credential for a speech-language pathologist (SLP) is a master's degree from an ASHA-accredited training program. The degree typically requires completion of a 2-year postbaccalaureate specialized program involving intensive training in diagnosis and treatment of speech, language, and swallowing disorders. At least 36 semester hours of graduate-level coursework are required, as well as 375 hours of supervised clinical fieldwork. For national certification, SLPs must pass a national examination in speech-language pathology and complete a supervised 9-month clinical fellowship. Figure 1-11 presents the steps for clinical certification by ASHA. The entry-level credential for a research or faculty-level position in speech-language pathology is typically a research doctorate (Ph.D.) in speech and hearing sciences, speech-language pathology, or a related field (e.g., psychology).

BOX 1-3 Spotlight on Research

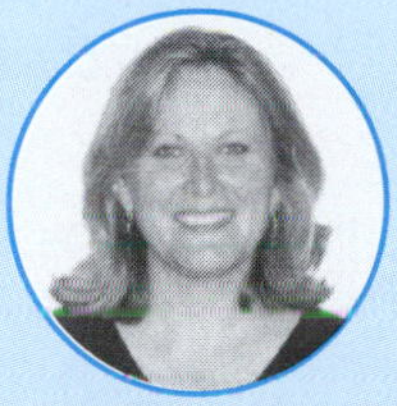

Erika M. Zettner, Ph.D., CCC-A
Associate Clinical Professor of Audiology, Joint Doctoral Program in Audiology at San Diego State University and the University of California, San Diego

Imagine the eyes emitting light and the nose emitting an aroma. Impossible, you say? Well, okay, that is a little far-fetched. However, the ears can emit sound! These noises are very soft and usually inaudible to others. Intensive investigation by dedicated researchers has led to the conclusion that the noises are serendipitously emitted as a result of normal inner-ear processes. I say serendipitously because although these sounds are not required for hearing, careful analysis has found that they reveal characteristics of the inner ear that we might not otherwise have known about. Recordings of these emitted sounds, called otoacoustic emissions, are now a standard part of hearing assessment. As a researcher, I focus on the question, "How can people hear even when there is loud background noise?" My current approach to this question is to measure otoacoustic emissions while introducing two or more sounds into the ear. These recordings tell me how the inner ear processes more than one sound at a time. This area interests me because being unable to hear when there is loud background noice is the most common complaint among individuals with hearing impairments. It is even a common complaint in people with normal hearing. Who would believe not only that sounds are emitted from the ears, but also that these sounds give clues about listening in noisy environments? Research provides opportunities to explore answers to questions like these that impact us all every day.

FIGURE 1-11 So you want to become a speech-language pathologist or audiologist . . . Here's how.

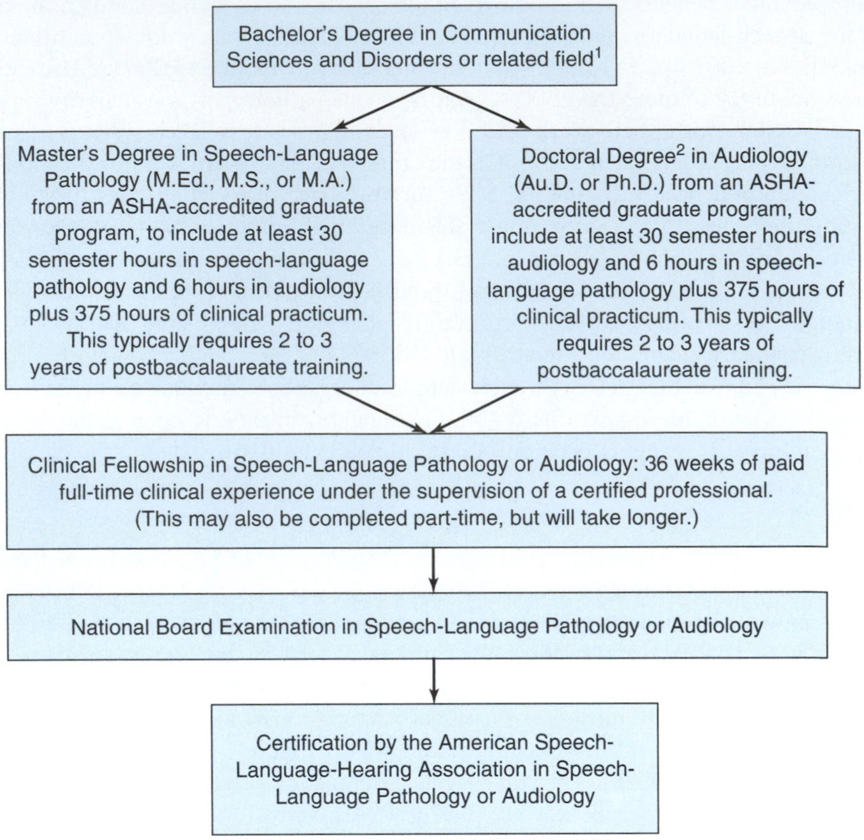

[1]This must include 27 credit hours in the basic sciences
[2]Doctoral degree required for people applying for certification in 2012 or later
Source: American Speech-Language-Hearing Association. (2005). Retrieved January 10, 2005, from http://www.asha.org/public/cert/

Audiology

Audiologists are specialists in identifying, assessing, and managing disorders of the auditory, balance, and other neural systems (ASHA, 1996). Primary roles involve prevention, identification, and management of hearing and balance system dysfunction. The scope of practice for audiologists is presented in Figure 1-12. These professionals work closely with SLPs when hearing affects an individual's communicative ability.

Employment Contexts

Audiologists work in many of the same settings as speech-language pathologists, including schools, hospitals, rehabilitation facilities, community and university clinics, private practices, and universities (ASHA, 2001). There are more than 12,000 audiologists currently working in the United States.

For the first decade of the 21st century, the occupational outlook for audiology is excellent. Audiology is ranked as one of the fastest growing professions for 2000–2010, with

BOX 1-4 Spotlight on Practice

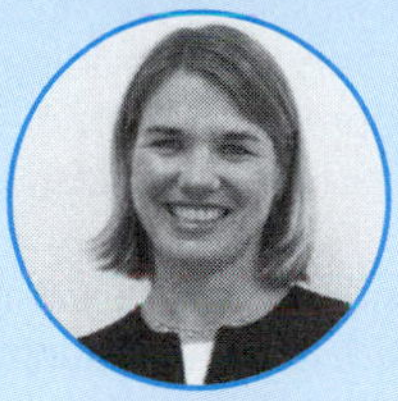

Rebecca Lower, M.Ed., CCC-SLP
Speech-Language Pathologist/
Clinical Instructor
University of Virginia Speech-Language-Hearing Center

During our nation's economic downturn, for much of the United States' workforce the prospect of going from the corner office to the unemployment line has become a real concern. Throughout this time, the number of positions for speech-language pathologists has not only remained stable, but has expanded, bolstered by ongoing changes in education and health care, two systems that drive how speech-language pathologists practice. Over the last several years, our scope of practice has grown beyond the bounds of traditional speech and language services in response to the medical community's call for services for individuals with swallowing difficulties and the education system's need for intervention for children struggling to read.

Although adapting to changes such as these can be stressful, I feel that it is a gift to have a career that challenges me and allows me to grow and solidify my place as an invaluable member of the community. Having practiced as a speech-language pathologist in many settings over the last decade—in a private pediatric practice (St. Petersburg, Florida), in children's health care (Atlanta, Georgia), in a child development center (Denver, Colorado), and in public schools (Santa Barbara, California)—I have now shifted to working indirectly with clients by training preprofessional speech-language pathologists at The University of Virginia's master's training program in communication disorders. Each semester, I supervise students in their initial forays into clinical practice. I find it especially exciting in my position at The University of Virginia to have the opportunity to work directly with our bright, young future professionals and to ensure the quality of our professional services.

FIGURE 1-12 Scope of practice in audiology.

Audiologists serve a diverse population and may function in one or more of a variety of activities. The practice of audiology includes the following activities.

1. Promotion of hearing wellness, prevention of hearing loss, and protection of hearing function by designing, implementing, and coordinating occupational, school, and community hearing-conservation and identification programs.
2. Identification of hearing problems by conducting activities that identify dysfunction in hearing, balance, and other auditory-related systems; supervising, implementing, and providing follow-up of newborn and school hearing-screening programs; screening for speech, language, and cognitive disorders; identifying populations and individuals who are at risk for hearing loss and other auditory or balance impairments; collaborating with speech-language pathologists to identify populations and individuals at risk for developing speech-language impairments.
3. Assessment of auditory performance to include the conduct and interpretation of methods to assess hearing, auditory function, balance, and related systems; measurement and interpretation of electrodiagnostic tests focused on neurophysiologic monitoring and cranial nerve assessment; evaluation and management of children with auditory-related processing disorders; performance of otoscopy; cerumen management; preparation of reports to interpret and summarize data; and referral to other professionals and agencies.
4. Rehabilitation of auditory performance to include evaluating, selecting, fitting, and dispensing hearing assistive technologies; assessing candidacy of persons for cochlear implants and providing habilitation for these devices; developing culturally appropriate audiological rehabilitative management plans; providing comprehension rehabilitation services for people with hearing loss that include communication

(*continued*)

FIGURE 1-12 *(continued)*

strategies, manual communication, and speech reading; consulting and providing vestibular and balance rehabilitation; participating in the development of individual education plans (IEPs) for school children; and measuring noise levels and monitoring environmental modification to reduce noise levels.

5. Advocacy and consultation for the communication needs of all individuals, including advocacy of specific issues that affect the rights of individuals with normal hearing; consultation to educators as a member of interdisciplinary teams; and consultation about accessibility for people with auditory dysfunction and hearing loss.
6. Education, research, and administration for audiology graduate and other professional education programs, to include measuring functional outcomes, consumer satisfaction, and the efficiency of practices and programs concerning the delivery of audiologic services, and the design of basic and applied audiologic research to increase the knowledge base and to develop new methods and programs related to audition and hearing.

Source: Adapted from the American Speech-Language-Hearing Association. (2004c). Scope of practice in audiology. *ASHA Supplement 24.* Rockville, MD: Author. Reprinted with permission.

a 45% increase in jobs anticipated during this time (Hecker, 2001). The reasons for this growth include advances in hearing technologies as well as the involvement of audiologists in providing services to a rapidly increasing older population.

The median annual salary for audiologists in 2002 was about $54,000, with a starting salary of about $42,000 (ASHA, 2002e). There is currently a shortage of practitioners and researchers in the audiology field. Like SLPs, audiologists also face challenges in the current health-care climate, in which professionals are asked to do more with less and regulations governing reimbursement change frequently. Audiologists advocate for their profession through their affiliation with state-level organizations and national organizations, including the American Academy of Audiology (AAA, or Triple A) and ASHA.

Credentials

The entry-level credential for a clinical audiologist is a master's degree from an ASHA-accredited graduate training program. The steps for becoming a certified audiologist are presented in Figure 1-11. At least 36 semester hours in communication science and disorders coursework is required at the graduate level, with 30 hours in the major area, and 375 hours of supervised clinical fieldwork. Beginning in 2012, a clinical doctorate (Au.D.) in lieu of a master's degree will be required for national certification. Audiologists also must pass a national examination in audiology and complete a supervised 9-month clinical fellowship. The entry-level credential for a research or faculty-level position in audiology is typically a research doctorate (Ph.D.) in speech and hearing sciences or audiology.

Allied Professions

Key partners in the assessment and treatment of communication disorders include special educators and many medical and allied health professionals, such as neurologists, occupational therapists, otorhinolaryngologists, pediatricians, and psychologists. Although the diagnosis and treatment of a communication disorder is usually the primary responsibility of speech-language pathologists and audiologists, these additional players have critical roles.

Special Educators

Special educators support the educational progress of children with communication disorders and often work closely with speech-language pathologists and audiologists. There are more than 300,000 special educators in U.S. schools (U.S. Department of Education, 1999). Serving primarily in public and private educational settings, special educators worked with nearly 6 million students in the year 2000 (Individuals with Disabilities Education Act [IDEA] Data, 2003). Early childhood special educators typically work with children who are 3 to 5 years of age, whereas special educators work with those between 6 and 21 years old and tend to specialize in a particular area (e.g., learning disabilities or behavioral disorders). More than 1.3 million 3- to 21-year-old children in U.S. public schools were identified as requiring speech-language services in 2000 (IDEA Data, 2003). Special educators are critical team members in designing special services for these children and in coordinating service delivery with parents, regular educators, and specialists. Special educators often collaborate with speech-language pathologists and other educators on eligibility, program, and placement decisions for students with communication disorders (Council for Exceptional Children, 2001). In working with families of children with communication disorders, special educators are often involved with activities associated with behavior management; career, vocational, and transitional planning; technology utilization; and promotion of independent living and community participation.

The field of special education is rapidly growing. In 2000, there were about 415,000 special educators working with exceptional children between the ages of 3 and 21 years. Licensure for special educators varies by state. The minimal requirement is typically a bachelor's degree from an accredited program, which involves specialized coursework in the characteristics of learners, individual learning differences, strategies for individualizing instruction, typical and atypical communication development, assessment, instructional planning, and collaboration. Almost 50% of special educators hold a graduate degree, and the majority are specially certified for their specific assignment (Boyer & Mainzer, 2003).

Occupational Therapists

Occupational therapists (OTs) deliver interventions to help people with disabilities, illnesses, or injuries develop or regain the activities of daily living (ADL), such as grooming, eating, and writing. OTs often work closely with infants, toddlers, and elderly people who are experiencing problems with feeding and swallowing.

Otorhinolaryngologists

Otorhinolaryngologists, or ear-nose-throat physicians (ENTs), collaborate with speech-language pathologists and audiologists in the diagnosis and management of communication disorders. ENTs work closely with people who have injury or illness of the ear, nose, or throat, performing surgery, prescribing medication, and conducting diagnostic investigations.

Neurologists

Neurologists help to identify the etiology of many communication disorders, particularly those involving nervous system dysfunction, such as autism, cerebral palsy, stroke, Alzheimer's disease, and Parkinson's disease.

Pediatricians

Pediatricians play an important role in early identification and ongoing treatment of communication disorders in children of all ages. Pediatricians, in collaboration with parents, provide referrals to speech-language pathologists and audiologists for speech, language, feeding, swallowing, and hearing assessments when warning signs are present.

Psychologists

Discussion Point: *Consider the cases discussed in Box 1-1: Anika, Mr. Shen, and Mrs. Parish. What is the role of the SLP and the audiologist in each of these cases?*

Psychologists are often involved in the evaluation and treatment of people with communication disorders, particularly when educational, behavioral, and emotional complications exist. Psychologists may complete diagnostic evaluations to include speech-language assessment and can help families cope with the challenges associated with communicative impairments.

CHAPTER SUMMARY

Communication is the sharing of information between two or more people. Humans communicate to achieve instrumental, regulatory, personal, heuristic, imaginative, and informative purposes. An effective communicator uses communication for these diverse purposes and is able to avoid communication breakdowns by providing and attending to feedback during the communication process.

Language, speech, and hearing are the essential ingredients of communication. Language is a socially shared, rule-governed symbol system used by humans to represent ideas about the world. Five domains of language include semantics, syntax, morphology, phonology, and pragmatics. Speech is a complex neuromuscular process that turns language into a sound medium that is transmitted to another person. Speech involves a three-stage process: conceptualization of a perceptual target, development of a motor schema, and speech output. Hearing is the perception of sound, and when applied to the communication process, refers specifically to the perception of speech. The acoustic process involves the creation of a sound source, the vibration of air particles, reception by the ear, and comprehension by the brain.

Significant, ongoing communication breakdowns may signal a communication disorder. Communication disorders are differentiated as language disorders (child language disorders, adult language disorders), speech disorders (articulation and phonology disorders, fluency disorders, voice disorders, motor speech disorders), hearing disorders (sensorineural hearing impairment, conductive hearing impairment, auditory processing disorder), and feeding and swallowing disorders (pediatric feeding and swallowing disorders, adult dysphagia).

The primary professionals who work with people who have communication disorders are speech-language pathologists and audiologists, both of whom are certified by the American Speech-Language-Hearing Association. Special educators, medical professionals, and members of the allied health professions also play key roles in diagnosis and remediation of communication disorders.

KEY TERMS

acoustics, p. 19
audition, p. 19
communication, p. 4
communication breakdown, p. 7
communication functions, p. 8
comprehension, p. 6
content, p. 13
extralinguistic feedback, p. 7
feedback, p. 6
form, p. 13
formulation, p. 5
frequency, p. 20
Grice's maxims, p. 9
intensity, p. 20
linguistic feedback, p. 7
metalinguistic awareness, p. 14
modality, p. 6
morphology, p. 14
nonlinguistic feedback, p. 7
paralinguistic feedback, p. 7
phoneme, p. 17
phonology, p. 14
pragmatics, p. 14
productivity, p. 12

reception, p. 6
semanticity, p. 12
semantics, p. 14
species specificity, p. 12
speech perception, p. 20
syntax, p. 14
transmission, p. 6
universality, p. 12
use, p. 13

ON THE WEB

Check out the Companion Website! On it, you will find:

- suggested readings
- reflection questions
- a self-study quiz
- links to additional online resources, including information about current technologies in communication sciences and disorders

An Overview of Communication Development

Khara Pence

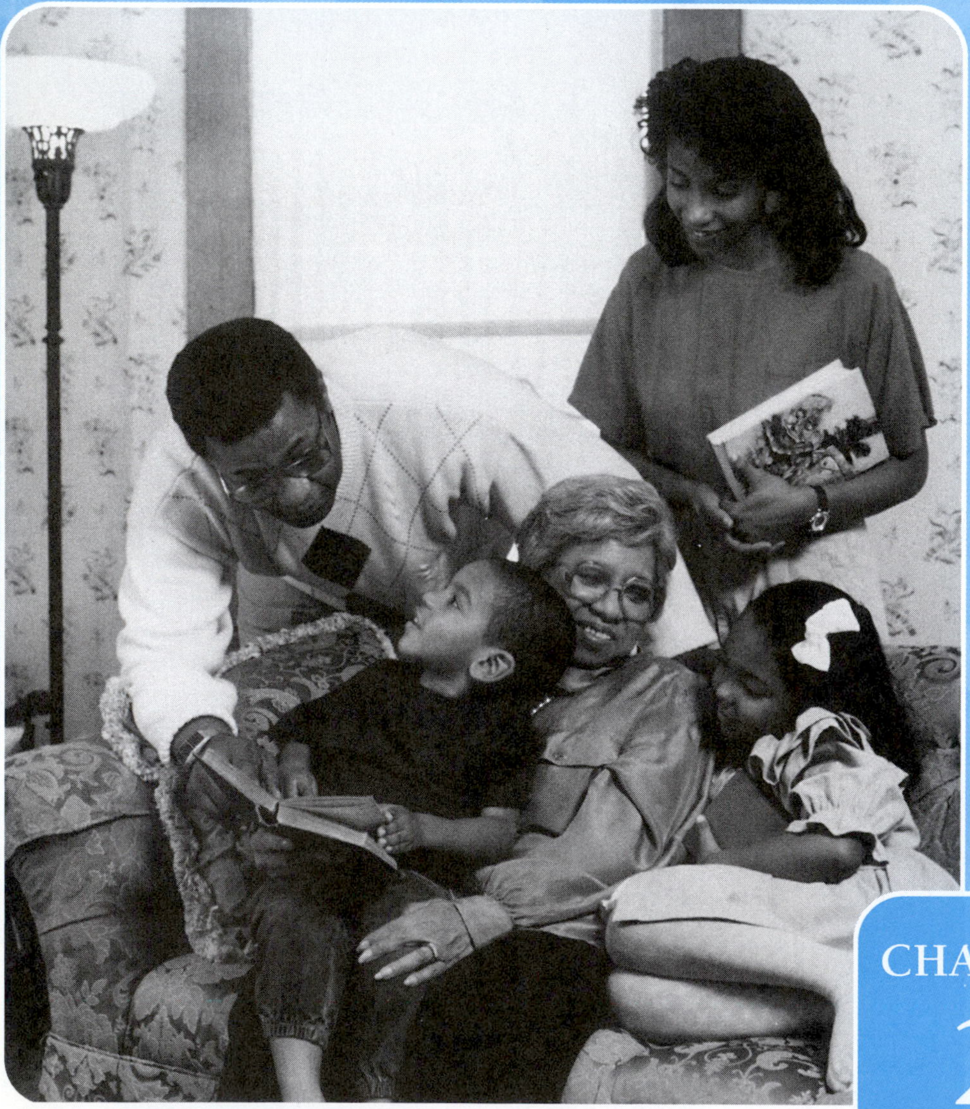

CHAPTER 2

FOCUS QUESTIONS

This chapter answers the following questions:

1. What is communicative competence?
2. What is the foundation for communicative competence?
3. What are major communicative milestones in infancy and toddlerhood?
4. What are major communicative milestones in preschool and school-age children?

INTRODUCTION

Before we can begin to understand disorders of communication, it is important to first understand how communication abilities develop in typical populations. This chapter provides an overview of communication development in typical populations. It defines communicative competence, describes the foundation for communicative competence, details some of the major milestones in language and speech development that take place between birth and adolescence, and considers some important multicultural issues in language and speech development. As you read this chapter, think about the development of communicative competence in some of the people you know. They could be your own children, nieces and nephews, brothers and sisters, or children you see on a regular basis. After reading this chapter, you may be surprised by the many capabilities we possess at birth, and you will gain a deeper appreciation for the rapid pace of communicative development and the qualitative differences in communication skills humans exhibit at various stages across the lifespan.

What Is Communicative Competence?

Definition

Communicative competence is the knowledge and implicit awareness that speakers of a language possess and utilize to communicate effectively in that language. Communicative competence entails much more than speaking in grammatically well-formed sentences; communicative competence is the speaker's skilled navigation of both linguistic and pragmatic elements of language that enables them to communicate successfully with other members of their speech community (Hymes, 1972). A speaker with communicative competence knows how, where, when, and with whom to speak.

Consider, for instance, how a speaker carefully modifies vocabulary choices, sentence structure, pitch and loudness, and body posture to simplify speech for an infant: "Addie go bye-bye!" Consider how this speech differs from speech to a peer: "Are you planning

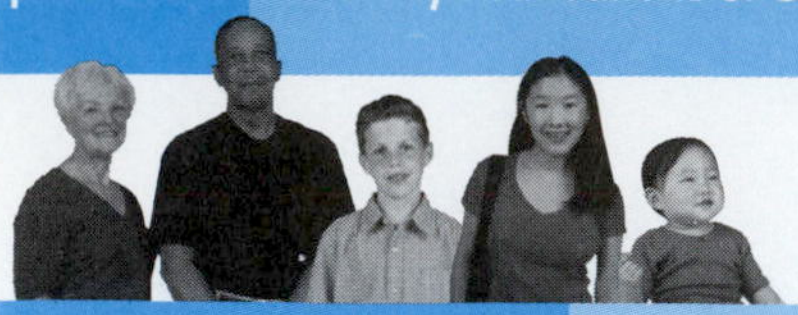

BOX 2-1 Communication Disorders Across the Lifespan: Case Examples

Leon is a 2-year-old child with a fraternal twin, Lionel. Lionel is talking in two-word sentences, but Leon is using only a few words. Leon and Lionel have a 6-year-old sister, Leona. These three youngsters are the children of a professional couple, Mr. and Mrs. Turner, residing in San Antonio, Texas. The Turners are concerned about Leon's speech and language development because it seems slow in comparison with his brother's. Leon does not inflect the verbs he uses ("Daddy ride bike"), and he speaks mostly in 2-word sentences ("Leon do"), whereas Lionel is beginning to inflect verbs ("Daddy's running"), and he uses more words in his sentences ("I want more juice"). Furthermore, both boys seem to be talking less than Leona did when she was 2. They seem to have more limited vocabularies and to ask fewer questions than Leona did. Mr. Turner conducted research on the Internet and found that 2-year-old children should be speaking in three- or four-word sentences, which heightened their concern. Mrs. Turner is taking Leon to the pediatrician next week for his 2-year well-child visit and plans to raise her concerns at that time.

Internet research

1. See what sources are available on the Internet concerning language milestones in young children. Evaluate the reputability of the resources you find.
2. Use the Internet to see what you can find out about language development in fraternal twins. Do twins usually develop language at the same rate?

Brainstorm and discussion

1. What are some possible reasons for the differences in the rate of language acquisition of Leon and Lionel?
2. The Turners are concerned because Leon and Lionel do not seem to be talking as much as their older sister did when she was their age. Do you think birth order has an impact on language development? Why or why not? Do you think gender has an impact on language development? Why or why not?

Reston is an 8-year-old boy who has struggled with speech and language development since he was a toddler. He is currently in the third grade at a public elementary school in northern Virginia. He receives speech and language therapy at his school for a language disorder, and he works with the learning disabilities specialist to help him with reading and writing. Reston still has difficulty recognizing how combinations of letters correspond to certain sounds in English. For example, he tries to decode, or sound out, words like *weigh* and *neighbor*. Reston also struggles with reading sentences fluently because he devotes so much of his attention to sounding out words. Reston's parents are concerned because at the end of the year Reston will be required to take the third-grade state-mandated achievement test. They do not think he will pass; moreover, they do not think he should have to take the test. Reston's parents are organizing a parent meeting at the school to discuss what they call high-stakes testing and whether it is appropriate for third graders in general as well as those with disabilities.

Internet research

1. What is a third-grade state-mandated achievement test?
2. Do all students have to take state-mandated achievement tests?
3. Why are these tests called high-stakes tests?

Discussion Point: *Think about the infant-directed speech that you use or that you have heard others use. How does infant-directed speech differ from the speech you use with your friends?*

on taking Adelaide with you to the picnic?" The former is an example of infant-directed speech, or the speech that we use when addressing young language learners, and it illustrates how communicative competence does not necessarily equate to using grammatically well-formed sentences. Instead, communicative competence allows a speaker to fine-tune language across different contexts and with different speakers to communicate most effectively.

Recall from chapter 1 that successful communication requires a sender to formulate and transmit a message and a receiver to receive and comprehend the message in the context of four communication processes (formulation, transmission, reception, and comprehension). Two aspects of communicative competence—linguistic and pragmatic—enable

Brainstorm and discussion

1. Should all students in public schools be required to take state-mandated tests of achievement? Why or why not?
2. Should students with disabilities be given modifications for these tests? If so, what kinds of modifications would be appropriate?

Sam Donalds is a 46-year-old man living in a small rural town in West Virginia. Sam, a coal miner, stopped working 3 years ago because of respiratory problems. He now receives disability benefits and is not employed. Sam has always had problems reading and has for the first time thought about going to school to try to improve his reading. He thinks that he may want to learn how to read better and then tutor students in elementary school. Sam has begun to attend a local adult literacy education program through his church. On Sam's first visit last week, his teacher, Ms. Lewis, gave him a basic assessment of word reading, which showed that he reads at a third grade level. This assessment also showed that Sam has significant problems with phonological awareness. For instance, Sam couldn't hear or make rhymes. Ms. Lewis did not think that Sam would be able to improve his reading skills to a large extent because of these problems. She is meeting with him this week to discuss other opportunities for volunteer work besides tutoring.

Internet research

1. What kinds of supports are available in your community for adults who want to learn to read?
2. What kinds of programs are available, according to Internet sources, to build phonological awareness?
3. To what extent is adult illiteracy a problem in the United States?

Brainstorm and discussion

1. What are your thoughts on Ms. Lewis's prognosis for Sam? Do you agree or disagree with her perspective?
2. Do you think it possible that problems in phonological awareness could be contributing to Sam's reading difficulties? Do you think these can be remediated?
3. What would *you* recommend if you were Sam's teacher?

humans to engage successfully in all four of these communication processes. Figure 2-1 provides a description of the different types of linguistic and pragmatic competencies that provide for successful communication.

Linguistic Aspects of Communicative Competence

Linguistic aspects of communicative competence relate to the nature and structure of language and include phonological competence, grammatical competence, lexical competence, and discourse competence.

FIGURE 2-1 **Linguistic and pragmatic aspects of communicative competence.**

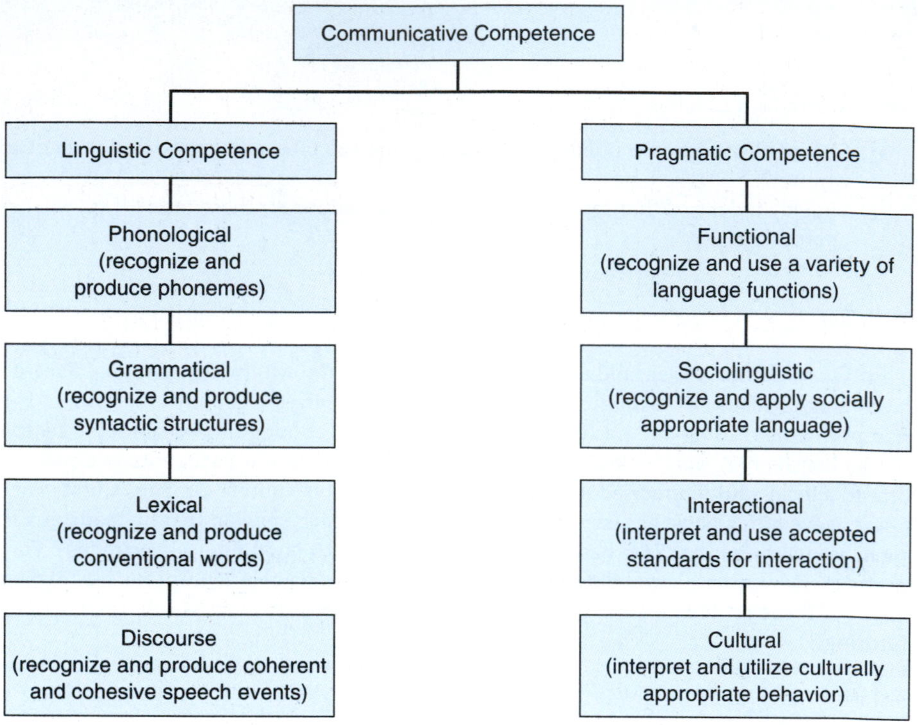

Phonological Competence. Phonological competence is the ability to recognize and produce the distinctive, meaningful sounds of a language, or phonemes. For English speakers, the consonant sounds /r/ and /l/ are phonemes, and changing these sounds in the context of other sounds would produce a change in meaning (*rip* and *lip* have different meanings, as do *rot* and *lot*). For speakers of some other languages, including Japanese, the consonant sounds /r/ and /l/ are not phonemic. As anyone who has studied another language knows, learning to distinguish and pronounce sounds that are not part of your native language's inventory is extremely challenging. Luckily, infants learning language for the first time are experts at dealing with fine phonemic contrasts.

Discussion Point: *Explain why it is so difficult to learn to speak a new language without an accent in light of what you now know about phonological competence.*

Infants are equipped to distinguish among the sounds of all the world's languages from birth. In the first few months of life, infants become attuned to the sounds they hear on a regular basis, and their ability to distinguish among sounds that are not in the phonemic repertoire of their own language diminishes. By the time infants reach their first birthday, they have become proficient in the sounds of their native language. At this time, children enter a period of vocabulary explosion; they begin to devote precious learning resources to the task of learning new words, at the expense of being able to make finer distinctions among sounds (Stager & Werker, 1997).

Although children's receptive phonological competence is achieved within their first year, competence in producing individual phonemes comes at a slower pace because it depends heavily on the development of the articulators. An infant's vocal tract is not a miniature version of an adult vocal tract; infants' vocal tracts more closely resemble the vocal tracts of nonhuman primates. The infant vocal tract is very small, and the larynx sits high in the throat. Only with development and time does the larynx drop lower to approximate its location in human adults.

Even as the vocal tract takes on its more adultlike shape, phonological competence does not magically appear. Although the articulators may be in place for children to produce the sounds of their native language, phonological errors that characterize children's expressive phonology often mask competence. In the field of language development, we call these errors phonological processes. **Phonological processes** are the normal phonological deviations that young children make in producing specific sounds and words. Phonological processes are context-specific processes, meaning that they occur in certain speech contexts. For example, consonants often take on features of sounds that follow them in words; thus, many young children produce the word *dog* as "gog", *cat* as "tat", or *yellow* as "lellow." In each case, the error occurs because of contextual influences in the word—for instance, the /d/ in *dog* becomes /g/ because of the influence of the /g/ at the end of the word. These naturally occurring processes should not be confused with an articulation disorder in which a child is physically unable to produce the /d/ or /k/ sounds in any context, or a phonological disorder in which these processes do not stop occurring at the appropriate age.

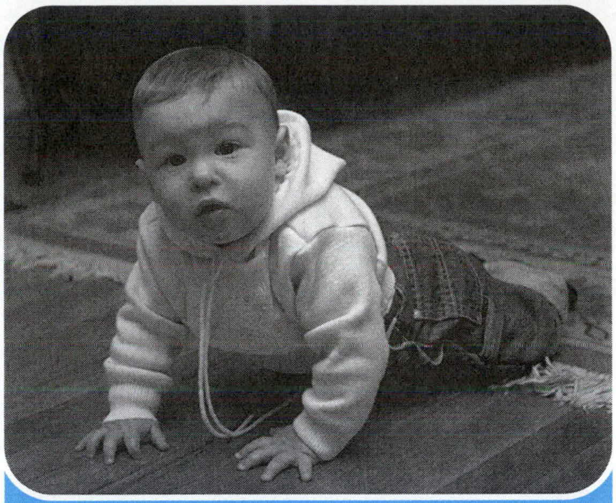

The infant vocal tract is not a miniature version of the adult vocal tract.

Grammatical Competence. The second linguistic aspect of communicative competence, grammatical competence, is the ability to recognize and produce the syntactic and morphological structures of a language effectively. For example, using their knowledge of word order, English speakers understand the sentence "Jim is hitting Bob" to mean that Bob is the recipient of Jim's unwelcome actions, and not the other way around. Infants demonstrate the ability to understand word order and know the difference between "Big Bird is tickling Cookie Monster" and "Cookie Monster is tickling Big Bird" by 16 months of age (Hirsh-Pasek & Golinkoff, 1996). In addition to using their knowledge of word order, English speakers utilize their knowledge of morphological structures to infer meaning. For example, English speakers understand that in the sentence "Jim is hitting Bob," the description of hitting and the act of hitting occur simultaneously because they recognize that /ing/ denotes continuous action. English-learning infants process these small but telling grammatical morphemes separately from the verbs on which they appear by 18 months of age (Addy et al., 2003).

Discussion Point: *Consider the case of Leon in Box 2-1. What evidence suggests that he is having some difficulty developing grammatical competence?*

Children's comprehension precedes production for grammatical competence. Although children understand the difference between "Big Bird is tickling Cookie Monster" and "Cookie Monster is tickling Big Bird" by 16 months of age, they might not produce such sentences until between 2 and 3 years of age. Likewise, children understand the meaning conveyed by the morpheme /ing/ by 18 months, but they do not produce this morpheme until about 24 months of age (Brown, 1973).

Lexical Competence. The third linguistic aspect of communicative competence is lexical competence. Lexical competence is the ability to recognize and produce the conventional words used by speakers of a language. Developments in this area occur early in the life of the language learner: infants usually understand their own names by about four months of age, understand the names of salient figures in their lives (e.g., *Mommy, Daddy*) by 6 months of age, and begin to comprehend other words shortly thereafter (e.g., *bottle, hug*). Interestingly, infants as young as 6 months who recognize their own names (or other highly salient and familiar names, such as *Mommy*) use this ability to their own advantage to learn new words. When infants hear their name embedded in continuous speech, they segment the word that follows it from the speech stream (Bortfeld, Rathbun, Morgan, & Golinkoff, 2003). So, an infant whose name is Annie who hears "Annie up" segments the *up* that follows *Annie,* which helps her to learn this new word. This early example of lexical competence shows how infants use their own names to get a foot in the door—once they learn to recognize their names as a unit of speech, they infer that the speech following it begins a new unit.

At all stages of life, lexical production follows lexical comprehension. For instance, although infants may understand a number of words at a very young age, they do not generally produce their first true word until 12 months of age. There are several possible reasons for why comprehension outpaces production (Golinkoff & Hirsh-Pasek, 1999). First, language comprehension requires only that we retrieve words, whereas language production requires that we assemble words. Second, with language comprehension, sentences are preorganized with lexical items, a syntactic structure, and intonation. Language production, however, requires that the speaker search for words, organize them, and place stress where required. Third, at least for infants and toddlers, language meant to be comprehended is usually highly contextualized, with many clues to aid comprehension. Children are generally at an advantage for comprehension because in most cases the words that are spoken to them have referents that are immediately available in the environment. In production, however, children must communicate a match between the context and language in order to express meaning.

Discourse Competence. Discourse competence, the fourth and final linguistic aspect of communicative competence, refers to the ability to fluently and coherently relay information to others. The speech event, rather than individual words or sounds, is the unit of analysis for discourse competence. People possessing discourse competence understand how to navigate ideas expressed across entire speech events when interpreting and producing extended conversation. For example, discourse competence allows listeners to assign reference to pronouns. Consider the following passage:

> My friend Jen once took a trip to the island of Corfu in Greece. While *there, she* joined her friends in swimming through a dark cave, which *they* later learned was called the "Canal D'Amour" because legend says that if a woman swims through *it* and passes a man swimming in the opposite direction, *they* will fall in love.

In order to successfully interpret each of the italicized words in the passage, the listener must rely on information given previously in the discourse. The word *there* refers to the island of Corfu, *she* refers to Jen, *they* refers to Jen's friends, and so forth. Likewise, the speaker navigates the expression of meaning over multiple sentences. For instance, the speaker identifies his or her friend Jen in the first sentence and then reverts to the pronoun *she* in future references.

Discussion Point: *Throughout this chapter, you have read that comprehension precedes production in several areas of communicative competence. What are some ways to test whether a child comprehends something that he or she is not yet producing?*

As with phonological, grammatical, and lexical competence, comprehension precedes production in discourse competence. Children who have not yet acquired discourse competence may fail to take the listener's perspective into account when using pronouns, for example. Preschool teachers frequently hear such exclamations as "He won't share with me," when the child speaking does not realize that he or she must introduce the conversational topic (in this case, name the offending child) before voicing the complaint.

Pragmatic Aspects of Communicative Competence

Pragmatic aspects of communicative competence relate to the social contexts in which language is used. People who possess competence in pragmatics take their conversational partner's attitudes, values, and beliefs into account when communicating. They also take the context of language into account and recognize that language can be used for a variety of purposes. Pragmatic aspects of communicative competence include functional competence, sociolinguistic competence, interactional competence, and cultural competence.

Functional Competence. Functional competence refers to the ability to communicate for a variety of purposes in a language. Recall from Chapter 1 that people share their thoughts and feelings for a variety of reasons; the three most basic functions are to request ("I'd like to try the red ones."), to reject ("No, thanks, these are too small."), and to comment ("I'll see if another store has my size."). As children develop, they communicate for an increasingly large set of purposes, such as reasoning, predicting, problem solving, and explaining.

Sociolinguistic Competence. Sociolinguistic competence is the ability to interpret the social meaning conveyed by language and to choose language that is socially appropriate for communicative situations. One important aspect of sociolinguistic competence is speech **register,** or the variety of speech appropriate to a particular speech situation. When talking with friends and family, informal registers are suitable ("Hey, how's it going?"), whereas conversations with, say, a prospective employer, call for a more formal register ("It is a pleasure to meet you."). The ability to switch among registers—for instance, to use a colloquial dialect with friends and a standard dialect with employees—is called code switching.

Interactional Competence. Interactional competence involves the ability to understand and apply implicit rules for interaction in various communication situations. Initiating and managing conversations appropriately are important skills for interactional competence, as is adhering to accepted standards for body language, eye contact, and physical proximity. These standards vary from culture to culture and even vary within cultures according to the communicative situation. To see how standards vary between cultures, we can compare two forms of interactional competence (initiating conversations and eye contact) in Japan and the United States. In Japan, children do not typically initiate conversations with adults, and people of all ages avoid direct eye contact. Conversely, in the United States, children frequently initiate conversation with adults, and Americans generally consider eye contact a sign of sincerity or confidence. To illustrate how standards for interactional competence differ within a culture according to the social context in which communication occurs, consider a new recruit in U.S. Army boot camp. It would be considered rude for the recruit to initiate conversation with the drill sergeant without first requesting permission to speak. Likewise, it would be considered inappropriate for the recruit to look the drill sergeant directly in the eye. Although these actions would be perfectly acceptable in other situations in American culture, the rules for this specific social situation dictate otherwise.

Cultural Competence. Cultural competence is the ability to function effectively in cultural contexts, both by interpreting behavior correctly and by behaving in a way that would be considered appropriate by the members of the culture. Cultural competence encompasses a wide variety of cultural understandings, including the attitudes, values, and beliefs of a culture's people. One mark of cultural competence is the ability to recognize expressions of emotion. For example, if we were to observe two people in close proximity to one another speaking in raised voices, we might infer that they were angry with one another or that they disagreed about something.

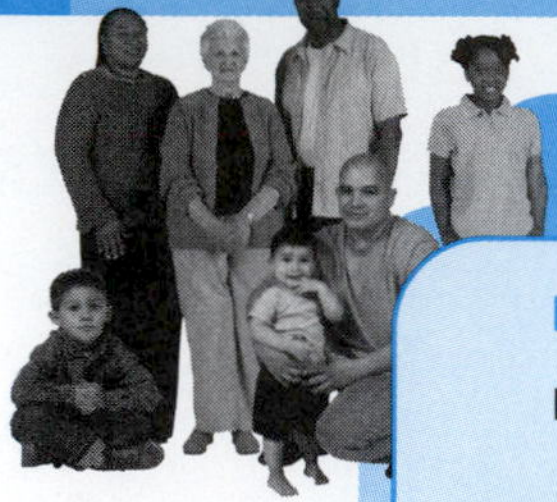

BOX 2-2 Multicultural Focus

Linguistic Variations

Language shapes the way we think, and determines what we can think about.

—Benjamin Lee Whorf

Is it possible that as we develop, the language we speak influences the way we think? This is exactly the theory proposed by Benjamin Whorf (1956), in what has come to be known as the **Whorf hypothesis.** The Whorf hypothesis proposes *linguistic determinism*, the idea that higher-order thinking is dependent on language. The Whorf hypothesis further proposes *linguistic relativism*, the notion that human experience is interpreted relative to language. The hypothesis essentially makes the argument that speakers of different languages experience the world differently.

Although many scholars believe that the Whorf hypothesis is not a valid way to consider the relationship between thought and language (see Gentner & Goldin-Meadow, 2003), the hypothesis is nonetheless helpful for explaining some recent research findings concerning how children categorize concepts cross-linguistically. For example, the English language distinguishes between actions that characterize containment (*put in*) and those that characterize support relationships (*put on*). The Korean language, on the other hand, distinguishes between tight-fit (*kkita*) and loose-fit, or contact relationships (various verbs) (Choi, McDonough, Bowerman, & Mandler, 1999). Children become sensitive to these language-specific spatial categories by 18 to 23 months, and Korean-learning infants of this age show evidence of classifying tight-fit relation events together. For instance, Korean-learning infants classify a book placed into a tightly fitting box and rings placed tightly on a pole similarly. English-learning infants, however, classify these two situations differently because they perceive one as representing a "put in" relation and the other as representing a "put on" relation. In other words, English-speaking infants do not categorize containment into loose versus tight fitting. Even at this young age, children are guided by their language in how they view certain spatial relations, a concept referred to as the *language as category maker hypothesis* (Bowerman & Choi, 2003).

Viewing children's native language as having a possible influence on the development of their cognition has important implications for understanding individual differences and diversity among children. Research shows, for example, that infants are sensitive to event concepts (e.g., the manner in which an object moves, the path that an object travels) that may later be labeled with verbs in their language (e.g., *spinning*) and that it is only as their vocabularies develop that their attention to event concepts not commonly labeled in their native language begins to diminish (Pulverman, Sootsman, Golinkoff, & Hirsh-Pasek, 2002). This and other research on the cognition-language relationship will inform understanding of linguistic variation across the world.

For Discussion

Do you agree with the Whorf hypothesis that language shapes thought? Have you ever experienced a thought or emotion that you just could not put into words? Do these types of experiences disprove or support the Whorf hypothesis? Many scholars have argued against the Whorf hypothesis as an ethnocentric hypothesis. It is a controversial idea. Why do you think it is so controversial?

Companion Website

To answer these questions online, go to the Multicultural Focus module in chapter 2 of the Companion Website.

What Is the Foundation for Communicative Competence?

The previous sections described the many areas of competence needed to achieve effective communication. This section describes the developmental pathways for these achievements from infancy to adulthood.

Earliest Foundations

We are not born with communicative competence. Rather, it takes time to acquire, and it is built on a host of early foundations. Several important early foundations are poured over the infant's first year, including joint reference and attention, rituals of infancy, caregiver responsiveness, and infant speech perception.

Joint Reference and Attention

Infancy is divided into three developmental phases (Adamson & Chance, 1998): (1) emergence to social partners, (2) emergence and coordination of joint attention, and (3) transition to language (see Figure 2-2).

Phase One: Birth to 6 Months. In the first phase, spanning from birth to about 6 months, infants develop patterns of attending to social partners. In these early months of life, infants value and participate in interpersonal interactions, learning how to maintain attention and be organized within sustained periods of engagement. Caregiver responsiveness is an important feature of this first phase; caregivers who are warm, sensitive, and responsive to their infants promote their children's ability and desire to sustain long periods of joint attention.

Phase Two: 6 Months to 1 Year. In the second phase, spanning from 5 or 6 months of age through about 1 year, children learn to navigate their attention between an object of interest and another person (Adamson & Chance, 1998, p. 18). This event signals the emergence of joint attention. **Joint attention** is the simultaneous engagement of two or more individuals in mental focus on a single external object. For example, members of the audience at a movie theater engage in joint attention as they focus on the movie. A baby and mother looking at a storybook are also engaged in joint attention. This seemingly simple activity symbolizes a critical avenue for early communication development, as periods of joint attention are the context in which children develop important communicative abilities. Children who engage in longer periods of joint attention with their caregivers have relatively larger vocabularies at 18 months compared with children who have fewer such experiences (Tomasello & Todd, 1983). Often, caregivers share much of the burden in sustaining periods of joint attention through a variety of techniques, such as using an animated voice, novel objects, and the like; this is called supported joint engagement. In supported joint engagement, the adult attempts to sustain the child's participation in a period of joint focus.

FIGURE 2-2 Three phases of infancy.

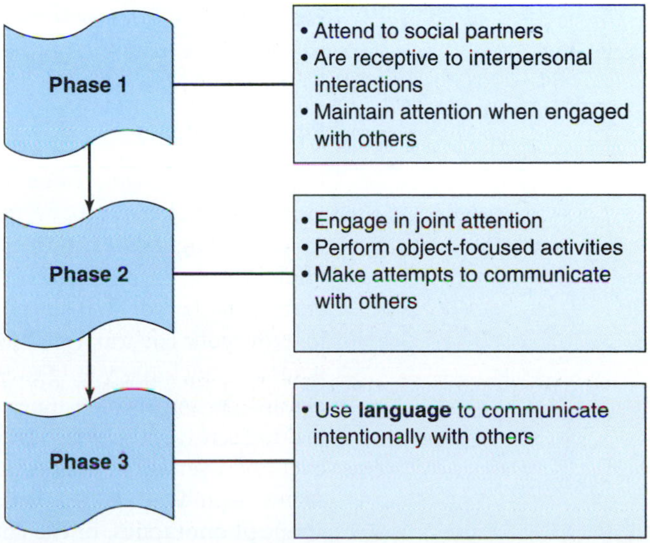
Phase 1
• Attend to social partners
• Are receptive to interpersonal interactions
• Maintain attention when engaged with others
Phase 2
• Engage in joint attention
• Perform object-focused activities
• Make attempts to communicate with others
Phase 3
• Use language to communicate intentionally with others

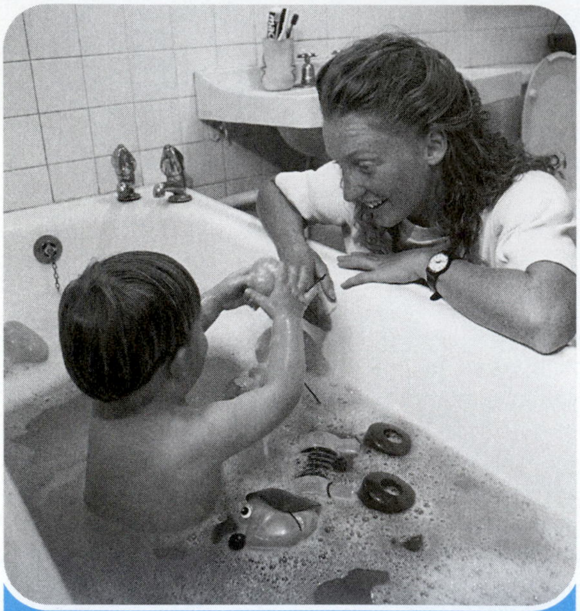

Episodes of joint attention help support young children's learning of new words.

Why is joint attention so important? In the absence of joint attention, infants miss out on word-learning opportunities and world-to-word mappings. Imagine a young infant being pushed in a stroller as his mother points upward and utters "Look at the birdie." Suppose the infant misses his mother's pointing gesture and hears the word *birdie* while he is focused intently on his new shoes. In this situation, mother and son are not jointly attending to the same entity in the world, making it unlikely that the baby will learn what the word *birdie* refers to. In the worst-case scenario, the baby might associate the word *birdie* with his new shoes. Luckily, by 18 months, infants use cues to support inferences about a speaker's referential intentions, including line of regard, gestures (e.g., pointing), voice direction, and body posture, and do not blindly associate the sounds they hear with the objects and events on which they are simultaneously focused.

Before infants can use cues to infer another's intentions, however, they must possess **intersubjective awareness,** or the recognition of when one shares a mental focus on some external object or action with another person. Only after infants realize that they can share a mental focus with other humans do they begin to interpret others' referential actions as intentional and use their own referential actions to point out objects and events of interest. An infant's attempt at deliberate communication with others is called **intentional communication.** Identifying when an infant's communicative behaviors are intentional or preintentional can be difficult unless you are familiar with some established guidelines. Indicators of intentionality include (a) the infant alternates eye gaze between an object and a communicative partner, (b) the infant uses ritualized gestures, such as pointing, and (c) the infant persists toward the goal by repeating or modifying gestures when communicative attempts fail (Bates, Camaioni, & Volterra, 1975).

Phase Three: 1 Year and Beyond. In phase three, children transition to using language within communicative interactions with others. With joint attention and intentionality well established, children shift to being able to engage socially with others and to use language to represent events and objects within these interactions.

Rituals of Infancy

Infants' lives are centered on feeding, bathing, dressing, and changing. These routines provide a sense of comfort and predictability to infants, and they also provide early opportunities for language learning. Consider dressing, for example. During this routine, parents often provide a commentary for their infants not unlike that of a sports commentator covering a baseball or football game. Babies hear such things as "Okay, let's put your right arm in. Now your left arm. Good job. Let's get these snaps. Snap! Snap! All done!" Although infants are much too young to learn about the concepts of right and left, they benefit from hearing the same words and phrases repeated each day. Infants are adept at computing and making sense of the statistical patterns they hear in speech. By hearing words and phrases over and over again, infants become attuned to where pauses occur, which helps them to segment phrases, clauses, and eventually words from the speech stream. They also learn about **phonotactics,** or the combinations of sounds that are acceptable in their language.

For example, English-learning infants quickly come to recognize that when they hear /ft/, as in *left,* the sounds preceding it belong to the same unit because they never hear /ft/ preceded by a pause.

In addition to the many linguistic patterns infants encounter in routines, they also have many opportunities to engage in episodes of joint attention with their caregivers. At bath time, for example, infants may look back and forth between their bathtub toys and the person who is bathing them, creating periods of joint attention where baby and adult are focused on the same entity in the world.

Discussion Point: *What are some rituals from infancy that you think would be particularly important for early language and communication development?*

Caregiver Responsiveness

Caregiver responsiveness refers to caregivers' attention and sensitivity to infants' vocalizations and communicative attempts. Caregiver responsiveness helps teach infants that their behaviors and communicative attempts are valued. Both the quality and the quantity of responsiveness by caregivers play a large role in early language development. Parents who are responsive and follow their children's leads foster greater occasions of joint attention and increase children's motivation to communicate, which results in more frequent initiations and bids for attention by children. More responsive language input by mothers is linked to children's language milestones, including saying the first word and producing two-word sentences (Nicely, Tamis-LeMonda, & Bornstein, 1999). Researchers Girolametto, Weitzman, and Greenberg (2000) described the following characteristics as key indicators of caregiver responsiveness.

1. *Waiting and listening:* Parents wait expectantly for initiations, use a slow pace to allow for initiations, and listen to allow the child to complete messages.
2. *Following the child's lead:* When a child initiates either verbally or nonverbally, parents follow the child's lead by responding verbally to the initiation, using animation, and avoiding vague acknowledgments.
3. *Joining in and playing:* Parents build on their child's focus of interest and play without dominating.
4. *Being face to face:* Parents adjust their physical level by sitting on the floor, leaning forward to facilitate face-to-face interaction, and bending toward the child when above the child's level.
5. *Using a variety of questions and labels:* Parents encourage conversation by asking a variety of Wh-questions (e.g., *who, where, why*), only using yes/no questions to clarify messages and obtain information, avoiding test and rhetorical questions, and waiting expectantly for responses.
6. *Encouraging turn taking:* Parents respond with animation, wait expectantly for responses, balance the number and length of adult to child turns, and complete their children's sentences only with children who are not yet combining words.
7. *Expanding and extending:* Parents expand and extend by repeating their child's words and correcting the grammar or by adding another idea, and use comments and questions to inform, predict, imagine, explain, and talk about feelings.

Infant Speech Perception and Categorization

Speech perception is the fuel for the child's language-learning system. Speech perception describes the child's attention to phonemes, rhythm, prosody, and lexical items. Children's perception of speech is categorical, meaning that children separate input into different categories. Much of language learning involves developing more precise categorization schemes. For instance, early in life children may categorize all animals by the term *cat.* As children

BOX 2-3 Spotlight on Research

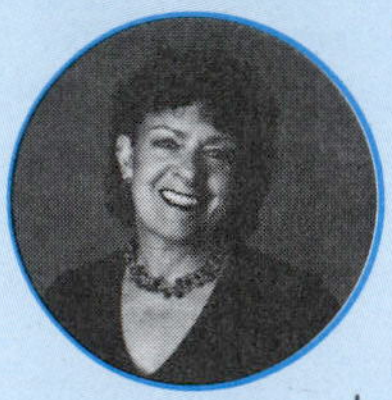

Roberta Michnick Golinkoff, Ph.D.
H. Rodney Sharp Professor,
School of Education
University of Delaware

Graduate school was a very interesting experience for me. I came in just as the field of language acquisition was being reinvented, influenced by the work of Noam Chomsky and George Miller, who "translated" Chomsky's work for the field of psychology. Eric Lenneberg was also at Cornell and was exploring the biological bases of language. So it was a very exciting time! I remember when Lois Bloom came to give a colloquium (she is now a dear friend), and we all so admired her approach of emphasizing that children had something to talk *about*, that they were struggling with expressing *ideas* in addition to using their burgeoning syntax. I studied concepts that underlie language use for my dissertation (agent and patient in events), and I am still doing that today! We have studies in our labs on manner—*how* an action is performed (the difference between "walk" and "run")—and *path*, or the trajectory over which an action takes place (such as "over" or "under" a figure). My work melds the study of cognitive, perceptual, and social development with the development of language. It examines the factors that become important to language acquisition at different points along the way in development. Since my work has continued in this vein for so long, I guess I'm consistent, if nothing else. One critical factor in the satisfaction and pleasure I take in my work has been a long-standing and very productive collaboration with Kathy Hirsh-Pasek of Temple University. We share much of our research program in common and our graduate students too! And I love working with students—doctoral as well as undergraduate. It is a great pleasure for me to work alongside my students and see dramatic growth in their thinking. I carry one of my former mentors around in my head—Eleanor Gibson ("Jackie")—and she was a wonderful model for me. If my students took from me just a fraction of what I got from Jackie, I would feel a great success!

Discussion Point: *What other categories come to mind when thinking about child language development? Explore how these might help children to divide and conquer as they develop as language learners.*

learn new labels (e.g., *dog, tail, soft, mouse*), new categories emerge. With speech perception, at the most general level, children categorize incoming sounds into speech and nonspeech. Later, children learn to categorize speech sounds into different phonemes and different words. Although the ability to perceive and categorize phonemes, rhythm, and prosody appears to be innate, the ability to perceive and categorize words depends on native language experience. The late Peter Jusczyk, one of the foremost researchers in infant speech

BOX 2-4 Spotlight on Practice

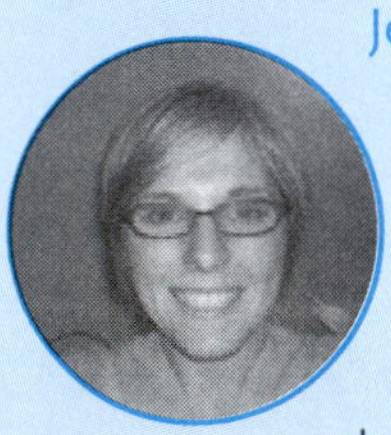

Jennifer L. Anderson, M.S.
Program Manager, Microsoft

As an undergraduate, I was always torn between math and psychology. I became bored with math classes because there was no human aspect; I became bored with psychology classes because there wasn't enough math. Finally though, I found my niche in linguistics and cognitive science. The blend of analysis and human development captured my interest.

After completing a B.S. in applied math with an emphasis in cognitive science, I studied cognitive science and linguistics in graduate school. My research focused on the acquisition of sounds by young infants. I found it fascinating that 8-month-olds could detect differences in sounds that adults weren't able to discriminate. How could an infant do what an adult couldn't?

My research led me to a related job in industry. Currently I am a program manager at Microsoft working on speech recognition software. Although acquisition by a machine is different from acquisition by a child, there is much overlap (in concepts and terminology) with human language acquisition.

When I began my career as a graduate student, I never imagined that I would work in the technology industry, given that I was studying language development. However, it is the perfect blend for my math and psychology interests. As you continue to study language development, I urge you to keep your mind open, as there are many careers available to you in addition to the academic and clinical paths that we typically consider.

perception and categorization, explained category development as providing children with a "divide and conquer strategy," that allows the child to "divide or partition the input . . . to detect the regularities that mark that particular native language" (Jusczyk, 2003, p. 43).

What Are Major Communicative Milestones in Infancy and Toddlerhood?

Chapter 1 described the universal nature of children's communicative achievements as a remarkable feature of language. Children achieve certain language and communication milestones at roughly the same age and in roughly the same order across the communities of the world. The sections that follow chronicle these achievements in a developmental fashion, beginning with the exploring infant.

Infancy: The Explorer

Infancy spans the period from birth to about 2 years of age, during which some of the most dramatic developments in communicative competence occur. We enter infancy essentially as helpless beings, unable to express anything beyond the most rudimentary calls for assistance. We leave infancy as intentional beings, well on our way to being competent communicators and able to express "No! Me do it!" with force and clarity. Infancy is indeed a period of exploration and discovery.

Stages of Vocal Development

Young children follow a fairly predictable pattern in their early use of vocalizations. Vocalizations are the sounds children produce; these are different from verbalizations, which refer to the words children use. The emergence of vocalizations is often viewed from a stage model, meaning that the emergence of certain vocalizations in children follows an observable and sequential pattern. These stages are presented in Figure 2-3 and are adapted from Vihman's (1998) writing on this topic.

FIGURE 2-3 Stages of vocal development.

Phonation Stage (0–1 month)	• Infants produce reflexive (e.g., crying) and vegetative sounds (e.g., coughs)
Gooing and Cooing Stage (2–3 months)	• Infants produce consonant-like and vowel-like sounds
Expansion Stage (4–6 months)	• Infants produce yells, growls, squeals, trills, raspberries • Infants produce marginal babbling, an early form of babbling
Canonical Babbling (6–8 months) and Variegated Babbling (8 months +)	• Infants use true consonants and true vowels in various combinations • No true words at this stage • Jargon emerges at end of this stage (about 1 year)

Sources: Oller (1980); Vihman (1998).

Phonation Stage (0–1 Month). The very first kinds of sounds infants produce are called **reflexive sounds.** These include sounds of distress (crying, fussing) and vegetative sounds produced during feeding (burping, coughing). Although neonates have no control for the most part over reflexive sounds, adults tend to respond as if these reflexes were true communication attempts. We hurry to babies' cribs when we hear them cry and use soothing voices in an attempt to alleviate their distress. It is only natural to interpret these early sounds as intentional. We might even ask, "Are you hungry? Does your diaper need to be changed?" although the child's vocalizations could mean something entirely different.

Gooing and Cooing Stage (2–3 Months). By 2 or 3 months, infants begin to produce gooing and **cooing sounds.** These are consonant-like sounds that infants produce when they are content ("kooooh," "gaaaa"). The consonants typically heard are the /g/ and /k/ sounds, which are produced far back in the oral cavity. These are easier for infants to produce than other sounds that require more precise manipulation of the tongue, lips, or teeth (/t/ and /b/, for instance).

Expansion Stage (4–6 Months). In the expansion stage, infants gain more control over the articulators. Their vocal repertoire increases as they begin to manipulate the loudness and pitch of their voices and to play with sounds. Infants at this stage begin to yell, growl, squeal, and make raspberries and trills. Also, marginal babbling emerges, an early type of babbling containing short strings of consonant-like and vowel-like sounds.

Canonical Babbling (6–8 Months) and Variegated Babbling (8 Months +). True babbling, which appears around 6 months, is distinguished from the earlier cooing, gooing, and marginal babbling by the child's production of authentic syllables. These vocalizations have a true consonant combined with a true vowel and are strung together to form chains: *ma-ma, di-di,* and *guh-guh,* for example. Often, parents view their children as beginning to talk when they begin to babble because of the resemblance of these syllable strings to the native language of the child. Canonical babbling consists of the single production or repetition of consonant-vowel sequences in which the same consonant-vowel sequence is repeated (*da-da-da-da*). Sequences of these canonical consonant-vowel repetitions are called **reduplicative babbling**. A mother should not fret when at 6 months her infant produces constant streams of *da-da-da-da.* It is not that the infant is favoring one parent over the other; it is more likely that the baby is just experimenting with sounds.

Variegated babbling emerges soon after infants begin to produce canonical babbling at about 8 months. Infants begin to use a wider range of sounds than in reduplicative babbling and begin to string together different consonant and vowel sequences (*da-bi, da-ma*). Across many languages, infants prefer the nasal consonants (*m*, *n*, and *ng*) and the stop consonants (*p*, *b*, *t*, *d*) in the variegated stage (Locke, 1983), combining these variously with vowels to produce long vocalized sequences. Many of the infant's early words, such as *Mommy* and *Daddy,* emerge directly from these variegated strings.

Jargon is a special type of babbling in which infants use the melodic patterns of their native language through a combination of rhythm, rate, stress, and intonation contours. Babies using jargon may sound as if they are producing questions, exclamations, or commands even in the absence of true words. Although vocalizations produced while babbling or when producing jargon may sound like short words or syllables, they are not considered true words because they are not referential, nor do they convey meaning.

Interestingly, babbling does not necessarily refer only to the spoken productions made by infants. Deaf babies and hearing babies born to profoundly deaf parents babble silently with their hands. In the same way that the vocalizations of babies exposed to oral language show sensitivity to specific rhythmic patterns that bind syllables, so, too, do the hand movements of babies born to deaf parents. Their hand movements have a slower rhythm than ordinary gestures and are produced within a tightly restricted space in front of the body (Petitto, Holowka, Sergio, & Ostry, 2001).

Emergence of Intentionality

Between 7 and 12 months, infants begin to communicate their intentions more clearly than before. Prior to this period, we consider children preintentional. Although infants may do things that are considered intentional (e.g., cry out in a certain way, babble), their intentions in these acts are inferred by the adults around them, as in the following:

Infant: (*squeal, smile*)

Father: Oh, you liked that!

Infant: (*burp*) Maa.

Father: You want more? You do, don't you? Yes, you do.

In this interaction, the infant produces preintentional behaviors that are ambiguous at best, but the father views these as intentional. The infant's intentionality comes not from within, but rather from the adult with whom the infant is interacting.

In the latter half of the first year of life, infants become increasingly interested in the people and objects around them, and they also become interested in intentionally communicating to people about objects and events. During this stage of development infants become attuned to the referential signals of others (e.g., pointing, eye gaze, line of regard), and they begin to incorporate their own intentional gestures to direct others' attention. This transition to intentionality is a particularly important event in the communication achievements of young children. With intentionality, children are well on their way to deliberately describing their needs, interests, and thoughts to the world around them, as in the following interaction:

Infant: Mama (looks at mother and raises arms).

Mother: Oh, you want me to pick you up?

Infants demonstrate evidence of intentionality through their communicative efforts toward others, by pointing to objects, showing objects, gesturing, and using eye contact.

Transition to Symbolic Representations

A word is a symbol, as it stands for and represents something else in the world. As infants approach their first birthday, they become aware of how sequences of sounds symbolize concepts in the world. Words are arbitrary symbols; with the exception of some onomatopoeic words (words, like *buzz* and *coo*, that sound like the concept they represent), they do not directly signal the concepts they represent. As infants develop, their **lexicons**, or mental dictionaries, develop as well. For each word they learn, infants create an entry in their lexicon, similar to the boldfaced words in dictionaries. The lexical entries are essentially a series of symbols. Each entry comprises the word, the sound of the word, the meaning of the word, and the word's part of speech (Pinker, 1999). Figure 2-4 shows the lexical representation for the word *money*.

FIGURE 2-4 Lexical entry for the word *money*.

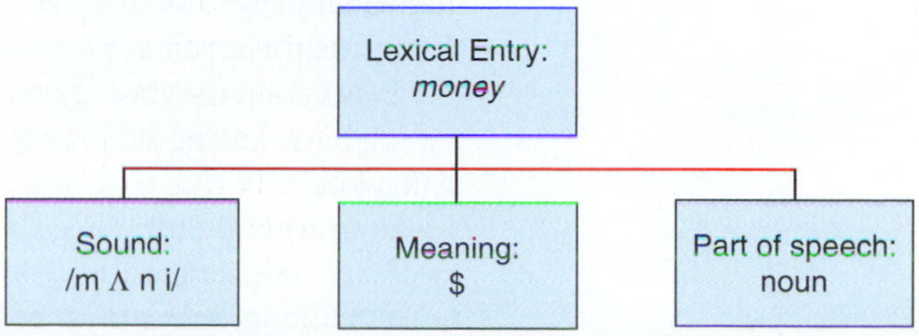

At roughly 1 year of age, children transition from using intentional communicative behaviors, including eye contact, gesture, and vocalizations, to using symbols, including words and gestures, to communicate. This 1-year mark signals an important and exciting transition for developing children. Although children at 1 year likely understand only a few words, parents often are quite gleeful when their children begin to use these understood words expressively.

Words are not the only types of symbols children use as they transition from nonsymbolic to symbolic communication. Children's use of referential gestures and words tends to emerge at roughly the same time. A referential gesture is a gesture that carries a fixed meaning, such as flapping the arms to refer to a bird (Iverson & Thal, 1998). It is different from a deictic gesture, such as pointing or waving, which is used to indicate or call attention to something. Referential gestures are symbolic and function much like words for young children; for instance, a young child waving her hand a particular way can clearly communicate to her parents her disdain for a particular food. As children develop their initial lexicons, the contributions of referential gestures should be recognized. Young children's use of referential gestures provides them a much larger communicative repertoire in their transition to symbolic communication than is possible with spoken words alone (Iverson & Thal, 1998).

We know from chapter 1 that adults communicate for three main reasons: to request, to reject, and to comment. Once intentionality emerges in infants, they, too, communicate for these same reasons, although the methods they employ are somewhat different. Prelinguistic infants may request a favorite toy by pointing to it. They may reject a not-so-favorite toy by pushing it away or hurling it across the room, and they may comment on a toy by holding it up for another person to see or even offering it to someone. When children begin to produce words, they use their first words for these same three communicative functions.

The First Word. Of all of the communicative milestones infants reach, none seems to be celebrated more than the first word. Infants utter their first true word at 12 months on average. First words usually refer to salient people and objects in infants' everyday lives, such as *mama, dada, doggie,* and the like. Researchers consider a vocalization a true word if it meets three important criteria.

First, words need to be uttered with a clear intention and purpose. When a baby says "doggie" while petting a dog, the baby undoubtedly has a clear intention and purpose of referring to the pet. If a baby is told by a parent to "say doggie, say doggie" and does so, the utterance is an imitation or repetition rather than a true word.

Second, a true word has a recognizable pronunciation. Obviously, 12-month-olds are not capable of producing all sounds accurately, but their first word should be a close approximation of the adult form and should be recognizable by others. Thus, the child's "doddie" for *doggie* is a close enough approximation that this can be considered a true word. However, if a child produces *doggie* as "oo-na"—even consistently and while clearly using this to refer to the family doggie—it is not considered a true word because it does not closely approximate the form adults use. The term *phonetically consistent form,* or *PCF,* describes these idiosyncratic, wordlike productions that are used consistently and meaningfully but do not approximate forms used by adults. Although not true words, these forms are important aspects of children's language development.

Third, a true word is one that a child uses consistently and extends beyond the original context. We would expect the baby who said "doggie" while petting the dog to use this word not only with that dog, but also for other people's dogs, pictures of dogs, and possibly even when hearing dogs barking in the distance. The extension of words across various contexts is related to the symbolic aspect of words and how one word can have many diverse referents across time and place. Children demonstrate the symbolic element of word use when they take a word and apply it to diverse contexts of use, even incorrectly, as in the child who calls every man "daddy" or all furry animals "cats."

Toddlerhood: The Experimenter

The word *toddlerhood* takes its name from children learning to walk, who take short, unsteady steps. Coincidentally, toddlers' achievements in communicative competence might also sound a bit clumsy to the naive listener. Have you ever heard a toddler say "I eated it all!" or "I have two mouses."? During this stage toddlers experiment with form, content, and use as they continue to acquire communicative competence.

Achievements in Form

From roughly 1 year to 18 months of age, children acquire an expressive lexicon of about 50 words. For approximately 6 months after the 50-word mark is reached (roughly from 18 months to 24 months), significant changes in children's communicative competence are evident. Children begin to show evidence of a rudimentary use of syntax, or language form, and begin to inflect words with grammatical morphemes. A grammatical morpheme is an inflection added to words to indicate aspects of grammar, such as the plural *s*, the possessive *'s*, the past tense *ed*, and the present progressive *ing*. These morphemes are an important aspect of grammatical development.

Children typically begin to move from single-word to multiword utterances between the ages of 18 and 24 months. During this time, parents begin to hear phrases such as "go bye-bye?" and "Mommy ball." It is at the two-word stage that children begin to acquire a sense of syntax, or language structure. They see the value that combining words has over using single words and can begin to use language for a greater variety of communicative functions. Some simple functions expressed at the two-word stage include commenting ("Daddy go."), negating ("No juice."), requesting ("More juice."), and questioning ("What that?").

When children move beyond one-word utterances to produce two- and three-word utterances, they begin to have a distinct grammar that governs the order of words. Recall from Chapter 1 that grammar, or syntax, refers to the rule system that governs the internal organization of sentences. When children produce only one-word utterances, there is no internal organization to consider. However, once children begin to link words to express ideas and desires ("Want go!"; "Me do it!"), then syntax emerges to govern how these words are organized.

Grammatical morphemes appear in children's speech when children are between 18 and 24 months of age, which is when expressive morphology can first be documented. When grammatical morphemes first emerge, language exhibits a *telegraphic* quality that results from the omission of key grammatical markers. For instance, the toddler's "Mommy no go." and "Daddy walking." are telegraphic reductions of "Mommy, don't go." and "Daddy is walking." The emerging use of grammatical morphemes signals the development of morphology and the gradual increase in grammatical precision by the child.

Roger Brown, a pioneer in early morphological development, isolated 14 grammatical morphemes and documented the ages at which children master these common morphemes as well as their order of acquisition (see Table 2-1). These grammatical morphemes develop in the same order and emerge at roughly the same time in all English-speaking children. The first grammatical morpheme that children use expressively is the present progressive form *-ing*, as in *doggie running*. Children begin to use this morpheme at around 18 or 19 months of age, with mastery by 28 months. Additional morphemes that appear during toddlerhood include the prepositions *in* and *on*, which children start to use at about 2 years of age (*in cup, on table*), the regular plural *s* (*babies eating*), the possessive *'s* (*kitty's bowl*), and the irregular past tense verb (*Dad broke it.*). Irregular past tense verbs, of which there are between 150 and 180, are verbs

TABLE 2-1 Acquisition of Brown's 14 grammatical morphemes

Grammatical Morpheme	Age (in months)	Example
Present progressive *-ing*	19–28	*mommy eating*
Plural *-s*	27–30	*baby shoes*
Preposition *in*	27–30	*hat in box*
Preposition *on*	31–34	*hat on chair*
Possessive *'s*	31–34	*baby's ball*
Regular past tense *-ed*	43–46	*kitty jumped*
Irregular past tense	43–46	*we ate*
Regular third person singular *-s*	43–46	*mommy drives*
Articles *a, the, an*	43–46	*the car*
Contractible copula *be*	43–46	*she's happy*
Contractible auxiliary	47–50	*she's coming*
Uncontractible copula *be*	47–50	*we were [we were here]*
Uncontractible auxiliary	47–50	*she was [she was coming]*
Irregular third person	47–50	*she did it*

Source: Brown (1973).

that must be memorized rather than formed by the addition of *-ed* (e.g., *eat/ate,* not *eat/eated*). Once children have acquired the regular past tense rule, they often overgeneralize its use to irregular verbs until they have had sufficient exposure to and practice with what Steven Pinker (1999) calls "words" (e.g., the irregular form of a verb) and "rules" (e.g., applying the past tense ending of a regular verb, *-ed*). There are other cases in language where children learn words and rules differently. For example, with contractions, children generally learn the word *won't* as a unit, rather than by combining the words *will not.* This likely occurs because the sound of the root (*will*) is not the same in the contracted form (*won't*).

Sentence forms appear awkward for the most part during the toddler years. Toddlers tend to use uninflected verb forms ("kitty eat") and to misuse or omit pronouns ("me go," "her do it"). Despite these awkward constructions, toddlers begin to use more adultlike forms for a variety of sentence types, including the yes/no question ("Are we going, Mommy?"), *wh*-questions ("What's that?"), commands ("You do it.") and negatives ("Me no want that.")

In addition to documenting grammatical morpheme usage, Roger Brown is well known for creating Brown's stages of language development, which characterize children's language achievements based on their ability to produce utterances of varying syntactic complexity (see Table 2-2). One of the defining characteristics of preschoolers' increasing language complexity is their **mean length of utterance (MLU).** MLU refers to the average length of children's sentence units, or utterances. Each utterance a child produces is broken into morphemes, which are the smallest units of meaning. MLU is calculated by counting the total number of morphemes used in a sample of 50 to 100 spontaneous utterances produced by a child and then dividing the total number of morphemes by the total number of utterances. The calculation is: *MLU = total number of morphemes/total number of utterances.*

During the toddler and preschool years, children's MLU demonstrates a systematic increase, as shown in Figure 2-5. The calculation of MLU is a common way to evaluate children's language skills against the expectations for their age. In order to achieve consistency in morpheme counts, researchers and practitioners should use Brown's rules for counting

TABLE 2-2 Brown's stages of language development

Stage	Age (upper limit)	MLU	MLU Range	Major Achievements
I	18 months	1.31	.99–1.64	• Single-word sentences • Uninflected nouns and verbs (*mommy; eat*)
II	24 months	1.92	1.47–2.37	• Two-element sentences • True clauses not evident (*Mommy up; Eat cookie*)
III	30 months	2.54	1.97–3.11	• Three-element sentences • Independent clauses emerge (*Baby want cookie*)
IV	36 months	3.16	2.47–3.85	• Four-element sentences • Independent clauses continue to emerge (*The teacher gave it to me*)
V	42 months	3.78	2.96–4.60	• Recursive elements predominate • Connecting devices emerge (*and, because*)
Post V	54 months	5.02	3.96–6.08	• Complex syntactic patterns • Subordination and coordination continue to emerge • Complement clauses used (*She's not feeling well*)

Source: Adapted from Kent, R. D. (1994). *Reference manual for communicative sciences and disorders: Speech and language.* Austin, TX: Pro-Ed; and Justice, L. M., & Ezell, H. K. (2002). *The syntax handbook.* Eau Claire, WI: Thinking Publications.

FIGURE 2-5 Age-related progression in mean length of utterance.

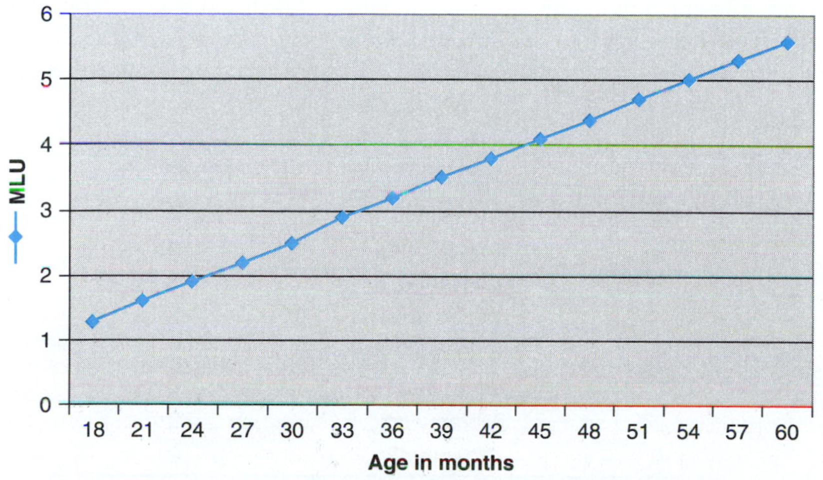

Source: Adapted from J. F. Miller and R. Chapman (1981). The relation between age and mean length of utterance in morphemes. *Journal of Speech and Hearing Research, 24,* 154–161. Reprinted with permission.

FIGURE 2-6 Brown's rules for counting morphemes.

1. Only fully transcribed utterances are used; none with blanks. Portions of utterances, entered in parentheses to indicate doubtful transcription, are used.
2. Include all exact utterance repetitions (marked with a plus sign in records). Stuttering is marked as repeated efforts at a single word; count the word once in the most complete form produced. In the few cases where a word is produced for emphasis or the like (*no, no, no*) count each occurrence.
3. Do not count such fillers as *mm* or *oh,* but do count *no, yeah*, and *hi.*
4. All compound words (two or more free morphemes), proper names, and ritualized reduplications count as single words. Examples: *birthday, rackety-boom, choo-choo, quack-quack, night-night, pocketbook, see saw.* Justification is that there is no evidence that the constituent morphemes function as such for these children.
5. Count as one morpheme all irregular pasts of the verb (*got, did, went, saw*). Justification is that there is no evidence that the child relates these to present forms.
6. Count as one morpheme all diminutives (*doggie, mommie*) because these children at least do not seem to use the suffix productively. Diminutives are the standard forms used by the child.
7. Count as separate morphemes all auxiliaries (*is, have, will, can, must, would*). Also all catenatives: *gonna, wanna, hafta.* These latter are counted as single morphemes rather than as *going to* or *want to* because evidence is that they function so for the children. Count as separate morphemes all inflections, for example, possessive {s}, plural {s}, third person singular {s}, regular past {d}, progressive {ing}.
8. The range count follows the above rules but is always calculated for the total transcription rather than for 100 utterances.

Source: Reprinted by permission of the publisher from A FIRST LANGUAGE: THE EARLY STAGES by Roger Brown, p. 54, Cambridge, Mass.: Harvard University Press, Copyright © 1973 by the President and Fellows of Harvard College.

morphemes, presented in Figure 2-6. MLU should be calculated using a language sample of at least 50 utterances for it to be valid and representative of what a child really does with language. For the sake of explanation, however, let's use the short sample that follows to demonstrate the use of MLU for a 2-year-old child.

	Utterance	Morphemes
1	Me do it.	3
2	No, me do it.	4
3	Eli want it.	3
4	Me go outside.	3
5	Outside.	1
6	What that?	2
7	Mommy do.	2
8	What that?	2

In this very brief transcript, the child produced eight utterances and a total of 20 morphemes, resulting in an MLU of 2.5. The norms presented in Table 2-3 show that the

TABLE 2-3 Normative references for interpreting MLU

Age (in months)	Predicted MLU	Predicted MLU +/− One Standard Deviation (68% of Population)
18	1.31	0.99–1.64
21	1.62	1.23–2.01
24	1.92	1.47–2.37
27	2.23	1.72–2.74
30	2.54	1.97–3.11
33	2.85	2.22–3.48
36	3.16	2.47–3.85
39	3.47	2.71–4.23
42	3.78	2.96–4.60
45	4.09	3.21–4.97
48	4.40	3.46–5.34
51	4.71	3.71–5.71
54	5.02	3.96–6.08
57	5.32	4.20–6.45
60	5.63	4.44–6.82

Source: Adapted from J. F. Miller and R. Chapman (1981). The relation between age and mean length of utterance in morphemes. *Journal of Speech and Hearing Research, 24,* 154–161. Reprinted with permission.

predicted MLU for a child who is 2 years of age is 1.92. Sixty-eight percent of children have scores within one standard deviation of 1.92, or between 1.47 and 2.37. If our sample is accurate, this child's MLU is higher than expected for his or her age.

Achievements in Content

Have you ever known parents to keep a diary or a list of words produced by their children? Parents who keep track of their children's new words generally begin to have trouble keeping up with the word-learning pace when their children are between 18 and 24 months of age. During the second half of the second year, or around the time when children have acquired 50 words, they often experience a **vocabulary spurt,** or word spurt (also called naming explosion), a remarkable increase in the rate of vocabulary acquisition. During the vocabulary spurt, children learn an average of seven to nine new words per day. Many parents of toddlers report that their children use new words out of the blue, words like *plenty, vent, dangerous, steep,* and so on.

During toddlerhood, substantial growth occurs in both the receptive and expressive lexicons. The receptive lexicon encompasses the words a person can comprehend, whereas the expressive lexicon refers to the words a person can produce. As previously mentioned, comprehension generally precedes production in language learning, and it does in the case of the receptive and expressive lexicons. Girls who are 18 months of age have an average of 65 words in their receptive vocabularies, but only 27 words in their expressive vocabularies; in comparison, boys of the same age understand an average of 56 words and produce an average of 18 (Fenson et al., 2000). The trend for a disparity between the size of receptive and expressive lexicons continues throughout toddlerhood, the school years, and into adulthood.

Although children learn about seven to nine new words per day between the ages of 18 and 24 months, they do not always use these words the way adults do. Children tend to use a new word cautiously at first. They apply newly learned words to specific referents rather than to a category of referents. This practice is called an **underextension.** For instance, children who have just learned the word *doggie* might use it only to refer to the family pet; or children might use their new word *cup* to refer only to their green sippie cup. A child might learn the word *yellow* for a specific shade of yellow and stoically refuse to consider this name for other variants of yellow.

Children also engage in a process called overextension, which is the opposite of underextension. **Overextension,** or overgeneralization, is when children use words in a wider set of contexts than considered appropriate by adults. Toddlers tend to overgeneralize about one-third of new words (Rescorla, 1980) on the basis of categorical, analogical, and relational similarities. A categorical overextension is when a child extends a known word to other referents because they are in the same category. For instance, a child may learn the color green and then call all colors (*red, blue, yellow*) by the word *green*. Likewise, a child may call all animals by the word *cat,* all liquids by the word *juice,* or all actions that involve clothing (buttoning, zippering, folding, etc.) by the word *snap*. An analogical overextension is when a child extends a known word to other referents because they have perceptual similarities. For instance, a child may use the word *ball* to describe anything that is round (e.g., a tire), or may use the word *ladder* to describe anything tall (e.g., a flagpole). A relational overextension is when a child extends a known word to other semantically related referents. For instance, the child may use the word *bird* to refer to both a bird feeder and birdseed.

Achievements in Use

In addition to acquiring new grammar and words as they transition from the single-word to the multiword stage, children acquire important new language functions and conversational skills. By the time children enter the multiword stage, they are capable of using a variety of language functions, including instrumental, regulatory, personal interactional, heuristic, imaginative, and informative functions (Halliday, 1978). Children can use requests to satisfy their own needs (instrumental), use directives to control the behaviors of others (regulatory), tell information about themselves and share feelings (personal interactional), request information and ask questions to learn and investigate the world (heuristic), tell stories to make believe and pretend (imaginative), and give information to communicate with others (informative). Children's success at using communication for a variety of purposes is one of the most important aspects of communicative development during toddlerhood. With their growing lexicon and sophisticated grammar, children use these resources for many purposes. When children's internal demand for speech—their desire to communicate various functions or intentions—exceeds their capacity, they can become frustrated.

One area in which toddlers are not highly skilled is conversation. Conversational skill requires being able to initiate a conversational topic, sustain a topic for several turns, and then appropriately take leave of the conversation. Those of us who have recently attempted to have a conversation with a young child know it is not usually very sophisticated:

Parent: What did you do at school today?

Toddler: Miss Sarah, Eli, Lila.

Toddlers may demonstrate some skill in starting a conversation, but cannot usually sustain a conversation for more than one or two turns. Typically, the adult has to provide a great deal of assistance to maintain a particular topic. Toddlers also have difficulty keeping their audience's needs in mind: they may use pronouns without appropriately defining to whom they refer, and they may discuss topics without ensuring that the listener has a frame of reference within which to understand them (Owens, 2001). Additionally, when asked a specific question or given an explicit opportunity to take a turn, toddlers do not always take advantage of the opportunity. They may simply not respond, or they may respond noncontingently (off the topic). Toddlers are not proficient at realizing when they are not following along in a conversation and thus are not likely to seek clarification.

Achievements in Speech

In the infancy period, children's vocal development undergoes considerable change as they move from reflexive sounds, like burping and coughing, to variegated babbling that sounds more like the language of their community. During the toddler years, children's development of phonology—their knowledge of the rules concerning the sound system—grows rapidly.

Expressive phonology refers to the observable sounds and sound patterns children use when producing syllables and words. When they speak, toddlers tend to use the sounds with which they are most skilled; because of this tendency, 2-year-old children correctly produce about 70% of the sounds they use (Stoel-Gammon & Dunn, 1985). Underlying every sound or sound pattern that a child produces is a *phonological representation,* a mental representation of a particular phoneme or sound pattern. These internal representations differentiate each phoneme in the child's repertoire from all of the other phonemes and provide children with the rules for combining sounds into different patterns. Together, these underlying representations form a child's phonological repertoire, or phonological system.

Attainment of Specific Phonemes. Published norms for phoneme acquisition are a common source for representing phonemic attainment in young children. Norm references consider when certain phonemes are mastered, as well as the order in which they are mastered. We interpret norm references with respect to the phonemic attainment of other children, rather than to an agreed criterion score. These references are derived from published studies that investigate the acquisition of phonology in large groups of children. Table 2-4 presents five sets of norms for the English consonants. These norms show the ages at which children typically acquire particular phonemes, providing a point of comparison for children of the same age. As shown in Table 2-4, however, these norms vary widely, depending on whether researchers elect to chart average ages of achievement of particular phonemes, or upper ages of achievement (e.g., the age at which 90% or 100% of a given sample produces adultlike phonemes). The data in Table 2-4 show, for instance, that children acquire /m/ sometime between 2 and 3 years of age.

The data in Figure 2-7 are probably the most widely used for determining when children can be expected to produce a particular sound correctly more often than they misarticulate or omit it (Sander, 1972), known as the customary age of production. The customary age of production differs from age of mastery, which is represented in Figure 2-7 as the right edge of the blue bars; this is the point at which 90% of all children are customarily using the phoneme.

Children are said to have mastered a consonant once they can produce the sound correctly in three different positions: in the initial position of a syllable (syllable initial, *b* in *bear*), in the middle position of a syllable (syllable medial, *r* in *berry*), and in the final position of a syllable (syllable final, *d* in *bread*). However, determining mastery is not as simple as it might seem. Consonant mastery is complicated when the influence of the consonants

TABLE 2-4 Normative references for phoneme acquisition

Consonant	Wellman et al. (1931)	Poole (1934)	Templin (1957)	Sander (1972)	Prather et al. (1975)
m	3	3½	3	before 2	2
n	3	4½	3	before 2	2
h	3	3½	3	before 2	2
p	4	3½	3	before 2	2
f	3	5½	3	3	2–4
w	3	3½	3	before 2	2–8
b	3	3½	4	before 2	2–8
ŋ		4½	3	2	2
j	4	4½	3½	3	2–4
k	4	4½	4	2	2–4
g	4	4½	4	2	2–4
l	4	6½	6	3	3–4
d	5	4½	4	2	2–4
t	5	4½	6	2	2–8
s	5	7½	4½	3	3
r	5	7½	4	3	3–4
tʃ	5		4½	4	3–8
v	5	6½	6	4	4
z	5	7½	7	4	4
ʒ	6	6½	7	6	4
θ		7½	6	5	4
ʤ			7	4	4
ʃ		6½	4½	4	3–8
ð		6½	7	5	4

Source: From Creaghead, Newman, & Secord, *Assessment and Remediation of Articulatory and Phonological Disorders* (2nd edition). Published by Allyn & Bacon, Boston, MA. Copyright © by Pearson Education. Reprinted/adapted by permission of the publisher.

Discussion Point: *What are some factors that contribute to a sound's being acquired earlier than other sounds? For instance, children master /b/ long before they master /r/ in English. What are some possible explanations for this?*

and vowels in the surrounding context are considered. For example, the production of syllable initial /t/ in the word *tip* differs from that of the initial /t/ in *trip* because we utter the latter with slight affrication (sounds more like /chrip/). A child may be able to produce syllable initial /t/ accurately in *tip* but not in *trip*.

While the exact age at which children have a particular phoneme varies across the norms, the order of acquisition—the order in which children tend to acquire the phonemes—is generally the same across the normative samples. As shown in Figure 2-7, /m/, /n/, /h/, and /p/ are early-acquired phonemes, and /v/, /z/, and /θ/ (as in *th*ink) are later-acquired phonemes. The data in Figure 2-7 identify the age range for attainment of the consonant phonemes; the left side of the bar shows when 50% of children use a consonant and the right side shows when 90% of children use it.

FIGURE 2-7 Sander's norms for age ranges of consonant development.

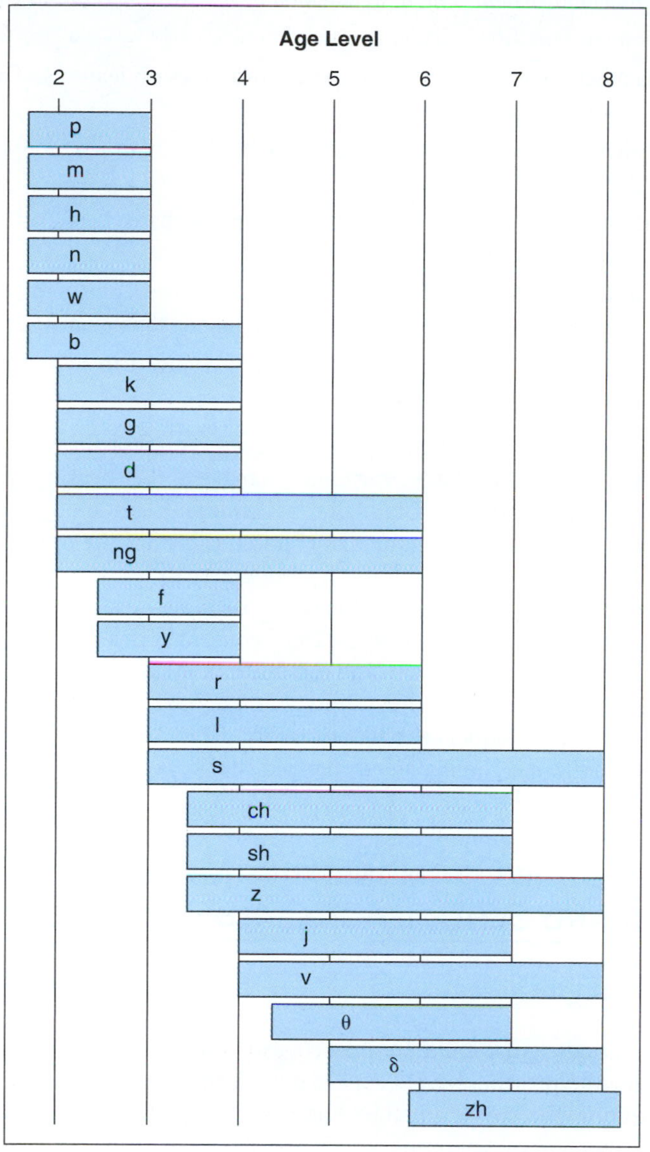

Source: From Sander, E. K. (1972). When are speech sounds learned? *Journal of Speech and Hearing Disorders, 37,* p. 62. Reprinted with permission.

Phonological Processes. As children develop their phonological prowess, they make a number of adjustments to the production of specific sounds and sound classes. These natural adjustments are called phonological processes; they are processes of sound change applied to words and syllables to simplify the child's phonological production. These processes reflect normal patterns of deviation from the adult phonology that will change as the child matures. These patterns are fairly universal across children. For instance, many preschool children say "doddie" for *doggie* and "tee" for *tree.* They say "jamas" for *pajamas* and "tum" for *thumb.* Adults who work often with young children expect to hear these systematic phonological patterns, or processes, in their speech.

Toddlers' expressive phonology exhibits a large variety of phonological processes. Common ones include:

1. *Final consonant deletion:* The final consonant of a word is omitted ("ca" for *cat*).
2. *Reduplication:* The first syllable in a word is repeated ("wa-wa" for *water*).
3. *Consonant harmony:* One consonant in a word takes on features of another consonant ("doddie" for *doggie*).
4. *Weak syllable deletion:* The unstressed syllable in a word is omitted ("jamas" for *pajamas*).
5. *Diminutization:* The second syllable in a word is changed to "ee" ("mommy" for *mother* and "blankie" for *blanket*).
6. *Cluster reduction:* A consonant cluster (two or more consonants that occur together, as in *st*ick or *cr*ayon) is reduced to a single consonant ("tick" or "cayon").
7. *Liquid gliding:* The consonants /l/ and /r/ are changed to *w* and *y* ("wabbit" for *rabbit* and "yove" for *love*). (Vihman, 1998)

These and many other types of phonological processes represent the systematic substitutions, omissions, and additions that young children make as they acquire the phonology of their language (Vihman, 1998). Gradually, as children's phonology matures, these processes undergo suppression, meaning that children exchange the immature production (e.g., liquid gliding) for the mature, adultlike production.

The suppression of processes tends to follow a general age-related pattern. For instance, of the processes listed previously, the first five (final consonant deletion, reduplication, consonant harmony, weak syllable deletion, and diminutization) are usually suppressed by age 3 (Stoel-Gammon & Dunn, 1985). Thus, although these processes may occur frequently in toddlers, they become less frequent as children age from 2 to 3 years. The last two processes, cluster reduction and liquid gliding, are suppressed later.

What Are Major Communicative Milestones in Preschool and School-Age Children?

Preschool Accomplishments

The preschool period, when children are between 3 and 5 years old, precedes formal schooling. During the preschool years, children overcome much of the language toddling of the experimenting phase of toddlerhood and truly begin to master form, content, and use in their development of communicative competence. By many accounts, language acquisition is nearly complete by the time children leave preschool. Those of you who have recently had a conversation with a 5-year-old child realize how true this is. The 5-year-old child has an amazingly large vocabulary, demonstrates skill (relatively speaking) in holding a conversation, and uses the syntax of an adult. From kindergarten on, achievements in language are subtle and protracted relative to the remarkable and rapid advances of the infancy, toddlerhood, and preschool years.

Achievements in Form

During the preschool years, children refine their syntax and morphology in significant ways. Noteworthy advances occur in children's increases in the use of grammatical and derivational morphology. Grammatical morphemes, discussed earlier, are the modifications to words that provide additional grammatical precision, such as pluralizing words (*cat/cats*) sand inflecting verbs (*go/is going*). Grammatical morphemes do not really carry meaning; rather, they provide grammatical detail. Derivational morphology is similar to grammatical morphology in that it modifies words structurally. However, derivational morphology refers to the addition of prefixes and suffixes that carry meaning and thus change a word's meaning and sometimes its part of speech. For instance, the suffix *-er* can be added to *work* to change its meaning and its part of speech from a verb to a noun (*worker*). The prefix *un-* can be added to *happy* to change its meaning. Additional common derivational morphemes include *pre-* (*preschool*), *super-* (*superman*), *-est* (*fullest*), *-ness* (*freshness*), and *-ly* (*slowly*). Morphological development is the ability to manipulate word structure by adding these and other prefixes and suffixes, allowing children to become increasingly precise and specific in their communication. Morphology allows children to magnify their basic word repertoire exponentially; for instance, from the word root *run* the child with well-developed morphology has access to numerous variations (*rerun, ran, running, runner,* etc.)

During the preschool years, children acquire additional grammatical morphemes, described by Brown (1973). For instance, children begin to use the articles *a, an,* and *the* to elaborate nouns (*a horse, an ant, the house*). The greatest area of development at this time is in verb morphology. Speakers of English inflect verbs to provide information about time (e.g., past, present, future). Often, the verb *be* serves as an important marker of time. When the verb *be* or one of its derivatives (*am, is, are, was, were*) is the main verb in a sentence, it is called a *copula,* as in *I am Paul.* When the verb *be* or one of its derivatives serves as a helping verb in a sentence, it is called an *auxiliary,* as in *I am hugging Paul.* The *be* copula and auxiliary forms can be contracted (*He's happy, I'm going*) or uncontracted (*He is happy, I am going*). During the preschool years children acquire many of the nuances about verb morphology, including mastering the variations of *be* as both copula and auxiliary. Delayed development of verb morphology is one of the major signs of a language disorder (Brackenbury & Fey, 2003). Major achievements in verb morphology that occur in children between the ages of 3 and 5 include mastering

Uncontractable copula (27 to 39 months): *be* copula that cannot be contracted, as in *Here she is* and *We were happy.*

Contractible copula (29 to 49 months): *be* copula that can be contracted, as in *Debbie's here.*

Uncontractible auxiliary (29 to 49 months): *be* auxiliary that cannot be contracted, as in *They were going* (note that if *were* were contracted, it would change the meaning).

Contractible auxiliary (30 to 50 months): *be* auxiliary that can be contracted, as in *Mommy's working.* (Owens, 2001)

In addition to major achievements in morphology, the preschool years shepherd in significant advances in sentence complexity. Preschoolers move from simple declarative subject-verb-object constructions (*Daddy drives a truck.*) and subject-verb-complement constructions (*Truck is big.*) to more elaborate sentence patterns, such as

- Subject-verb-object-adverb (*Daddy's hitting the hammer outside.*)
- Subject-verb-complement-adverb (*Baby is sleepy now.*)
- Subject-auxiliary-verb-adverb (*Baby is eating now.*) (Justice & Ezell, 2002)

Children at this time begin to embed phrases and clauses in their sentences to create complex and compound sentences. Children also use coordinating (e.g., *and, or, but*) and subordinating conjunctions (e.g., *then, when, because*) to connect clauses. By the end of the preschool period, children produce compound sentences, as in *I told Daddy, and Daddy told Mommy,* as well as complex sentences with embedded clauses, as in *I told Daddy, who told Mommy* (see Justice & Ezell, 2002).

Achievements in Content

The preschool period represents an active and rich period of lexical development in which children build the content of their language. Two areas of preschool content achievements warrant discussion. First, preschoolers show rapid expansion of their receptive and expressive lexicons. Second, preschoolers increase their ability to use decontextualized language.

The Lexicon. Children learn an average of 13,000 words by the time they enter kindergarten! Children's learning of new words during the preschool period appears to occur through *incidental exposures,* or situations in which children informally experience new words within contexts of use. Preschool children show remarkable talent in their ability to effectively and efficiently acquire new words within a variety of daily activities (Brackenbury & Fey, 2003).

Only one exposure is often adequate for giving children a general sense of a novel word. However, children's vocabulary acquisition is a gradual process. Children's initial word representations progress from an immature and incomplete representation to a mature and accurate representation. The initial exposure to a word accompanied by the rapid acquisition of a general sense of its meaning is called fast mapping (Carey & Bartlett, 1978; McGregor, Friedman, Reilly, & Newman, 2002). These initial representations are then refined over time with repeated exposure to the concept over multiple contexts.

Curtis (1987) describes children's vocabulary development as a four-stage process. In stage 1 a child has no knowledge of a word ("I've never heard it"), in stage 2 a child has emergent knowledge of a word ("I've heard of it, but I don't know what it means"), in stage 3 a child has contextual knowledge of the word ("I recognize it in context. It has something to do with . . ."), and in stage 4 a child has full knowledge of the word ("I know it") (p. 43). During the preschool period, children's vocabularies include words at each of these stages: some are quite familiar, consistent with full knowledge, whereas others are fairly rudimentary, with emergent and contextual knowledge.

Decontextualized Language Skills. Preschool-age children begin to make an important shift from being highly contextualized in their language skills to being decontextualized. Contextualized language is rooted in the immediate context: the here and now. Contextualized language aids understanding through the incorporation of and reliance on shared knowledge, gestures, intonation, and immediately present situational cues. A child using contextualized language might say "Gimme that." while pointing to something in the listener's hands or might refer to a "Superman cake" in the context of a birthday party.

Decontextualized language is appropriate and necessary for discussing events and concepts beyond the here and now. These events may have occurred long ago or might occur in the future; they may be occurring in the next room or only in an abstract realm. Sometime during the preschool years, children become able to use language in a decontextualized manner. Decontextualized discourse relies heavily on the language itself in the construction of meaning. Decontextualized language may not contain context cues and does not assume shared background knowledge or context as does contextualized language. A child using decontextualized language might ask a parent for something in another room of the house ("Can you get the blocks down from my bookshelf?") or might describe a Superman cake to someone after the birthday party has taken place ("My mom made a Superman cake for my birthday party."). The child cannot rely on context to help in the communication with the mother; as with all types of decontextualized discourse, the child must use highly precise syntax and vocabulary to represent events that are beyond the here and now.

The ability to engage in decontextualized discourse is fundamental to academic success, as nearly all the learning that occurs in schools focuses on events and concepts beyond the classroom walls. This ability develops during the preschool years as children learn to use grammar and vocabulary in a highly precise manner.

Achievements in Use

Use is how language is applied functionally for meeting personal and social needs. During the preschool years, children begin to master several new discourse functions, improve their conversational skills, and use narratives.

Recall that as toddlers enter the two-word stage, they are already capable of using language to satisfy six different communicative functions (instrumental, regulatory, personal interactional, heuristic, imaginative, and informational). Preschoolers begin to use language for an even greater variety of discourse functions, including interpretive, logical, participatory, and organizing functions (Halliday, 1975, 1977, 1978). Interpretive functions are those that interpret the whole of one's experience. Logical functions express logical relations between ideas. Participatory functions express wishes, feelings, attitudes, and judgments. Organizing functions organize discourse. As the number of discourse functions grows, so, too, do preschooler's conversational skills.

One mark of an effective conversationalist is the ability to take turns in a conversation. Preschool-age children quickly become adept at turn taking. Preschoolers can maintain a conversation for two or more turns, particularly when the topic is their favorite: themselves! While they still have some difficulties understanding when communication breakdowns occur and giving listeners the appropriate amount of information to facilitate understanding, preschoolers are increasingly sophisticated conversationalists. They understand that they should respond to questions, and they discover that speaking at the same time as another person makes for ineffective communication.

Children also begin to hone their narrative skills in the preschool years. "Hey, Mom, guess what happened on the bus today?" is one way in which a preschooler might begin a narrative. Narratives are essentially decontextualized monologues. They are decontextualized in that rather than describing the here and now, they often focus on people or characters not immediately present or on events removed from the current context. Narratives are monologues in that they are largely uninterrupted streams of language, unlike conversations, in which two or more people share the linguistic load.

In a narrative, the speaker presents a topic and organizes the information pertaining to that topic in such a way that the listener can assume a relatively passive role, providing only minimal support to the speaker. Two important types of narratives are the personal narrative, in which an individual shares a factual event of his or her life, and the fictional narrative, in which an individual shares a made-up event. Usually, both types of narratives are threaded by an explicit sequence of events that are either causally or temporally related. A causal sequence unfolds following a cause-and-effect chain of events (e.g., Jesse didn't want to go to school . . . so Jesse told his mom he was sick.). A temporal sequence unfolds over time (e.g., First we went to the store. Then we told the clerk what we wanted.). In producing narrative—whether personal or fictional—the speaker must negotiate a complex set of linguistic skills, including syntax for ordering words and ideas, verb morphology for signaling the time of events, vocabulary for precisely representing events and people, and pragmatics for knowing how much information to share with the listener.

Although narrative skills begin to develop as early as age 2, most children are not able to construct true narratives until around age 4. Children's early narratives may include only a minimal description of the participants, time, and location relevant to the event. In some cases, this information may be omitted altogether. So, for example, when listening to a 3-year-old narrate a story, it may be necessary to ask such questions as "You said Dominick scratched you—is he your brother or your cat?" and "Did that happen on TV?" to get a better picture of what the child is trying to express. Importantly, narratives become clearer for the listener as children's ability to consider the listener's perspective emerges. Children's repertoire of linguistic devices, including adverbial time phrases (e.g., *yesterday,*

TABLE 2-5 Major achievements in narrative

Approximate Age of Emergence	Narrative Stage	Characteristics
2 years	Heaps	• Few links from one sentence to another • Organization based on immediate perception
2–3 years	Sequences	• Superficial but arbitrary time sequences • No causal links between events
3–4 years	Primitive Narratives	• Have a concrete core surrounded by a set of clarifying or amplifying attributes
4–4½ years	Unfocused Chains	• Story as a whole loses its point and drifts off
5 years	Focused Chains	• A main character experiences a series of events, but no true concept is present
5–7 years	True Narratives	• Has a theme or moral • Concrete, perceptual, or abstract bonds hold the story together

Source: Adapted with permission from Hughes, D., McGillivray, L., & Schmidek, M. (1997). *Guide to narrative language: Procedures for assessment.* Eau Claire, WI: Thinking Publications.

this morning) and verb morphology (signaling the time of activities) also grows, thus increasing the comprehensibility of their narratives.

Discussion Point: *Children of lower socioeconomic status generally have a more difficult time producing fictional narratives (Shiro, 2003). Why do you think this might be so?*

Narrative skills are an important area of mastery for preschoolers. Narrative skills have been found to be one of the best predictors of later school outcomes for preschoolers at risk for late developing language skills (Paul & Smith, 1993). The decontextualized language inherent in narratives may be the critical link to the acquisition of early literacy skills and subsequent school achievement (Peterson, Jesso, & McCabe, 1999). Table 2-5 summarizes these major achievements in narrative and shows how children move from "heaps" and descriptive sequences to well-rounded, complex stories ("true narratives") in the elementary years.

Achievements in Speech

During the preschool years, children continue to expand and stabilize their sound repertoires. By the end of the preschool period, children are likely to have mastered nearly all of the phonemes in their native language. Children aged 4 and 5 typically exhibit only lingering difficulties with a few of the later-developing phonemes, including *r* (*row*), *l* (*low*), *s* (*sun*), *ch* (*cheese*), *sh* (*shy*), *z* (*zoo*), and *th* (*think, though*). Difficulties with some of the earlier acquired sounds may persist in complex multisyllabic words (*daffodil*) or in words with consonant clusters (*split*). However, at the end of the preschool period children are highly intelligible, and their expressive phonemic repertoire is nearly as extensive as an adult's.

As mentioned earlier, phonological processes refer to the systematic deviations children make in their expressive phonology. In the preschool years, nearly all processes are suppressed as children's phonological systems stabilize. The greatest rate of suppression occurs at 3 to 4 years of age (Haelsig & Madison, 1986). Weak syllable deletion and cluster reduction may occur with 4-year-olds, but are usually suppressed by 5 years of age. Two patterns that may persist past the fifth birthday include liquid gliding (substituting *y* and *w* for *l* and *r*) and *th* substitution (substituting *d* and *t* for *th*).

Receptive phonology also continues to develop during the preschool years. The achievement of these internal phonological representations is very important. Reading development—discussed later in this chapter—requires that a child have robust phonological representations in order to make sense of the alphabetic principle, or the relationship between letters (graphemes) and sounds (phonemes). Environmental and biological factors can impact the development of adequate phonological representations. For instance, children who receive little linguistic stimulation and children who have ongoing middle-ear infections are at risk for delays in the development of solid phonological representations (Nittrouer, 1996). The quality and quantity of phonological stimulation relates to children's development of robust phonological representations.

Achievements in Emergent Literacy

The preschool period marks several critical achievements in young children's development of literacy. Between ages 3 and 5, children begin to make sense of reading and writing in a rudimentary way (Justice & Ezell, 2001). They learn how print works, they begin to play with the sound units that make up words, and they develop an interest in reading and writing. Researchers refer to this earliest period of learning about reading and writing as emergent literacy. Emergent literacy encompasses children's developing knowledge about reading and writing conventions. While children at this time are not yet reading and writing in a conventional sense, their emerging knowledge about print and sounds forms an important foundation for the reading instruction that commences in kindergarten (Justice & Pullen, 2003).

Emergent literacy achievements depend largely on metalinguistic ability, or the child's ability to view language as an object of attention. Emergent literacy involves the child's engagement in activities in which oral or written language is the object of scrutiny, such as pretending to write, looking at words in a storybook, or making up rhyming patterns (Chaney, 1998). Being able to engage with language at a metalinguistic level is an important achievement of the preschool period that correlates well with the likelihood that children will later succeed at writing and reading instruction, which depend on the child being able to focus on language as an object of attention (Justice & Ezell, 2004).

The two most important metalinguistically governed achievements in emergent literacy for preschoolers are print awareness and phonological awareness. **Print awareness** describes the young child's understanding of the form and functions of written language. **Phonological awareness** describes the young child's understanding of and sensitivity to the sound units of oral language, namely, the series of larger and smaller units that make up speech (phonemes, syllables, words).

Print awareness includes a number of specific achievements that children generally acquire along a developmental continuum (Justice & Ezell, 2004): (1) print interest, (2) print

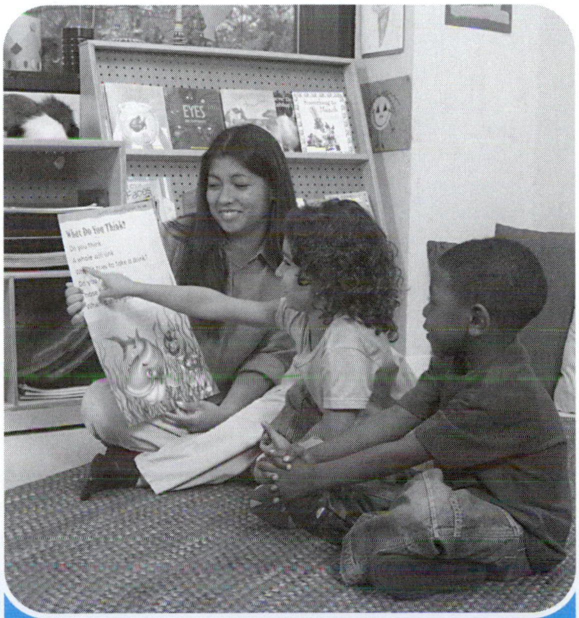

Pointing to print while reading to preschoolers can help foster print awareness.

FIGURE 2-8 Major achievements in print awareness during the preschool years.

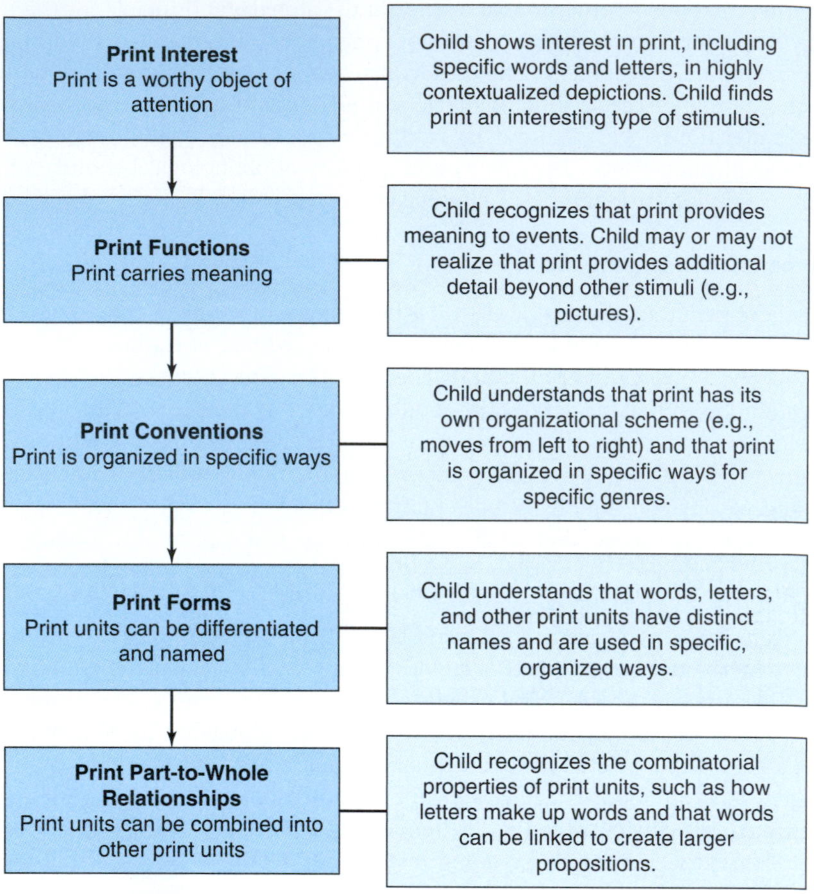

Source: Justice, L. M., & Ezell, H. K. (2004). Print referencing: An emergent literacy enhancement technique and its clinical applications. *Language, Speech, and Hearing Services in Schools, 35,* 185–193. Reprinted with permission.

functions, (3) print conventions, (4) print forms, and (5) print part-to-whole relationships (see Figure 2-8). First, young children develop an interest in and appreciation for print. Children recognize that print is a specific type of stimulus in the environment and in books. Second, they begin to understand that print conveys meaning, that it has a specific type of function. Third, children develop an understanding of specific print conventions, such as how print moves left to right and top to bottom. Fourth, children learn the language that describes specific print units, such as words and letters. Fifth, children learn the relationship among different print units, such as how letters combine to form words. Influences on children's development of these abilities include their home environment as well as their general oral language ability. Although many children enter kindergarten with sophisticated levels of print awareness, other children enter school at a significant disadvantage (Boudreau & Hedberg, 1999).

Phonological awareness is the child's sensitivity and access to the sound structure of spoken words. Phonological awareness emerges incrementally, beginning around 2 years of age, moving from a shallow level of awareness to a deep level of awareness (Stanovich, 2000)

TABLE 2-6 Achievements in phonological awareness

Phonological Awareness Skill	Description	Level	Developmental Expectation
Word awareness	Segment sentences into words	Shallow	Early to middle preschool
Syllable awareness	Segment multisyllable words into syllables	Shallow	Early to middle preschool
Rhyme awareness	Recognize when two words rhyme; produce pairs of words that rhyme	Shallow	Early to middle preschool
Onset awareness	Segment the beginning sound (onset) from the rest of a word; blend the beginning sound (onset) with the rest of a word	Shallow	Late preschool
Phoneme identity	Identify sounds at beginning and end of word; identify words that start with the same sound	Shallow	Late preschool, early kindergarten
Phoneme blending	Blend phonemes to make a word	Deep	Early kindergarten
Phoneme segmentation	Segment a word into its phonemes	Deep	Middle to late kindergarten
Phoneme counting	Identify the number of phonemes in a word	Deep	Late kindergarten to end of first grade
Phoneme manipulation	Delete, add, and rearrange phonemes in a word	Deep	Elementary grades

Source: From Kaderavek, J., & Justice, L. M. (2004). Embedded-explicit emergent literacy: II Goal selection and implementation in the early childhood classroom. *Language, Speech, and Hearing Services in Schools, 25,* 212–228. Reprinted with permission.

(see Table 2-6). Children possessing shallow levels of phonological awareness show an implicit and rudimentary sensitivity to large units of sound structure. They are able to hear and produce rhymes, segment sentences into words and words into syllables, and detect beginning sound similarities across words (e.g., *sing, sack, sun*). Children develop these shallow sensitivities during the preschool years, from roughly 3 to 5 years of age. Children with a deep level of phonological awareness demonstrate an explicit and analytical knowledge of the smallest phonological segments of speech, representing the phoneme. They are able to count the number of phonemes in words (e.g., *wig* has three sounds, and *spray* has four sounds), segment words into their constituent phonemes (e.g., *big* can be broken into /b/ + /I/ + /g/), and manipulate the phonological segments contained within words (e.g., deleting the first sound in *spray* and moving it to the end of the word, for *prays*) (Justice & Schuele, 2003).

Discussion Point: *Based on what you know about phonological awareness, describe what kinds of activities might support Sam, introduced in Box 2-1, as he tries to improve his reading ability?*

School-Age Accomplishments

You may wonder what language and communication achievements remain for school-age children to master. So much of the research concerning language development focuses on the achievements of infants and young children that it is tempting to equate language development with the very young child, overlooking the accomplishments of the older child.

Yet substantial development and refinement in the areas of syntax, pragmatics, and semantics occur throughout adolescence. The following sections discuss the most important aspects of communicative development among school-aged children, which include functional flexibility, reading and writing, literate language, and form and content refinements.

Functional Flexibility

Functional flexibility refers to the ability to use language for a variety of communicative purposes, or functions. This flexibility is increasingly important for school-age children who are asked to compare and contrast, to persuade, to hypothesize, to explain, to classify, and to predict. Figure 2-9 provides a more complete list of language functions required of school-age children, attesting to the importance of flexibility in language for children of this age.

Each function requires a distinct set of linguistic, social, and cognitive competencies, all of which develop over the school-age years and must be integrated by the child for communicative competence. For example, according to Nippold (1998), students must integrate seven skills in order to use language to persuade:

1. Adjust to listener characteristics (e.g., age, authority, familiarity)
2. State advantages as a reason to comply
3. Anticipate and reply to counterarguments
4. Use positive techniques such as politeness and bargaining as strategies to increase compliance
5. Avoid negative strategies such as whining and begging
6. Generate a large number and variety of different arguments
7. Control the discourse assertively

Students who cannot use language flexibly are more likely than other students to have difficulty with the academic and social demands of elementary, middle, and high schools.

FIGURE 2-9 **Language functions required of school-age children.**

1. *To instruct:* To provide specific sequential directions
2. *To inquire:* To seek understanding through asking questions
3. *To test:* To investigate the logic of a statement
4. *To describe:* To tell about, giving necessary information to identify
5. *To compare and contrast:* To show how things are similar and different
6. *To explain:* To define terms by providing specific examples
7. *To analyze:* To break down a statement into its component parts, telling what each means and how they are related
8. *To hypothesize:* To test a statement's logical or empirical consequences
9. *To deduce:* To arrive at a conclusion by reasoning; to infer
10. *To evaluate:* To weigh and judge the relative importance of an idea

Source: From Bereiter, C., & Engelmann, S. (1966). *Teaching disadvantaged children in the preschool.* Published by Allyn and Bacon, Boston, MA.

Reading and Writing

Reading and writing are two major achievements that take place during the school-age years. Success at learning to read requires the child's unlocking of the alphabetic principle, as to read English, children must learn how the orthography of letters (graphemes) corresponds to the phonology of sounds (phonemes). Children's success with grapheme–phoneme correspondence rests on their achievement of print awareness and phonological awareness in the preschool period. Children who enter school with skills in these areas are more likely than others to succeed at beginning reading instruction (Chaney, 1998).

Children learning to read generally progress through a predictable series of stages that span the period between preschool and adulthood (Chall, 1996). The preschool years correspond to an emergent literacy or prereading stage, during which the most critical developments consist of oral language, print awareness, and phonological awareness. Children then progress through five stages that build on this early foundation, as presented by Chall (1996).

Stage 1, *Initial Reading, or Decoding,* covers the period between kindergarten and first grade, when children are between 5 and 7 years of age. During this stage, children learn to associate letters with the sounds they represent and attend to sound-spelling relationships as they begin to decode words. The focus at this stage is learning to read, or the development of decoding skills and the untangling of the alphabetic principle.

Stage 2, *Confirmation, Fluency, and Ungluing from Print,* covers the period between second and third grade, when children are between 7 and 8 years of age. During this stage, children hone their decoding skills and develop strategies for comprehending what they read. Children gradually transition from learning to read to reading to learn.

Stage 3, *Reading for Learning the New,* lasts from grades 4 to 8, when children are between 9 and 13 years of age. Children read to gain new information and are solidly using reading to learn. Reading during this stage helps expand children's vocabularies, build background and world knowledge, and develop strategic reading habits.

Stage 4, *Multiple Viewpoints: High School,* covers the high school period from the age of 14 to the age of 18. During stage 4, students learn to handle increasingly difficult concepts and to read the texts that describe them. Students learn to analyze texts critically and to understand multiple points of view.

Stage 5, *Construction and Reconstruction—a World View: College,* occurs from age 18 on. During this stage, the linguistic and cognitive demands placed on readers continue to increase, and readers are able to construct understanding by analyzing and synthesizing text.

Discussion Point: *Using what you know about Reston, introduced in Box 2-1, do you predict that he would also exhibit difficulties with reading comprehension? Why or why not?*

Literate Language

An earlier section of this chapter described the difference between contextualized and decontextualized language. When children enter school, language becomes increasingly decontextualized—removed from the here and now. Literate language is the term used to describe language that is highly decontextualized. The literate language style characterizes language that is used to "monitor and reflect on experience, and reason about, plan, and predict experiences" (Westby, 1985, p. 181). Literate language refers to the child's ability to use language without the aid of context cues for supporting meaning; the child must rely on language itself to make meaning. Developing a literate language style, or progressing from contextualized to decontextualized language, is crucial for children's participation in the type of discourse that occurs in school settings. Imagine the following conversation taking place between 4-year-old Amber and her 8-year-old sister, Kristy:

Amber: I want that crayon!

Kristy: No way! You wrote on the wall with my crayons the other day while I was at school and I got in trouble.

Discourse development lies along a continuum reflecting oral language on one end and literate language on the other (Westby, 1991). In our example, Amber's and Kristy's utterances represent opposite ends of this continuum. At the lower level of the discourse continuum lies *oral language,* or the linguistic aspects of communicative competence necessary for communicating very basic desires and needs (phonology, syntax, morphology, and semantics). Westby describes children at this end of the continuum as "learning to talk." Children learning to talk are able to satisfy some basic language functions, including requesting and greeting. They can also produce simple syntactic structures. English speakers, for example, can form yes or no questions by inserting *do* before the subject (*You like ice cream* becomes *Do you like ice cream?*) and can mark the past tense by adding *ed* or by retrieving the appropriate irregular past tense verb. The most salient characteristic of oral language is its highly contextualized style. Highly contextualized language is language that depends heavily on the immediate context and environment. Markers of highly contextualized language include referential pronouns, or pronouns that refer to something physically available to the speaker ("I want *that.*"), as well as gestures and facial expressions. Only when children have mastered oral language can they begin to "talk to learn," or to use language to reflect on past experiences and to reason about, predict, and plan for future experiences using decontextualized language (Westby, 1991).

Children who talk to learn represent the literate language end of the continuum. At this end, children use language chiefly as a way to communicate higher-order cognitive functions (e.g., reflecting, reasoning, and planning). Highly specific vocabulary and complex syntax that express ideas, events, and objects beyond those of the present typify literate language. Some specific features of literate language that children learn to use include the following (Curenton & Justice, 2004):

1. Elaborated noun phrases: Groups of words consisting of a noun and one or more modifiers that provide additional information about the noun, including articles (e.g., *a, an, the*), possessives (e.g., *my, his, their*), demonstratives (e.g., *this, that, those*), quantifiers (e.g., *every, each, some*), *wh*-words (e.g., *what, which, whichever*), and adjectives (e.g., *tall, long, ugly*).
2. Adverbs: Syntactic forms used to modify verbs, which enhance the explicitness of action and event descriptions. Adverbs provide additional information about time (e.g., *suddenly, again, now*), manner (e.g., *somehow, well, slowly*), degree (e.g., *almost, barely, much*), place (*here, outside, above*), reason (*therefore, since, so*), and affirmation or negation (e.g., *definitely, really, never*).
3. Conjunctions: Words or phrases that organize information and clarify relationships among elements. Coordinating conjunctions include *and, for, or, yet, but, nor,* and *so*. Subordinating conjunctions are more numerous and include *after, although, as, because,* and *for,* among others.
4. Mental/linguistic verbs: These verbs refer to various acts of thinking and speaking. Mental verbs include *think, know, believe, imagine, feel, consider, suppose, decide, forget,* and *remember*. Linguistic verbs include *say, tell, speak, shout, answer, call, reply,* and *yell*.

Consider these structures in the following example of decontextualized language:

> Last night, after I got home, I was wondering how to occupy myself when I decided that I would rearrange my kitchen cabinets. You see, I was quite bored, given all that had transpired. I started to pull cans off the top shelf, at which point I came upon something quite odd. Now, before I tell you what I found . . .

This author paints a picture for the listener by using a variety of techniques that transcend vocabulary and syntax. Specificity is provided lexically by elaborated noun phrases (*my kitchen cabinets, the top shelf*), adverbs (*last night, now*), and mental/linguistic verbs (*wondering, decided, tell*). Conjunctions and conjunctive adverbs are spread liberally across the story to weave together events in a causal and temporal manner (e.g., *at which point, now*). These devices provide context that is not otherwise available to the listener, or in this case, the reader. As children move through the elementary grades into adolescence and high school, we expect them to be able to use literate language structures to create context for readers and listeners.

Discussion Point: *Describe in writing what you did last night. Document the use of literate language features in this written sample. Which features occur most frequently? Least frequently?*

Form and Content Refinements

Form Refinements. As students move through the elementary grades into high school, form achievements progress slowly and subtly. Because many of the syntactic skills that children exhibit are only rarely used in conversation, such as the passive voice, these form accomplishments can be hard to witness. The most important achievements in form for school-age children are in the area of complex syntax. Complex syntax refers to developmentally advanced grammatical structures that mark a literate language style (Paul, 1995). These structures occur relatively infrequently in spoken language, but when used in written language indicate more advanced levels of grammar. Examples of complex syntax include noun phrase postmodification with past participles (*a tree called the willow*), complex verb phrases using the perfective aspect (*They have driven a long way*), and adverbial conjunctions (e.g., *only, consequently*).

The development of syntax over the school-age years is most easily visible in students' writing. Persuasive writing in particular is a vehicle for the expression of more complex syntax. Persuasive writing, according to Nippold (2000), is a challenging communicative task, yet it is an important skill developed in the school-age period. Persuasive writing requires an awareness of what others believe and value and the ability to present one's ideas in a logical sequence. Syntactic complexities arise in persuasive writing as children must produce "longer sentences that contain greater amounts of subordination and stronger linkages between sentences, attainments that are partially achieved through the proper use of adverbial connectors" (Nippold, 2000, p. 20).

Context Refinements. The typical school-age child makes considerable gains in developing the lexicon. These gains occur primarily from reading books, an activity that provides students with access to words and concepts that are not typically the topic of everyday conversations. The receptive and expressive vocabularies of school-age students continue to expand so that by the time they graduate from high school, they will have command of over 60,000 words (Pinker, 1994). One reason for this significant advance is that school-age children are able to use the context surrounding new words to infer their meanings.

Three areas of notable content development for school-age students are (1) understanding multiple meanings, (2) understanding lexical ambiguity, and (3) understanding figurative

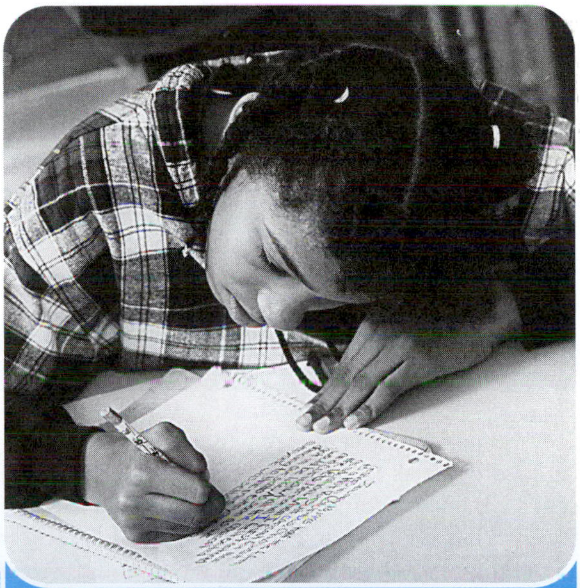

Mastering the art and skill of persuasive writing is one linguistic challenge school-age children face.

language. As children's lexicons grow and children encounter more and more words, they realize that many words have more than one meaning. Students become able to provide multiple definitions for words that have several common meanings. Doing this requires not only lexical knowledge, but also metalinguistic knowledge, both of which are necessary to achieve full competence at the literate end of the oral-literate language continuum.

The understanding of lexical ambiguity is a second and related area of notable content achievement for school-age children. Lexical ambiguity occurs for words with multiple meanings, as in "That was a real bear," in which the meaning of "bear" is ambiguous. Lexical ambiguity regularly fuels the humor in jokes, riddles, comic strips, newspaper headlines, and advertisements (Nippold, 1998), as in the joke "Is your refrigerator running?" (You'd better go catch it!). When students come across words that are ambiguous, they must first notice the ambiguity, and then they must scrutinize the words to arrive at the appropriate meaning. Students with weak oral language skills are often not very adept at noticing lexical ambiguities and are less likely than other students to seek clarification for an ambiguity when they do notice one. The result can be a communication breakdown (Paul, 1995).

A third semantic refinement that occurs over the school-age years is the ability to use and understand figurative language. Figurative language is the use of words, phrases, symbols, and ideas in a nonliteral and often abstract way to evoke mental images and sense impressions. Of the different types of figurative language, including similes, metaphors, oxymorons, hyperboles, and proverbs, Nippold (2000) reports that proverbs are one of the most difficult types to master. Proverbs serve a variety of communicative functions, such as

- Commenting (Blood is thicker than water.)
- Interpreting (His bark is worse than his bite.)
- Advising (Don't count your chickens before they hatch.)
- Warning (Better safe than sorry.)
- Encouraging (Every cloud has a silver lining.) (Nippold, 2000)

Nippold reports that proverb understanding improves gradually during the adolescent years and that the presence of a supportive linguistic environment can facilitate the process. Proverb understanding has been correlated with measures of academic success in literature and mathematics in adolescents (Nippold, 2000), likely because proverb understanding reveals a student's ability to contend with abstract and metalinguistic aspects of language.

CHAPTER SUMMARY

Communicative competence refers to the understandings and abilities that speakers of a language must possess and utilize in order to communicate effectively in that language. Communicative competence is acquired at two main levels, linguistic and pragmatic. Linguistic aspects include phonological competence, grammatical competence, lexical competence, and discourse competence and are related directly to the nature and structure of language. Pragmatic aspects of communicative competence include functional competence, sociolinguistic competence, interactional competence, and cultural competence and relate to the social contexts in which language is used. Communicative competence develops along a fairly predictable trajectory across the life span, with major milestones achieved in roughly the same order and at roughly the same ages across cultures. Communicative competence is constructed on some innately given abilities and early foundations and continues to develop throughout toddlerhood, the preschool years, the school-age years, and into adulthood.

KEY TERMS

communicative competence, p. 39
cooing sounds, p. 52
intentional communication, p. 48
intersubjective awareness, p. 48
jargon, p. 52
joint attention, p. 47
lexicon, p. 53
mean length of utterance (MLU), p. 56
overextension, p. 60
phonological awareness, p. 69
phonological processes, p. 43
phonotactics, p. 48
print awareness, p. 69
reduplicative babbling, p. 52
reflexive sounds, p. 52
register, p. 45
underextension, p. 60
variegated babbling, p. 52
vocabulary spurt, p. 59
Whorf hypothesis, p. 46

ON THE WEB

Check out the Companion Website! On it, you will find:

- suggested readings
- reflection questions
- a self-study quiz
- links to additional online resources, including information about current technologies in communication sciences and disorders

Anatomical and Physiological Bases of Communication and Communication Disorders

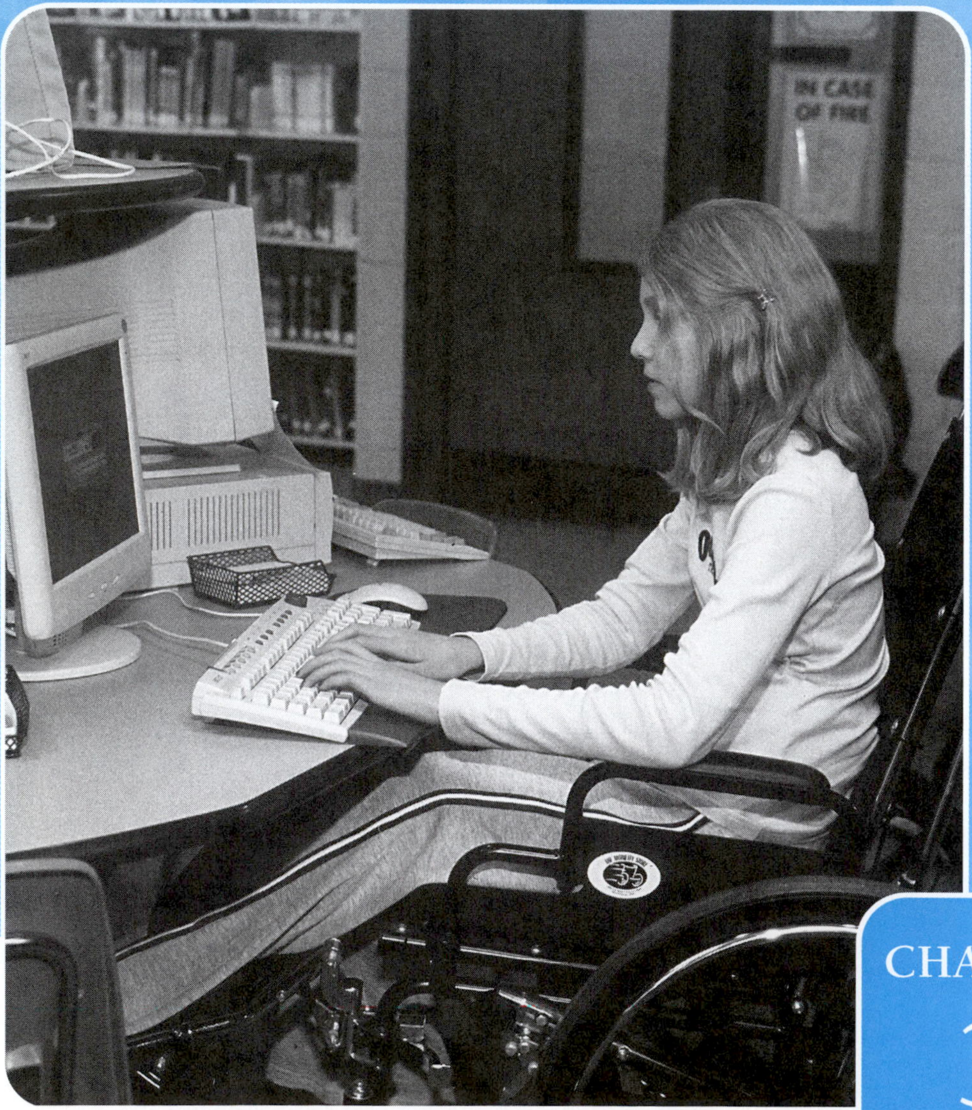

CHAPTER 3

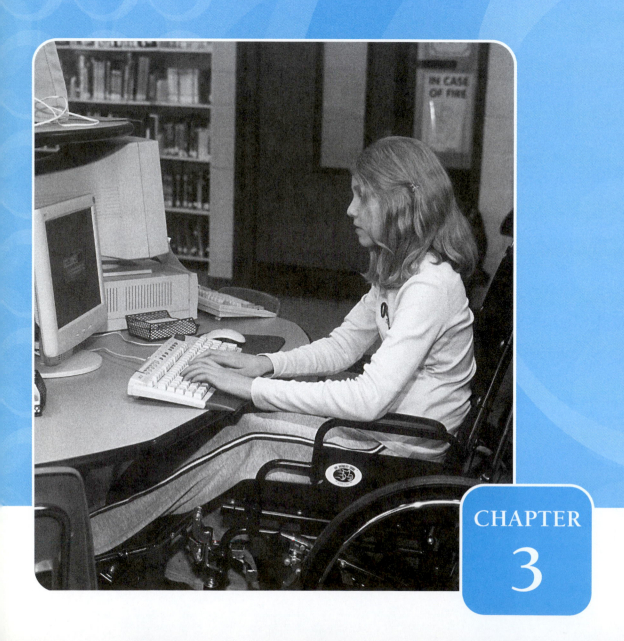

FOCUS QUESTIONS

This chapter addresses the following topics:

1. Neuroscience and human communication
2. Anatomy and physiology of speech
3. Anatomy and physiology of hearing
4. Anatomy and physiology of swallowing

INTRODUCTION

Human communication involves the complex interaction of many systems of the human body. People involved in the assessment and treatment of communication disorders require a sophisticated understanding of the functions and structures of these systems. This chapter provides a basic introduction to the anatomy, physiology, and neuroscience involved with speech, language, hearing, and swallowing.

Anatomy and physiology together form the branch of science concerning the description of body structures (anatomy) and the functions of those structures (physiology) (Zemlin, 1988). To understand the process of human communication, we need to consider both structure and function—to understand not only the specifics of a particular anatomical structure, including how it relates to other structures and forms an anatomical system, but also how a structure works both by itself and in concert with other structures as a physiological system.

Anatomy and physiology are ancient sciences dating back many centuries. The Greek physician Hippocrates (c. 460–377 B.C.E.) is considered the father of medicine as well as the father of anatomy as a science. Hippocrates' work provided an important impetus for centuries of inquiry into how the human body is organized and how its parts work (or do not work) when in a state of health or disease. Inquiries into the anatomy and physiology of speech, language, hearing, and swallowing date back hundreds of years.

Neuroscience is a particular branch of science that focuses on the anatomy and physiology of the nervous system, including the brain (Bhatnagar & Andy, 1995). It is a relatively new science characterized by rapid and remarkable advances in new technologies, such as magnetic resonance imaging (MRI), positron emission topography (PET), and computed tomography scan (CTS). These technologies are able to provide detailed images of both the anatomy and the physiology of the brain. The brain is the intermediary, or mediator, of the body's sensory and motor systems, including the systems involved with speech, language, hearing, and swallowing. Therefore, interest in how the brain works has consumed many researchers and practitioners in the discipline of communication sciences and disorders in recent decades.

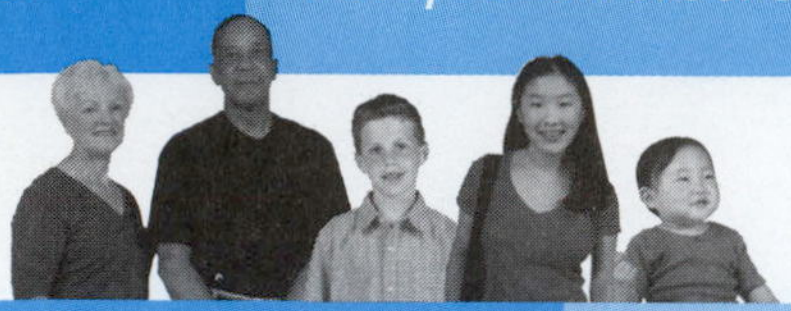

BOX 3-1 Communication Disorders Across the Lifespan: Case Examples

Timmy Sullivan is a 60-year-old, thrice-divorced man living in Washington, D.C. Timmy is a Vietnam veteran who, near the end of his 2-year tour of duty in 1968, experienced a severe head injury, for which he received a silver star. Specifically, during combat, shrapnel pierced Timmy's left forehead and lodged in his frontal lobe. Surgery was performed within hours to remove the shrapnel, and after a 1-month rehabilitation and recuperation period, Timmy was discharged from active service. Timmy has not sought any additional rehabilitation for his injury in the years since discharge, and he does not feel that he shows any symptoms related to his 35-year-old brain injury. Timmy has not had a regular job in the last 10 years, but brings in some income by doing odd jobs in his neighborhood. His friends and ex-wives describe Timmy as fun loving, energetic, and warm, but erratic, irresponsible, and disorganized in his behavior.

Internet research

1. What kind of assistance is available for military personnel who have experienced brain injuries?
2. How common are brain injuries among active-duty military personnel today? How do these figures compare with corresponding figures from the Vietnam era?
3. What is the Vietnam Head Injury Study?

Brainstorm and discussion

1. Brainstorm some possible short- and long-term repercussions of a serious injury to the frontal lobe.
2. What kinds of supports should be made available to military personnel who experience brain injuries during active duty?

Patricia is a 3-year-old girl recently adopted by Mr. and Dr. Franklin of Cincinnati, Ohio. Patricia's birth parents died in a car accident when she was only 12 weeks old. From the age of 12 weeks to the age of 18 months, Patricia lived with a foster family, where she was allegedly physically and mentally abused by two older foster siblings. Patricia was removed from this foster home and lived in a second foster home until she was 3 years old, when she was adopted by the Franklins. Mr. and Dr. Franklin are concerned about Patricia's history of abuse, although she appears to have no symptoms associated with abuse and seems to be a well-adjusted and happy child. Mr. Franklin is a stay-at-home dad; Dr. Franklin is a neuroscientist who studies the effects of early maltreatment on the brain development of rodents at the University of Cincinnati. She is familiar with research showing that early abuse and maltreatment can affect brain physiology in rodents. The Franklins are thus seeking assistance through an early intervention program in Cincinnati to have Patricia comprehensively evaluated for social, emotional, cognitive, and linguistic development. However, the early intervention program is balking at covering the cost of the assessment given that Patricia shows no apparent signs of developmental difficulties due to abuse.

Neuroscience and Human Communication

Terminology

Descriptions of anatomy and physiology often utilize a specific terminology, or nomenclature. Much of this terminology has its roots in ancient Latin and Greek. It is essential for the student of communication sciences and disorders to be familiar with the terminology associated with positions and directions. Common positional terms used to describe aspects of anatomy and physiology include **anterior** (toward the front) and **posterior** (toward the back); **superior** (toward the top) and **inferior** (toward the bottom); **external** (toward the outside) and **internal** (toward the inside); and **proximal** (toward the body)

Internet research

1. What is early intervention?
2. How common are maltreatment and abuse among young children in the United States?
3. Is there evidence showing that early childhood abuse can have a negative impact on brain development?

Brainstorm and discussion

1. Should a developmental assessment be provided to Patricia even if she displays no outward signs of developmental difficulties?
2. What are some possible repercussions of early abuse on brain development?

Hortencia Rivera is a 16-year-old adolescent in San Diego, California. From birth to 6 years of age, Hortencia had recurrent seizures. At age 5, she was diagnosed with a right temporal lobe ganglioglioma, a type of brain tumor that has been linked to seizure disorder. At age 6, Hortencia underwent a temporal lobectomy, during which her entire right temporal lobe was removed along with the tumor. In the 10 years since surgery, Hortencia has been seizure free, and there has been no recurrence of the brain tumor. There appear to be no negative repercussions from the loss of the right temporal lobe.

Internet research

1. How common is temporal lobectomy?
2. Why would a tumor in the temporal lobe result in seizures?
3. What is the likelihood of having complete resolution of seizures *and* no apparent long-term side effects following temporal lobectomy?

Brainstorm and discussion

1. From a parent's perspective, discuss the pros and cons of having your child undergo a temporal lobectomy versus living a life with seizures.
2. How is it possible that the complete loss of one's temporal lobe can have no negative repercussions? Brainstorm some possibilities.

and **distal** (away from the body) (Zemlin, 1988). Two directional terms often used to describe organization of the nervous system and neuroscience include **afferent** (towards the nervous system) and **efferent** (away from the nervous system).

Becoming knowledgeable about neuroscience and, specifically, neuroanatomy, can be challenging. Many of the terms and concepts may be new to students. Nonetheless, knowledge about neuroanatomy is crucial both for professionals who work with people who have communication disorders and for those who conduct research in speech, language, hearing, and swallowing disorders. This knowledge base helps professionals and researchers to (1) better understand and identify the neurological causes of communication disorders, (2) recognize signs and symptoms associated with specific neurological pathologies, and (3) find solutions to neurological problems, resulting in improved interventions for children and adults (Bhatnagar & Andy, 1995).

FIGURE 3-1 The central and peripheral nervous systems.

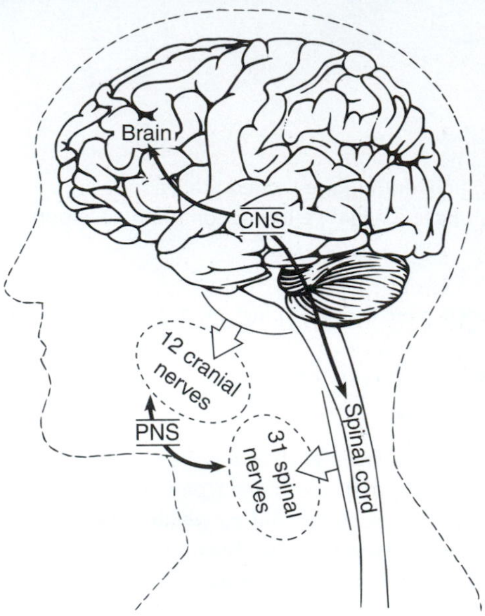

FIGURE 3-2 The neuron.

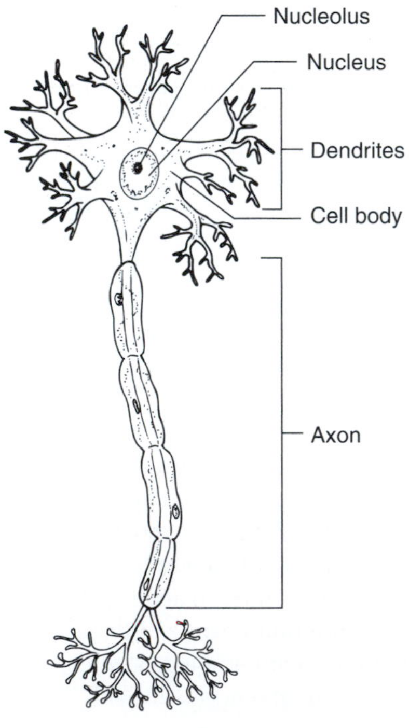

The Nervous System

The human nervous systems mediate nearly all aspects of human behavior. The human body has two major nervous systems: the central nervous system (CNS) and the peripheral nervous system (PNS). The CNS consists of the brain and the spinal cord. The PNS consists of the nerves that emerge from the brain and the spinal cord to innervate the rest of the body. In neuroscience the term *innervate* describes the supply of nerves to a particular region or part of the body. The 12 pairs of nerves that emerge from the brain are the **cranial nerves.** The 31 pairs of nerves that emerge from the spinal cord are called **spinal nerves.** The cranial and spinal nerves carry information back and forth between the brain, the spine, and the rest of the body. This information includes sensory information carried to the brain and motor information carried away from the brain. Figure 3-1 illustrates the major structures in the CNS and PNS.

Neurons

The highly specialized cells that make up the nervous system and carry its sensory and motor information are **neurons.** The brain is made up of billions of neurons. A neuron consists of a cell body and two extensions that receive and transmit information in the form of electrical-chemical nerve impulses to and from the cell body, as shown in Figure 3-2. The two types of neural extensions are dendrites and axons. **Dendrites** are afferent extensions, meaning that they bring nerve impulses into the cell body. **Axons** are efferent extensions, meaning that they take nerve impulses away from the cell body. Electrical-chemical nerve impulses move from one neuron to another, traveling down one neuron's dendrite and into its cell body, and then along the axon to another neuron's dendrite. The **synapse** is the space where two neurons meet (see Figure 3-2). For the two neurons to communicate, the nerve impulse must cross the synapse. **Neurotransmitters** are chemical agents that help to carry information across the synaptic cleft, which is the minute space between the axon of the transmitting neuron and the dendrite of the receiving neuron.

Neurons are sheathed in a coating called **myelin**. The myelin sheath contributes importantly to the rapid relay of nerve impulses; this sheath also helps to protect the neuron. Myelinization, the growth of the myelin sheath, is a slow process that is not complete until late in childhood. Incomplete myelinization or the loss of myelin can result in serious neurological problems. For instance, multiple sclerosis (MS), a degenerative motor disease, results from the loss of myelin.

Central Nervous System

The CNS consists of the brain and the spinal cord. The brain is essentially the chief operator of the entire CNS: the brain initiates and regulates virtually all motor, sensory, and cognitive processes (Bhatnagar & Andy, 1995). The CNS carries sensory information from the body to the brain via afferent pathways, and motor commands from the brain to the rest of the body via efferent pathways.

The CNS is what makes humans human. Accordingly, damage to the CNS—the brain or spinal cord—can result in grave consequences. Damage to the brain, as occurs with a traumatic brain injury, can completely alter a person's personality because the brain is where all the components of personality are stored. Serious brain damage can also disable many of the cognitive acts that make humans what they are—rational and thoughtful problem solvers. Damage to the spinal cord can severely restrict a person's ability to perform both essential and nonessential physical functions, such as breathing, swallowing, walking, and writing.

Many of us know or know of a person who has experienced significant damage to the CNS. Christopher Reeve, an actor who played Superman in several movies, is one such well-known person. Reeve sustained serious spinal cord injury in 1995 in a horse-riding accident and passed away in 2004 due to complications from this injury. He worked tirelessly to find a cure for paralysis. Our familiarity with such cases may make it seem as though the CNS is particularly vulnerable to injury. To the contrary, the CNS is designed to be resistant to damage. Think of all the times you have hit your head or fallen on your back without sustaining serious injury. This is possible because the CNS has a series of three protective shields that help keep it from being damaged.

Discussion Point: *What are some common activities in which persons engage that could result in CNS injuries?*

The first shield is bone. Both the brain and the spinal cord are protected by bone; the skull covers the brain, and the vertebral column covers the spinal cord. The second shield is a series of three layered membranes, the **meninges**, that completely encase the CNS. The inside layer of membrane, called the pia mater, tightly wraps around the brain and spinal cord and holds the blood vessels that serve the brain. It is a thin, transparent shield that gives the brain its bright pink color. The second layer is the arachnoid mater. The third and outermost layer is the dura mater (literally, "hard mother"). The dura mater consists of thick fibrous tissue that completely encases the brain and the spinal cord. Finally, the third shield protecting the CNS is a layer of fluid, specifically, cerebrospinal fluid (CSF). CSF circulates between the innermost two layers of the meninges, the pia mater and the arachnoid mater. CSF carries chemicals important to metabolic processes, but it also serves as an important buffer for any jolts to the CNS.

Brain

The brain is the commander-in-chief, or mediator, of the entire human body. Of all the structures of the human body, the human brain has changed the most in our recent evolutionary history. The most marked change has been in its size and weight. Our ancestor of approximately 3.5 million years ago, *Australopithecus africanus,* had a brain vault roughly the size of a chimpanzee's, weighing about 14 ounces. At that time in our history, the brain was approximately 1% of our body weight. In comparison, the modern human brain averages about 46 to 49 ounces in weight (about 3 pounds), constituting roughly 2.5% of our body weight (Sears, 2003). The greatest change in the human brain, accounting for these increases in weight and mass, has been the enlargement of the cerebrum. The cerebrum is one of three major parts of the brain. The two other major parts are the brain stem and the cerebellum (see Figure 3-3).

FIGURE 3-3 The human brain.

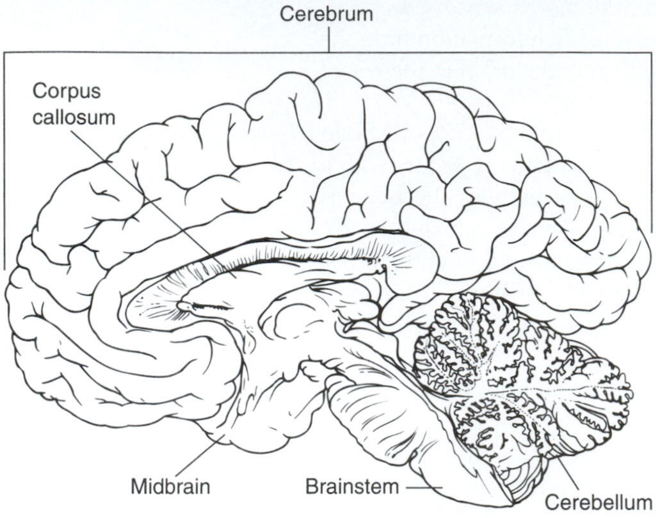

Brain Stem. The **brain stem** sits directly on top of the spinal cord and serves as a conduit between the rest of the brain and the spinal cord. The brain stem consists primarily of nerve tracts that carry sensory information to the brain and motor information away from the brain. It is a major relay station for nerves supplying the head and face and for controlling the visual and auditory reflexes. The brain stem structures and functions are also associated with metabolism and arousal. Three major reflex centers are located in the brain stem: the cardiac center, which controls the heart; the vasometer center, which controls the blood vessels; and the respiratory center, which controls breathing.

Cerebellum. The **cerebellum** is an oval-shaped "little brain" that sits posterior to the brain stem. The cerebellum is primarily responsible for regulating motor and muscular activity and has little to do with the part of the brain that involves conscious planning and responses. The motor-monitoring functions of the cerebellum include coordination of motor movements, maintenance of muscle tone, monitoring of movement range and strength, and maintenance of posture and equilibrium (Bhatnagar & Andy, 1995).

Discussion Point: *Consider the case of Timmy in Box 3-1. To what extent do you think it likely that his brain damage is linked to the personality qualities his friends describe?*

Cerebrum. The **cerebrum**, or cerebral cortex, is the part of the brain that governs the unique human qualities of thinking, problem solving, planning, creating, and rationalizing. Of the three major divisions of the brain—brain stem, cerebellum, and cerebrum—the cerebrum is the largest. The cerebrum consists of two mirror-image hemispheres, the right hemisphere and the left hemisphere. The two hemispheres are separated by a long cerebral crevice, or fissure, called the longitudinal fissure. The **corpus callosum** is a band of fibers that connects the two hemispheres, serving as a conduit for communication between the hemispheres.

The cerebrum is organized into six lobes of four different types: one frontal lobe, two temporal lobes, two parietal lobes, and one occipital lobe. Figure 3-4 shows the lobe locations.

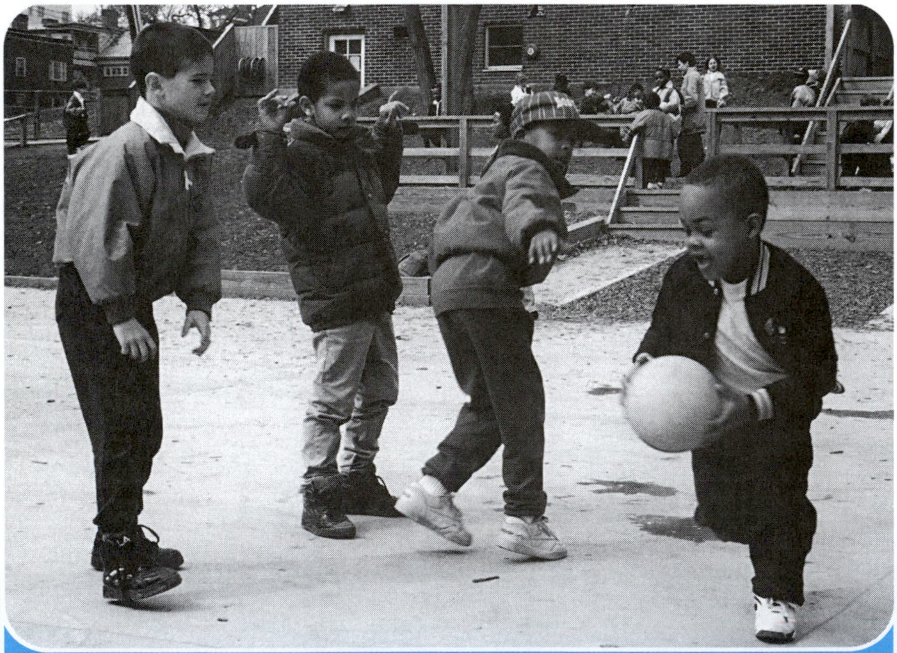

The cerebellum is responsible for motor and muscular activity.

FIGURE 3-4 Lobes of the brain.

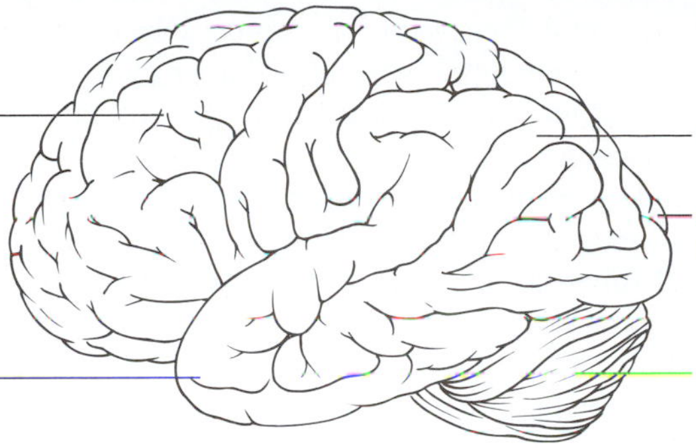

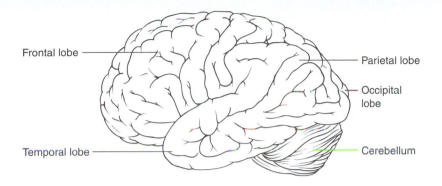

The **frontal lobe** is the largest lobe; it sits in the most anterior part of the brain, behind the forehead. Two key functions of the frontal lobe are (1) activating and controlling both fine and complex motor activities, including the control of speech output, and (2) controlling human executive functions. **Executive functions** include problem solving, planning, creating, reasoning, decision making, social awareness, and rationalizing. These unique and important human qualities represent executive functions because they describe the organized, goal-directed, and controlled execution of critical human behaviors. The executive functions are what allow humans to "override or augment reflexive and habitual reactions in order to orchestrate behavior in accord with our intentions" (Miller, 2000, p. 59). Executive functions are what allow you to keep your arm from reaching for a second piece of chocolate cake (if you really want to!).

Within the frontal lobe sits the prefrontal cortex, which is the part of the brain that has evolved most recently and that is most developed in humans relative to other species (Miller, 2000). The prefrontal cortex is connected with all other sensory and motor systems of the brain, allowing it to synthesize the vast stores of information needed for complex, goal-directed human behavior (Miller, 2000). As noted by Miller, people with damage to the prefrontal cortex may superficially appear quite normal (e.g., they can carry on a conversation, they can perform well on perceptual and memory tests)

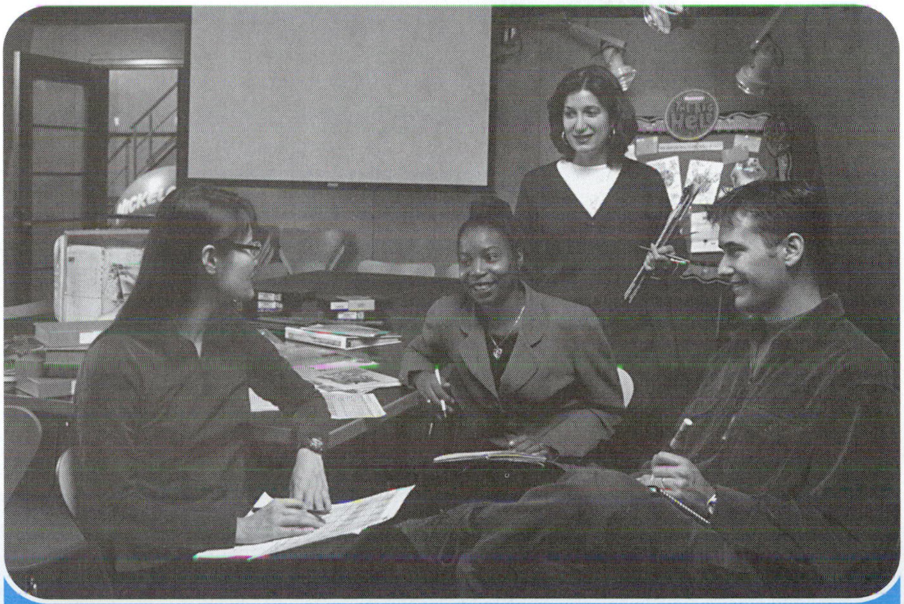

The frontal lobe controls human executive functions, such as planning, reasoning, and decision making.

Discussion Point: *Consider the case of Timmy in Box 3-1. If he did haves serious frontal lobe damage, what might be some characteristics of this damage?*

but can have profound difficulties with organization, self-control, and goal-oriented tasks. Accordingly, the prefrontal cortex represents the seat of the executive functions.

The frontal lobe is also the home to **Broca's area**, an important region of the brain for communication. Situated in the left part of the frontal lobe, Broca's area is responsible for the fine coordination of speech output. It is named after the French physician Paul Broca, who was among the first to recognize the functional specializations of the brain in the mid-1800s. Broca's discovery stemmed from his curiosity about a patient who lost the ability to speak following brain damage. When he performed an autopsy on the patient, Broca found damage to the area subsequently named after him.

The two **parietal lobes** sit posterior to the frontal lobe on the left and right sides, above the ears. Key functions of the parietal lobes include (1) perceiving and integrating sensory and perceptual information and (2) comprehending oral and written language and calculation for mathematics.

The two **temporal lobes** also sit posterior to the frontal lobe, but inferior to the parietal lobes (behind the ears). The left temporal lobe is an important site for human communication. The left temporal lobe contains the auditory cortex, also known as **Heschl's gyrus**, which interprets auditory information received from both ears. (Richard Heschl was an Austrian pathologist who in the mid-nineteenth century identified critical functions of the auditory area of the temporal lobe.) The left temporal lobe also contains **Wernicke's area**, which is a critical site for language comprehension. (Carl Wernicke was a German psychiatrist who studied language disorders in adult populations in the mid-1800s.) Heschl's gyrus first processes spoken language, and then Wernicke's area takes over for further linguistic processing. Damage to either Heschl's gyrus or Wernicke's area can result in significant problems in understanding language.

The single **occipital lobe** sits at the rear of the cerebral cortex, in front of and above the cerebellum. The occipital lobe receives and processes visual information.

Organizational Principles of the Human Brain. To help you understand how the human brain works and make sense of its critical role in communication function and dysfunction, this section presents five key principles governing the brain's organization. These principles are derived from Bhatnagar and Andy's text on neuroscience (1995), and appear in Figure 3-5.

1. *Interconnectedness.* The brain functions and structures are highly interconnected. The two hemispheres and their combined six lobes constantly interact via a rich weaving

FIGURE 3-5 **Organizational principles of the human brain.**

Interconnectedness	All brain functions and structures are highly interconnected, interacting via a rich, complex web of brain fibers.
Hierarchy	The central nervous system is arranged hierarchically, with lower-level functions managed by the spinal cord and higher-level functions managed by the brain.
Specialization	Each area of the brain is highly specialized to perform specific functions.
Plasticity	The human brain has the capacity to organize and re-organize itself as a result of experience.
Critical Period	Certain periods of development correspond to rapid structural and functional growth in the brain.

Source: Adapted from Bhatnagar & Andy (1995).

of brain fibers. Thus, while one area of the brain might be recognized as critical for a particular brain function (e.g., Wernicke's area for language comprehension), the reality is that brain activity reflects the ongoing and intricate integration of information from across the brain's regions.

2. *Hierarchy.* The central nervous system is organized hierarchically. Although all human behavior passes through the central nervous system—and indeed no two body parts are able to communicate without involvement of the CNS—lower-level functions can be directed by the spinal cord, whereas higher-level functions require mediation by the brain's cerebral cortex. The more sophisticated or complex the behavior, the greater the involvement of the brain.

3. *Specialization.* The brain is organized into two hemispheres that communicate via the corpus callosum. Although the two brain hemispheres are mirror images in appearance, they are quite different functionally. In fact, each area of the brain is highly specialized for particular functions. The nerve cells within specific brain areas are specialized to process particular types of information—for example, about touch, temperature, incoming auditory information, or outgoing motor movement. All areas of the brain are connected by highly specialized motor and sensory pathways, which are designed to carry very specific types of information.

4. *Plasticity.* **Plasticity** refers to change, and in neuroscience this term describes the remarkable ability of the brain "to reorganize and modify functions and adapt to internal and external changes" (Bhatnagar & Andy, 1995, p. 5). From birth, the human brain has the important capacity to organize and reorganize itself as a result of experience. Because of plasticity, children who lose their sight early in life become able to process auditory information better than children with sight as the brain reorganizes itself to compensate for the visual deprivation caused by blindness (Bavelier & Neville, 2002). However, plasticity describes not only changes in the brain following accidents or injuries, but all changes that occur in the brain. Developmental plasticity describes neural organization that is stimulated by sensory experiences in the environment, as when young children hear the language of their parents. Learning plasticity describes the way the brain changes as a result of instruction and learning. Learning plasticity explains why the auditory cortex of musicians is better tuned than that of nonmusicians to complex harmonic sounds (Münte, Altenmüller, & Jäncke, 2002). Injury-induced plasticity describes the way the brain reorganizes and even regenerates itself following injury (Kandel, Schwartz, & Jessell, 2001). Similar processes underlie all three types of plasticity. Furthermore, the human brain demonstrates plasticity across its lifespan, which has important implications for the promise of therapeutic interventions for restoring communicative abilities following injury.

5. *Critical period.* A critical period is a period of time during which growth in a particular function or structure in the developing brain is most rapid. During a critical period, specific neurons grow rapidly and forge important neural pathways. In the earliest critical period of brain development, 3 to 4 weeks after conception, neurons migrate from their place of origin through a process called neural migration to form the inner structures and functions of the brain. Neurons glide along pathways to their final destiny, at which point they forge connections associated with their ultimate function (Brain Briefings, 1995). During this early critical period of brain development, various prenatal influences, such as drug abuse by a mother, can impact neural migration and misplace neurons, resulting in significant developmental disabilities, such as epilepsy.

The critical period for the development of language, extending from the prenatal period approximately through puberty, is well established (Moskovsky, 2001) and involves three phases:

1. *Sensory learning:* developing an internal representation (or template) of one's native language through exposure

2. *Sensorimotor output:* producing language and gradually matching one's own performance to a stored template of mature language through internal and external feedback
3. *Stabilization:* stabilizing of mature language patterns due to loss of plasticity and maintenance through use (Brainard & Doupe, 2000)

Discussion Point: *The critical period is an important concept in language acquisition. What have you heard about it? How does the critical period concept apply to the cases of Patricia and Hortencia described in Box 3-1?*

The critical period for development of speech and language in humans corresponds to that in many other species as well. For instance, songbirds must be exposed to the songs of their own species, even if it is via audiotape, during a critical period early in life in order to be able to produce those songs themselves later (Brainard & Doupe, 2000).

Speech and Language in the Human Brain. The brain contains the essential architecture of human communication. Key centers of the brain involved in communication include Broca's area, Heschl's gyrus, and Wernicke's area, as shown in Figure 3-6.

These three sites sit near to one another in the left hemisphere of the brain, allowing for close communication among the centers. Broca's area is the primary center for fluent expression of speech and language. It is located in the posterior portion of the left frontal lobe. Heschl's gyrus is the primary center for auditory perception and sensation. Located in the superior portion of the left temporal lobe, Heschl's gyrus is responsible for the interpretation of all types of sounds, not just speech and language. It is connected via a band of fibers to Wernicke's area, the primary center for language comprehension, which is located just posterior to Heschl's gyrus in the left temporal lobe. In Wernicke's area, meaning is attributed to the linguistic stimuli sent forth from Heschl's gyrus. Thus Wernicke's area is where language comprehension takes place.

These three centers for communicative processes share information with many other parts of the brain during the processes associated with speech, language, and hearing. For instance, in comprehending linguistic information, Wernicke's area corresponds with regions of the frontal lobe involved with higher-order functions, such as problem solving, reasoning, and planning. Likewise, in interpreting auditory information, Heschl's gyrus utilizes memory stores from throughout the brain. Thus, while it is important to understand brain specializations in speech, language, and hearing, it is also necessary to recognize the integrative linkages across the brain that are critical in human communication.

Peripheral Nervous System

The CNS comprises the brain and the spinal cord and represents the central mediator of all human thought and behavior. The peripheral nervous system, or PNS, is the system of nerves connected to the brain stem and the spinal cord. The PNS carries sensory information to the CNS and motor commands away from the CNS, controlling both voluntary and involuntary activity.

FIGURE 3-6 **Language centers of the brain.**

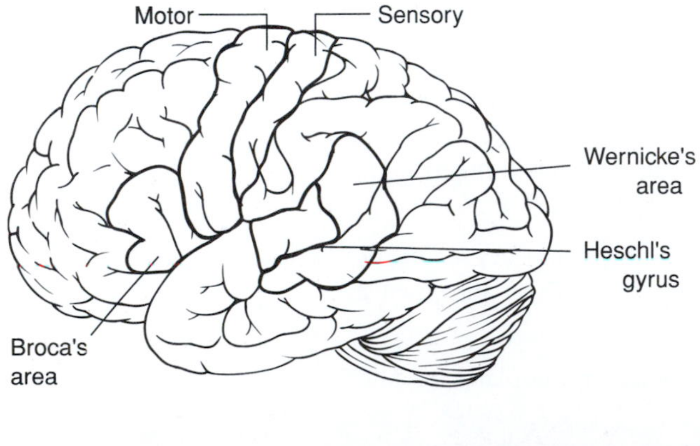

The PNS consists of cranial nerves and spinal nerves. The 12 pairs of cranial nerves run between the brain stem and the facial and neck regions and are particularly important for speech, language, hearing, and swallowing. The cranial nerves carry information concerning four of the five senses to the brain: vision, hearing, smell, and taste. Importantly, the cranial nerves also carry the motor impulses from the brain to the muscles of the face and neck, including those activating the tongue and the jaw, both of which are involved with speech.

The seven cranial nerves most closely involved with communicative functions and the functions they are related to are

- Trigeminal (V): Facial sensation; jaw movements, including chewing
- Facial (VII): Taste sensation; facial movements, including smiling
- Acoustic (VIII): Hearing and balance
- Glossopharyngeal (IX): Tongue sensation; palatal and pharyngeal movement, including gagging
- Vagus (X): Taste sensation; palatal, pharyngeal, and laryngeal movement, including voicing
- Accessory (XI): Palatal, pharyngeal, laryngeal, head, and shoulder movement
- Hypoglossal (XII): Tongue movement

The 31 pairs of spinal nerves run between the spinal cord and all peripheral areas of the human body, including the arms and legs. These spinal nerves mediate reflexes and volitional sensory and motor activity.

Anatomy and Physiology of Speech

The production of spoken language involves the complex interaction of three interrelated systems of human anatomy and physiology: respiration, phonation, and articulation (see Figure 3-7).

Respiration

The evolution of spoken language as the essential act of being human did not require the creation of any new body structures. Rather, the evolution of spoken language efficiently made use of many body structures that had already been developed to serve other purposes. Respiration is an excellent example. Respiration is the system of the human

FIGURE 3-7 **Respiration, phonation, and articulation.**

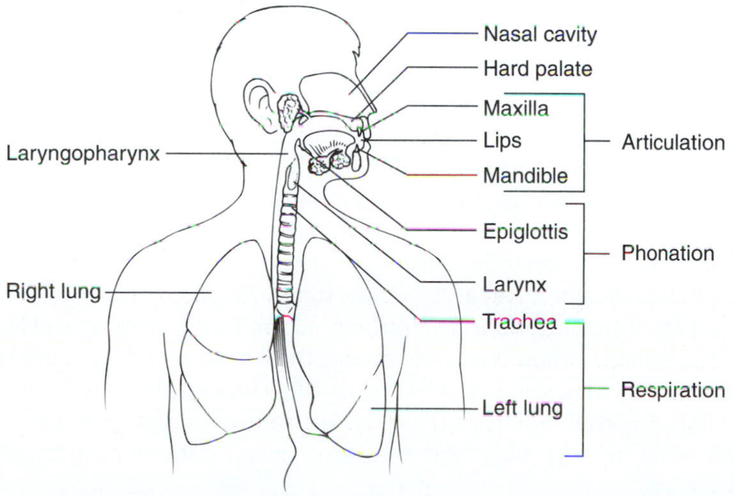

FIGURE 3-8 The respiratory system.

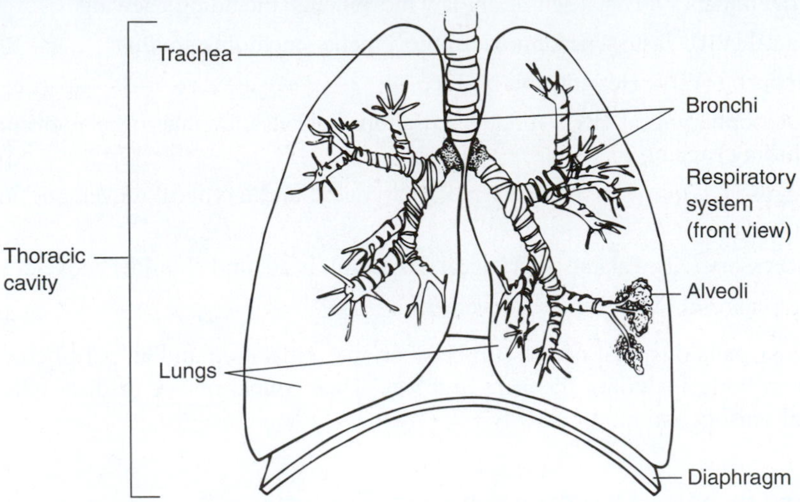

body that controls breathing; its purpose is to draw oxygen from the air into the blood and to exchange it with carbon dioxide. The major respiratory organs are the lungs. The human respiratory system has undergone few modifications in the several million years of our existence, with the exception of its being borrowed to serve as the power supply for speech.

Many key structures are involved in the respiratory process and, therefore, in human speech production. The respiratory system is divided into a lower and upper respiratory system (see Figure 3-8). The lower respiratory system comprises the lungs, bronchi, and alveoli; the upper respiratory system comprises the trachea, larynx, and oral and nasal cavities.

The thorax is the skeleton of the chest, which houses the structures of the lower respiratory system. The thoracic skeleton consists of the rib cage in the front connected to the vertebral column in the rear. The thoracic skeleton creates a thoracic cavity, housing the heart and lungs, which work in concert to exchange oxygen from the air and carbon dioxide from the blood. The diaphragm, a large muscle that contracts and expands with breathing, forms the bottom of the thoracic cavity. The lungs—of which there are two, a right and a left—sit within the **pleura**, a thin sac that attaches to the inner side of the thorax and the outer side of the lungs. Both lungs contain an intricate web of bronchi and alveoli. Air enters the lungs through two main bronchi, one for each lung. The bronchi divide into smaller and smaller tubes, ending in small sacs called alveoli. Oxygen from the air and carbon dioxide from the blood are exchanged in the alveoli.

Respiration is controlled in the brain stem and is typically an involuntary activity. However, respiratory control can be voluntary, as those of us know who have learned to use deep breathing as a relaxation technique.

The respiratory system serves as the power supply for speech production through the inhalation and exhalation of air during breathing. To produce speech, one inhales and then exhales air. The exhaled airflow is sent up through the larynx, over the vocal folds, and into the oral and nasal cavities, where it is manipulated to make different speech sounds (see Figure 3-9). Good speech requires a strong energy source: inhalation must bring an adequate supply of air into the lungs, and exhalation must be strong enough to propel this supply upward and outward.

Respiration for breathing, or passive respiration, differs from respiration for speaking in several key ways (Borden, Harris, & Raphael, 1994). First, more air is inhaled and then exhaled for speech respiration than for passive respiration. To illustrate, speak the sentence, "Hi, my name is Alfred Peterson, and I am a college student." You will note that you inhale and exhale a greater volume of air than you do when simply breathing for the purpose of staying alive. Second, the inhalation-exhalation process involved in speech is subject to greater voluntary control than the process involved in normal breathing. Passive respiration is controlled reflexively—we usually don't think too much about it. In contrast, when we are usurping respiration for speech production, we take greater control of the activity, manipulating inhalation and exhalation to serve the dynamics of speech. For instance, in responding to the query, "Can I have the rest of your chocolate brownie?" the breath supply to produce a vehement "Absolutely not!" is manipulated in a particular way to get the unequivocal message across. Third, speech respiration differs from passive respiration in the ratio of inhalation to exhalation in one respiratory cycle. A respiratory cycle comprises one inhalation and one exhalation. In respiration for breathing, a cycle is about 40% inhalation and 60% exhalation. During speech the ratio is about 10% inhalation to 90% exhalation—exhalation dominates the cycle because it is the part that is used for producing speech.

FIGURE 3-9 Exhalation for speech.

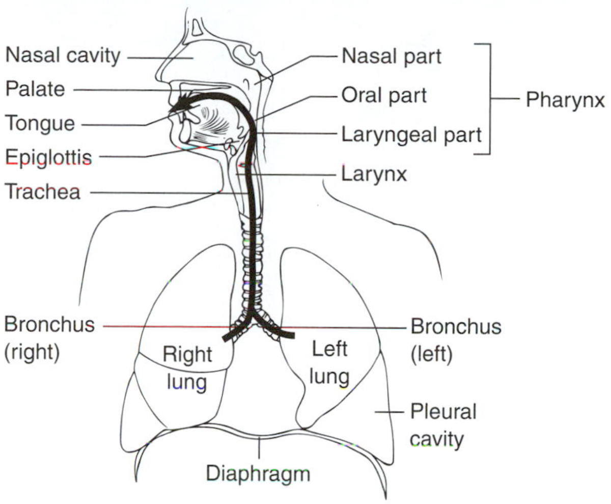

Discussion Point: *How long is a typical breath cycle in passive respiration? Work with a partner and a stopwatch to find out. Then, contrast your finding with a breath cycle in speech: Tell what you did last night using just one breath cycle, and calculate the length of exhalation.*

Phonation

The energy source provided by the respiratory system must be converted to speech; otherwise, it is just another breath of air. Two additional systems, the phonatory and articulatory systems, carry out this process. The phonatory system takes the energy that is sent upward from the lungs and further modulates the airflow to convert the energy into sound.

Key structures in phonation include the pharynx, the trachea, and the larynx. The **pharynx** is a mucosa-lined muscular tube that runs from the nasal cavity, through the rear of the oral cavity, to the entrance of the larynx and the esophagus. The pharynx can be divided into three sections: the nasopharynx, the oropharynx, and the laryngopharynx, as depicted in Figure 3-9. The **nasopharynx** is a posterior continuation of the nasal cavity. The **oropharynx**, or throat, is the length of the pharynx that connects with the oral cavity. The **laryngopharynx** is the most inferior portion of the pharynx, a small portion of tube that opens in the anterior to the larynx and in the posterior to the esophagus.

The **larynx** is a cartilaginous box that sits at the front of the neck on top of the trachea, or windpipe. The trachea leads from the larynx to the lungs. The primary function of the larynx is to protect the trachea by keeping out everything but air. Within the laryngeal box sit the vocal folds, which close tightly to prevent foreign matter from descending into the trachea. In addition to serving as a protective seal, the vocal folds vibrate to produce the voice; hence the larynx—home to the vocal folds—is also known as the voice box.

The larynx is suspended from the **hyoid bone**, a horseshoe-shaped bone that floats horizontally at the base of the neck. The larynx is made up of cartilages that are connected through muscle and ligament: one cricoid cartilage, one thyroid cartilage, two arytenoid cartilages, and the epiglottis cartilage (see Figure 3-10). The cricoid cartilage is a ring of cartilage that forms the base of the larynx and sits at the top of the trachea. Superior to the

FIGURE 3-10 The larynx.

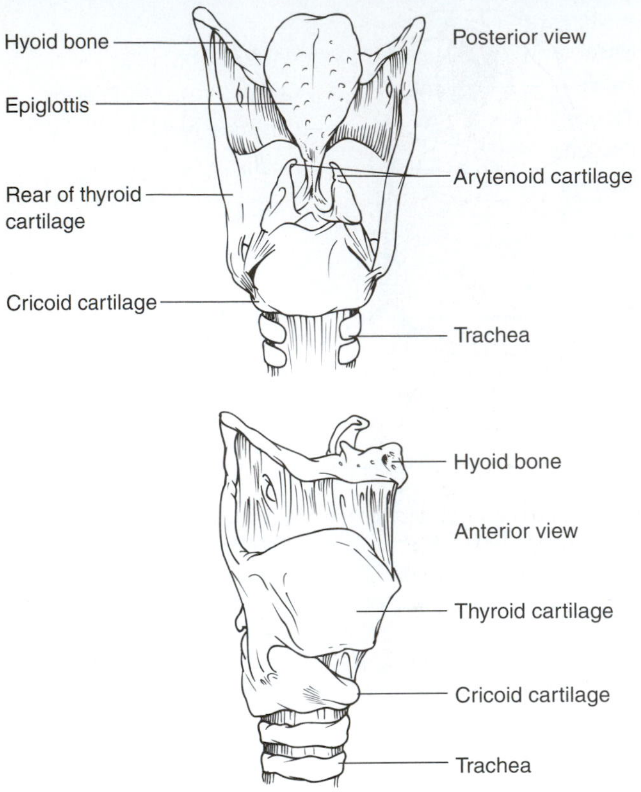

cricoid cartilage is the thyroid cartilage, the largest of the laryngeal cartilages. The thyroid cartilage looks like two shields fused together; you can feel the two shields by pressing your fingers softly against the front of your neck. The ridge where the two shields come together is sometimes called the Adam's apple; the V-shaped opening above it is the thyroid notch. Two tiny arytenoid cartilages, small, pyramid-shaped structures, attach to the top posterior portion of the cricoid cartilage and form anchors for the vocal folds. The epiglottis, a leaf-shaped cartilage, is attached anteriorly to the top of the thyroid cartilage, running up against the hyoid bone and to the back of the tongue. The epiglottis is able to drop over the larynx, helping to protect it from penetration by unwelcome substances.

The vocal folds stretch horizontally from the arytenoid cartilages in the back to the thyroid cartilage in front. The **vocal folds**, or vocal cords, are two thin sheets of tissue connected on their outer edge to the inside of the thyroid cartilage. Figure 3-11 provides a sketch of the vocal folds looking down into the larynx. Lying within the tissue of the vocal folds is a thin layer of muscle called the vocalis muscle, and along the internal edge of each tissue is a vocal ligament. As noted, the vocal folds can close tightly to protect the trachea and lungs from foreign matter. When the vocal folds are brought together, they are said to be approximated. The sequence in Figure 3-12 shows the vocal folds open for breathing (top left and bottom right) and approximated for voicing (top right and bottom left).

At some point in the evolution of humans, the vocal folds began to be utilized for creating voice. **Voice** is the creation of sound by vocal fold vibration. When air is exhaled from the lungs and sent up through the larynx, the vocal folds can be set into rapid vibration to create voice. Humans can speak without voicing, by whispering, but using one's voice has clear advantages, as anyone knows who has experienced laryngitis, in which the ability to produce voicing is lost.

The **trachea** is the cartilaginous tube that runs from the oral cavity down to the lungs, where it separates into the two bronchi. The trachea is about 28 centimeters (cm; 11 in.) long and 5 cm (2 in.) wide. The trachea's principle function is to transport air between the environment and the lungs. The trachea should not be confused with the esophagus, another tube that sits behind the trachea and transports food and water from the oral cavity to the stomach. Air, water, and food all enter via the same cavity—the mouth—and need to be directed to the appropriate channel: the trachea for air to the lungs, or the esophagus for water and food to the stomach.

FIGURE 3-11 The vocal folds.

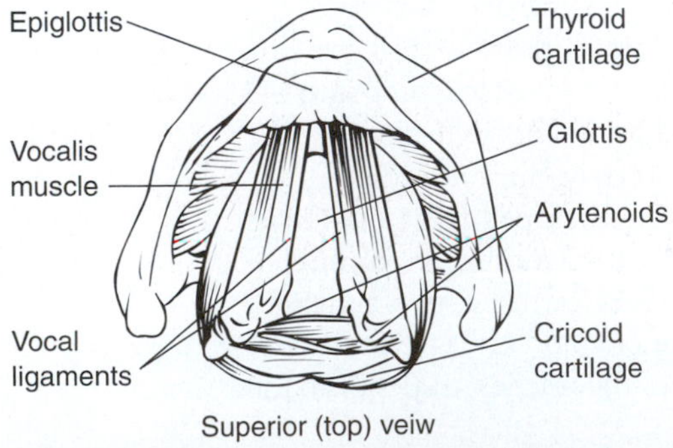

The pharynx, larynx, and trachea constitute the phonatory system, which plays three important roles in speech production. First, these structures together form the essential pathway for the energy supply of speech. They channel the air supply from the lungs into the oral and nasal cavities.

Second, the vocal folds in the larynx turn the airflow into voice through their vibration. The number of times the vocal folds vibrate in a second (the cycles per second) relates to the frequency of a person's voice. Female vocal folds vibrate roughly 240 times per second, translating to a fundamental frequency of 240 hertz (or Hz, cycles per second). The fundamental frequency is the lowest, or base, frequency of a complex sound wave. Male vocal folds vibrate at a slower rate, roughly 130 hertz. These differences relate to the mass of the vocal folds; women's vocal folds are smaller and shorter than those of men, and thus they vibrate at a higher rate.

Third, the pharynx provides a resonating chamber for the airflow. Resonance describes the airflow's ongoing vibration as it moves through the pharyngeal tract. Airflow resonates along the laryngopharynx, oropharynx, and nasopharynx and provides an added fullness to speech. To understand resonance and its influence on vocal quality, think about the last time you had a stuffy nose. When the nose is stuffed up, the nasopharynx is not available as a resonating chamber for the airflow, which impacts the quality of speech.

FIGURE 3-12 Vocal fold movement.

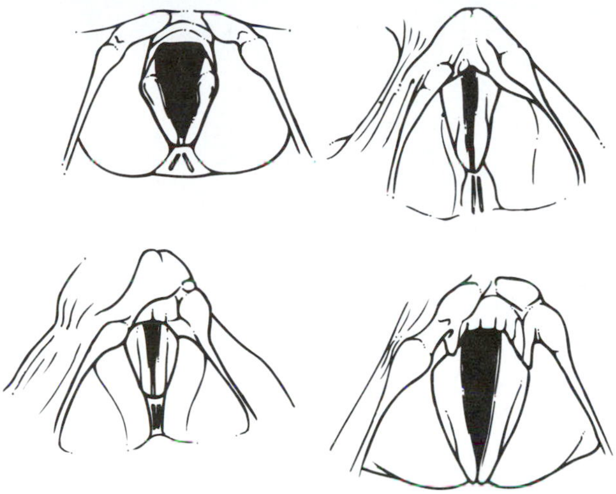

Vocal fold cycle: breathing (*top left*), start of phonation (*top right*), end of phonation (*bottom left*), and breathing (*bottom right*).

Discussion Point: *Sometimes a girl's voice may be indistinguishable from her mother's or sister's voice. What is the explanation for this?*

Articulation

The column of air that is channeled through the phonatory system is further modulated by the articulatory system. The role of the articulators is best illustrated by an activity:

> Produce a continuous "ahhhh."
>
> After 3 seconds, change "ahhh" to "eeee."
>
> After 3 more seconds, change "eeee" to "seee."

How does "ah" become "ee" and "ee" become "see?" Articulation. Articulation is the act of manipulating the airflow submitted by the phonatory system to create highly precise speech sounds. In Standard American English, there are

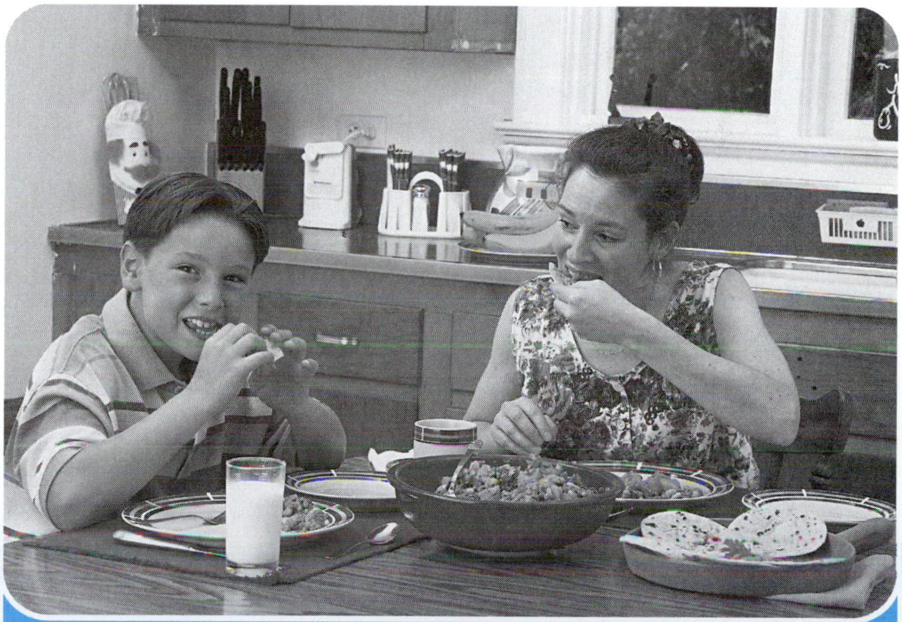

Air, food, and water, once entering through the mouth, need to be directed to the appropriate channel.

FIGURE 3-13 The articulators.

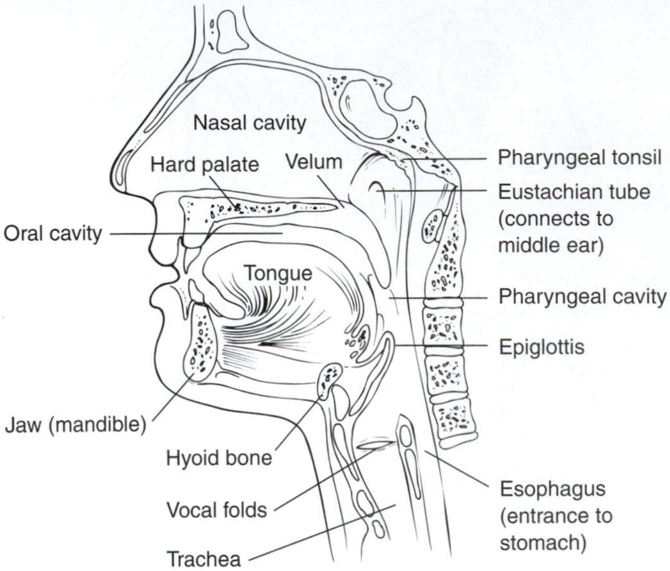

around 40 speech sounds, or phonemes, depending on the particular dialect. The chief manipulators—or articulators—involved with the precise production of these phonemes include the maxilla and mandible, lips, teeth, hard and soft palates, and tongue (see Figure 3-13). These articulatory structures were not evolved for the purpose of speech; rather, they are principle organs for tasting, chewing, and swallowing. However, in developing the capacity for speech, humans have usurped the articulators for key and critical functions.

The maxilla and mandible are the upper and lower jaws, respectively. Although the maxilla does not move during speech production, the mandible is able to open and close and move side to side, actions important for production of specific speech sounds. To illustrate, note the position of the mandible when you produce the sound "ee," as in *meet,* and then when you produce the sound "ah," as in *hot.* The lips are also important for articulation. For some sounds, the lips are brought tightly together (e.g., /b/) and then are popped open, and for other sounds (e.g., /s/) the lips are drawn widely open. The teeth are articulators used for the production of several sounds (e.g., /f/ and /s/), although for other sounds (e.g., /m/) they have little articulatory role. The palate, or roof of the mouth, is another articulatory structure. The palate includes the hard palate and the soft palate. The hard palate spans from the alveolar ridge (the hard bump right behind the upper teeth) back to the end of the bony part of the roof of the mouth. (Draw your tongue back from the alveolar ridge until the roof of your mouth becomes soft. This signals the end of the hard palate.) The soft palate, or velum, is the roof of the mouth that extends from the hard palate back to the uvula—the portion of the soft palate that hangs like a teardrop in the back of the oral cavity. The hard and soft palates play important roles for a number of speech sounds. For instance, /t/ and /d/ are made by striking the tip of the tongue against the alveolar ridge of the hard palate; /k/ and /g/ are made by lifting the root of the tongue up against the soft palate. Additionally, for several sounds (e.g., /m/ and /n/), the soft palate is raised to block off the oral cavity and channel air into the nasal cavity. Of all the articulators, the tongue is probably the most important, as it is manipulated in some principle way for all sounds. The tongue consists of the tip, blade, and root. The tip is the endmost portion (apex) of the tongue; the blade is the front body of the tongue that sits under the palates; and the root, or dorsum, is the part of the tongue that sits deep within the mandible.

Although each speech sound has a shared source of energy, each also has its own distinct articulatory gesture, or pattern, which describes how the airflow is manipulated within the oral and nasal cavity to produce the sound. For instance, the gesture for the speech sound /b/ involves a complete closure of the lips followed by an opening of the lips in which the sound is forced out. The gesture for /b/ is the same gesture as that for /p/; /b/ and /p/ are distinct speech sounds because they differ in their voicing. In the production of /b/, the vocal folds vibrate, whereas in the production of /p/, the vocal folds do not vibrate. Each sound, or phoneme, that we use in speech has its own unique articulatory pattern. Take a moment to think about how the following pairs of sounds are different: "ee," as in *beet,* versus "ai," as in *bait;* "t," as in *tan,* and "f," as in fan; and "sh," as in *ship* and "ch," as in *chip.* Think about whether the energy source for each sound is unvoiced or voiced; also think about how the articulators are positioned for the production of each sound. (Chapter 5 presents an in-depth description of the articulatory pattern that characterizes each English speech sound.)

Anatomy and Physiology of Hearing

The human ear plays an essential role in communication involving spoken language. While the sense of hearing, or audition, provides humans access to diverse auditory stimuli from the environment—from the rustle of leaves to the cry of a baby to the thunderous boom of jet engines—it also provides the means for spoken language to enter the sensory system and then to be delivered to the brain. Spoken language is essentially a series of rapidly changing, complex sound waves. These sounds waves—acoustic energy—are received by the outer portion of the human hearing apparatus and subsequently transformed into mechanical energy, then hydraulic energy, and finally neural energy. The neural energy is interpreted by specific brain centers to identify the linguistic meaning of spoken language.

To accommodate all these energy transformations, the human ear is a complex organ. The portion of the ear that we can see sticking out from both sides of our head belies the complexities of the ear inside. The human ear consists of three distinct sections: the outer ear, the middle ear, and the inner ear. The auditory nerve runs from the inner ear to the auditory centers of the brain, where auditory stimuli are interpreted. Figure 3-14 depicts major structures along the pathway of audition: outer ear, middle ear, inner ear, auditory nerve, and auditory brain center.

FIGURE 3-14 The auditory pathway.

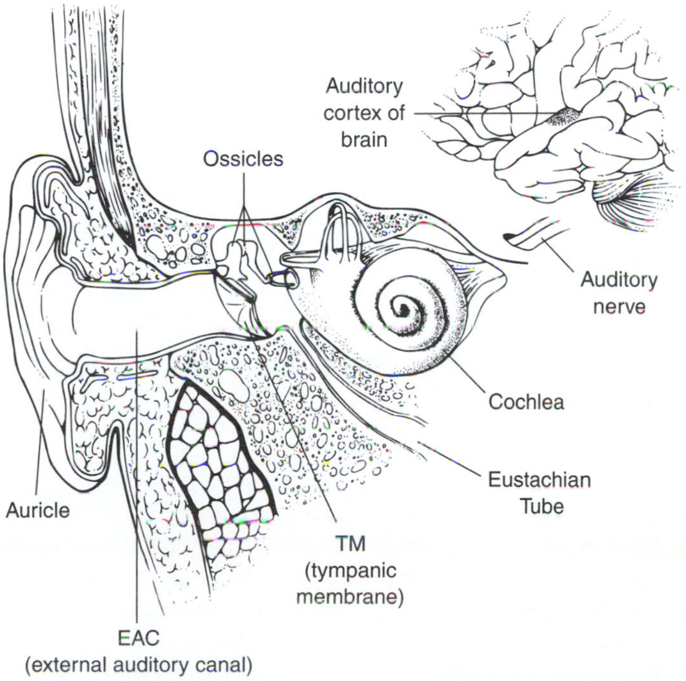

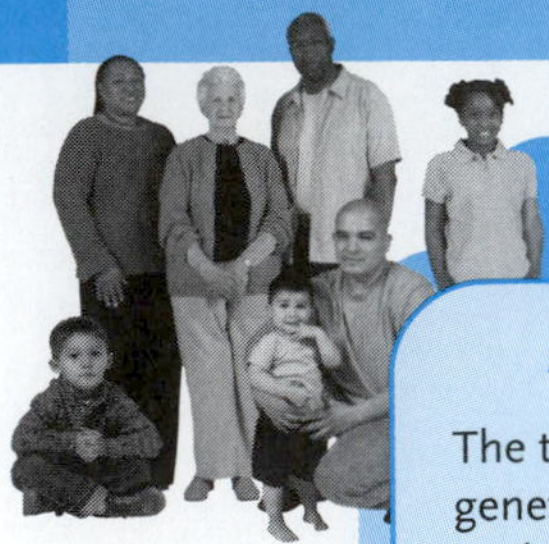

BOX 3-2 Multicultural Issues

Anatomy, Physiology, and Race

The term *race* is often used in discussions of multicultural issues. It refers to an individual's genetic heritage, which is identified by tracing one's ancestry to a specific location of origin, such as China, Scotland, or India. In the United States, the term *African American* refers to people whose ancestry originated in Africa, and the term *European American* refers to people whose ancestry originated in Europe. Race is technically an objective term used to identify human diversity, but because of the historical subjugation of people in the United States and elsewhere specifically because of race, conversations that focus on race require the sensitivity and openness of all involved.

In the study of human communication sciences and disorders, race is a variable that requires consideration. Because of differences in genetic history, human races may vary in important anatomical and physiological ways that provide important insights into communicative processes. Consider, for instance, the genetic history of a race with origins in a region where a particular disease was prevalent. The current members of this race most likely have a genetic disposition that is geared toward protecting against that disease, whereas members of other races probably do not have this genetic protection. This genetic difference explains why some races show higher or lower prevalence rates for particular diseases.

Anatomy also comes into play in understanding differences across races in the prevalence of certain pathologies and in how these pathologies are manifested. For instance, the width and height of the palate in the oral cavity differs across races. Studies of the palates of African Americans and European Americans in the United States show differences in the width and height of palatal structures (Burris & Harris, 1998). Interestingly, research in forensic science has proved useful in understanding the anatomical and physiological differences of these two races—the two largest racial groups in the United States. Research on the height and width of the palate, for instance, is informative for medical professionals who must sometimes identify the race of an individual with serious bodily damage, such as might be sustained in a car accident. In addition, such information enables us to consider the influence of anatomical and physiological differences across races on communication processes and pathologies, furthering our knowledge in this area.

For Discussion

Consider other ways in which an individual's racial history might influence anatomical and physiological characteristics associated with communication development and communication disorders.

This box discussed race, which is different from ethnicity. What is ethnicity? How might ethnicity influence communication processes and disorders?

Companion Website

To answer these questions online, go to the Multicultural Focus module in chapter 3 of the Companion Website.

Outer Ear

The **outer ear** is the outermost portion of the human ear. It comprises the auricle, the external auditory canal, and the tympanic membrane. The outer ear serves as the entry point into the human hearing apparatus for sound waves. The funnel shape of the outer ear helps gather sound waves and channel them inward. The outer ear also helps protect the interior of the hearing apparatus from damage.

The visible portion of the outer ear is the **auricle**, sometimes referred to as the pinna. The auricle consists of cartilage covered by skin. Key parts of the auricle include the earlobe, or lobule, which is the fleshy skin hanging from the bottom of the auricle; the tragus, which is the hard, cartilaginous triangle that protrudes over the entrance to the auditory canal; and the helix, which is the outer body of the auricle.

Discussion Point: *Push your tragus in so that it lies over the external auditory canal. Have a conversation with someone nearby. Why does that person sound softer, but you sound louder?*

Opening from the auricle is the **external auditory canal**, or EAC. The role of the EAC is to conduct sound waves inward toward the brain. The EAC is a short tube, about 2.5 cm (1 in.) in length, that is shaped as a loose S. In children, the EAC curves downward, whereas in adults the EAC curves upward. The outermost portion of the EAC, nearest the auricle, passes through cartilage and is lined with skin, hair follicles, and glands that produce cerumen, or earwax. The hair follicles and cerumen serve as protective devices for trapping dust and other matter, preventing them from entering inner portions of the hearing apparatus. The innermost portion of the EAC passes through bone and is thus called the bony portion of the EAC. There are no cerumen-secreting glands or hair follicles in the bony portion.

Middle Ear

The EAC ends at the tympanic membrane, or eardrum. The **tympanic membrane** (TM) is a very thin, concave membrane that stretches across the bony portion of the EAC. The TM, when healthy, is pearly white and translucent. Although tiny—roughly 0.75 cm^2—the TM plays a large role in the hearing process, serving as a "miniature loudspeaker" (Zemlin, 1988, p. 437). When sound waves travel through the EAC, they reach and strike the TM. The TM is highly sensitive to pressure, and its vibrations replicate the auditory information carried in the sound wave.

The TM serves as the boundary between the outer ear and the middle ear. The **middle ear** is an air-filled, bony cavity sometimes called the tympanic cavity. The eustachian tube runs from the middle ear to the pharynx and serves as a pressure-equalizing tube (PET) for the middle ear space. The middle ear cavity is small, about 2 cm^3, and holds the three smallest bones of the human body: the malleus, the incus, and the stapes. These three bones are called ossicles and form a linked chain, the **ossicular chain**.

The first of the three bones in the ossicular chain, the malleus, looks like a mallet, or hammer, with a long handle and head. The handle of the malleus is attached to the inside of the TM, and its head is attached to the second ossicle, the incus. In turn, the incus is attached to the stapes. When the TM is struck by sound waves traversing the EAC, it vibrates, transporting all the auditory information of those waves. The vibrations of the TM set in motion the conversion of the acoustical energy (sound waves) in the outer ear to mechanical energy in the middle ear. The vibrations are carried along the three ossicles as mechanical energy. The ossicular chain is shown in Figure 3-15.

Discussion Point: *The Valsalva maneuver is when you hold your nose shut and push, as you might to relieve pressure in your ears when flying in an airplane. What is happening physiologically when you perform the Valsalva?*

Inner Ear

Our look at the major structures and functions of the auditory pathway has so far included the auricle, the external auditory canal, the tympanic membrane, and the ossicles. In the outer ear, the auditory information is in the form of acoustical energy, or sound waves. In the middle ear, the auditory information is in the form of mechanical energy that travels along the ossicles. Next on the auditory pathway is the inner ear, which houses the cochlea. Here, the auditory information is converted from mechanical energy to hydraulic energy, as shown in Figure 3-16.

The **inner ear** is a fluid-filled cavity that resides deep inside the temporal bone behind the eye socket. It is sometimes called the "bony labyrinth" because it consists of a complex system of canals and cavities (Zemlin, 1988, p. 459). The inner ear contains three major

FIGURE 3-15 The middle ear.

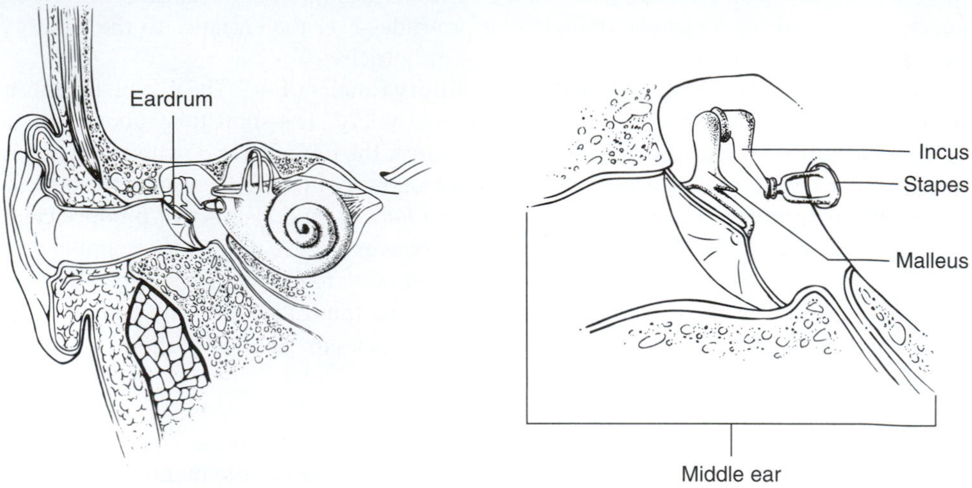

cavities: the vestibule, the semicircular canals, and the cochlea. The vestibule is the central portion, or entryway, of the inner ear that sits between the cochlea and the semicircular canals. The semicircular canals open off one side of the vestibule and consist of three canal systems that serve as the organs of balance. The **cochlea** opens off the other side of the vestibule and consists of a single, fluid-filled canal that serves as the organ of hearing. The cochlea is a relatively long (3.5 cm; about 1.4 in.) bony canal, coiled two and a half times into a snail shape. Along the inner length of the cochlea sits the basilar membrane, an important membrane that contains the **organ of Corti**, essentially a long row of hair cells which together form the hearing organ.

Discussion Point: *Repeated exposure to loud noise can lessen the sensitivity of the organ of hearing. What are some professions in which repeated noise exposure is common? How can workers in these professions protect themselves?*

Auditory information is transported from the middle ear to the organ of Corti in a series of small but important gestures. The stapes, the third ossicle in the middle ear, is shaped like a stirrup. The footplate of the stirrup sits in a window of the inner ear's vestibule, called the oval window. When the ossicular chain vibrates, the footplate of the stapes vibrates in and out of the oval window. On the other side of the oval window is the fluid-filled vestibule. The in-and-out movement of the stapes's footplate sets the fluid of the vestibule in motion. The fluid waves carry the auditory information transmitted by the motion of the stapes, now transformed into hydraulic energy, into the cochlea. The fluid waves moving through the cochlea stimulate the basilar membrane, which in turn stimulates the hair cells of the organ of Corti. These hair cells interpret the auditory information coming from the fluids of the cochlea and turn the information into neural energy that is transported from the cochlea along the auditory nerve to the brain.

FIGURE 3-16 Energy transformations in the auditory pathway.

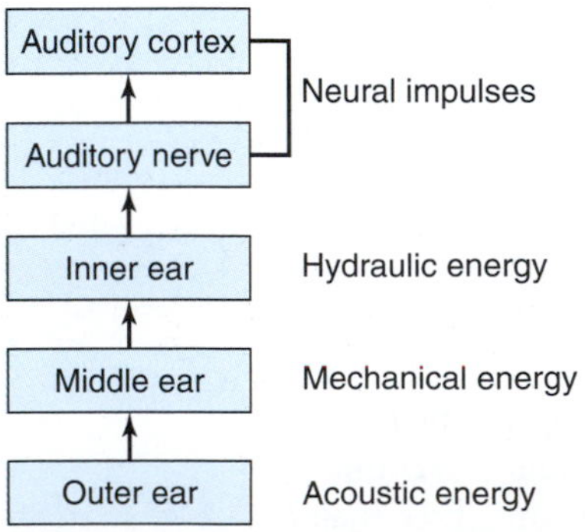

The Auditory Nerve

The auditory information carried in the moving fluids of the cochlea is interpreted by the hairs of the organ of Corti. These hairs are connected to a bundle of nerve fibers that exits the cochlea and travels to the brain. This bundle is the auditory nerve, or the VIIIth cranial nerve. It transports the auditory information, now in the form of neural energy, from the cochlea to the brain stem, the midbrain, and finally to the cerebrum. The temporal lobe of the cerebrum houses the auditory center of the brain.

Auditory Brain Center

Recall from our earlier discussion that the left temporal lobe contains the auditory cortex, also known as Heschl's gyrus. Heschl's gyrus receives information carried along the auditory pathway and analyzes it for frequency, loudness, timing, location, and so forth. A bundle of nerve fibers that runs between Heschl's gyrus and Wernicke's area helps interpret auditory stimuli that carry linguistic information.

Anatomy and Physiology of Swallowing

Within the last few decades, disorders of swallowing have increasingly been considered within the scope of practice of speech-language pathologists. The act of swallowing—**deglutition**—involves many of the same neuroanatomical and anatomical structures involved in speech. When deglutition is inefficient or unsafe, a disorder of swallowing called dysphagia may be present.

It was previously noted that the evolution of speech by the human species did not require the creation of any new body structures. Rather, as speech evolved it made use of many existing body structures, primarily those involved with deglutition. The chief

BOX 3-3 Spotlight on Research

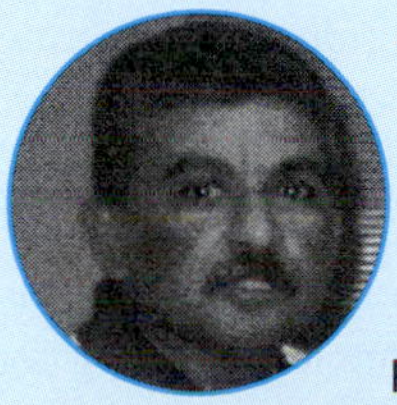

Ananthanarayan (Ravi) Krishnan, Ph.D., CCC-A, FAAA
Associate Professor of Audiology/Hearing Science
Purdue University

Ravi Krishnan has been an associate professor of Audiology and Speech Sciences at Purdue University, where he directs research in the Auditory Electrophysiology Laboratory, since 1998. Dr. Krishnan's area of expertise is in auditory electrophysiology. This research evaluates the nature of neural representation of speechlike sounds in normal-hearing and hearing-impaired individuals to determine the perceptual consequences of degraded neural representation that result from cochlear impairment and adverse listening conditions. To date, our knowledge about neural representation of speech sounds is solely derived from animal experiments that are not readily applicable to humans. Auditory electrophysiology provides a noninvasive window into the physiological mechanisms underlying the processing of speech sounds in normal-hearing individuals and how hearing impairment and adverse listening conditions could alter this mechanism. Knowledge about the characteristics of neural representation of speech in normal-hearing and hearing-impaired individuals may shed light on the acoustic features of speech sounds that are important for their identification.

Dr. Krishnan collaborates with Drs. Glenis Long at the City University of New York and Jeff Lucas and Todd Freeberg in Biological Sciences at Purdue University to focus on electrophysiologal measures of auditory sensitivity in different species of birds. They hope to determine whether there are species differences in hearing and, if there are, the implications for the development of communication calls in various birds.

Dr. Krishnan is also collaborating with Dr. Jack Gandour (Audiology and Speech Sciences) on a research project evaluating the evoked potential correlates of voice pitch in English and Chinese speakers. The goal is to determine whether language-relevant information is contained in FFR for listeners with a native tonal language (Chinese) versus nontonal language listeners (English). The initial results appear to suggest that language-relevant processes may already be operating at the brainstem level. Dr. Krishnan's research work has been supported by grants from the National Institute of Health and the National Organization for Hearing Research.

BOX 3-4 Spotlight on Practice

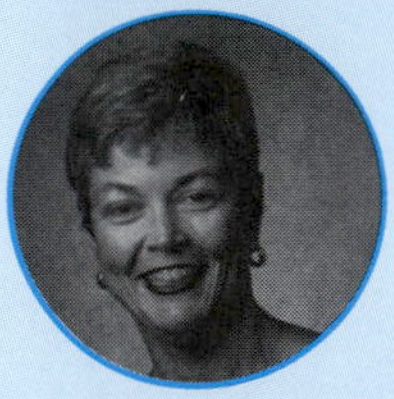

Davida Parsons, M.A., CCC/SLP
Coordinator of Clinical Services
College of Health and Human Services, Ohio University

Many clients have touched my heart over the years, but I will always remember the first day of school the first year I was a public school speech-language pathologist. I was working in one of my four assigned elementary buildings when I received an urgent call from a kindergarten teacher in another building. The caller asked that I come quickly and do what I could for a little girl in her class that no one at school, including the teacher, could understand. As it turns out, no one at home could understand her either. She could correctly produce vowel sounds, but she could not produce any consonant sounds correctly. She cried and stopped talking to others from the frustration of not being understood by the important people around her. At the first parent meeting, her mother also expressed frustration with the situation, stating, "I have to come to this meeting with you (the speech-language pathologist) and sign these papers for my daughter to attend speech therapy because she is the stupid one, unlike her brother, who is the smart one." From that moment I became committed to both mother and child. They needed my skills as a speech-language pathologist. Five years later, following the parent meeting held at the completion of successful speech therapy, the mother grabbed my hand and, with tears in her eyes, thanked me for the gift of communication she now had with her daughter and for being patient with her earlier misunderstandings of her daughter's communication disorder. This is one example of why I am very proud to be a speech-language pathologist. I believe a speech-language pathologist can make a remarkable contribution to the quality of an individual's life and to the people who love them.

I have worked in public schools, medical settings, and out-patient rehabilitation. Currently, I am the Coordinator of Clinical Education for the School of Hearing, Speech and Language Sciences at Ohio University and a member of the Ohio Board of Speech-Language Pathology and Audiology. I am committed to the needs of individuals with communication disorders who may not have a voice to advocate for themselves and the training of the professionals who will serve them. I am extremely fortunate to have the opportunity to do what I love and to serve others in the process.

articulators—including the maxilla and mandible, lips, teeth, hard and soft palates, and tongue—are all essential deglutition structures. When used for deglutition, the function of these structures shifts from speech production to delivering food or drink for sustenance and survival.

The overlap in the anatomical functions and structures involved with speech and deglutition can have some grave repercussions. For instance, we all know we should not talk when we have food in our mouth. This is not simply an issue of manners. Rather, when we have food in our mouth the body is focused on propelling that food from the pharynx to the stomach. When we eat and drink the airway is closed to protect the respiratory system from penetration. When we talk, the body is focused on coordinating respiration and phonation to produce speech, which requires the airway to be open. If we try to talk and eat at the same time, food can enter the wrong tube—the larynx and trachea rather than the esophagus. When food or drink enters the laryngeal area, it is called penetration. If food or drink gets beyond the larynx and into the lungs, it is called aspiration. Coughing is a reflex that occurs with penetration to protect the larynx; a cough is often enough to propel foreign matter up and out of the laryngeal area. However, if the penetrating item is large enough, choking can occur, effectively shutting off the channel through which oxygen arrives to the lungs. Even if the item is not large enough to cause choking, or if drink is involved, penetration can result in small bits of food or drink entering the lungs, which can cause pneumonia and other serious respiratory problems. Thus, while the sharing of functions and structures for speech and deglutition keeps us from having to drag around extra body parts evolved just for talking, it also introduces some dangers of which we all need to be aware.

Discussion Point: *It is considered good manners not to eat and talk at the same time. From a physiological perspective, explain why this is an important lesson to learn as children.*

FIGURE 3-17 Three phases of deglutition.

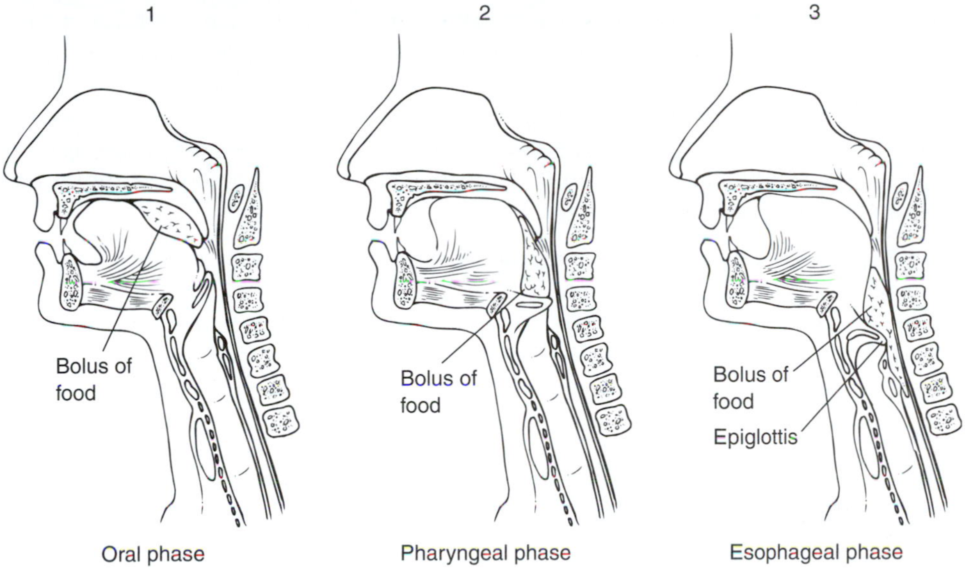

Three Phases of Swallowing

Deglutition is a carefully orchestrated three-phase process whose function is to move a bolus from the lips to the stomach and to keep it from penetrating the larynx and respiratory system. *Bolus* is the term to describe the food or liquid matter that is being transported. Figure 3-17 depicts the three phases of deglutition. The first phase is the oral phase. In this phase, the bolus is prepared for transport and then propelled toward the stomach via a swallow. The oral phase is voluntary; we are able to control it. The second phase is the pharyngeal phase. In the pharyngeal phase, the bolus is propelled into the oropharynx toward the entrance to the esophagus. The pharyngeal phase is involuntary. The third phase is the esophageal phase, which is also an involuntary phase. In this phase, the bolus enters and then is pushed through the long muscular esophageal tube. The esophagus runs from the inferior part of the pharynx to the entrance to the stomach below the lungs and diaphragm. Speech-language pathologists are concerned with disordered swallowing primarily in the oral and pharyngeal phases.

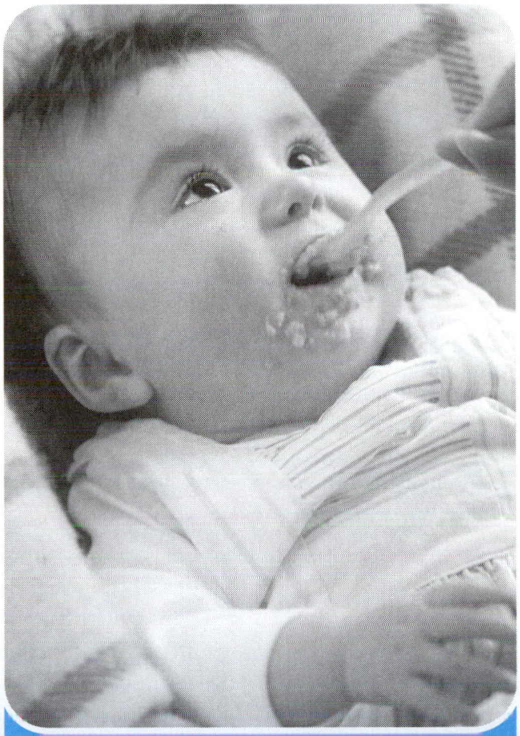

Swallowing involves the oral phase, the pharyngeal phase, and the esophageal phase.

Oral Phase

The foods humans eat come in many textures—mashed potatoes are soft, gumdrops are chewy, beef jerky is tough, pudding is creamy, pretzels are crunchy, and so on. Even liquids can vary, from the thin consistency of lemonade to the thick consistency of a milkshake. In the oral phase of deglutition, the bolus is manipulated and modified into a form that can be readily transported through the pharynx and esophagus to the stomach. Preparation of the bolus often requires mastication—chewing and grinding to break the bolus down. Some boluses require considerable mastication (e.g., popcorn), others require a moderate amount of mastication (e.g., rice), and others require little or no mastication (e.g., yogurt). The oral phase involves two stages: the oral preparatory stage and the oral transport stage. In all, the oral phase of swallowing takes about 1 second, although age, disease, and various disorders can slow the swallowing process (Blonsky, Logemann, & Boshes, 1975).

Oral Preparatory Stage. The oral preparatory stage consists of two activities: (1) bolus preparation, and (2) bolus placement (Perlman & Christensen, 1997). Bolus preparation is needed for any food item that requires reduction to a more transportable and digestible form (e.g., popcorn, walnuts, rice). When the bolus enters the oral cavity, the tongue moves the bolus to the middle of the cavity so that it sits on the blade of the tongue between the molars. Here the bolus is broken down through a chewing and grinding process using the molars. Saliva secreted by the salivary glands moistens the bolus to help reduce it. Saliva also has antifungal, antibacterial, and antiviral properties that protect the oral cavity from invading pathogens (National Institute of Dental and Craniofacial Research, 2003). After the bolus is appropriately masticated, it is again placed on the blade of the tongue between the molars, where it waits for transport via a swallow.

Key structures involved in the oral preparatory stage include the lips, the mandible and the maxilla, the teeth, the tongue, and the palate. When a bolus enters the oral cavity, the lips and jaws (mandible and maxilla) open and then close quickly. The lips are held tightly together, helping to create a pressure vacuum for easy movement and control of the bolus. The teeth and tongue are important for positioning the bolus so that it can be masticated. At the same time, the palate—particularly the back portion of the palate, the soft palate—descends to make contact with the rear third of the tongue, or the tongue base. This action seals off the oral cavity from the nasal passage so that the person can breathe while masticating. The seal also keeps the bolus from exiting the oral cavity during its preparation.

Oral Transport Stage. The oral transport stage begins once the bolus is fully prepared for propulsion. Note that for a swallow to be safely executed, breathing must stop. A swallow can be thought of as a "single pressure-driven event" (Perlman & Christensen, 1997, p. 18). To understand the process, try initiating a swallow using saliva as the bolus (or, if you have something nearby to drink or eat, take a sip or bite). Notice that in producing a swallow, the oral cavity is tightly sealed to create a pressure vacuum, and your tongue arches up to propel the bolus out of the oral cavity into the pharynx. There are four essential acts in the initiation of a swallow: (1) the soft palate elevates, effectively closing off the nasal cavity, (2) the lips contract, creating a tight oral seal, (3) the tongue blade drops, with the bolus descending slightly back into the oral cavity, and (4) the tongue tip rises to press against the hard palate (Perlman & Christensen, 1997). With all systems go, the muscular tongue arches to propel the bolus onward into the pharynx. In addition, during the execution of a swallow, the vocal folds close tightly within the larynx to protect the lungs from penetration by the bolus.

In both stages of the oral phase the chief structure involved is the tongue. Normal tongue movement and sensation are needed to move a bolus to the appropriate place for preparation and then to transport the bolus from the oral cavity to the pharynx. The front two-thirds of the tongue help in preparation and then propulsion; the back one-third of the tongue makes contact with the velum (soft palate) to seal off the nasal cavity at the time of transport.

Pharyngeal Phase

The pharyngeal phase begins when the bolus reaches the tonsils. The tonsils are a ring of tissue around the entrance to the pharynx from the oral cavity. At about this time, the epiglottis drops to protect and seal the larynx from the bolus. From the tonsil ring in the rear of the oral cavity the bolus descends into the pharynx. The pharynx has been called "the gateway to the gut" (Sicher & DuBrul, 1975), although it is also the gateway to the lungs. The pharynx is lined with a series of constrictor muscles. The bottom-most constrictor muscles blend into the muscles of the esophagus (Zemlin, 1988). The muscles lining the pharynx constrict during the pharyngeal phase to propel the bolus to the entrance of the esophagus. The entire pharyngeal phase lasts approximately 0.8 seconds (McConnel, Cerenko, Jackson, & Guffin, 1988).

Esophageal Phase

The esophagus is a long tube of muscle that runs from the bottom of the pharynx to the entrance of the stomach. The esophagus is about 25 cm (10 in.) long (Curtis & Barnes, 1989) and features two sphincter muscles, one at its upper end (the upper esophageal sphincter) and one at its lower end (the lower esophageal sphincter). The sphincters aid in propelling the bolus through the esophagus via a series of involuntary, wavelike contractions called peristalsis. Eventually, the bolus reaches the stomach and the intestines for digestion.

CHAPTER SUMMARY

The human body consists of two major nervous systems: the central nervous system (CNS) and the peripheral nervous system (PNS). The CNS comprises the brain and spinal cord; the PNS comprises the cranial nerves and spinal nerves, which carry information to and from the CNS. The brain is the commander-in-chief of the entire human body; it consists of the cerebrum, the brain stem, and the cerebellum. The lobes of the cerebrum include the frontal lobe, two temporal lobes, two parietal lobes, and the occipital lobe. The frontal lobe controls the executive functions and is home to Broca's area; the parietal lobes control sensory and perceptual processing; the temporal lobes contain the hearing and language centers; and the occipital lobe controls vision.

The production of spoken language involves respiration, phonation, and articulation. Respiration provides the power supply for speech through exhalation of air from the lungs. The power supply is sent from the lungs through the trachea to the larynx, which contains the vocal folds to create voice. The air supply further resonates in the pharynx and is articulated in the oral cavity to produce the variety of speech sounds.

The hearing process involves seven main areas: the outer ear, which serves as the entry point for sound; the external auditory canal, which channels sound inward; the tympanic membrane, which vibrates; the ossicular chain, which carries the sound as mechanical energy; the cochlea, which contains the organ of hearing and receives the sound as hydraulic energy; the auditory nerve, which transports neural energy from the cochlea to the brain; and the auditory center of the brain, which interprets the sound.

Deglutition refers to the three-phase act of swallowing. In the oral phase, the bolus is received and prepared through mastication for further transport. The bolus is then placed on the middle of the tongue and propelled backward toward the pharynx with the initiation of a swallow. In the brief pharyngeal phase, the bolus moves from the oral cavity to the base of the pharynx. In the esophageal phase, the bolus traverses the esophageal tube to arrive at the stomach for digestion.

KEY TERMS

afferent, p. 81
anterior, p. 80
auricle, p. 97
axons, p. 82
brain stem, p. 84
Broca's area, p. 86
cerebellum, p. 84
cerebrum, p. 84
cochlea, p. 98
corpus callosum, p. 84
cranial nerves, p. 82
deglutition, p. 99
dendrites, p. 82
distal, p. 81
efferent, p. 81
executive functions, p. 85
external, p. 80
external auditory canal, p. 97
frontal lobe, p. 85
Heschl's gyrus, p. 86
hyoid bone, p. 91
inferior, p. 80
inner ear, p. 97
internal, p. 80
laryngopharynx, p. 91
larynx, p. 91
meninges, p. 83
middle ear, p. 97
myelin, p. 82
nasopharynx, p. 91
neurons, p. 82
neurotransmitters, p. 82
occipital lobe, p. 86
organ of Corti, p. 98
oropharynx, p. 91
ossicular chain, p. 97
outer ear, p. 96
parietal lobes, p. 86
pharynx, p. 91
plasticity, p. 87
pleura, p. 90
posterior, p. 80
proximal, p. 80
spinal nerves, p. 82
superior, p. 80
synapse, p. 82
temporal lobes, p. 86
trachea, p. 92
tympanic membrane, p. 97
vocal folds, p. 92
voice, p. 92
Wernicke's area, p. 86

ON THE WEB

Check out the Companion Website! On it, you will find:

- suggested readings
- reflection questions
- a self-study quiz
- links to additional online resources, including information about current technologies in communication sciences and disorders

Communication Assessment and Intervention

Principles and Practices

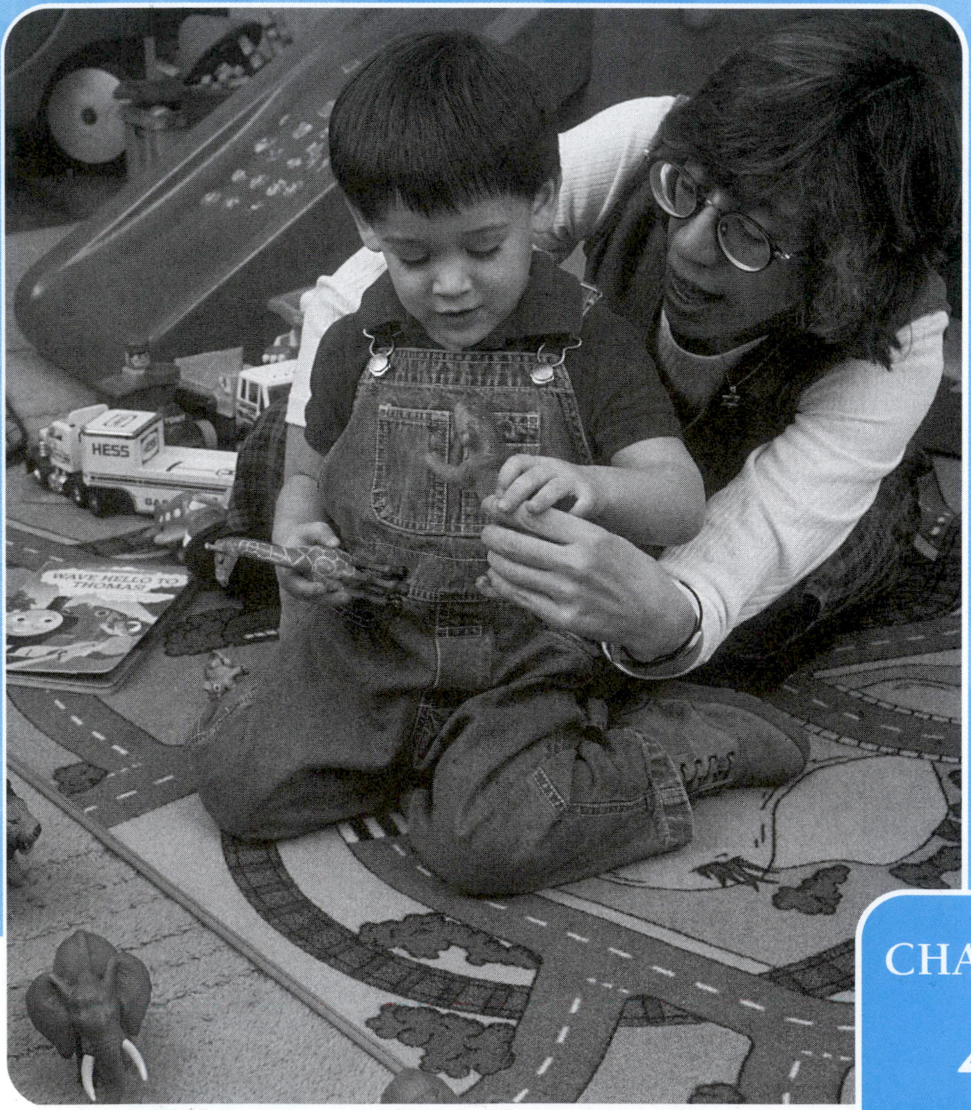

CHAPTER 4

FOCUS QUESTIONS

This chapter answers the following questions:

1. What is assessment?
2. How are assessment instruments categorized?
3. What is intervention?
4. How are interventions categorized?

INTRODUCTION

People are drawn to the discipline of communication sciences and disorders for diverse reasons. Students often come to an introductory course in communication disorders with some general impressions of the field derived from interaction with family members who have worked as speech-language pathologists, audiologists, or special educators. Some students have had direct experience of the field when a family member or friend required evaluation or treatment for a communication disorder. Through direct exposure or indirect impression, many students are already aware of three benefits of a profession in communication sciences and disorders: (1) the opportunity to make a difference in the lives of others, (2) the potential to have a job that offers significant challenges and the promise of day-to-day variability, and (3) the excitement of working in a dynamic field in which new discoveries are constantly informing and enhancing practice. These features make the communication disorders disciplines highly desirable to many traditional university students who are looking toward their professional futures as well as to many nontraditional students who are considering reentry into the workforce or a change in their profession.

Although people in the communication disorders professions fill a variety of roles—from university faculty, to administrators, to consultants—the majority of them are direct service providers, working as therapists or educators. The key responsibilities of a direct service provider are assessment and intervention, or diagnosis and treatment. The daily responsibilities of assessment and intervention are what make it possible for these professionals to make a difference in the lives of others, to have a job that offers great challenges, and to ensure attention to new scientific discoveries that can inform and enhance our practice.

Because there are many varieties of communication disorders, there is great variability in the assessment and intervention techniques and tools used by professionals. This chapter provides an overview of terminology related to assessment and intervention, as well as key principles and practices associated with these two aspects of service delivery. The content of this chapter serves as a foundation for many of the concepts discussed in chapters 5 through 15, which provide more detailed content on assessment and intervention as they relate to the disorders discussed in the chapters.

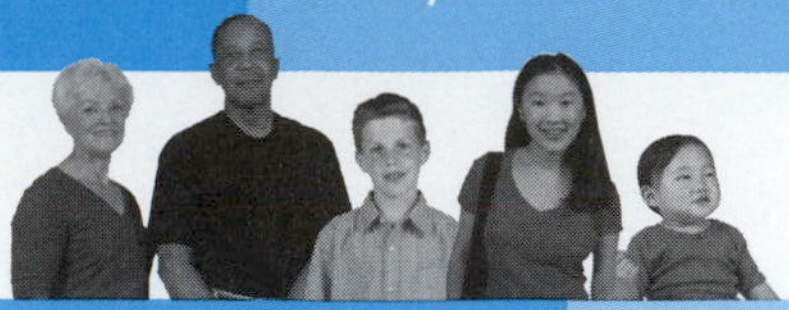

BOX 4-1 Communication Disorders Across the Lifespan: Case Examples

Lila is a 7-year-old who lives in St. Louis, Missouri. She entered first grade at a public elementary school this past fall. A routine developmental screening conducted at that time indicated that Lila might be showing some stuttering behaviors. Lila rarely speaks in class. During a recent round-robin reading activity in which the children took turns reading from their literature book, Lila got stuck on the first sound in a word four times in the first short paragraph she was asked to read. Her teacher, Mr. Kendall, stopped Lila in the middle of her turn because Lila seemed to be about to cry and the other children were giggling. Mr. Kendall referred Lila to the school speech-language pathologist, Ms. Tyler, for a comprehensive evaluation. Ms. Tyler, however, does not want to do an evaluation because her caseload is too large; she currently serves 72 children in the elementary school.

Internet research

1. What is the typical caseload for a speech-language pathologist in an elementary school in St. Louis, Missouri? See what you can find out. Compare this to the caseload sizes recommended by the American Speech-Language-Hearing Association.
2. Mr. Kendall is using the Internet to find some suggestions for helping Lila in the classroom. What kind of materials will he find? How can he differentiate between good information and bad information?

Brainstorm and discussion

1. Ms. Tyler has agreed to interview Lila's mother to gather more information about Lila. What are some questions she will likely ask?
2. If Ms. Tyler decides to conduct an evaluation, what would be the goal of the evaluation?
3. If intervention is warranted, would it be considered prevention, remediation, or compensation?

Mr. Mykel is the director of an adult literacy center located in a Detroit public housing neighborhood. The average income for neighborhood households is $9,000 annually. The families are primarily Spanish speaking, and the majority (72%) of households are headed by single mothers. Mr. Mykel has formed a collaboration with several nurses in the area who are interested in working with mothers in this neighborhood to promote early language development. Mr. Mykel and the nurses have received a local grant for $3,000 for pilot work.

Internet research

1. Use the Internet to find descriptions of programs used with low-income parents to promote their children's language development. What types of programs did you find?

What Is Assessment?

Definition

Assessment is the systematic process of gathering information about an individual's background, history, skills, knowledge, perceptions, and feelings. In the field of communication disorders, assessment focuses on comprehensively understanding processes and abilities in one or more of the following areas: language, speech, cognition, feeding, swallowing, voice, fluency, and hearing. Assessment is often a **multidisciplinary** process involving many professionals who bring their diverse knowledge, skills, and experiences to the assessment. It is also a systematic process that follows certain procedures so that its outcome will be

2. Find out the current poverty threshold for families in the United States. How many families are living in poverty?
3. To what extent are communication disorders more prevalent among lower-income families?

Brainstorm and discussion

1. What are some techniques that might be used for outreach to the neighborhood mothers?
2. What are some strategies that might be used to help these mothers foster early language development in their children?
3. What might some barriers be to the success of this program?

Mr. Stevens is a morbidly obese man with diabetes who is unable to leave his home because of complications associated with these conditions. Mr. Stevens has vocal nodules, a voice disorder often characterized by hoarseness and breathiness. He is no longer able to use the telephone because his voice quality is too poor for him to be understood. Mr. Stevens lives in a rural and remote area of Wyoming and does not have access to speech-language pathologists who might be able to work with him directly in his home. He has been referred to a telehealth model of voice therapy that is delivered using remote video teleconferencing from the Tripler Army Medical Center in Honolulu, Hawaii (Mashima et al., 2003).

Internet research

1. What is teleheath?
2. What kinds of medical conditions are currently treated using telehealth models?
3. For people who live in remote areas, what are options for treating communication disorders other than telehealth?

Brainstorm and discussion

1. In what ways does Mr. Stevens's communication disorder negatively impact his quality of life?
2. To participate in the Tripler Army Medical Center's telehealth program, a comprehensive interview will be conducted to judge the likelihood that Mr. Stevens will complete the voice therapy program. What kind of questions do you think will be included in this interview?

comprehensive, nonbiased, and valid. Assessment is more than testing. A test is the administration of one task to examine a person's skills or knowledge in a particular area. A test might be part of an assessment, but a test alone is not assessment.

Purposes of Assessment

Assessment has four purposes, as shown in Table 4-1. The first purpose is to identify skills that a person has and those that a person does not have in a particular area of communication. This information determines whether an individual's performance is consistent with a disorder. For instance, the assessment for 2-year-old Marcus, brought by his father to a speech-language pathologist (SLP) because he is not yet talking, focuses on identifying the

TABLE 4-1 Four purposes of communication assessment

Purpose	Application
1. To identify skills that a person does and does not have in a particular area of communication	To determine whether a person's performance indicates presence of a disorder
2. To guide the design of intervention for enhancing a person's skills in a particular area of communication	To identify specific short- and long-term goals and specific learning targets and to identify strategies and contexts for addressing these goals
3. To monitor a person's communicative growth and performance over time	To determine progress made in intervention and whether specific outcomes are reached and to monitor progress after discharge
4. To qualify a person for special services	To determine whether a person meets the eligibility requirements to receive coverage of educational and therapeutic services for a particular governing organization or institution

language skills that Marcus does have as well as those that Marcus does not have. The SLP carefully studies Marcus's skills to determine whether a disorder is present. The SLP may conclude that Marcus has a communication disorder and recommend treatment. Conversely, the SLP may conclude that Marcus's language skills are appropriate for his age and background, and thus not recommend therapy.

The second purpose of assessment is to guide the design of intervention for enhancing a person's skills in a particular area of communication. This purpose focuses on people who have an identified communication disorder, although it may also focus on people who do not have a disorder but would nonetheless benefit from some type of assistance, such as a prevention program designed to lower an individual's risk for developing a communication problem. In building a program of intervention for a particular individual, assessment enables the SLP to identify (1) specific short- and long-term goals and (2) strategies and contexts for addressing those goals. For Marcus, the assessment process identifies the language goals that are most appropriate for him at this time and how those goals should be addressed. Specifically, through the assessment the SLP finds that Marcus is not yet using communication to meet his needs at home or at day care and identifies (among others) the following short-term goal:

- Marcus will use gestures and single words to ask for objects and actions in interactions with his father and the day care provider.

Marcus's SLP considers information gained from the assessment process in making decisions about where and when intervention will take place, identifying the people who will be involved in delivering the intervention, and determining the types of techniques likely to be most effective for helping Marcus meet his communication goals.

The third purpose of assessment is to monitor a person's communicative growth and performance over time. Assessment measures progress made in intervention and reveals whether specific outcomes have been reached. Assessment is also used to periodically monitor people following their discharge from intervention or people for whom no intervention is provided but periodic assessment seems warranted. Assessment used for this purpose permits practitioners to be highly flexible in their intervention. Periodic assessments enable practitioners to change goals, modify treatment schedules, change treatment settings, and shift treatment approaches. For instance, after a 3-month period of implementation of techniques to facilitate Marcus's use of single words and gestures for requesting, the SLP used a reassessment to study Marcus's communication skills at home and at day care. This assessment showed that Marcus was frequently using gestures and single words to meet his needs. The SLP used this information to revise Marcus's goals and strategies.

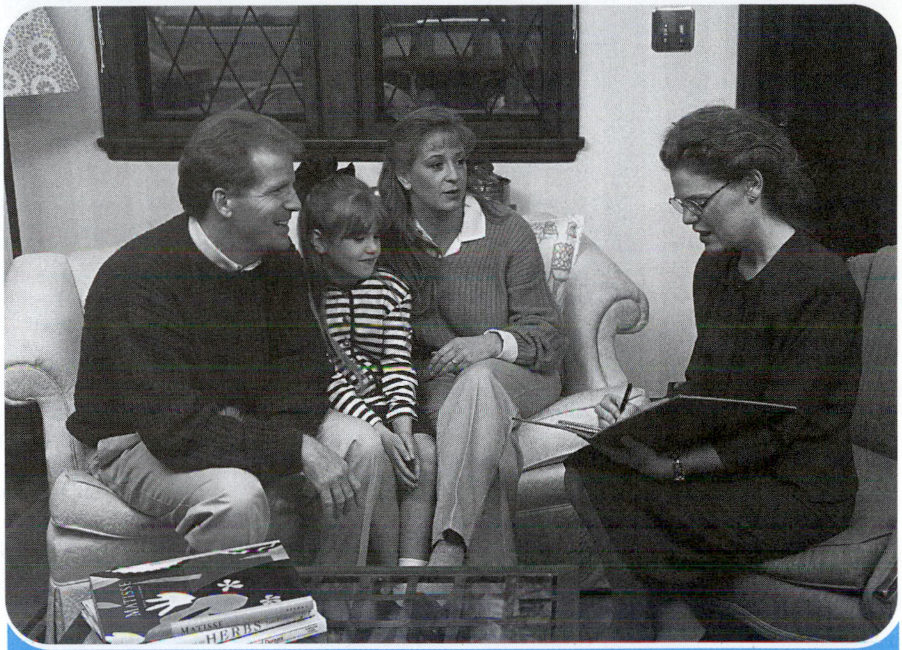

Assessment may take place in a client's home to see how communication occurs in the home environment.

The fourth purpose of assessment is to qualify a person for special services. Treatments for communicative impairments are often expensive, although treatment benefits usually outweigh the costs. Whereas some people pay for communicative therapies out of their own pockets, often these services are paid for by public school divisions, Medicaid and Medicare, and private-pay health insurance. These organizations and institutions often have strict regulations governing what coverage they will provide. For instance, school districts are required by law to pay for a student's communicative therapies only if the communicative impairment has a measurable impact on educational achievement. School districts have considerable discretion both in how they determine whether a communicative impairment has a negative educational impact and in determining the level of impairment that must be exhibited for services to be provided. Nonetheless, the assessment process must document the adverse effects of a communication disorder on educational achievement for a child to qualify for special services. Federal health-care coverage through Medicare and Medicaid as well as private-pay insurance agencies also set their own guidelines concerning eligibility for communication-related services. The purpose of assessment thus often includes determining whether an individual meets the eligibility requirements of a particular governing organization for speech, language, or hearing services.

Discussion Point: *Consider the case of Lila in Box 4-1 and these four purposes of assessment. Which of the four purposes are most relevant to her current needs?*

The Assessment Process

The assessment process is a systematic, comprehensive activity that includes a six-stage scope and sequence (see Figure 4-1): screening and referral, designing the assessment protocol, administering the assessment protocol, interpreting assessment findings, developing an intervention plan, and monitoring progress and outcomes.

FIGURE 4-1 Scope and sequence of communicative assessment.

1. Screening and referral
2. Designing the assessment protocol
3. Administering the assessment protocol
4. Interpreting assessment findings
5. Developing an intervention plan
6. Monitoring progress and outcomes

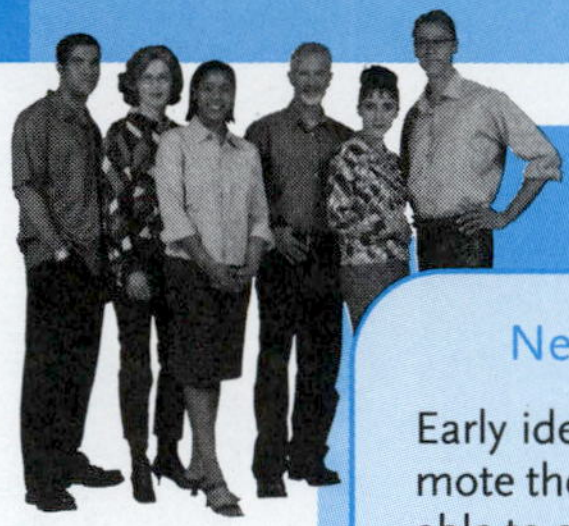

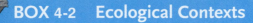

BOX 4-2 Ecological Contexts

Newborn Hearing Screening

Early identification of hearing loss is critical for providing early intervention services that promote the positive outcomes of children. With early identification, children with hearing loss are able to achieve their full potential at home and school. In 35 states, all infants are administered a hearing screening within a few days of birth. Universal newborn hearing screening was legislated in these states because it is seen as the most efficient way to identify significant hearing problems in infants (De Michele & Ruth, 2003). Other states provide screening only to infants who show obvious risk factors according to the high-risk register, a list of ten variables that are most closely linked to hearing loss in infants (Joint Committee on Infant Hearing, 1995), such as bacterial meningitis, use of medications that damage the ear, and parental concern about the child's hearing. The most recent publication of the high-risk register by the Joint Committee on Infant Hearing (2000) argues for the use of physiological measures to screen all newborn infants, rather than screening only those with certain risk factors, as data suggest that as many as 50% of children do not meet the screening criteria of the high-risk register (De Michele & Ruth, 2003). Thus, without universal screening, the average age at which children are identified as having a significant hearing problem is 2 to 4 years, and valuable language-learning years are lost. The costs of screening all infants at birth pale in comparison to the costs associated with allowing hearing problems to go undetected during this valuable language-learning time.

For Further Discussion

1. Which states do not mandate universal newborn hearing screening? Why would some states not adopt this program?
2. What are some risk factors that you would expect to see on the high-risk register?
3. The description of the Joint Committee on Infant Hearing's most recent position is available online at the organization's website: http://www.jcih.org/. How have the organization's positions on the use of newborn hearing screening changed over the last decade?

To answer these questions online, go to the Ecological Contexts module in chapter 4 of the Companion Website.

Screening and Referral

Both screening and referral are used to identify people who may require a more comprehensive communicative assessment.

Screening. **Screening** is the delivery of a test or task that provides a quick check of an individual's performance in a particular area. For instance, an infant's hearing skills may be screened to identify early hearing loss (see Box 4-2). Most readers have probably had an audiological screening at some point to check their hearing. This procedure provides a quick and relatively inexpensive probe of an individual's hearing at key levels, as shown in Figure 4-2. A pass on a screening such as this precludes the need for a lengthier, more expensive, and professionally administered audiological assessment.

Screening differs in several important ways from assessment. First, screening probes an individual's skills broadly, whereas assessment examines an individual's skills in a focused, in-depth manner. Second, screening is conducted in just minutes, whereas assessment may take several hours. Third, screening typically costs just dollars per individual screened, whereas assessment may cost hundreds or even thousands of dollars per individual. Fourth, screening can be conducted by a person with relatively little training, whereas assessment is conducted only by highly qualified individuals.

Screening for communicative skills is typically done at key developmental junctures in a person's life; hence it is referred to as **developmental screening**. For many children,

FIGURE 4-2 Hearing screening protocol.

Name:	Date:
Date of Birth:	Age:
Screening Site:	Examiner:
Patient Background	
___history of hearing loss	___ear infections
___earaches	___ringing in the ears
___head trauma	___medications
___noise exposure	___chronic disease
Comments:	
Screening Results	
dB level (circle one) 25dB 30dB 35dB	
Right	Left
___1000 hz	___1000 hz
___2000 hz	___2000 hz
___4000 hz	___4000 hz
___Pass ___Fail	
Notes:	
Referral:	

developmental screening starts at birth and continues with every visit to the pediatrician through their first 5 years. The newborn hearing screening described in Box 4-2 is an example of developmental screening.

Screening is also routinely used to identify the extent of an illness or injury; this is called **injury-related screening**. For example, a person who has had a stroke is screened for communication because stroke is a leading cause of adult speech and language disorders. Likewise, a child who has a chronic history of middle ear infections is routinely screened for hearing to establish the effects of the illness and the potential need for a more in-depth hearing evaluation.

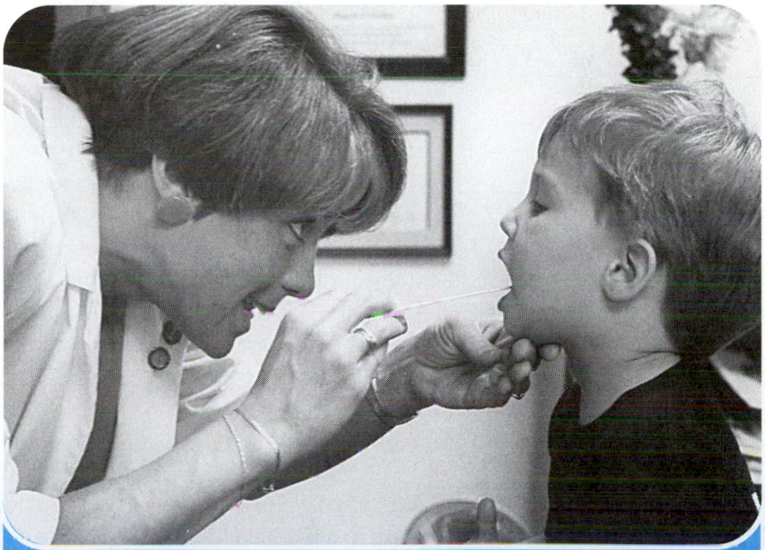

Development screening takes place at critical junctions in life.

Referral. **Referral** often accompanies screening and describes the process by which the involvement of speech, language, and hearing professionals is formally requested. Referrals are typically made by parents or other caregivers, and educational and health-care professionals. For example, young children routinely see their pediatricians at regular

FIGURE 4-3 Signs and symptoms of swallowing problems: indicators for dysphagia referral and assessment.

Drooling
Coughing, choking, or gagging
"Wet" quality of voice after drinking/eating
Food falling out of mouth
Frequent throat clearing
Pocketing of food in cheeks
Changes in eating patterns
Severe weight loss
Frequent respiratory infections
Excessive length of chewing or mealtimes
Drink held in mouth for 5 seconds or longer before swallowing
Nasal regurgitation
Excessive tongue movement

Sources: American Speech-Language-Hearing Association (2000); Best practice: Evidence-based practice information sheets for health professionals (2000); Shipley & McAfee (1998).

Discussion Point: *What factors might influence the likelihood of a physician referring a patient to a speech-language pathologist or audiologist?*

intervals over the first few years of life. At each visit, the pediatrician screens the child's communication skills, either by using a formal screening instrument or by informally questioning the parent and interacting with the child. If the pediatrician has concerns about any aspect of a child's communicative abilities, he or she is likely to refer the child to a speech, language, or hearing professional for a comprehensive assessment. As another example, nurses who provide care for people following stroke carefully observe their patients for signs of swallowing problems, as shown in Figure 4-3. If a patient shows evidence of a swallowing problem, the nurse will confer with the patient's physician to discuss the need for a referral to a speech-language pathologist. Once a referral is made, the speech-language pathologist will determine whether a more comprehensive swallowing assessment is warranted.

Designing the Assessment Protocol

The screening and referral process typically identifies a specific area of concern for a particular individual. For instance, a speech-language pathologist may receive a referral from a physician that requests "diagnosis and treatment for hoarse vocal quality" or "assessment for possible stuttering." Professionals use their clinical skills and knowledge of current research to design a highly individualized assessment for each client that is sensitive, comprehensive, and nonbiased.

A sensitive protocol is one that accurately identifies whether a problem is present and characterizes the severity of the problem. A sensitive protocol is not affected by a false positive (the assessment reveals a problem when there is no problem) or a false negative (the assessment shows no problem when there is a problem).

A comprehensive protocol is one that accurately identifies all the dimensions of the problem. A comprehensive protocol characterizes the influences of the problem on diverse aspects of a person's life and skills, including how the problem affects daily living activities at home, school, and work.

A nonbiased protocol is one that accurately characterizes communicative performance regardless of a person's race, ethnicity, gender, socioeconomic background, culture, or native language.

In designing the assessment protocol to meet these specifications, the professional uses many different techniques and materials to obtain information about areas of concern. Common techniques and materials include chart review, interviews, systematic observation, questionnaires and surveys, testing, and instrumentation.

Chart Review. A **chart review** is the systematic examination of an individual's developmental, educational, and medical history that has been collected by other professionals. Chart review provides the professional with access to other practitioners' opinions and diagnoses, previous test results evaluating broad aspects of health and development, and descriptions of outcomes from other interventions. For professionals working with children who have received special services through state agencies, a chart review includes examining the family's Individualized Family Service Plan (IFSP) and the child's Individualized Education Plan (IEP). An IFSP is a document used to identify services and outcomes for infants and toddlers; an IEP is a document used to identify services and outcomes for children aged 3 and older. IFSPs and IEPs are federally required plans that identify specific goals for children and specific strategies for addressing these goals. The clinician's careful review of chart information, when available, provides an important vehicle for getting to know a client and his or her unique developmental, educational, and medical history.

Discussion Point: *Consider the case of Mr. Stevens in Box 4-1. A chart review will be conducted in consideration of his candidacy for the Telehealth Voice Therapy Program. What kind of information might be useful in determining whether he is an appropriate candidate for this program?*

Interview. An interview is a unique vehicle for collecting information from individuals, their families and caregivers, and other professionals that can aid in understanding the nature, history, and extent of the problem. An interview provides indispensable information about the impact of a disorder on a person's life at home, at school, at work, and in the community. It may also reveal how the characteristics of a disorder have evolved and changed over time. Examples of interview questions used to collect information from people receiving a voice evaluation are presented in Figure 4-4.

Discussion Point: *Consider the case of Lila in Box 4-1. If you were to interview her mother, what questions would you include?*

Systematic Observation. Systematic observation is the process of observing how an individual uses communication for functional purposes in real-life, authentic activities. Systematic observation allows a professional to examine an individual's communicative performance at home, at school, at work, and in the community. The observational protocol presented in Figure 4-5 is used by speech-language pathologists to observe students' understanding of directions within the classroom. Figure 4-6 presents a sample instrument used to observe a caregiver-child interaction for a child with a language impairment. This same assessment strategy could be used to study how people with other types of communicative impairments, such as language disorder following stroke, interact with others in real-life contexts. Language

FIGURE 4-4 **Sample interview questions for voice evaluation.**

1. What specifically is bothering you about your voice?
2. Please describe the onset of your voice problem.
3. What do you think may be the cause of this problem?
4. Tell me how the voice problem progressed after you first noticed it.
5. How is your voice different now from before the onset of problems?
6. What terms would you use to describe your voice now?
7. Can you identify any environmental factors that may make your voice problems worse or improved?
8. In what ways does your voice problem affect your life at home and at work?
9. How important to you is it that your voice problem be resolved?

Sources: Awan (2001); Stemple, Glaze, & Gerdeman (1995); Verdolini (2000).

FIGURE 4-5 Sample items from systematic observation to assess student performance in classroom discussion.

Classroom Discussion Behaviors	0 Never	1 Sometimes	2 Often or Always
1. Difficulty paying attention	0	1	2
2. Difficulty understanding abstract concepts	0	1	2
3. Difficulty answering questions from peers	0	1	2
4. Difficulty answering questions from teachers	0	1	2
5. Difficulty asking for help or clarification	0	1	2
6. Difficulty providing details	0	1	2
Notes:			

FIGURE 4-6 Systematic observation of child communication initiations during caregiver-child conversation.

	Intervals									
	1	2	3	4	5	6	7	8	9	10
Communication Behavior Gesture (G) Eye Contact (E) Vocalization (Vo) Verbalization (Ve)										
Communication Intent Request Action (RA) Request Object (RO) Comment (C) Reject (R) Imitate (I) Other (O)										
Observations:										
Directions: Complete this checklist in a 20-min. observation of child engaged in play-based interactions with primary caregiver. Watch continuously for a 1-min. period and then code for 1 min. all behaviors observed in child. Repeat this process for a total of 10 intervals (1-min. observation followed by 1 min. of coding).										

sampling, or conversational sampling, refers to the process of collecting samples of language or conversation during functional activities. As described more fully in Chapter 7, the clinician transcribes the language an individual produces and then analyzes it carefully for content, form, and use to determine which skills are and are not present.

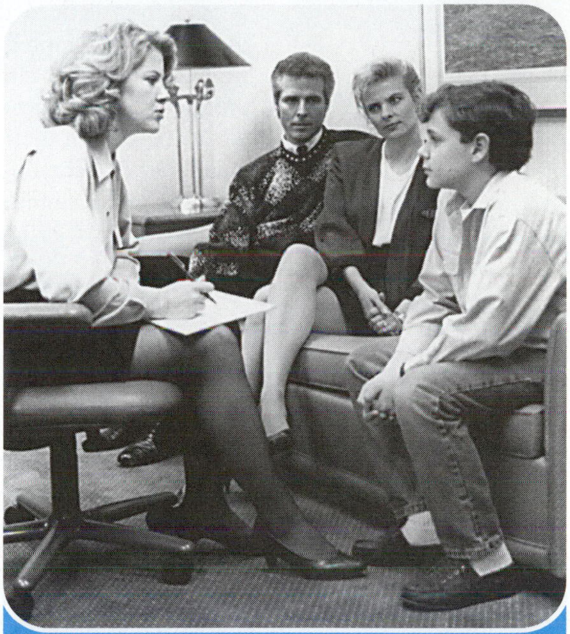

With language sampling, the clinician transcribes the language an individual produces for later analysis.

Questionnaire/Survey. Questionnaires and surveys are formal mechanisms for gathering information on particular topics. They are administered to individuals, their family members, and relevant professionals to gather input. For instance, a speech-language pathologist might ask a client to complete a self-rating scale to describe his voice quality (loudness, shakiness, hoarseness, monotone) (Fox & Ramig, 1997). Or, a special educator might ask a pupil's parent to complete the Social Skills Rating System (Gresham & Elliot, 1990), on which parents rate their children's skills in cooperation, empathy, assertion, self-control, and responsibility. Questionnaires and surveys like these provide useful information about clients that might be difficult to collect through other avenues.

Questionnaires and surveys are also valuable for gathering information following a course of intervention. For instance, researchers at the University of Sydney in Australia used a survey to determine parents' satisfaction following use of a stuttering program with their children (Lincoln, Onslow, Lewis, & Wilson, 1996). This program featured parental praise of children's stutter-free speech and correction of their children's stuttering during conversation. The parental survey, administered 12 months after the end of the program, showed that parents were very satisfied with the outcomes of this treatment. Data provided through questionnaires and surveys are a useful way to determine the success of treatments and the extent to which results are maintained over time.

Testing. Professionals often use formal, commercial tests to evaluate a person's communicative skills in a standardized manner. A standardized test is given in a highly specific and uniform way so that its administration does not influence the individual's performance. With stringent rules governing administration, the results of a standardized test presumably can provide unbiased information about a person's achievements in a particular aspect of communication or can compare a person's achievement to that of a more general population. Principles associated with formal testing are discussed later in this chapter.

Instrumentation. Assessment for many types of communication disorders relies heavily on technological instrumentation. An individual's swallowing performance, for instance, can be evaluated using video-fluoroscopic barium swallow studies, in which a person swallows food mixed with barium and the swallow is followed from the oral cavity through to the esophagus. An individual's vocal fold appearance and movement is evaluated using video stroboscopy, in which a long, flexible endoscopic tube is threaded through the nose into the pharynx to look down onto the vocal folds. The individual is instructed to make certain sounds, and the professional can watch the vocal fold movement either through an eyepiece or on a video monitor.

Technological innovations are useful for evaluating online performance in communication. **Online performance** refers to studying a communicative process as it happens (Shapiro, Swinney, & Borsky, 1998). Clinicians often use assessment tasks that study communicative processes after they happen; this is called offline assessment. For instance, if a clinician asks an adult patient to point to a picture of an umbrella from an

Discussion Point: *Some professionals might fear that technology will take over the assessment of communication disorders, making the clinician superfluous. How important, in your opinion, is the human factor in medical and educational assessments?*

array of four pictures, the pointing behavior (whether successful or not) occurs only after the client has comprehended the information. Many technological innovations now provide the means for clinicians to look at the process of communication, rather than the product. For instance, with technology we are able to examine a person's vocal folds while the person is talking and observe a person's brain while it is processing a command. Other technological innovations that influence communication assessments range from the use of computer software to evaluate language samples collected from children to the use of eye-gaze analyses to study comprehension in adults following stroke.

Interpreting Assessment Findings

When the assessment process is complete, the results must be interpreted. The first step, diagnosis, is to determine from the assessment findings whether a disorder is present and if one is, to identify it. Diagnosis is based on the preponderance of evidence from a variety of tools and techniques. Generally speaking, a disorder is diagnosed when the assessment shows that a particular aspect of communication is markedly discrepant from what is observed in the typical population or from what is expected in the individual being assessed. Also, there must be some adverse effect on the person's functional activities at home, at school, at work, or in the community.

Discussion Point: *Consider the cases of Lila and Mr. Stevens in Box 4-1. What are some ways that stuttering and voice disorders can affect a person's functional activities at home, at school, at work, and in the community?*

Accurate diagnosis requires the clinician to engage in a process called **differential diagnosis**, or solving "diagnostic dilemmas" (Philips & Ruscello, 1998, p. 2). Sometimes it is difficult to differentiate disorders that share symptoms and causes. Differential diagnosis is the process of systematically differentiating a disorder from other possible alternatives to arrive at the most accurate diagnosis.

Once the presence of a disorder is confirmed, the clinician uses the available evidence to determine the severity of the disorder. Severity ranges along a continuum of *very mild, mild, moderate, severe,* and *very severe* (e.g., Wingate, 1976). As an example, the American Speech-Language-Hearing Association (1998) provides guidelines for differentiating the severity of disorders on a 7-point scale, shown in Table 4-2, for adult language disorders.

Finally, the clinician characterizes the client's prognosis, or changes expected as a result of treatment. Prognosis statements are subjective predictions made by clinicians that are influenced by characteristics of the disorder (severity and cause) and characteristics of the client (age, family supports, motivation, general health, etc.).

Developing an Intervention Plan

The clinician uses the assessment process to develop an intervention plan based on the individual's strengths and needs in communication. Development of the plan involves identifying treatment goals, describing the possible length and frequency of treatment, and describing treatment contexts and activities. The goals that are identified vary with different types of communicative disorders. For instance, for a person with a swallowing disorder, goals are likely to focus first on ensuring safety while swallowing and second on improving quality of life. For a child with a disorder of speech production, goals may focus first on developing other means of communication so the child's needs can be made known and met and second on improving speech intelligibility.

All goals identified through the assessment process should exhibit the following characteristics:

1. *Functional:* Goals should directly improve the client's life in some way.
2. *Measurable:* Goals should link directly to some aspect of measurement so that progress toward the goal can be documented.
3. *Attainable:* Goals should be realistic and achievable for the client so that progress, however incremental, is possible.

TABLE 4-2 Severity classifications for adult language disorders

Severity	Description
Level 1	Individual is alert, but unable to follow simple directions or respond to yes/no questions, even with cues.
Level 2	With consistent, maximal cues, individual is able to follow simple directions, respond to simple yes/no questions in context, and respond to simple words or phrases related to personal needs.
Level 3	Individual usually responds accurately to simple yes/no questions. Individual is able to follow simple directions out of context, although moderate cueing is consistently needed. Accurate comprehension of more complex directions/messages is infrequent.
Level 4	Individual consistently responds accurately to simple yes/no questions and occasionally follows simple directions without cues. Moderate contextual support is usually needed to understand complex sentences/messages. Individual is able to understand limited conversations about routine daily activities with familiar communication partners.
Level 5	Individual is able to understand communication in structured conversations with both familiar and unfamiliar partners. Individual occasionally requires minimal cueing to understand more complex sentences/messages. Individual occasionally initiates the use of compensatory strategies when encountering difficulty.
Level 6	Individual is able to understand communication in most activities but some limitations in comprehension are still apparent in vocational, avocational, and social activities. Individual rarely requires minimal cueing to understand complex sentences. Individual usually uses compensatory strategies when encountering difficulty.
Level 7	Individual's ability to independently participate in vocational, avocational, and social activities is not limited by spoken language comprehension. When difficulty with comprehension occurs, the individual consistently uses a compensatory strategy.

Source: American Speech-Language-Hearing Association (1998). *National outcomes measurement system.* Reprinted with permission.

Monitoring Progress and Outcomes

Assessment is not a one-shot deal that stops when the diagnosis is made. Rather, assessment is an ongoing process that monitors progress and outcomes for the client. Assessment is used to monitor a client's progress during treatment, to modify the treatment plan as progress is made, and to determine when a client should be discharged from treatment. The use of assessment to guide intervention is a natural part of the treatment process for experienced clinicians. During every treatment session, the experienced clinician probes the client's skills and progress, making adjustments to the treatment process to enhance the effectiveness of the session and the overall treatment plan.

How Are Assessment Instruments Categorized?

Professionals use a variety of instruments to identify an individual's strengths and needs in communication and to develop an assessment protocol that is sensitive, comprehensive, and nonbiased. A variety of instruments is necessary because no one assessment instrument fulfills all these characteristics.

Validity and Reliability

All assessment instruments should exhibit two critical qualities: validity and reliability. **Validity** is the extent to which a particular instrument measures what it says it measures. For instance, a test purporting to evaluate the oral language skills of Spanish-speaking children in the United States for the purpose of identifying children with a language disorder has questionable validity if it was designed based on English-language developmental data (Restrepo & Silverman, 2001). The validity of an instrument relates to the design and content of the instrument's tasks (McCauley & Swisher, 1984). Three types of validity especially important to clinicians when selecting instruments include construct validity, face validity, and criterion-related validity (McCauley & Swisher, 1984).

Construct validity is the extent to which an instrument examines the underlying theoretical construct it was designed to examine. For instance, the items on a newly designed test of intelligence should clearly reflect what experts know about intelligence and how it can be measured. For a test to have construct validity, it must measure a defined construct, or a definable aspect of knowledge or ability. In the field of communication sciences and disorders, important constructs include speech, language, cognition, communication, swallowing, and hearing. It is often hard to get experts to agree on the parameters and definitions of these and other important constructs. As expert opinion redefines or refines certain constructs, the tests used to measure these constructs change as well.

Face validity is the extent to which an instrument appears superficially to test what it purports to test. If you watch an experienced audiologist examine a client's auditory discrimination skills, it should be fairly obvious to you that the test is examining some aspect of auditory discrimination.

Criterion-related validity is the extent to which the outcomes of an instrument reflect the outcomes from other instruments measuring the same construct. There are two types of criterion-related validity. **Concurrent validity** describes how an instrument's outcomes relate to outcomes on other, similar measures. For instance, the results of a new test that examines adults' language comprehension after brain injury should be similar to those of prevailing tests. **Predictive validity** describes how performance on an instrument predicts future performance in the area examined. Many of you reading this text have taken the SAT. The SAT was designed to predict the likelihood that a particular student would be successful in the first year of university studies. If the SAT did not have adequate predictive validity, it would not

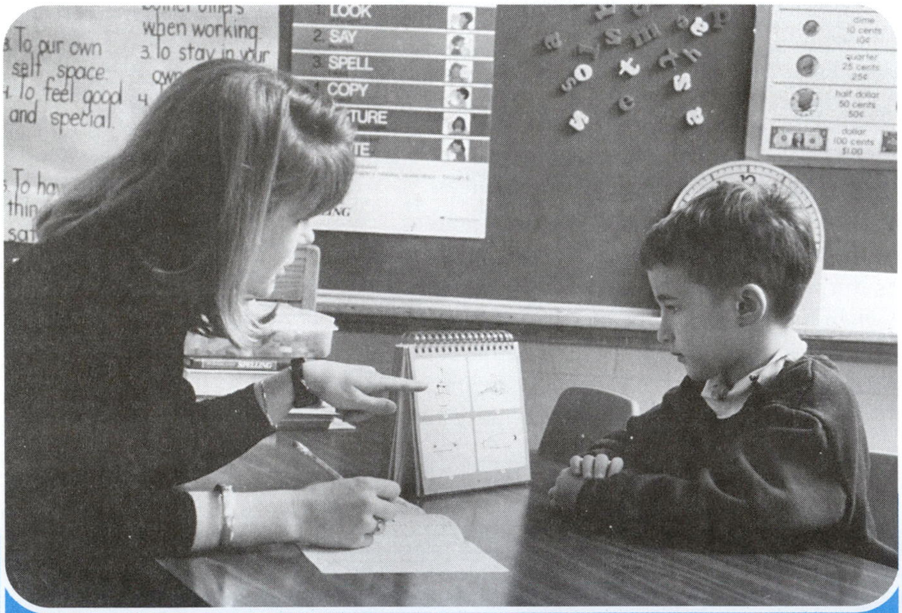

Test-retest reliability refers to the stability of test scores over time.

make sense for so many high school students to take it. The same is true for all instruments used for evaluative purposes: tests should be able to reasonably predict future performance.

Reliability is another important concept related to assessment and testing. **Reliability** is the extent to which a particular instrument is consistent in its measurement of a particular skill, behavior, area of knowledge, perception, or belief. For instance, if a person took a personality test on a Monday and was classified as outgoing and bold, and then took the same test the following Friday and was classified as shy and introverted, we would question the test's reliability, or consistency. Slight variation can be expected as a result of any number of factors (e.g., fatigue on one day); however, test outcomes should be fairly consistent. Two important types of reliability are test-retest reliability and inter-rater reliability (McCauley & Swisher, 1984).

Discussion Point: *What are some tests you have taken in the last few years? Think about a particular test and consider its validity. What was the purpose of the test? What did it purport to measure?*

Test-retest reliability describes the stability of an individual's test performance over time. A test has test-retest reliability when scores are similar over repeated administrations. In the example just cited, the personality test did not have test-retest reliability. In the field of communication disorders, test-retest reliability is crucial because clinicians use tests to make important diagnostic decisions. For example, if a voice assessment shows that a person has a significant voice disorder, but the assessment instrument has inadequate test-retest reliability, the diagnosis may be in error.

Discussion Point: *Describe a task that you believe would not have good test-retest reliability. Why is it unreliable?*

Inter-rater reliability describes the consistency of assessment outcomes over multiple observers. This type of reliability is particularly important for assessments that involve any level of subjective scoring. For instance, in administering a vocabulary comprehension test that involves pointing to pictures (such as might be given to an elderly person who has had a stroke), will two observers reliably score the client's pointing behaviors as correct or incorrect? In using a stuttering observation assessment to evaluate the stuttering behaviors of a young boy, will two observers reliably rate the stuttering as mild, moderate, or severe? If both observers consistently scored behaviors the same way, these tests would have inter-rater reliability. Assessment instruments need to be carefully designed to ensure that all observers of an individual's test performance will see the same thing.

Types of Assessment

Four categories of assessment instruments are used by speech, language, and hearing professionals: norm-referenced, criterion-referenced, performance-based, and dynamic instruments. These four types of instruments vary primarily on the basis of their outcome goals: What is it the instrument was designed to accomplish? Table 4-3 provides a description of these major types of instruments.

Norm-Referenced Instruments

The goal of **norm-referenced assessment** is to compare an individual's performance in a particular area of communication to that of his or her same-age peers. To achieve this goal, norm-referenced tests share three important qualities: (a) standardization, (b) normative sample, and (c) standard scores.

Standardization. **Standardization** means that the test must be given in a uniform and scripted manner so that it is given in exactly the same way to everyone who takes it. To accurately achieve the test's goal of comparing one person's performance to that of others, all test takers must be tested in the same way.

Normative Sample. With norm-referenced testing, an individual's test performance can be compared to that of a **normative sample**. The normative sample is a group of individuals who were given the test to identify standards of performance at specific age levels. For instance, in

TABLE 4-3 Major types of assessment instruments

Type of Instrument	Purpose and Description
Norm-referenced	Compares an individual's performance to that of same-age peers. Often required to establish an individual's eligibility for special services for organizations (e.g., school districts, insurance companies). Administered according to standardized guidelines; results interpreted against a normative sample to derive standard scores and percentile ranks.
Criterion-referenced	Determines an individual's level of achievement or skill in a particular area of communication. Individual's performance on a set of tasks is evaluated against a clear standard of performance. May use questionnaires, surveys, formal tests, informal tests, and observation.
Performance-based	Describes an individual's skills or behaviors within their actual contexts of use. Studies communicative performance across contexts that vary in the demands of the situation. May use questionnaires, surveys, observation, and collection of artifacts in portfolios for portfolio analysis.
Dynamic assessment	Identifies how much and what types of support are needed to bring an individual's communicative performance to a higher level. Uses graduated prompting after independent level of skill is identified to see how performance changes through interaction and assistance.

developing an assessment of vocal quality to be used with adults aged 21 through 100, test developers would gather a normative sample of individuals representing the characteristics of the people who will ultimately be given the test. A normative sample ideally resembles those for whom the test is designed in terms of geographic residence, socioeconomic status, dialect, and disability status (McCauley & Swisher, 1984). In our example, the normative sample would be likely to comprise about 800 people, 100 from each major age band (21–30 years, 31–40 years, 41–50 years, etc.). When the test becomes commercially available, it will be able to compare a 45-year-old person's vocal quality to the vocal quality observed in the comparable age group of the normative sample.

When professionals use norm-referenced tests, they must ensure the appropriateness of comparing a client's performance to that of the normative sample. It may not be appropriate, for instance, to use a norm-referenced language test with adolescents with traumatic brain injuries if people with brain injuries were not included in the normative sample (Turkstra, 1999). Similarly, it may not be appropriate to use norm-referenced tests for members of particular ethnic or racial groups if their ethnic or racial peers were underrepresented in the test's normative sample (Laing & Kamhi, 2003).

Standard Scores. The use of a standardized, norm-referenced test results in a **standard score**, the index that identifies how a person's test performance compares to that of their normative peers. Standard scores are frequently used by speech, language, and hearing professionals to determine whether a person has a disorder and whether a person qualifies for intervention services. Many public school special education programs depend on standard scores to determine whether a student qualifies for special education.

To understand standard scores, it is necessary to understand what happens when a person is administered a norm-referenced test. Let's take 8-year-old Garcia, who is administered a norm-referenced test of speech intelligibility. On this test, Garcia is asked to say

20 words; the number of speech-sound errors is counted for each word. Garcia makes 32 speech-sound errors; this is Garcia's raw score. A **raw score** is the number of items scored as incorrect or, on some tests, the number of items scored as correct. Because this is a norm-referenced test, we want to compare Garcia's performance to that of other 8-year-old children. The raw score is not helpful in this regard. Although we know that Garcia made 32 errors, we do not know how this compares to the number of errors made by other 8-year-old children. Thus, we must turn to the normative references gathered by testing a large number of children across the country. Normative references are available in the test manuals of standardized, norm-referenced tests. For Garcia, we look for the table describing performance of 8-year-old males, which indicates 71 as the standard score correlate of a raw score of 32.

Now that we have a standard score, we need to interpret it. It is easier to interpret a standard score than a raw score because standard scores are derived from the same standard metric: the standard normal distribution. The **standard normal distribution** is derived from mathematical models of probability regarding how scores will range for a skill or aptitude that is assumed to be normally distributed within the population. The standard normal distribution assumes that certain percentages of the population will perform at particular levels; for instance, really poor scores on a test of speech intelligibility will be seen only for about 2% of 8-year-old children. Standard scores are mathematically arranged along a standard normal distribution, or **normal curve**, to approximate these probabilistic expectations.

The standard normal distribution is defined by two parameters: a mean of 100 and a standard deviation of 15. **Mean** refers to the average score, which in the standard normal distribution is a standard score of 100. **Standard deviation** (*SD*) refers to the spread of scores; on a normal curve, standard deviation units work their way outward from the mean, and scores are characterized in terms of how many standard deviation units they lie away from the mean. Figure 4-7 shows the parameters of the standard normal distribution: a score of 70, for instance, is 2 standard deviation units below the mean (−2 *SD*); a score of 110 is within 1 standard deviation unit of the mean; and a score of 149 is more than 3 standard deviation units above the mean (+3 *SD*). Standard deviation units are relative to the mean score expected for a person's age. On the basis of the normal distribution, we can expect that

- 68.3% of scores will be between 85 and 115, often referred to as "within normal limits"
- 13.6% of scores will be between 116 and 130, often referred to as "above average"

FIGURE 4-7 Standard normal distribution.

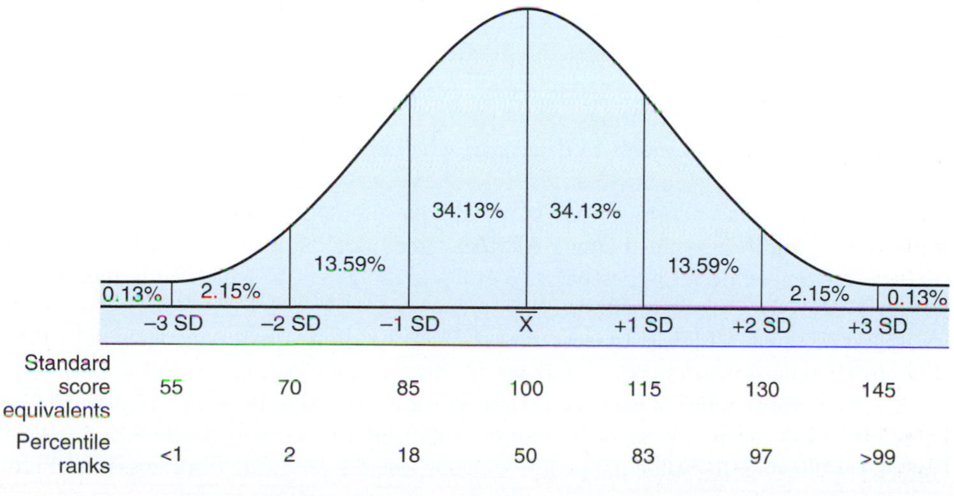

- 13.6% of scores will be between 70 and 84, often referred to as "below average"
- 2.3% of scores will be 131 or higher, often referred to as "significantly above average," with 0.13% of scores over 145 ("truly extraordinary")
- 2.3% of scores will be below 69, often referred to as "significantly below average," with 0.13% of scores under 55 ("severely/profoundly depressed")

To return to our example, Garcia's standard score of 71 on the norm-referenced measure of speech intelligibility is significantly below average relative to the scores of his peers.

In addition to standard scores, the outcome of a norm-referenced test provides several types of derived scores—scores that are derived from raw scores. A **percentile rank**, often used in conjunction with a standard score to interpret an individual's performance (see Figure 4-7), indicates the percentage of people in the normative reference group whose scores were at or below a given point. For instance, Garcia's percentile rank on the test of speech intelligibility was 6: only 6% of children within Garcia's age group received a score at or below Garcia's standard score of 71. Conversely, 94% of 8-year-old children in the normative sample had scores higher than 71.

Discussion Point: *Consider the case of Lila in Box 4-1. How useful would a norm-referenced test be in an assessment of her communicative abilities?*

An **age-equivalent score** provides an age-based reference for an individual's test performance. For instance, Garcia's age-equivalent score was 3-8, or 3 years, 8 months, meaning that Garcia's score was similar to that achieved by children aged 3 years and 8 months. However, many experts believe that the way in which age-equivalent scores are derived from normative data is flawed and that these scores misrepresent an individual's test performance (McCauley & Swisher, 1984). Professionals sometimes use age-equivalent scores to describe a child's performance as a number of years behind, as in "Garcia is 5 years behind in his speech skills." This is an inaccurate interpretation, however. An age-equivalent score does not indicate how far behind a child is; it is an indication only that a score is similar to the mean of children of that age. The standard score, which compares a child's performance to that of same-age children, is a more useful measure. Professionals should use age-equivalent scores sparingly and cautiously.

Criterion-Referenced Assessment

The goal of **criterion-referenced assessment** is to determine an individual's level of achievement or skill in a particular area of communication. The term *criterion* means that the individual's performance is judged against a particular standard (criterion). For example, audiologists often use criterion-referenced instruments to evaluate hearing acuity. These tests are designed to determine whether an individual can hear at a level considered adequate for daily living activities. If not, amplification, such as a hearing aid, may be indicated.

Criterion-referenced instruments are useful for probing intensively at what a person can do in a specific aspect of communication and are often used to document treatment progress. For instance, after fitting a client with a hearing aid, the audiologist uses several criterion-referenced instruments to determine whether the client's hearing has improved. These might include systematic observation of how the client performs in a conversation with his or her spouse, administration of several questionnaires and checklists, and evaluation with clinical instrumentation. All these methods of evaluation are considered criterion-referenced because the goal is to evaluate the extent to which an individual has achieved established standards for hearing.

Criterion-referenced instruments are defined by three important qualities. First, criterion-referenced instruments require establishment of a clear standard of performance. The standard against which a person's performance is evaluated must be carefully defined. As an example, let's consider swallowing disorders and the use of criterion-referenced tasks to evaluate swallowing. In evaluating people with suspected swallowing disorders, it is of little relevance how they compare against normative references. What is important is whether their swallowing skills are consistent with a standard, which is based on knowing the standard level of skill needed to safely execute a swallow. Minimally, the standard requires a swallow to be coordinated and executed in a way that prevents any threat to nutrition or the airway.

Second, criterion-referenced instruments require design of specific tasks that reliably document an individual's performance against the standard. These instruments may include observation, questionnaires and surveys, formal tests, informal tests, and instrumentation. Continuing with the swallowing example, any one of these types of instruments may be used to document a person's performance against a standard. For instance, the professional might observe the client swallowing a variety of foods and liquids and watch for indicators that the standard of a safe swallow is not met.

Third, criterion-referenced instruments must provide clear guidelines for interpreting performance and determining whether an individual has achieved the standard. For instance, many toddlers and preschoolers go through a period in which they show stuttering behaviors, or dysfluencies. Criterion-referenced procedures for identifying a child's rate of stuttering must provide clear guidelines that enable professionals to determine whether the rate of dysfluencies observed is significantly higher than would be expected and thus whether some type of intervention is needed.

Discussion Point: *Describe a criterion-referenced task that would document a student's participation in your class. What does the task look like? How is it scored? How could you determine its validity and reliability?*

Performance-Based Assessment

Performance-based assessment (PBA), also called authentic assessment, describes an individual's skills or behaviors within authentic contexts of use, such as at home, in the workplace, in the classroom, or in the community (Secord & Wiig, 2003). One rationale for using PBA is that communicative skills are highly influenced by context and therefore vary across different situations (Klein & Moses, 1999). For communication assessment to be valid, it should document an individual's communicative performance in a variety of real contexts that have different performance demands. A second rationale for using PBA is that traditional models of assessment, namely, norm-referenced instruments, are of limited use in planning treatments. Whereas norm-referenced assessment is useful for making diagnoses, assessing severity, and recommending treatments, the outcomes from such assessment cannot be used directly to inform the design of treatments (Secord & Wiig, 2003). With PBA, by documenting the strengths and limitations of individuals' skills and behaviors within the contexts of their lives, professionals are better able to design interventions that promote functional, meaningful outcomes.

Several techniques are available for conducting PBA. These include many of the techniques already described, such as systematic observation, surveys, and questionnaires. For PBA, these techniques are employed within actual contexts. For instance, to study how well 10-year-old Adele is able to meet the communicative demands of the curriculum, a speech-language pathologist may use systematic observation to code and analyze her communication behaviors within the classroom. An important aspect of PBA is studying *how* an individual performs in relation to the context. In assessing Adele's communication in the classroom, PBA documents key features of the environment that relate to her performance, such as classroom organization and the teacher's instructional approaches.

An additional technique used in PBA is **artifact analysis**, or collection and analysis of communicative samples produced by an individual, such as a spelling test, a thank-you note, or a grocery list (Secord & Wiig, 2003). Often, artifacts are collected and maintained in portfolios for **portfolio analysis**. Professionals analyze the portfolio to identify patterns of communicative strengths and weaknesses across different contexts. This analysis is used to select communication targets and to identify contexts requiring intervention.

Discussion Point: *What kind of information does a portfolio provide about a person that might not be available through other types of assessment?*

FIGURE 4-8 Description of graduated prompting.

One common type of dynamic assessment is *graduated prompting,* in which the professional studies how an individual's performance changes as interactive supports are gradually introduced. Prompts are graduated in that they are arranged hierarchically in their intensity of support. For instance, the following hierarchical prompts might be used to examine how much support is needed to assist an adult to say his or her name:

Prompt 1: Ask client to say name ("Tell me your name.")
Prompt 2: Provide an auditory model ("Tell me, 'Will.'")
Prompt 3: Provide a visual model ("Look in this mirror. Try to say 'Will.'")
Prompt 4: Provide a starter ("Let's make the first sound: /w/.")

With this approach, the professional can determine how much and what type of assistance is needed to improve performance. For example, if Will can produce his name following prompt 3 (use of a mirror and a model), this type of support is most beneficial to Will and this response provides information that is useful to designing his treatment program.

Source: Gutiérrez-Clellen & Peña (2001).

Dynamic Assessment

Dynamic assessment analyzes how much and what types of support or assistance are needed to bring an individual's communicative performance to a higher level. This approach is sometimes described as interactive assessment or mediated learning (Justice & Ezell, 1999), as it examines how interaction and mediation influence an individual's ability to complete a task (see Figure 4-8).

Dynamic assessment has its roots in the theories of Lev Vygotsky, a Russian psychologist who believed that the best indicator of a person's **learning potential** was how much he could achieve with the assistance of another (Vygotsky, 1978). As an example, consider two 20-month-old children—Danielle and Eli—who are at the single-word stage of language development. Neither child spontaneously produces two-word utterances (e.g., "doggie up."), but both can produce two-word utterances given some level of adult mediation. Danielle produces a two-word utterance following an adult model:

Adult: doggie up
Danielle: doggie up

Eli produces a two-word utterance only when an adult breaks the two words into a succession of single words:

Adult: doggie up
Adult: tell me doggie
ELI: doggie
Adult: up
ELI: up

Assessment techniques that focus on what a person can do *independently* would characterize both children similarly as being at the one-word utterance stage of language development. Dynamic techniques that focus on what a person can do *dependently* (within the context of assistance) differentiate the children by their learning potential. In our example, Danielle's language skills are more advanced than Eli's, as Danielle is able to perform at a higher level within the context of adult assistance. As this example suggests, we cannot document learning potential without considering how an individual performs with assistance. Dynamic assessment differs from other assessment approaches that withhold assistance to the individual to focus only on what the individual can do independently.

Dynamic assessment complements norm-referenced, criterion-referenced, and performance-based measures. Professionals may use dynamic assessment after other techniques have identified an individual's independent level of skill (the level achieved without any assistance) to identify the type of supports needed to bring performance to higher levels. Dynamic assessment is particularly valuable for use with people from culturally and linguistically diverse populations, as traditional methods of assessment may underrepresent their abilities and learning potential (Laing & Kamhi, 2003; Peña, Iglesias, & Lidz, 2001).

The Assessment Protocol

The four types of assessments described here—norm-referenced, criterion-referenced, performance-based, and dynamic—have distinct and complementary purposes. Together they fulfill the four fundamental purposes of assessment: (1) identifying skills that a person does and does not have in a particular area of communication, (2) informing a program of intervention that is designed to enhance a person's skills in a particular area of communication, (3) monitoring a person's communicative growth and performance over time, and (4) qualifying a person for special services. Professionals utilize a wide variety of instruments to achieve these purposes and to ensure that the assessment protocol is sensitive, comprehensive, and nonbiased.

What Is Intervention?

Definition

The term **intervention** in the field of communication disorders refers to the implementation of a plan of action to improve one or more aspects of an individual's communicative abilities (Klein & Moses, 1999). Professionals may also use the terms *treatment, therapy,* and *remediation* to refer to this plan of action. Important considerations in designing and implementing interventions are effectiveness, efficiency, and adherence. Effectiveness is the likelihood that an intervention will have the expected outcome. An effective intervention has been shown by scientists to have value for a certain population. Efficiency is the time it takes for an intervention to result in change. An efficient intervention is one that effects change relatively quickly compared to other treatment options. Adherence is a person's implementation of an intervention following the professional's prescription; adherence is highly influential in treatment outcomes. When selecting interventions, professionals must consider the likelihood that an individual will show fidelity to a recommended course of treatment.

Discussion Point: *In your opinion, what characteristics of an individual are most influential in determining whether that individual will adhere to a prescribed course of treatment?*

There is no "one size fits all" intervention that will meet the communicative needs and values of all people with communication disorders. In fact, for one category of disorder, such as stuttering, there may be dozens of treatment variations from which to choose. Professionals must be knowledgeable about the many treatment options for different types of communication disorders and about related issues of effectiveness, efficiency, and adherence.

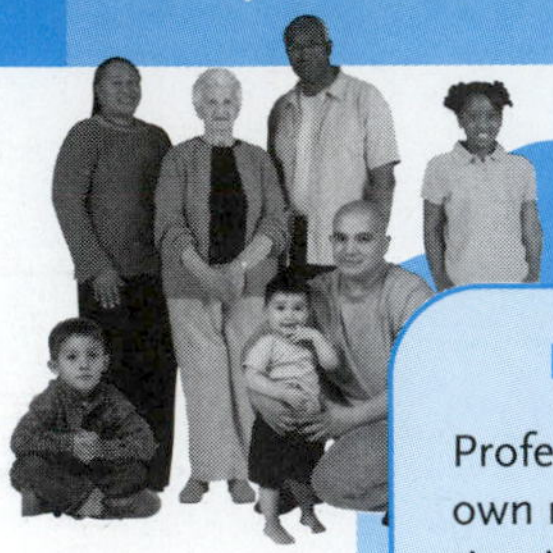

BOX 4-3 Multicultural Focus

Multicultural Issues

Professionals who work with children and families whose cultural backgrounds differ from their own must be aware of how culture influences child-rearing behaviors and practices. Communication interventions for young children often focus on parent-child interactions as a means for improving language achievements, as emphasized in Mr. Mykel's case (described in Box 4-1). Mr. Mykel and his nursing colleagues want to work with parents to facilitate children's early language achievements so as to prevent delays. Many of the families in the neighborhood are Hispanic and speak Spanish. Although Mr. Mykel and his nurse collaborators are not Hispanic and do not speak Spanish, they recognize that their outreach efforts and the design of their program must be culturally sensitive, particularly given the powerful interactions between culture and the nature of parent-child interaction.

Studies show that culture influences parental beliefs about child rearing. For instance, Rodriguez and Olswang (2003) studied parents' beliefs about child rearing for 30 Mexican American and Anglo-American mothers. The Mexican American mothers in this study either were born in Mexico or were first-generation Mexican Americans. Each of the Mexican American and Anglo-American mothers had one child receiving speech therapy in the public school system. Rodriguez and Olswang surveyed each mother to study her beliefs about child rearing and parenting. Their findings include the following:

- Mexican American mothers held more traditional and authoritarian educational beliefs than did Anglo-American mothers. Mexican American mothers viewed schools as having greater responsibility for the education of their children, and they viewed their own roles in their children's education as subservient to those of the schools and teachers. However, Mexican American mothers held progressive educational beliefs concerning the importance of their own roles in teaching their children at home to foster their school success.
- Mexican American mothers placed higher value on teaching their children characteristics of conformity—being polite, being a good student, and obeying elders—than of self-direction. The mothers viewed the characteristics of conformity as being very important to their children as learners.

Making Treatment Decisions: The Knowledgeable Clinician

Some professionals work in a setting in which they treat only one type of communication disorder; for example, clinicians who work in a cleft palate clinic likely see only children with cleft palate. Many professionals, however, work in settings in which they serve a more diverse clientele. For instance, in any given week in a communication disorders outpatient clinic, a professional might treat children with communicative impairments associated with autism, apraxia, mental retardation, and vocal nodules and adults with communicative impairments associated with stroke, traumatic brain injury, dementia, and hearing loss. Being a competent clinician requires, more than anything else, a solid knowledge base that drives ongoing decision making with diverse clients. The knowledgeable clinician is one who can make sound treatment decisions for any client by integrating four areas of knowledge:

1. *Theoretical knowledge* about typical communication and how a particular disorder impacts communication
2. *Empirical knowledge* derived from the scientific literature on the disorder, including knowledge of the effectiveness and efficiency of different treatment options

- Mexican American mothers were more likely than Anglo-American mothers to view children's communicative difficulties as resulting from external causes, such as the home or school environment. In contrast, the Anglo-American mothers emphasized intrinsic causes of communication problems, such as medical conditions and family history.

Two important points made by Rodriguez and Olswang warrant note. First, these experts saw considerable intracultural diversity among the mothers they studied. The Mexican American mothers, for instance, varied widely in their perspectives on parenting. This is significant. Whereas professionals must be sensitive to the cultural backgrounds of the families with whom they work, they must also avoid stereotypes and find a way to emphasize the "significance of each family's beliefs and values in developing culturally relevant intervention programs" (p. 459). Second, Rodriguez and Olswang noted significant differences when comparing the parenting beliefs of the Mexican American mothers with those of the Anglo-American mothers in the study. This finding emphasizes the need for professionals to be sensitive to the values and practices of the families with whom they work and to take time to understand each family uniquely. Rodriguez and Olswang comment:

> The diversity of cultural beliefs and values should be viewed as a strength on which [professionals] can draw to design culturally relevant assessment and intervention services and to maximize the benefits to families and children. Mothers' beliefs and values can shape the nature of their involvement in the assessment and intervention process, influence the selection of intervention goals and objectives, and have an effect on the selection of effective service delivery models. (2003, p. 459)

For Discussion

What are some possible explanations for cross-cultural differences in parents' beliefs about child rearing?

Survey your classmates to discuss their beliefs about child rearing. What do they think about conformity, politeness, discipline, and the like? How much similarity and difference is there among the classmates you surveyed?

Companion Website

To answer these questions online, go to the Multicultural Focus module in chapter 4 of the Companion Website.

3. *Practical knowledge* gained through clinical experience with other clients with this disorder
4. *Personal knowledge* of the client's values and needs

Evidence-based practice is the process by which the clinician integrates these four areas of knowledge to arrive at the best plan of action for a particular client. The term *evidence-based practice* emphasizes the use of empirical (scientific) literature for making treatment decisions, but also recognizes the roles of theoretical knowledge, practical knowledge, and personal knowledge in designing interventions. Evidence-based practice provides a means for guarding against the use of fringe therapies—treatments for which there is no scientific evidence of validity. Fringe therapies are often inconsistent with theoretical models of communication and communication disorders. Many fringe therapies are touted as viable treatments for certain communication disorders despite these scientific and theoretical shortcomings. They may become popular through testimonials, which are easily disseminated through word-of-mouth and the Internet. Often, the authors of fringe therapies make statements that the therapy will "cure" a disorder and that "scientific evidence" has shown this to be so. Fringe therapies presented in this way frequently appeal to the families of people with communication disorders, particularly when the disorder has no known cure and treatment progress is slow.

BOX 4-4 Spotlight on Practice

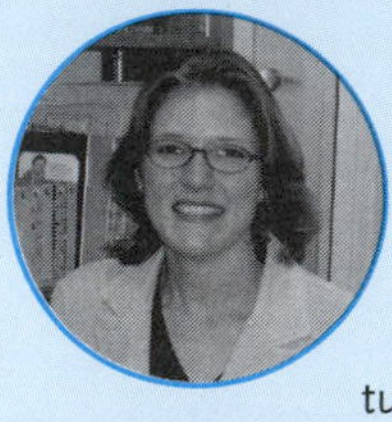

Angela Beckman, M.S., CCC-SLP
Doctoral Student, Curry School of Education
University of Virginia

Working at a specialized private preschool in D.C. afforded me the opportunity to work closely with children who were deaf and hard of hearing and users of hearing aids and cochlear implants. In this unique setting, I collaborated in the classroom with early childhood educators to facilitate participation and learning for all children. The program was designed to provide a naturalistic setting in which the deaf children could learn to understand and use oral language.

Working in this environment was an excellent learning experience, as I was responsible for teaching both typically developing children and those who required hearing-related services for hearing loss. This environment helped me to better understand what typical developmental milestones looked like and what steps needed to be taken to facilitate learning for children who were delayed in meeting those milestones. Also, sharing teaching responsibilities with a master's level educator provided for ongoing learning opportunities as we shared our background knowledge and experiences with each other. Being in the classroom all day was a challenging experience, as my training had primarily been in one-on-one and small-group therapy, but as I adapted to this new environment, I grew to enjoy it, particularly for the naturalistic opportunities it provided to address speech, language, and auditory goals.

I recently enrolled in a Ph.D. program in the McGuffey Reading Center at the University of Virginia to broaden my scope of knowledge in the literacy field. In addition, I continue to be involved in the field of speech-language pathology by supervising master's level clinicians and by administering assessments, conducting research, and teaching courses in the areas of language and literacy.

BOX 4-5 Spotlight on Research

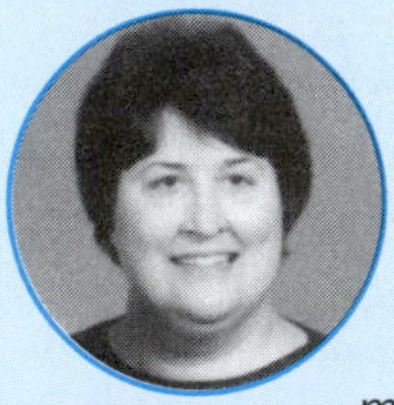

Adele W. Miccio, Ph.D.
The Pennsylvania State University, University Park, PA

My interest in child phonology grew during my master's program at the University of Northern Colorado and my later experiences as a speech-language pathologist in the public schools of rural Colorado. Since earning a Ph.D. in Speech and Hearing Sciences at Indiana University-Bloomington, I have worked at Penn State, where I am Associate Professor of Communication Sciences and Disorders and Applied Linguistics and teach courses in clinical phonetics and phonology.

In my research I ask questions about the effects of phonological intervention for young children, particularly the role of *stimulability* for particular sounds and how this predicts children's growth during treatment. I am also very interested in the study of speech development in children at risk. I have, for example, conducted longitudinal studies of phonological development in infants and toddlers with chronic middle-ear infections. We are finding that although the phonological systems of most children with otitis media develop typically, this is not necessarily the case for children who have early and high incidences of middle-ear infections, whose speech development seems compromised.

A third area of interest is the relationship between phonological development and literacy abilities in bilingual children. We are conducting a longitudinal investigation of language, phonology, and literacy development of bilingual children in Head Start to show how the developmental paths of children with early second language acquisition differ from those of children with first language bilingual acquisition. More details on these and other studies are seen in:

Miccio, A. W. (2005). A treatment program to enhance stimulability for phonological acquisition. In A. Kamhi & K. Pollock (Eds.); *Phonological disorders in children: Clinical decision making in assessment and intervention.* Baltimore: Brookes Publishing Co.

Miccio, A. W. (2002). Clinical problem solving: Assessment of phonological disorders. *American Journal of Speech-Language Pathology, 11*, 221–229.

Miccio, A. W., Yont, K. M., Clemons, H. L., & Vernon-Feagans, L. (2002). Otitis media and the acquisition of consonants. In F. Windsor, M. L. Kelly, & N. Hewlett (Eds.), *Investigations in clinical phonetics and linguistics* (pp. 429–438). Mahwah, NJ: Lawrence Erlbaum.

Purposes of Intervention

Intervention has three primary purposes: (1) prevention, (2) remediation, and (3) compensation. **Preventive interventions** attempt to prevent a disorder from emerging. They typically target all people who are considered at risk for developing a particular communicative disorder but who do not yet show signs of the disorder. Here are three examples:

Adelaide: At Adelaide's routine 12-month checkup, the pediatrician instructed Adelaide's mother to read storybooks to her daily. This is a preventive intervention designed to stimulate Adelaide's early language and literacy development and thereby reduce her risk for developing a language or literacy disorder.

Alfonso: Alfonso is a construction worker who builds office buildings in urban settings. Each worker in Alfonso's company is required to take an annual 2-hour hearing protection seminar designed by an audiologist and receives ear protectors to wear while working at sites with high levels of construction noise. This is a preventive intervention designed to reduce Alfonso's risk for developing hearing loss.

Matthew: Matthew is a professional opera singer who engages in vocal exercises daily. A speech-language pathologist designed these vocal exercises to strengthen Matthew's vocal cords and other muscles of the larynx. This is a preventive intervention designed to reduce Matthew's risk for developing a vocal disorder and experiencing vocal strain.

One challenge to delivering effective preventive interventions is outreach. Outreach is the process of identifying people who are at risk of developing a particular disorder and ensuring that they have access to the preventive intervention. Because these people do not have signs of the disorder, they may be hard to find, and they may not view themselves as in need of intervention. Also, outreach efforts can be expensive. To justify their implementation, the potential benefits must outweigh the possible costs.

Discussion Point: *Mr. Mykel, described in Box 4-1, needs to think of strategies for effective outreach. What are some approaches you think would be effective?*

Remediation interventions are clinical or educational interventions designed to slow the progress or reverse the course of a disorder once it has emerged. These are delivered to people who have been diagnosed with a communicative disorder. Here are three examples of remediation interventions:

Breah: For reasons unknown, 30-month-old Breah is producing very few words, although she seems to understand everything that is said to her. She has been diagnosed with an expressive language impairment. She sees a speech-language pathologist (SLP) twice weekly in individual sessions to promote expressive language skills; the SLP also provides Breah's mother with training in specific techniques to use at home. This is a remediation intervention designed to slow or reverse the course of Breah's expressive language impairment.

Maurice: Maurice is a second-grade teacher in a rural elementary school who has been diagnosed with vocal nodules resulting from overuse and misuse of the vocal cords. Maurice's voice is hoarse and breathy. Maurice is seeing a speech-language pathologist for intervention for a voice disorder. The remediation intervention is designed to eliminate the cause and symptoms of the vocal disorder by retraining Maurice to use his voice properly.

Tenard: Tenard is a 4-year-old boy who has mild hearing loss and is experiencing a delay in language development. Tenard's audiologist helps his preschool teacher use sound-field amplification in large- and small-group activities in the classroom. This intervention is designed to speed up Tenard's learning and remediate early delays.

Remediation interventions, in contrast to preventive interventions, are delivered to people who show clear signs of having a disorder. These interventions are delivered with much greater intensity than are preventive interventions, and often at much greater cost.

Interventions designed for **compensation**, or compensatory interventions, are clinical interventions that help a person cope with a disorder whose symptoms are not likely to dissipate. Compensatory interventions are used when significant communicative difficulties remain after a course of remediation intervention, when a disorder is not amenable to remediation, and when it is unlikely that the progression of a disorder will be reversed. Here are three examples of compensatory interventions:

Riz: Sixty-year-old Riz had his larynx removed as a result of cancer. During the laryngectomy, Riz was fitted with a voice valve that allows him to speak by diverting air from the lungs to the back of the throat. Riz is working with a therapist to learn how to create voice using the valve. This is a compensatory intervention that will help Riz contend with a disorder that is not going away. Riz will learn a series of compensatory techniques that will allow him to be a functional communicator.

Quinton: Quinton is a 42-year-old surgeon. He has stuttered for as long as he can remember and has not received any intervention since middle school. Because his work increasingly requires him to speak publicly at conferences and training sessions, Quinton has sought the help of a speech-language pathologist to lessen the frequency of his stuttering during public speaking. This is a compensatory intervention: Quinton's stuttering is unlikely to go away, but he can be helped to manage his stuttering with specific compensatory techniques.

Leia: Leia is a high school student who has severe hearing loss resulting from use of a prescription drug during cancer treatment. Leia is working with the deaf-and-hard-of-hearing teacher at her school to learn how to use her residual hearing in the classroom in combination with her hearing aids. This is a compensatory treatment, as Leia's hearing loss is not going to go away. However, intervention will help her compensate for this loss and to participate more fully in educational activities.

Discussion Point: *Consider the three types of interventions and then study the cases in Box 4-1. Think about the purpose of the interventions discussed for Lila, Mr. Mykel, and Mr. Stevens.*

Compensatory interventions help people who have disorders that significantly affect their communication and that are not likely to be resolved. Like remediation interventions, compensatory interventions often require a significant investment of time by both clinician and client.

Intervention Planning

An array of professionals who are vested in preventing the emergence of communicative disorders, such as nurses, teachers, physicians, human resource managers, psychologists, and social workers, deliver preventive interventions, whereas speech-language pathologists, audiologists, and special educators are most intimately involved with the design and delivery of remediation and compensatory interventions. Preventive interventions often use a "one size fits all" approach, delivering the same intervention to everyone. In contrast, remediation and compensatory interventions are highly individualized to meet the unique needs and strengths of a particular client through the careful selection of goals and procedures (Klein & Moses, 1999).

An **intervention goal** is the targeted communication achievement of an individual, and an **intervention procedure** is the clinician's plan of action (Klein & Moses, 1999). The professional sets both short- and long-term goals and identifies specific procedures for achieving these goals. Intervention planning involves three decision-making phases, as described by Klein and Moses (1999).

In phase 1, the professional sets long-term goals for a client, the anticipated outcomes of therapy. The long-term goals identify the "best performance that can be expected of an individual in one or more targeted areas of communication within a projected period of time" (Klein & Moses, 1999, p. 98). This phase involves specifying the general area of communication skill targeted, the time frame of the intervention, and the performance outcome anticipated. Examples include the following:

- Jason will achieve normal swallowing functions.
- Heather will be fully intelligible during conversations.
- LeShawn will use his voice appropriately in all speaking situations.
- Ava will exhibit expressive language skills that are consistent with her age.

In phase 2, the professional sets the short-term goals that will lead to the desired long-term goals. Typically, sequential short-term goals are identified that will lead to achievement of the long-term goal. For instance, a special educator sets the following sequence of short-term goals for Jequan, an eighth-grade student whose long-term goal stipulates that he "will produce complex fictional narratives linked to classroom literature" (Merritt, Culatta, & Trostle, 1998):

1. Retell a one-episode story while looking at a story map.
2. Retell a one-episode story following a peer model.
3. Answer questions about a two-episode story within class discussions.
4. Fill in character maps related to characters' motives and feelings from two-episode stories.

By achieving competence in each of these short-term goals, Jequan moves toward the long-term goal of producing complex fictional narratives.

In setting short-term goals, professionals use their knowledge of normal and disordered communication development to identify the steps needed to achieve desired long-term outcome. Professionals place priority on short-term goals that are achievable and linked to real-life communicative needs, as in the example of Jequan, for whom the short-term goals are directly linked to academic performance.

In phase 3, the professional sets session-level goals for a client that are written in measurable and observable terms (Klein & Moses, 1999). Session-level goals are addressed in a specific therapy session and over time lead to the attainment of the short-term and long-term communicative goals. Session goals are observable behaviors that represent "an act of learning" that presumably will lead to the acquisition of a communicative goal (Klein & Moses, 1999, p. 174). For example, consider the following three session goals for Gabby, a child with a feeding disorder. Gabby's long-term goal is to discontinue tube feeding, and a short-term goal is for her to "chew food on her own during each of three meals in a day":

1. Gabby will sit upright with her head and trunk remaining stable at the kitchen table for a continuous 10-minute meal.
2. Gabby will follow cues for tongue and lip movement with at least 90% accuracy prior to eating.
3. Gabby will swallow at least 5 ounces of rice cereal with jaw support assistance.

These three session goals identify clearly observable behaviors that are linked to both short- and long-term goals for Gabby. The goals are functional, measurable, and presumably achievable. Importantly, these goals also reflect specific behaviors that are believed by the therapist to represent acts of learning. Through participation in this session, Gabby will make incremental improvements in feeding skills, particularly those associated with positional stability, muscle tone, and sensory experiences (Kedesdy & Budd, 1998).

Intervention Models

The design and delivery of effective interventions for people with communication disorders often requires the expertise and involvement of many professionals. Their involvement may be direct or indirect. Direct service is when the professional provides services directly to the individual who has the disorder; indirect service is when the professional serves as a consultant. Collaborative intervention is when two or more professionals work together to deliver an intervention. Common models in the design and delivery of communication interventions include the following:

- **Pull-Out/Direct Service:** A therapist or an educator provides an intervention to an individual or small group. This is one of the most common types of service delivery, and is used in almost all clinical settings (e.g., schools, clinics, hospitals, nursing homes).
- **Co-Teaching/Parallel Instruction:** Two or more therapists or educators work together to provide intervention to an individual or group. This collaborative model is becoming increasingly common in early intervention and school-based programs.
- **Intervention Consultation:** The therapist or educator provides guidance to other professionals or to family members concerning assessment data and intervention approaches, but does not work directly with the individual. This model is prevalent in many clinical settings. (DiMeo, Merritt, & Culatta, 1998; Meyer, 1997)

How Are Interventions Categorized?

The intervention approach used with a client is uniquely designed to meet that client's needs and strengths in communication. Recall from earlier in this chapter that decisions involved in designing and delivering interventions are based on the clinician's combined theoretical knowledge, empirical knowledge, practical knowledge, and personal knowledge. Interventions are typically categorized on the basis of theoretical knowledge of how communication change is facilitated through intervention. Four prevalent models of intervention are behaviorist approaches, linguistic-cognitive approaches, social-interactionist approaches, and information-processing approaches. An approach that combines two or more of these models is called a hybrid approach (Fey, 1986).

Behaviorist Approaches

Behaviorist approaches are based on classic learning theory, which emphasizes the importance of the environment for shaping behavior and in particular, the influence of consequences on behavioral change. Behaviorist approaches view communication as a behavior that is amenable to change through operant conditioning—the modification of behavior by environmental reinforcers, both positive and negative. Behavior that is positively reinforced improves, whereas behavior that is negatively reinforced is extinguished.

Inherent to behaviorist approaches is a focus on observable and measurable behaviors as the units of change and the use of systematic, hierarchical sequences of goals to structure and deliver intervention (Mercer, 1997). In behaviorist approaches to intervention, a particular target behavior, or terminal behavior—the behavior that the clinician wants the client to achieve—is broken down into its smallest components. Examples of terminal behaviors in communication disorders include: (1) saying one's own name fluently, (2) executing a swallow, (3) asking for help, (4) listening to conversational speech, and (5) understanding three-step directions.

FIGURE 4-9 Behaviorist-oriented approach for training more appropriate voice volume.

Terminal Behavior: Use of appropriate volume in all situations with self-monitoring	
Specific Competency	Mastery Required
Appropriate volume in quiet room: monitor by clinician	Maintains for 30 minutes continuously
Appropriate volume in quiet room: monitor by client	Maintains for 30 minutes continuously
Appropriate volume in noisy setting: monitor by clinician	Maintains for 30 minutes continuously
Appropriate volume in noisy setting: monitor by client	Maintains for 30 minutes continuously
Appropriate volume with people talking: monitor by client	Maintains for 30 minutes continuously
Appropriate volume with people talking in noisy setting: monitor by client	Maintains for 30 minutes continuously

Source: Adapted from S. Goldberg, *Clinical intervention: A philosophy and methodology for clinical practice*. Published by Allyn and Bacon, Boston, MA. Copyright © 1993 by Pearson Education. Reprinted/adapted by permission of the publisher.

Terminal behaviors are subjected to task analysis to identify all of their smaller components. Task analysis identifies the skills needed to perform a terminal behavior and determines the order of instruction for these component skills (Mercer, 1997). These components are then arranged into a systematic, hierarchical sequence of goals. In communication interventions, the client is gradually led to mastery in each of these components—a process called shaping—based on the assumption that mastery of each of the parts will lead to mastery of the whole. Figure 4-9 illustrates the behaviorist approach as applied to voice therapy; note the discrete, measurable objectives and the level of mastery required in each for an individual to progress to the next objective.

Behaviorist approaches to intervention tend to emphasize the role of the clinician over that of the learner or client in the intervention process, as it is the clinician who is responsible for organizing the environment and learning tasks to shape the learner's achievements toward mastery. Therefore, these approaches are referred to as clinician directed or trainer oriented, meaning that the clinician maintains a high degree of control in the implementation of the intervention. The clinician is responsible for (1) identifying observable and measurable goals arranged in a hierarchy, (2) specifying the level of mastery at each goal needed to move to the next level, (3) controlling each intervention session to focus systematically on the appropriate goal in the hierarchy, and (4) collecting data in each session to determine progress toward the targeted goal.

Linguistic-Cognitive Approaches

Linguistic-cognitive approaches are based on theories of developmental psychology and cognitive science, which emphasize the developmental sequences and underlying rule-governed organization of communicative behavior (Klein & Moses, 1999). These approaches view communication development as the individual's achievement of a set of highly specific rules that inform different categories of communication. For instance, children learn the underlying rule for how to make requests (a category of communication) by combining the verb *want* with any number of actions or objects (e.g., want go, want car, want eat). The linguistic-cognitive perspective suggests that children do not need to be taught every possible way to produce a request; rather, they need only learn the general underlying rule governing this communicative category. This approach is influenced by the work of Noam Chomsky, a linguist who described the underlying grammatical rules of language acquisition, and Jean Piaget, a cognitive psychologist who described the developmental organization of early cognition.

Unlike behaviorist approaches, cognitive-linguistic interventions emphasize the role of the learner over that of the clinician in the intervention process. The learner's interaction with the environment is integral to the process of learning, as it is through interactions with the environment that an individual acquires new rules about effective communication. The extent to which these interactions enhance or accelerate learning is influenced by how the learner perceives, organizes, and interprets new information (Mercer, 1997). The role of the clinician is to study how learners interact with their environment in the learning process and to enhance the environment to promote rule-governed learning.

Linguistic-cognitive approaches to intervention are defined by three general parameters. First, the goals of communicative interventions are derived from knowledge of normal communication development, particularly *when, how,* and *why* individuals use communication. Professionals select and organize goals based on the normal process of communication acquisition and emphasize the interaction between an individual and the environment during communication.

Second, communicative goals focus on helping the individual learn the rules that underlie successful communication. By focusing on general rules rather than a smaller set of highly specific behaviors, linguistic-cognitive approaches attempt to induce an underlying change in communication that can then be applied to a wide variety of situations.

Third, the learner is engaged fully in the intervention process. Cognitive-linguistic approaches emphasize that learning takes place within an individual and that the role of the clinician is to structure the environment to facilitate the individual's induction of rules that govern successful communication. The interventionist's role is to study how an individual perceives, organizes, and applies new information and to guide the learner to more efficient learning (Mercer, 1997).

The delivery of cognitive-linguistic interventions tends to be more client-directed than the delivery of interventions. In client-directed approaches, the client and clinician share control over the materials and the general structure of intervention. The emphasis on greater learner control is consistent with the cognitive-linguistic belief that learners themselves (rather than the clinician) are the critical agents in determining the effectiveness of communicative interventions.

Social-Interactionist Approaches

Social-interactionist approaches are based on theories of developmental psychology, which emphasize the importance of social interactions among individuals as a critical means for development and learning. This approach is strongly influenced by the work of Lev Vygotsky, a Russian psychologist who believed that children's development and learning proceed from a social plane to a psychological plane (see Justice & Ezell, 1999). The **social plane** is the knowledge contained within the interaction between two individuals, whereas the **psychological plane** is the knowledge that one possesses internally and independently.

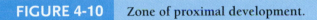

FIGURE 4-10 Zone of proximal development.

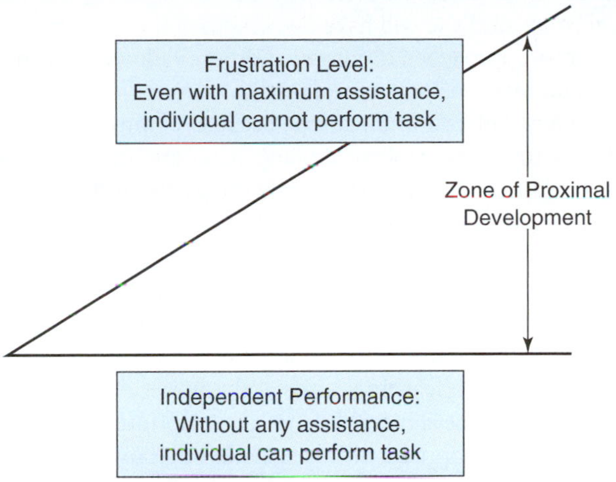

According to Vygotskian theory, all knowledge exists initially on a social plane (in the interactions between two people), and then proceeds to the psychological plane. A concept must first be introduced to an individual on the social plane within the context of social interaction; only after this introduction can a concept move inward to the psychological plane.

Two additional important concepts of Vygotsky's theory that are relevant to communicative interventions are the zone of proximal development, depicted in Figure 4-10, and scaffolding. The **zone of proximal development** refers to the range between an individual's independent performance of a particular skill or behavior (what he or she can do by himself or herself) and the person's level of performance when aided by another person (what he or she can do with assistance). The zone of proximal development represents the skills and knowledge in the process of maturation, or **learning potential. Scaffolding** is the assistance provided by another person to raise an individual's level of performance. Scaffolding provided within an individual's zone of proximal development is a primary vehicle of learning and is viewed as the essential mechanism for social-interactionist interventions.

As an illustration of these three key social-interactionist concepts—social and psychological planes, zone of proximal development, and scaffolding—let's consider a child's knowledge of the linguistic term *in*. How does the child learn the meaning of this term? According to social-interactionist theory, the child is first introduced to the term within an interaction with a more knowledgeable person, such as a parent or older sibling. The child's knowledge of the concept *in* exists at first only within the social plane:

Jen (sibling): Erin, put the candy *in* the box. Put it *in* the box. Like this (puts one piece of candy into the box).

Erin complies, putting one piece of candy into the box.

Jen: Good, Erin. You put it *in*. Now do this one.

Jen probably doesn't know it, but she is providing scaffolding within Erin's zone of proximal development. Erin does not know the term *in* independently—she can't say it, and she doesn't quite understand it—but with help Erin shows knowledge of this term by appropriately acting out its usage with candy and a box. Jen uses a variety of scaffolds to aid Erin's performance: she uses a slow pace with generally simple grammar, she repeats herself, and she emphasizes the key term *in* by increasing her pitch and loudness. Also, she praises Erin's performance and explains to Erin what it is she accomplished. Thus, within the context of this social interaction with her more knowledgeable sibling, Erin is able to comprehend the concept *in*. Importantly, Erin's knowledge of *in* at this point is socially dependent, evident *only* within the social plane. With time, however, Erin's knowledge of *in* will work its way inward to the psychological plane, and she will have ownership of the concept.

Social-interactionist approaches to intervention are defined by three general parameters. First, the goals and methods of communicative interventions emphasize the function, purpose, and social nature of communication. Because communication skills are seen to advance from the social to the psychological plane, goals and methods used in intervention emphasize the social plane as a context for facilitating communication change. Goals are organized to emphasize an individual's engagement with others in socially relevant communication.

Second, communication interventions emphasize the importance of the zone of proximal development as the area in which learning is maximized and hence as the target for intervention. Goals at the lower end of the zone—the person's independent level—are too easy and will not result in much learning; goals at the upper end of the zone—the frustration level—are too hard and not achievable. The clinician must carefully identify an individual's zone of proximal development and ensure that therapy goals are within this zone, called the instructional level because it is where learning takes place.

Third, social-interactionist interventions emphasize the clinician's use of scaffolding as an essential ingredient to delivering effective interventions. Scaffolding allows a learner to perform skills that are within the zone of proximal development, but beyond the level of independent skill. Scaffolds are the nonverbal and verbal support provided by professionals to help the learner complete learning tasks that cannot be achieved independently.

Information-Processing Models

Information-processing approaches are derived from theories of cognitive science, which emphasize how the brain processes information and the interactions between brain processing and various aspects of communication, known as the brain-behavior relationship (Klein & Moses, 1999). The brain-behavior relationship suggests that communication problems are rooted in specific processing limitations. The processing of auditory and linguistic information during communication relies on many cognitive processes, including "encoding, organizing, storing, retrieving, comparing, and generating or reconstructing information" (Chermak & Musiek, 1997). Bottom-up processes are involuntary processes involved with moving perceptual information from the sensory systems toward the brain. Top-down processes are voluntary executive and self-regulatory strategies used to monitor information that has been received from the senses. A limitation in any of these basic processes can undermine effective communication.

During the last several decades, our understanding of how humans process information and how brain injuries or abnormalities affect this processing has advanced considerably. The literature on the processing of auditory information has been particularly influential in the design and delivery of speech, language, and hearing interventions. For instance, speech-language pathologists, audiologists, and special educators now have access to several computer programs designed specifically to help individuals learn to process auditory information in more efficient ways (e.g., Merzenich et al., 1996). However, these programs are not without controversy (Gillam, 1999). A major criticism is that our theoretical knowledge of how the brain processes certain types of information is incomplete and may even be erroneous in some cases (Nittrouer, 1999).

As our understanding of brain processing and neurological organization improves, information-processing approaches are likely to become more influential in the treatment of communication disorders. These approaches focus on identifying the processing limitations that result in communication limitations (Torgesen, 1993) and then enhancing these processes. Remediation is directed to improving specific bottom-up processing abilities of the brain, such as the retrieval of words, discrimination of sounds, or auditory memory. Remediation is also directed to improving top-down processing, such as how to monitor one's own comprehension during communicative interactions. Improvement of bottom-up and top-down processing can be accomplished in several ways, including using technologies or programs designed to promote specific processing skills, heightening an individual's awareness of his or her own processing abilities (and disabilities), and manipulating the environment to improve processing.

CHAPTER SUMMARY

Assessment is the methodological process of gathering information about an individual's background, history, skills, knowledge, perceptions, and feelings. It has four purposes. The first purpose is to identify skills that a person does and does not have in a particular area of communication. The second purpose is to inform a program of intervention designed to enhance a person's skills in a particular area of communication. The third purpose is to monitor a person's communicative growth and performance over time. The fourth purpose is to establish eligibility for special services.

There are six stages of scope and sequence in the assessment process: screening and referral, design of the assessment protocol, administration of the assessment protocol, interpretation of assessment findings, development of an intervention plan, and monitoring of progress and outcomes. Tools for design and administration of the assessment protocol include chart review, interviews, systematic observation, questionnaires and surveys, testing, and instrumentation. The professional's responsibility is to use a variety of instruments so that the assessment protocol is sensitive, comprehensive, and nonbiased.

Intervention is the implementation of a plan of action to improve some aspect of an individual's communicative abilities and includes preventive, remediation, and compensatory approaches. Four categories of intervention, based primarily on theoretical perspectives of communicative development and disorders, include behaviorist, linguistic-cognitive, social-interactionist, and information-processing approaches. Behaviorist approaches, based on classic learning theory, emphasize environmental consequences for influencing change in observable behavior. Linguistic-cognitive approaches are derived from an understanding of normal developmental sequences in communicative acquisition and the underlying rule-governed organization of communication. Social-interactionist approaches are based on the belief that all human communication moves from a social to a psychological plane and that skills emerge through socially meaningful interactions between two or more people. Information-processing approaches focus on the underlying processing mechanisms responsible for communication. Intervention that combines two or more approaches is considered a hybrid approach.

KEY TERMS

age-equivalent scores, p. 124
artifact analysis, p. 125
assessment, p. 108
behaviorist approaches, p. 134
chart review, p. 115
compensation, p. 132
concurrent validity, p. 120
construct validity, p. 120
co-teaching/parallel instruction, p. 134
criterion-referenced assessment, p. 124
criterion-related validity, p. 120
developmental screening, p. 112
differential diagnosis, p. 118
dynamic assessment, p. 126
evidence-based practice, p. 129
face validity, p. 120
information-processing approaches, p. 138
injury-related screening, p. 113
inter-rater reliability, p. 121
intervention, p. 127
intervention consultation, p. 134

intervention goal, p. 132
intervention procedure, p. 132
learning potential, pp. 126, 137
linguistic-cognitive approaches, p. 135
mean, p. 123
multidisciplinary, p. 108
normal curve, p. 123
normative sample, p. 121
norm-referenced assessment, p. 121
online performance, p. 117
percentile rank, p. 124
performance-based assessment, p. 125
portfolio analysis, p. 125
predictive validity, p. 120
preventive intervention, p. 131
psychological plane, p. 136
pull-out/direct service, p. 134
raw score, p. 123
referral, p. 113
reliability, p. 121
remediation, p. 131
scaffolding, p. 137
screening, p. 112
social plane, p. 136
social-interactionist approaches, p. 136
standard deviation, p. 123
standard normal distribution, p. 123
standard score, p. 122
standardization, p. 121
test-retest reliability, p. 121
validity, p. 120
zone of proximal development, p. 137

ON THE WEB

Check out the Companion Website! On it, you will find:

- suggested readings
- reflection questions
- a self-study quiz
- links to additional online resources, including information about current technologies in communication sciences and disorders

PART II

Communication Disorders Across the Lifespan

Phonological Disorders

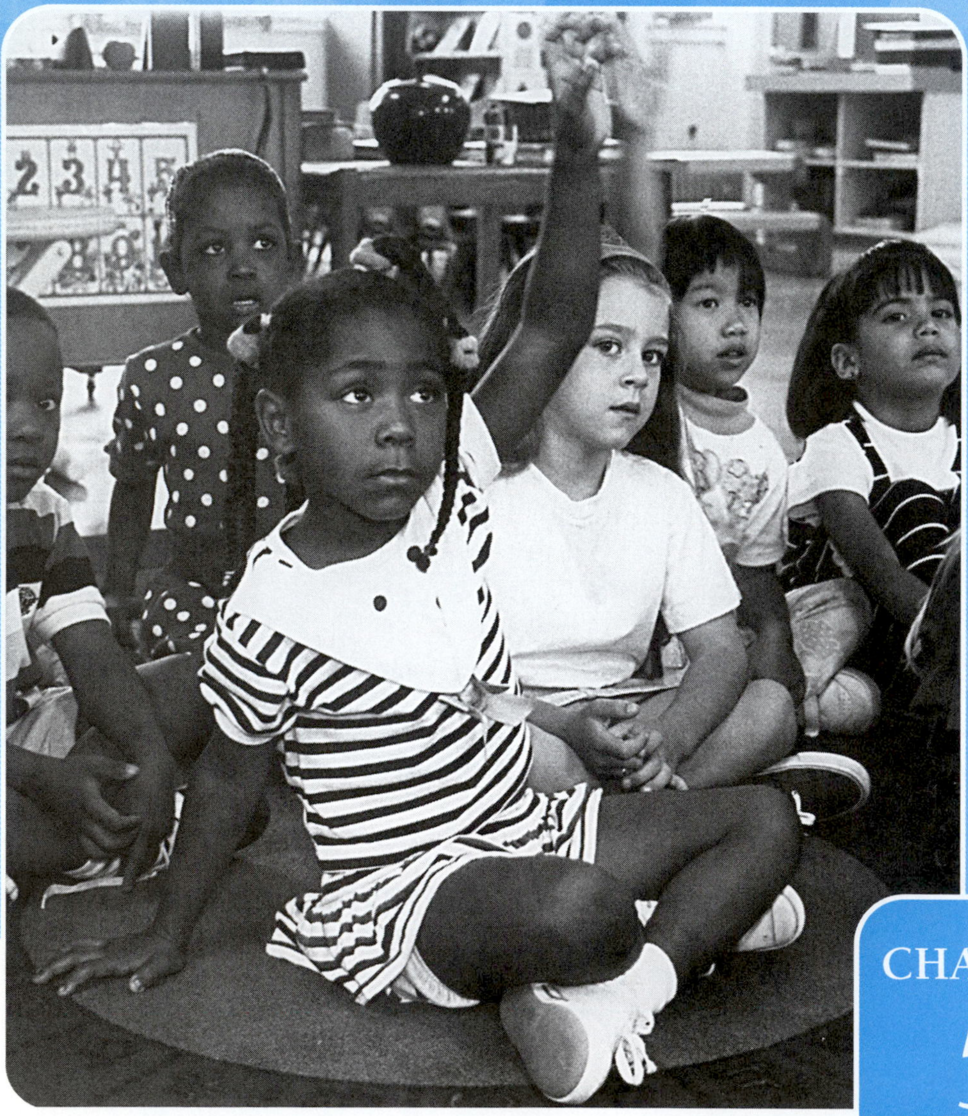

CHAPTER 5

FOCUS QUESTIONS

This chapter answers the following questions:

1. What is a phonological disorder?
2. How are phonological disorders classified?
3. What are the defining characteristics of phonological disorders?
4. How are phonological disorders identified?
5. How are phonological disorders treated?

INTRODUCTION

Phonological disorders are one of the most prevalent types of communication impairment among children. Children with phonological disorders have difficulty developing and using the sounds of their native language, a problem commonly known as **speech delay**. These children make multiple errors in the articulation of specific sounds and sound patterns and are often unintelligible because they produce few words accurately. Unintelligibility can cause marked frustration in very young children because they are unable to communicate their needs and interests to important people in their lives. Consider, for instance, the following interaction between Julie and her mother:

Julie: e-uh an I o-ah mo-y e ou a be

Mother: What? Say it again.

Julie: e-uh an I o-ah mo-y e ou a be

Mother: You want the ear? The mirror? Honey, what?

Julie starts crying and lies down on the floor.

In older children, phonological disorders can affect the ability to communicate effectively with peers and teachers and can undermine the ability to learn critical literacy skills, including reading and spelling.

A phonological disorder becomes evident during the developmental period for speech-sound acquisition, from birth through 9 years of age (Shriberg, 1997). During this period, children develop a keen sensitivity to the rules that govern the phonology of their native language and learn to articulate all the sounds of their language to intelligibly produce words and sentences. As children's phonological growth progresses, they often produce imaginative renditions of words and sounds that display their yet-to-be-perfected phonological and articulation skills. It would not be surprising, for instance, to hear a 2-year-old refer to a computer as a *moocuter* and a tomato as a *motito,* or to hear a 3-year-old say *lellow tun* for "yellow sun" or *over dey-ah* for "over there." Four- and five-year-old children might say *dat* for "that" and *wabbit* for "rabbit." Errors such as these are normal and mark children's ongoing quest

Discussion Point: *Young children's speech is characterized by a number of typical developmental errors in the production of specific sounds. Think about the consonants used by children you know. Which sounds seem to be the hardest for children to develop?*

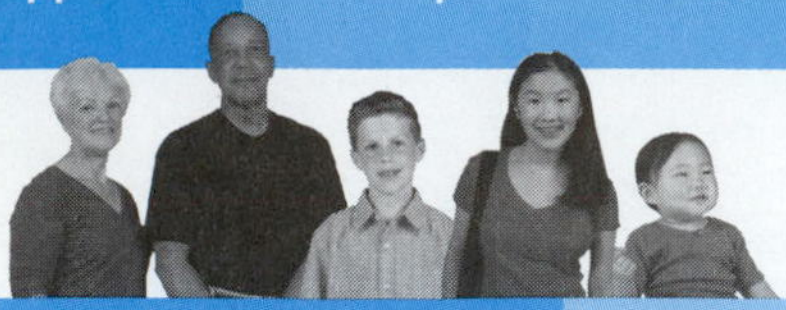

BOX 5-1 Phonological Disorders in Early and Later Childhood: Case Examples

Octavio is a 5-year-old student in Ms. Hudson's kindergarten classroom in San Diego, California. Octavio has only limited proficiency in English as he comes from a home in which Spanish is spoken exclusively. Octavio speaks few words in English in the classroom and does not interact at all with his peers. Octavio works with an English as a Second Language (ESL) teacher, Mr. Peras, who is bilingual in Spanish and English. Both Mr. Peras and Ms. Hudson are concerned about Octavio's speech-sound production, noticing that in both Spanish and English he is very hard to understand. In English, for instance, he says *obby* for doggy and *aa-oo* for "bathroom." Mr. Peras and Ms. Hudson have asked the speech-language pathologist to come to the kindergarten classroom and observe Octavio for an evaluation. They have also called for a child study meeting to begin the process of referral for a formal speech-language evaluation.

Internet research

1. What proportion of children in California's schools speaks Spanish as a first language?
2. Octavio's ESL teacher is bilingual, but his teacher is not. How likely is it that a teacher in an American elementary classroom of primarily Spanish-speaking children would not speak Spanish?

Brainstorm and discussion

1. What strategies can be used to identify whether Octavio's suspected phonological difficulties are the result of a speech difference or a speech disorder?
2. What are some strategies Ms. Hudson might use in the classroom to promote Octavio's successful communication with his classmates?

Emily is a 9-year-old who has received speech-language therapy for as long as she can remember. She has always struggled with producing certain sounds, and still has problems producing /l/ and /r/. Emily has always valued working with the speech-language pathologist at her school and feels that she is making good, although slow, progress. This year, Emily's drama teacher is encouraging her to audition for a role in the school play, *Much Ado about Nothing.* Emily is hopeful that by the time auditions come around her speech problems will be completely resolved. Recently, Emily's parents were informed that Emily was no longer eligible for speech services at school as her speech problems did not impact her educational performance. School officials explained that they could not provide services unless the effects of Emily's speech difficulties had clear educational impact. Emily has asked her parents if she can see a speech-language pathologist privately, but they cannot afford it, and their insurance will not cover it. Emily is very concerned about her upcoming audition and is considering backing out.

Internet research

1. How many children receiving special education services at school participate in extracurricular activities such as school plays?
2. What percentage of children in the early elementary grades qualify for special education services? What amount of the federal budget for education is directed toward special education services for children?
3. What does the term *educational impact* mean in schools when determining whether a child is eligible for special education services?

toward mastery of phonology and articulation. Such errors are systematic, predictable, and typical for this important period of speech-sound development. For roughly 90 to 95% of young children, they do not impact speech intelligibility, nor do they cause breakdowns in children's communication with others.

For a small but consequential portion of children, phonological development proceeds much more slowly, and early achievements in phonology and articulation are marked by great difficulty and unintelligibility. When children's speech is unintelligible, their ability to

Brainstorm and discussion

1. What does the term *educational impact* mean to you? What are some obvious and less obvious ways that a communication disorder can affect a child's educational performance?
2. Emily's parents are considering appealing to the school to pursue her right to special education services. Do you think they will be successful in their appeal? What factors might affect the likelihood of success?

Barcley is a 22-year-old single mother in St. Louis, Missouri. Barcley is attending the local Adult Education Literacy Center (AELC) as part of a social services program in which she participates. Barcley goes to AELC three nights a week for 2 hours and works on developing basic reading skills. She has considered herself dyslexic her whole life and has always had problems with even basic skills, like remembering the names of the letters of the alphabet. When she was a child, she also had lots of problems talking, and she recalls seeing a speech therapist to work on making different sounds. A new teacher in the center, Ms. Shan, was formerly a reading specialist in the city school system. Ms. Shan has been working with Barcley for the last 2 weeks on learning the alphabet letters and practicing the sounds that go with the letters. Ms. Shan believes that Barcley might have a serious problem with phonological awareness, and she gave Barcley a few tasks to test her hypothesis, like making rhymes *(cat, hat)* and identifying when two words share the same first sound *(hat, hope)*. Barcley could not do any of these activities and told Ms. Shan that she had "never been able to rhyme." Ms. Shan has a program she used to use with first graders that helped them develop phonological awareness, and she wants Barcley to go through the 36 lessons of this program. Barcley is definitely game and hopes to start next week.

Internet research

1. What proportion of adult Americans are unable to read at a basic level?
2. What types of community resources are commonly available for adults who cannot read?

Brainstorm and discussion

1. What might the connection be between Barcley's early problems with speech production and her current problems with reading?
2. What kinds of activities might be included in Barcley's phonological awareness training program? What is the goal of such a program?
3. In your opinion, how likely is it that Barcley will become a reader at age 22? What factors will most affect the likelihood of her success?

communicate with those in their lives is compromised, and there can be long-standing consequences for literacy and social performance when they enter school. Although phonological disorders often accompany physical and developmental disabilities, such as hearing impairment and mental retardation, for the majority of children with significant phonological disorders the cause is unknown. Chapter 5 provides an overview of the characteristics of phonological disorders and describes assessment and treatment options for children with these disorders.

What Is a Phonological Disorder?

Definition

A **phonological disorder** is an impairment of an individual's phonological system resulting in a significant problem with speech-sound production that differs from age- and culturally based expectations. The onset of the disorder occurs prior to 9 years of age, and its cause may be known or unknown (Shriberg, Kwiatkowski, & Gruber, 1994). The term **articulation disorder**, often used interchangeably with the term *phonological disorder*, emphasizes the impact of the disorder on an individual's ability to articulate certain speech sounds effectively (Bauman-Waengler, 2004). The term *phonological disorder* is the preferred term to emphasize that the articulation disturbance results from an impaired phonological system.

Recall from chapter 1 that phonology is the part of the language system that governs its sound structure. Phonology includes the inventory of sounds used in a particular language and the set of rules governing how these are combined to make meaningful units (e.g., syllables and words) (Bauman-Waengler, 2004). As their phonological systems develop, children acquire a representation of each phoneme in their native language as well as the rules that govern how these phonemes are arranged into syllables and words. Children develop boundaries around each phoneme that differentiate the phonemes from one another in the phonological system. For instance, in English, /r/ and /l/ have boundaries that separate them, whereas in Mandarin Chinese there is no such boundary, and these are considered a single phoneme.

Two important aspects of phonological development are therefore (1) developing a representation for each phoneme in one's language and (2) developing a solid (or crisp) boundary around each phoneme to make it distinct from the other phonemes. The boundary is particularly important for phonemes that are similar, such as /t/ and /d/ and /f/ and /v/. The boundary between these **cognates**—two phonemes that differ by only one characteristic (voicing for these examples)—needs to be especially solid for their differentiation.

If the phonological system develops too slowly, children experience a delay in the acquisition of internal phonological representations and have difficulty creating boundaries between phonemes (Nittrouer, 1996). These problems with the phonological system can result in mild to profound problems producing individual speech sounds and using these speech sounds in syllables and words for conversational speech. The most common symptom of this disorder is unintelligibility.

Prevalence and Incidence

Prevalence and *incidence* are epidemiological terms used to describe the number of cases of a condition among the population. *Prevalence* describes the percentage of persons who have exhibited a disorder in their lifetime, whereas *incidence* estimates the percentage of persons who exhibit a disorder at a given time.

Estimates of the prevalence of phonological disorders indicate that 4% to 13% of children are affected, with recent research supporting the lower estimate of about 4 in 100 children (Shriberg, Tomblin, & McSweeney, 1999). Phonological disorders affect boys at slightly higher rates than girls, 4.5% versus 3%. Estimates also suggest that African American children exhibit phonological disorders at slightly higher rates (5.3%) than do European American children (3.8%) (Shriberg et al., 1999). In the majority of cases (60%), the phonological disorder cannot be attributed to any known cause; about 40% of cases are associated with recurrent middle-ear infections, developmental motor speech disorders (described in Chapter 6), and other developmental disorders, such as Down syndrome (Shriberg, 1997).

Discussion Point: *Young boys are affected with phonological disorders at slightly higher rates than are girls. Brainstorm some possible explanations for this phenomenon.*

Terminology

Phonological versus Articulation Disorders

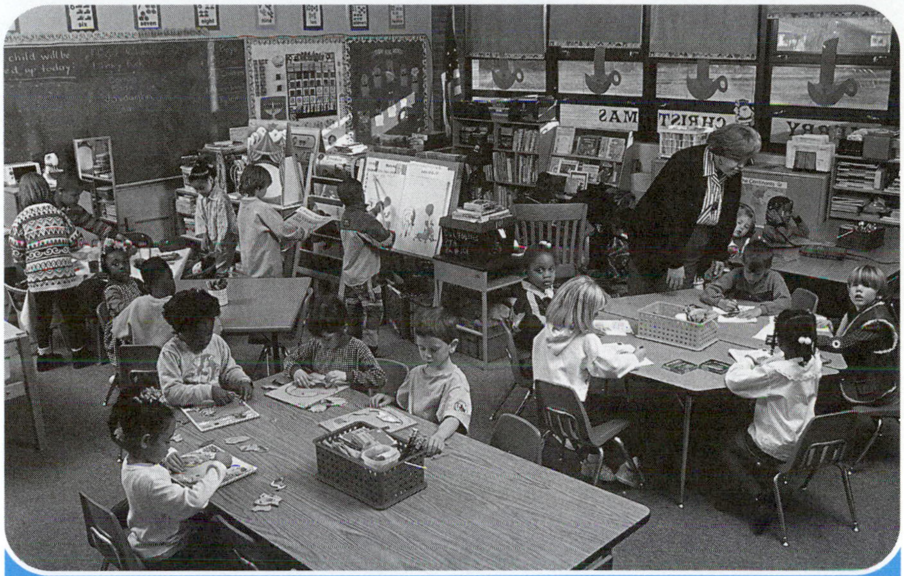

Phonological disorders affect boys at slightly higher rates than girls.

Speech-language pathologists (SLPs) were historically called speech teachers because of their focus on treating speech-sound problems. Although much has changed in the treatment of communication disorders over the last several decades, treatment of speech-sound problems remains one of the most common activities of speech teachers, now called speech-language pathologists. Because of their prevalence, speech-sound problems are also one of the most heavily researched childhood communication disorders.

Changes in the terminology used to describe speech-sound problems mirrors our increasing knowledge about the bases for speech delays. Until recently, the terms *articulation disorder* and *speech disorder* prevailed in the literature describing significant speech-sound problems in children, and these terms are still often used. The use of the term *articulation* emphasized the perspective that speech-sound problems resulted from a motor problem affecting the positioning of the articulators (tongue, lips, teeth, etc.). Consequently, traditional approaches to treatment focused on speech correction—helping children to improve their articulatory patterns by remediating one sound at a time (van Riper, 1963).

Research in the 1970s increasingly emphasized a linguistic perspective that viewed articulation problems as rooted in the phonological system specifically and the language system more generally (Elbert, 1997). Figure 5-1 provides a contemporary model of speech production that depicts the link between phonological representations and speech output, or articulation. A linguistic perspective of disordered speech views the problem as emerging from the level of phonological representation. Children's faulty phonological representations result in immature but systematic phonological productions. Although on the surface such children have difficulties articulating sounds, the problem results from delays in the maturation of the underlying phonological system. This perspective emphasizes the importance of considering both the **surface representation** and the **underlying representation** of phonology—what we produce (articulation) and the underlying representation (phonology). Increasingly, treatment for phonological disorders focuses on building and reorganizing children's phonological representations rather than improving the surface articulation of specific speech sounds.

These shifting perspectives have influenced the terminology used to describe significant speech disorders affecting children. *Phonological disorder, developmental phonological disorder,* and *phonological impairment* are the current preferred terms (Shriberg, 1997). Likewise, terms used to describe assessment and treatment for speech-sound disorders also emphasize a phonological perspective. These include *phonological assessment* and *phonological analysis,* which describe clinical tools to evaluate the organization of an individual's phonological system, and *phonological remediation* and *phonological intervention,* which describe the process clinicians use to bring about change in an individual's phonological system.

FIGURE 5-1 Model of speech production.

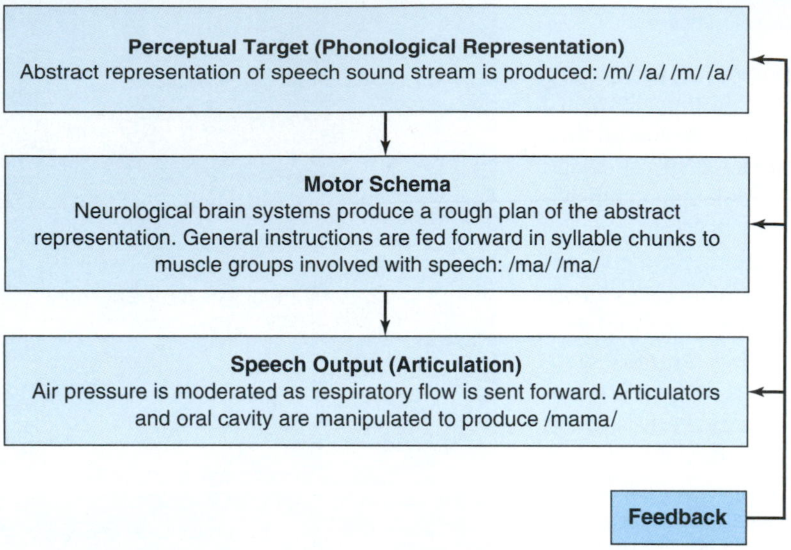
Perceptual Target (Phonological Representation)
Abstract representation of speech sound stream is produced: /m/ /a/ /m/ /a/
Motor Schema
Neurological brain systems produce a rough plan of the abstract representation. General instructions are fed forward in syllable chunks to muscle groups involved with speech: /ma/ /ma/
Speech Output (Articulation)
Air pressure is moderated as respiratory flow is sent forward. Articulators and oral cavity are manipulated to produce /mama/
Feedback

Source: Adapted with permission from Borden, G. J., Harris, K. S., & Raphael, L. J. (1994). *Speech science primer: Physiology, acoustics, and perception of speech* (3rd ed.). Baltimore: Williams & Wilkins.

The term *phonological disorder* does not capture all varieties of speech-sound problems in children. Chapter 6 describes two other prevalent childhood disorders that impact the production of speech sounds: apraxia and dysarthria. Unlike phonological disorders, apraxia and dysarthria are disorders of the motor functions that affect articulation planning and delivery; thus, these are considered motor speech disorders rather than phonological disorders.

Describing Phonology and Articulation

Knowledge of a number of key concepts is necessary to discuss phonological disorders and their impact on articulation. These are presented next.

Phonemes as Contrasts

Recall from Chapter 1 that every language has a relatively small number of sounds, called phonemes, and that Standard American English (SAE) uses about 40 phonemes to create its thousands of words. SAE speakers actually use many more sounds, but these sounds are not considered phonemes. For instance, the /p/ in *pig* is subtly different from the /p/ in *map*. Despite being produced differently, however, these two variations of /p/ are not different phonemes; rather, they are allophones. **Allophones** are the variations of a single phoneme.

__Discussion Point:__ This chapter describes the abstract concept of phonological representation, which is a difficult concept for some students to understand. Spend a few moments creating your own definition of this term, and share it with a peer.

To be considered a phoneme, a speech sound must be able to signal a contrast in meaning between two words of a language. This property of phonemes is called contrastiveness. We know, therefore, that /b/ and /p/ are two different phonemes in English, as they signal a meaning contrast in words that share all other sounds, such as *bat* and *pat*, *big* and *pig*, and *rip* and *rib*. During the developmental period of speech-sound acquisition, children form an underlying representation of each phoneme—a phonological representation—that establishes its contrast to other phonemes.

The International Phonetic Alphabet

Any discussion of speech sounds and phonological disorders requires at least a basic knowledge of the International Phonetic Alphabet (IPA). The **IPA** is a phonetic alphabet that describes and classifies each speech sound on the basis of how and where it is produced in the speech mechanism. The IPA is the most commonly used system to represent the phonemes making up the world's languages. It is used by SLPs, linguists, educators, and others to transcribe children's speech patterns.

The IPA represents each phoneme used in the world's languages—both vowels and consonants—as a specific symbol. When IPA symbols are used to transcribe an individual's speech production, each sound is represented by a symbol and the transcription is usually placed between slashes (e.g., /bIg/ for *big*). The IPA is presented in Figure 5-2. Each of the consonant phonemes is presented in the top chart, and the vowels are presented in the lower left-hand corner. Figure 5-3 provides a list of the IPA symbols used to transcribe the American English consonants.

Articulatory Phonetics

Examination of the IPA chart may reveal some unfamiliar terms, such as *bilabial, labiodental, fricative,* and *trill*. These terms characterize and classify the articulatory features of different phonemes. An articulatory feature serves as a road map to what the articulators are doing when a phoneme is produced. The classification of speech sounds in this way is called **articulatory phonetics**.

One important articulatory feature of a speech sound is whether it is a vowel or a consonant. Vowels and consonants differ primarily in the extent of constriction in the oral cavity when the sound is produced. With a **vowel**, there is relatively little constriction against the airflow in the oral cavity, whereas with a **consonant**, the airflow is constricted in some way—this is their defining feature. For instance, with /t/ and /d/, the constriction occurs when the tongue strikes against the alveolar ridge. With /m/, /b/, and /p/, the constriction occurs when the top and bottom lips press together. With /h/, the constriction occurs in the glottal area near the vocal folds.

Vowels. Each vowel is characterized by three articulatory features:

1. *Height:* How high is the tongue placed when the vowel is produced? Vowels are classified as high, mid, or low.
2. *Frontness:* How far forward is the tongue placed when the vowel is produced? Vowels are classified as front, central, or back.
3. *Roundness:* Are the lips rounded when the vowel is produced? Vowels are classified as rounded or unrounded. Only vowels characterized as back on the frontness dimension are rounded. (Lowe, 1994)

For example, the features for /I/ (as in *pin*) are (1) the tongue is high in the oral cavity, (2) the tongue is forward in the oral cavity, and (3) the lips are unrounded. Table 5-1 describes these characteristics for each vowel in the Standard American English vowel system.

Consonants. Consonants are also characterized by three key articulatory features, although the dimensions by which they are classified differ from those of vowels.

1. **Place of articulation:** Where in the oral cavity or vocal tract is the constriction when the consonant is produced? Consonants are classified as bilabial, labiodental, interdental, alveolar, palatal, velar, or glottal.

FIGURE 5-2 The International Phonetic Alphabet.

CONSONANTS (PULMONIC)

	Bilabial	Labiodental	Dental	Alveolar	Postalveolar	Retroflex	Palatal	Velar	Uvular	Pharyngeal	Glottal
Plosive	p b			t d		ʈ ɖ	c ɟ	k g	q ɢ		ʔ
Nasal	m	ɱ		n		ɳ	ɲ	ŋ	ɴ		
Trill	ʙ			r					ʀ		
Tap or Flap				ɾ		ɽ					
Fricative	ɸ β	f v	θ ð	s z	ʃ ʒ	ʂ ʐ	ç ʝ	x ɣ	χ ʁ	ħ ʕ	h ɦ
Lateral fricative				ɬ ɮ							
Approximant		ʋ		ɹ		ɻ	j	ɰ			
Lateral approximant				l		ɭ	ʎ	ʟ			

Where symbols appear in pairs, the one to the right represents a voiced consonant. Shaded areas denote articulations judged impossible.

CONSONANTS (NON-PULMONIC)

Clicks		Voiced implosives		Ejectives	
ʘ	Bilabial	ɓ	Bilabial	ʼ	as in:
ǀ	Dental	ɗ	Dental/alveolar	pʼ	Bilabial
ǃ	(Post)alveolar	ʄ	Palatal	tʼ	Dental/alveolar
ǂ	Palatoalveolar	ɠ	Velar	kʼ	Velar
ǁ	Alveolar lateral	ʛ	Uvular	sʼ	Alveolar fricative

VOWELS

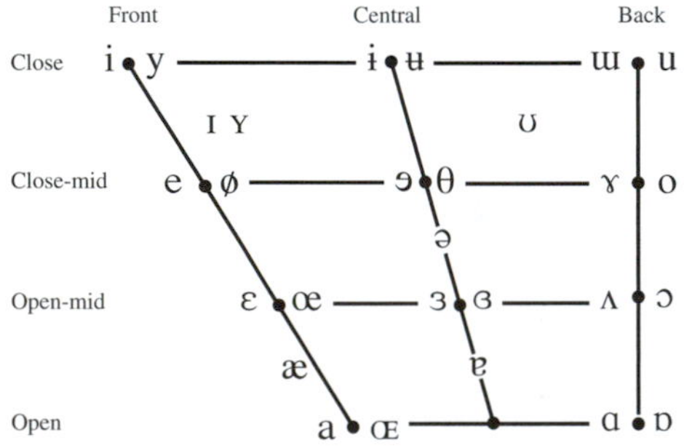

Where symbols appear in pairs, the one to the right represents a rounded vowel.

OTHER SYMBOLS

ʍ	Voiceless labial-velar fricative
w	Voiced labial-velar approximant
ɥ	Voiced labial-palatal approximant
ʜ	Voiceless epiglottal fricative
ʢ	Voiced epiglottal fricative
ʡ	Epiglottal plosive
ɕ ʑ	Alveolo-palatal fricatives
ɺ	Alveolar lateral flap
ɧ	Simultaneous ʃ and x

Affricates and double articulations can be represented by two symbols joined by a tie bar if necessary.

k͡p t͡s

SUPRASEGMENTALS

ˈ	Primary stress	ˌfoʊnəˈtɪʃən
ˌ	Secondary stress	
ː	Long	eː
ˑ	Half-long	eˑ
˘	Extra-short	ĕ
.	Syllable break	ɹi.ækt
|	Minor (foot) group	
‖	Major (intonation) group	
‿	Linking (absence of a break)	

TONES & WORD ACCENTS

LEVEL			CONTOUR		
e̋ or	˥	Extra high	ě or	˩˥	Rising
é	˦	High	ê	˥˩	Falling
ē	˧	Mid	e᷄	˦˥	High rising
è	˨	Low	e᷅	˩˨	Low rising
ȅ	˩	Extra low	e᷈	˧˦˧	Rising-falling etc.
↓		Downstep	↗		Global rise
↑		Upstep	↘		Global fall

DIACRITICS

Diacritics may be placed above a symbol with a descender, e.g. ŋ̊

◌̥	Voiceless	n̥ d̥	◌̤	Breathy voiced	b̤ a̤	◌̪	Dental	t̪ d̪
◌̬	Voiced	s̬ t̬	◌̰	Creaky voiced	b̰ a̰	◌̺	Apical	t̺ d̺
ʰ	Aspirated	tʰ dʰ	◌̼	Linguolabial	t̼ d̼	◌̻	Laminal	t̻ d̻
◌̹	More rounded	ɔ̹	ʷ	Labialized	tʷ dʷ	◌̃	Nasalized	ẽ
◌̜	Less rounded	ɔ̜	ʲ	Palatalized	tʲ dʲ	ⁿ	Nasal release	dⁿ
◌̟	Advanced	u̟	ˠ	Velarized	tˠ dˠ	ˡ	Lateral release	dˡ
◌̠	Retracted	i̠	ˤ	Pharyngealized	tˤ dˤ	◌̚	No audible release	d̚
◌̈	Centralized	ë	◌̴	Velarized or pharyngealized ɫ				
◌̽	Mid-centralized	e̽	◌̝	Raised	e̝ (ɹ̝ = voiced alveolar fricative)			
◌̩	Syllabic	ɹ̩	◌̞	Lowered	e̞ (β̞ = voiced bilabial approximant)			
◌̯	Non-syllabic	e̯	◌̘	Advanced Tongue Root	e̘			
˞	Rhoticity	ɚ	◌̙	Retracted Tongue Root	e̙			

Source: Reprinted with permission from The International Phonetic Alphabet (updated 1996). Copyright 1996 by International Phonetic Association, http://www.arts.gla.ac.uk/IPA/ipa.html.

FIGURE 5-3 IPA symbols for consonant phonemes of Standard American English.

b	bat	r	rose
p	pat	s	sun
d	dip	ʃ	shine
t	tip	t	toast
g	give	tʃ	church
h	hot	θ	think
j	yes	ð	that
k	cat	v	vet
l	lot	w	wash
m	mine	z	zag
n	nose	ʒ	treasure
ŋ	ring	ʤ	jail

2. **Manner of articulation:** How is the consonant produced and/or how is the airflow manipulated by the articulators? Consonants are classified as stop, nasal, fricative, affricate, liquid, or glide.
3. **Voicing:** Are the vocal folds vibrating during production of the consonant? Consonants are characterized as voiced or unvoiced.

Table 5-2 depicts the consonants of Standard American English on these features, and Figure 5-4 is a guide to thinking about these characteristics for the consonant /s/.

TABLE 5-1 Vowels, characterized by three articulatory features

Vowel Symbol	Example	Articulatory Features
i	feet	high, front, unrounded
I	fit	high, front, unrounded
e	make	mid, front, unrounded
ɛ	bet	mid, front, unrounded
æ	cat	low, front, unrounded
a	father	low, front, unrounded
u	blue	high, back, rounded
ʊ	hoof	high, back, rounded
ɔ	bought	mid, back, rounded
o	go	mid, back, rounded
ɑ	box	low, back, unrounded
ʌ	bug	mid, central, unrounded
ə	around	mid, central, unrounded
ɝ	bird	mid, central, unrounded
ɚ	father	mid, central unrounded

TABLE 5-2 Place, manner, and voicing features of consonants

Consonant Feature	Categories	Description	Examples in English
Place of Articulation			
	Labial	Lips are site of constriction	/b/, /m/, /w/
	Dental	Teeth are site of constriction	/f/, /ɵ/ð
	Alveolar	Alveolar ride is site of constriction	/s/, /t/, /n/
	Palatal	Hard palate is site of constriction	/ʃ/, /j/
	Velar	Soft palate is site of constriction	/k/, /g/, /ŋ/
	Glottal	Glottis in the vocal fold area is site of constriction	/h/
Manner of Articulation			
	Stop (Plosive)	Airflow is completely stopped somewhere in the vocal tract; air pressure builds up to be released in a quick burst; also called plosives.	/p/, /b/, /t/k
	Fricative	Airflow is continually forced through a tiny fissure in the vocal tract	/f/, /z/, /s/, /h/ð
	Nasal	Airflow is channeled into the nasal cavity by lowering the velum (soft palate)	/m/, /n/, /ŋ/
	Affricate	Airflow is completed stopped in the vocal track; air pressure is build up and then released in a continuous stream through a tiny fissure in the vocal track (a stop followed by a fricative)	/tʃ/, /ʤ/
	Glide	Articulators are held more open than for other consonants; in their production, articulators glide from a constricted to a more open position; also called approximants	/w/, /j/
	Liquid	Tongue is held tight at midline with openings laterally; airflow moves around the sides of the tongue.	/l/, /r/
Voicing			
	Voiced	The vocal folds vibrate during when airflow is pushed over the vocal folds during speech.	/z/, /b/, /v/, /r/
	Unvoiced	The vocal folds do not vibrate and are held open (are approximated) when airflow is pushed over the vocal folds during speech.	/s/, /p/, /f/, /t/

FIGURE 5-4 Thinking about place, manner, and voicing for consonant production.

1. Locate the place of articulation for /s/, or where the constriction occurs in the vocal tract when /s/ is produced. Produce a few other sounds, such as /m/ and /g/, to think about where different sounds are produced. Note then that the constriction for /s/ occurs at the site where the tongue rests against the alveolar ridge. (By comparison, the constriction for /m/ occurs forward at the lips, and for /g/ occurs back on the hard palate.) Sounds that are created at the alveolar ridge are called *alveolars;* accordingly, /s/ is an alveolar phoneme. Can you think of any other sounds in English that are created by making a constriction at the alveolar ridge?
2. Identify the manner of articulation for /s/, or how it is produced. It might be helpful to compare the production of /s/ with other sounds, such as /t/ and /m/. Notice that when producing /s/, a tight constriction is formed in the mouth and the airflow is channeled through this constriction. (By contrast, /t/ is produced by forcing a complete stoppage of air followed by a quick release, whereas /m/ is produced by forcing a vibrating column of air into the nasal cavity.) Sounds that are produced this way are called *fricatives,* of which /s/ is one.
3. Determine whether your vocal folds are vibrating for /s/. Is it a voiced sound? Or is it unvoiced? The easiest way to identify whether /s/ is voiced or unvoiced is by holding your palm across the front of your throat and producing a long "ssss." In doing so, you will not feel any vibration of the vocal folds, showing /s/ to be an unvoiced consonant. By contrast, produce a long "zzzz" to feel the vocal folds' vibration, and note that /z/ is a voiced sound.

Now, do the same activity for several more phonemes. Work with a peer to describe place, manner, and voicing for /d/, /m/, and /t/. Do you arrive at the description provided in Table 5-2 for these consonants?

Children's Acquisition of Consonants

Children follow a fairly predictable path in acquiring the English phonemes, as discussed in Chapter 2 and shown in Table 5-3. The 24 consonant phonemes of English can be further divided into three groups on the basis of when they are typically acquired: Early 8, Middle 8, and Late 8 (see Table 5-4) (Shriberg, Kwiatkowski, & Gruber, 1994). Children who are developing

TABLE 5-3 Development of the phonemic inventory during early childhood

	Groups of Sounds		
Period of Development	**Labial and Dental Consonants**	**Alveolar Consonants**	**Palatal and Velar Consonants**
18 months to 24 months	m p b w	n t d	
24 months to 30 months	m p b w	n t d	h k g ŋ
30 months to 42 months	m p b w f	n t d s	h k g j ŋ
42 months to 54 months	m p b w f v w	n t d s z l	h k g j ʃ ŋ
54 months and older	m p b w f v w θ ð	n t d s z l r	h k g j l ʃ ŋ ʤ ʒ tʃ

Source: Adapted with permission from Grunwell, P. (1987). *Clinical phonology* (2nd ed.). Baltimore: Williams & Wilkins.

their phonology normally master the Early 8 phonemes by about 3 years of age, the Middle 8 phonemes by about age 4, and the Late 8 phonemes by age 6½. For children exhibiting speech delays, progress is much slower; for instance, although typically developing children have mastered the Early 8 phonemes by about 3 years of age, children with phonological disorders may not achieve mastery until age 7 (Shriberg, Kwiatkowski, & Gruber, 1994).

Sounds and Syllables

Assessment and treatment of phonological disorders often focus on describing how a child produces (or doesn't produce) individual sounds, but it is also necessary to consider how sounds are used in syllables, words, and sentences. This is the context, or the phonological environment in which a sound is used. Often, the context in which a sound is used influences how it is produced. For instance, the /t/ in *tea* is produced differently than the /t/ in *too;* note how the /t/ in *tea* is produced with the lips drawn back into a smile (influenced by the high, front, unrounded features of the vowel), whereas the /t/ in *too* is produced with rounded lips (influenced by the high, mid, rounded features of the vowel). These two variations of the /t/ phoneme occur because of coarticulation. **Coarticulation** explains how the articulatory characteristics of phonemes vary according to context and how sounds overlap one another during articulation (Liberman, 1998). Although we might think that speech production involves the production of a series of discrete, individual sounds (e.g., /t/ + /I/ + /p/) that are linked to make words, in articulation these sounds do not exist as discrete entities; rather, the individual sounds are smeared across the entire word (Liberman, 1998).

Assimilation is another concept important to understanding phonology, and it also describes a phenomenon involving the influence of context on the production of specific sounds. **Assimilation** describes how the features of one sound take on the features of neighboring sounds. In the word *man*, for instance, the vowel /æ/ is influenced by the nasal features of the surrounding /m/ and /n/, and it becomes nasalized. When children are developing their phonology, they make many errors that are attributable to assimilation, such as saying *goggy* for "doggie" and *lellow* for "yellow". The sound substitutions (/g/ for /d/ and /l/ for /j/) mirror other sounds in the words—the result of assimilation.

Phonology and Literacy

To learn to read, children must unlock the alphabetic code that forms the basis for written English. The **alphabetic code** is the symbolic relationships between letters of the alphabet and the sounds of spoken language that they represent. The sound-symbol relationship between letters and sounds (for instance, the letter *k* and the sound it makes, /k/) is called **grapheme-phoneme correspondence**. The instruction children receive to help them learn about sound-symbol relationships is called **phonics**. Phonics is a necessary part of a balanced literacy program and is particularly critical for children who have difficulties unlocking the alphabetic code on their own.

TABLE 5-4 Three groups of phonemes

		Age of Mastery for Group	
Phoneme Group	**Phonemes**	**Typical Children**	**Speech Delay**
Early 8	m, b, j, n, w, d, p, h	3 years	7 years
Middle 8	t, ŋ, k, g, f, v, tʃ, ʤ	4 years	8 years
Late 8	ʃ, s, z, ɵ, ð, r, ʒ	6.5 years	>12 years

Source: Adapted with permission from Shriberg, L. D., Kwiatkowski, J., & Gruber, F. A. (1994). Developmental phonological disorders: II Short-term speech-sound normalization. *Journal of Speech and Hearing Research, 37,* 1127–1150.

Phonics instruction typically begins in kindergarten and continues into first and second grade. It gives children the tools they need to decode words. Decoding is the child's use of knowledge about grapheme-phoneme correspondence to read words. To profit from phonics instruction, children must have adequate sensitivity to the phonology of their language, and they must have knowledge of the print system used to represent that phonology, which for English is the alphabet. **Phonological awareness** is the child's awareness of how running speech can be broken into smaller phonological components (Justice & Schuele, 2004). For instance, the spoken string *I am hungry* consists of three words, four syllables, and eight phonemes. At about 3 or 4 years of age, children become sensitive to the word and syllable segments of speech. For instance, a 3-year-old child might break the word *butterfly* into three syllables, showing awareness of phonological units of words. At about 5 or 6 years of age, children recognize the phonemic nature of spoken language—that words and syllables can be broken into phonemes (e.g., *cat* is made up of three sounds). Children with underdeveloped phonological awareness often struggle during phonics instruction and consequently develop reading skills more slowly than other children. This puts children at risk for reading disabilities and academic difficulty (Torgesen, Wagner, & Rashotte, 1994).

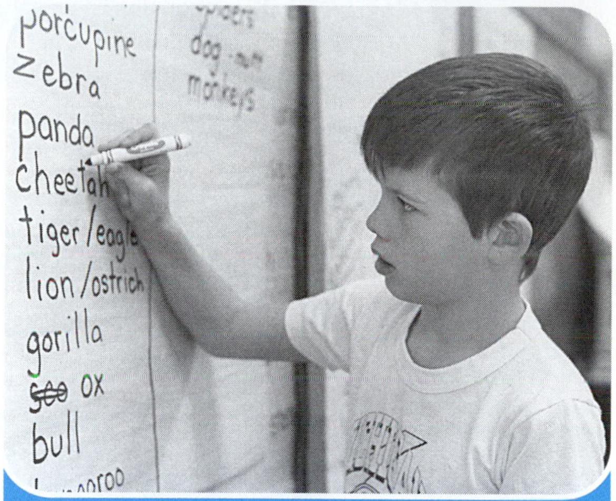

The phonological system enables children to unlock the alphabet code.

The relationship among phonological disorders, problems with speech-sound production, and difficulties with phonological awareness is not straightforward. On the one hand, some children with phonological disorders do not have problems developing phonological awareness. On the other hand, some children have difficulties with phonological awareness but do not have a problem with speech-sound production (Dodd et al., 1995). Despite the lack of clear overlap between these two types of developmental challenges, both stem from an underlying problem with the development of phonological representations. In some cases, the weak phonological representations result in a problem with speech-sound production; in others, they produce a problem with phonological awareness. For some children, problems in both areas occur. Monitoring the development of phonological awareness for all children, including those with phonological disorders, is important for ensuring that children are able to develop reading skills and phonics knowledge as effortlessly and fluently as possible.

Discussion Point:
Phonological disorders and reading problems appear to co-occur in a number of children. Consider the case of Octavio in Box 5-1. If he has a phonological disorder, how would you expect it to impact his reading development in kindergarten and first grade?

How Are Phonological Disorders Classified?

Differentiating Phonological Disorders from Other Speech-Sound Disorders

The primary symptom of many communication disorders is a problem with speech-sound production. Not all instances of speech-sound problems result from a faulty phonological system; some speech-sound problems result, for instance, from motor and muscular disturbances. The two major indicators of a defective phonological system are

1. Immature or inaccurate representations of individual phonemes or groups of phonemes
2. Immature or ineffective organization of phonemes within the larger phonological system

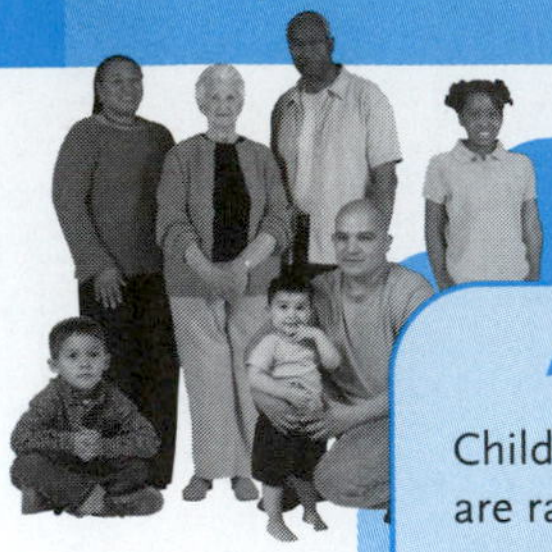

BOX 5-2 Multicultural Focus

Assessing Phonology In Bilingual Children

Children in the United States are a uniquely diverse group both culturally and linguistically. They are raised in homes that vary widely in their values, practices, beliefs, customs, dialects, and languages. One goal of U.S. education is to ensure that all schoolchildren, regardless of cultural and linguistic background, develop a basic level of English proficiency in speaking, listening, reading, and writing to ensure their success at home, at school, and in the larger community. Developing the English communication skills of children who come to school speaking languages other than English is a challenge for educators, particularly when those children have disabilities that affect their ability to communicate, such as phonological disorders.

When working with culturally and linguistically diverse youngsters and their families to develop intervention programs, educators must focus on understanding families' strengths, needs, and beliefs. Special attention is directed toward three areas: (1) emphasizing family strengths and natural support networks, (2) understanding families' perceptions of disability and communication, and (3) ensuring the flexibility of the design of the educational program. The concepts described in the following sections are derived from suggestions and questions provided by Bennett, Zhang, and Hojnar (1998).

Emphasize family strengths and natural support networks. The strengths and natural supports available to families must be reflected in the educational plans developed for culturally and linguistically diverse children with phonological disorders. Questions educators should ask include (1) Does the educational plan respect the family's existing family structure (e.g., single-parent family, extended family under one roof)? and (2) Does the educational plan build on informal support networks available to the family (e.g., multigenerational relationships)?

Understand the families' perceptions of disability and communication. How a communicative disability, such as phonological impairment, is viewed by a family should be carefully considered when developing educational plans. Perspectives of communicative proficiency and disability are highly influenced by one's cultural background. When devising educational plans for culturally

Obviously, we cannot look at the representations and organization of the phonological system as they are deeply hidden within the brain and are only discernable with complex technologies. Thus, we must look for four major symptoms often associated with a faulty phonological system.

1. **Expressive phonology:** Difficulties producing specific speech sounds or groups of speech sounds and delays suppressing the normal errors (phonological processes) of early phonological production. These problems result in decreased intelligibility and are a hallmark of a phonological disorder.
2. **Phonological awareness:** A lack of sensitivity to the phonological units of spoken language, such as how syllables make up words and how phonemes make up syllables. This problem undermines a child's ability to learn to read (Christensen, 1997).
3. **Verbal working memory:** Difficulties processing and storing linguistic information, such as temporarily holding a sentence in working memory so that its meaning can be processed. This difficulty may impact language comprehension and production (Liberman, 1998; Weismer, Evans, & Hesketh, 1999).
4. **Word learning and word retrieval:** Problems accessing and retrieving words from one's language system in which words are organized as phonological

and linguistically diverse children with phonological disorders, educators should ask such questions as (1) Does the educational plan take into account the family's perspective of communicative disability, health, and healing? and (2) Does the educational plan take into account the family's priorities?

Ensure the flexibility of the design of the educational program. When designing educational programs that respect and involve culturally and linguistically diverse families, the program design and the professionals involved in its design must be flexible and adaptive: "The ongoing and dynamic nature of [building educational plans] requires professionals to modify and change their practices according to the individual families' changing characteristics and needs" (Zhang & Bennett, 2004). Questions educators must ask include (1) Is the educational plan built on trust, reciprocity, honesty, and respect? (2) Does the educational plan reflect family input at all stages? and (3) Does the educational plan identify roles of family members based on their identification of the roles?

For Discussion

What are some examples of family strengths that would enhance a child's ability to progress rapidly in an intervention program?

What are some examples of an intervention program that would not be flexible and adaptive to meet the individual needs of children and families of culturally and linguistically diverse backgrounds?

Individuals' beliefs about disability can vary tremendously, as they reflects one's culture. Explore with your classmates your own perspectives of disability, such as: How would you feel if you had a child with a disability? Why? Should children with disabilities receive their education in the regular classroom with typically developing kids? Why or why not? Do any of your friends have significant disabilities? If not, how come?

Companion Website

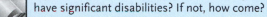

To answer these questions online, go to the Multicultural Focus module in chapter 5 of the Companion Website.

representations. Problems with the phonological system can slow a child's learning of new words (word learning) and can affect the ability to efficiently retrieve words from the language system (word retrieval) (Storkel & Morrisette, 2002).

Children who show speech-sound production problems (symptom 1) but who do not show any of the other three signs of a faulty phonological system may not have a phonological disorder. Rather, these children may have a motor-speech disorder (see Chapter 6) or they may have an articulation disorder resulting from a structural problem with the articulators (e.g., palate or teeth).

Speech Disorders Classification System

The Speech Disorders Classification System (SDCS; Shriberg, Austin, Lewis, McSweeney, & Wilson, 1997b) is one system commonly used to classify children's speech-sound disorders. It is also used for differentiating phonological disorders from other speech-sound disorders. As shown in Figure 5-5, the SDCS at its most global level differentiates developmental phonological disorders from nondevelopmental speech disorders and speech differences.

A developmental phonological disorder, called phonological disorder in this chapter, is an impairment of the phonological system sufficient to impact speech intelligibility

FIGURE 5-5 Speech Disorders Classification System (SDCS).

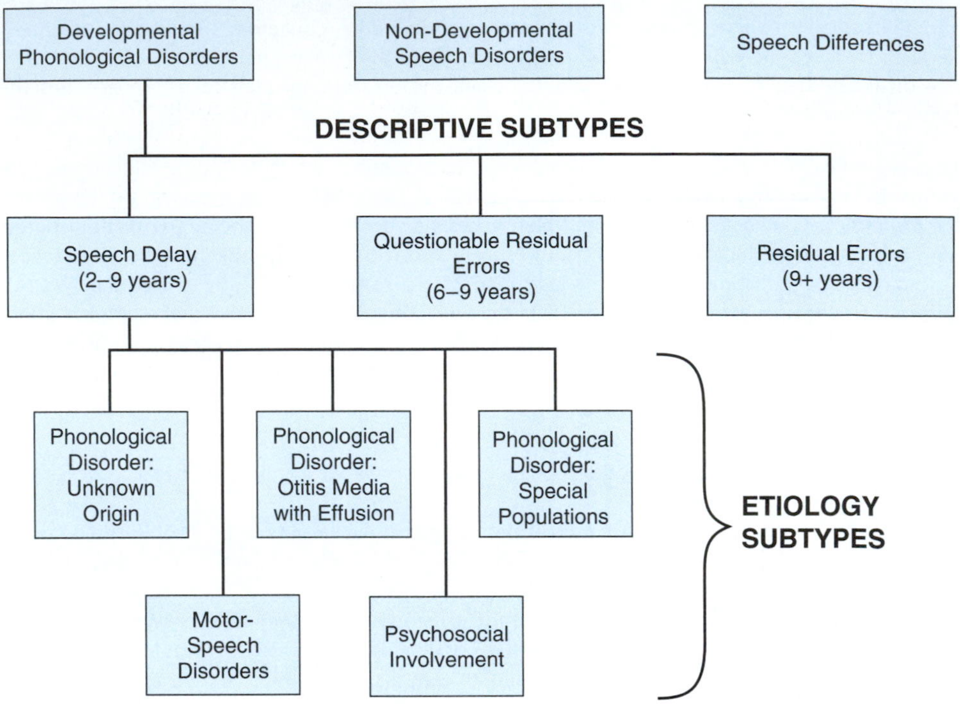

Source: Adapted with permission from Shriberg, L. D., Austin, D., Lewis, B. A., McSweeney, J. L., & Wilson, D. L. (1997b). The Speech Disorders Classification System (SDCS): Extensions and lifespan reference data. *Journal of Speech-Language-Hearing Research, 40*, 723–740. Reprinted with permission.

Discussion Point: *The SDCS differentiates at the most global level developmental phonological disorders, nondevelopmental phonological disorders, and speech differences. Consider the case of Octavio in Box 5-1. Of these three categories, which two might explain his speech challenges?*

with onset prior to 9 years of age. A phonological disorder causes problems with expressive phonological production—the production of speech sounds—and the underlying phonological representations that may potentially impact phonological awareness, verbal working memory, and word learning and retrieval. In contrast, a nondevelopmental speech disorder is a disorder of speech production occurring after 9 years of age, perhaps as a result of illness, trauma, or accident. A speech difference refers to speech-sound distinctions attributable to linguistic or cultural factors (Shriberg et al., 1997b). Speech differences are the speech patterns of an individual that reflect a native language or a regional or cultural dialect. In the United States, many regional and cultural dialects vary from the Standard American English dialect, including the regional dialect of Appalachia and the dialects of some African American communities. These should not be mistaken for speech disorders, as they represent naturally occurring cultural or geographic variations of a language.

Descriptive Subtypes

The SDCS classifies developmental phonological disorders into three descriptive subtypes and five etiology subtypes, as shown in Figure 5-5.

Speech Delay. This subtype describes children between 2 and 9 years of age who show low intelligibility and a high frequency of errors in their speech production. Although children less than 2 years of age can show delayed speech development, and such delays are important indicators of later risk for phonological disorder, children are typically not diagnosed as truly delayed in speech development until age 2. About 75% of children diagnosed with speech delay will develop normal speech production by age 6 (Shriberg, 1997).

Questionable Residual Errors. This subtype describes children who, between 6 and 9 years of age, continue to show subtle errors in speech production. These errors do not typically affect intelligibility. They include sound substitutions, such as using /w/ for /r/, and sound omissions, such as dropping one or more sounds in consonant clusters (e.g., the /r/ in *strong*).

Residual Errors. This subtype describes children older than 9 who persist in making errors in speech production, many of whom have a history of speech delay. **Residual errors** include distortions of sounds, omissions of sounds, and substitutions of sounds, particularly for late 8 sounds presented in Table 5-4.

Etiology Subtypes for Speech Delay

Phonological Disorder: Unknown Origin. This subtype describes children with phonological disorders for which there is no known cause, also called functional phonological disorders. This is the most prevalent type of phonological disorder, accounting for about 60% of cases of childhood speech delay (Shriberg, 1997). As many as 40% of children in this subtype may have a genetically based vulnerability for phonological problems. Children with an affected immediate family member are five to six times more likely than other children to develop a phonological disorder (Felsenfeld, McGue, & Broen, 1995).

Phonological Disorder: Otitis Media with Effusion. Chronic infections of the middle-ear cavity, particularly those that involve the persistent presence of a thick, serous fluid within the middle-ear space, can delay children's phonological development (Nittrouer, 1996). Otitis media with effusion (OME) is caused by such microorganisms as pneumococcus, *Hemophilus influenzae,* and streptococcus, which infect and inflame the middle-ear space via the Eustachian tube, typically the result of a respiratory infection (Hall & Mueller, 1997). Phonological development can be impaired when children have recurrent infections during infancy and toddlerhood (Shriberg, 1997).

However, the relationship between chronic OME and difficulty with phonological development is not straightforward. Many well-conducted studies have failed to find a direct causal relationship between early chronic OME and an increased risk for speech delay and phonological problems in young children (Micchio, Yont, Clemons, & Vernon-Feagans, 2002; Shriberg, Flipsen, Kwiatkowski, & McSweeney, 2003). Although the current body of science on ear infections and phonology suggests an increased rate of speech deficits in children with histories of chronic OME (Shriberg, Flipsen, et al., 2003), not all children with chronic OME will experience phonological difficulties.

Discussion Point: *The occurrence of otitis media among young children appears to be increasing. Brainstorm some reasons that might explain why this is happening.*

Phonological Disorder: Special Populations. Phonological disorders are a common symptom of several developmental disorders that affect the language system, the hearing system, or both. Three special populations of children in which the phonological system appears particularly vulnerable include children with hearing impairment, children with Down syndrome, and children with cleft palate.

Children with hearing impairment have an organic disorder of the hearing system resulting in mild to profound hearing loss. The impact of this loss on the acquisition of phonology can range from minimal to severe. Children with Down syndrome often have significant delays in the development of phonology as Down syndrome frequently affects both the language system, of which phonology is a part, and the hearing system. Hearing

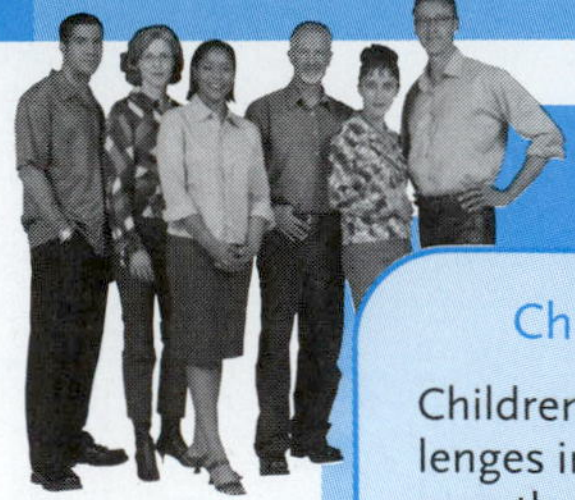

BOX 5-3 Ecological Contexts

Children with Phonological Disorders at Home and at School

Children with phonological disorders are more likely than other children to experience challenges in learning to read when they enter school. One way to help these youngsters is to prepare them early for a successful transition to kindergarten. This transition is difficult for many children as they adjust to being a learner in a school. Whereas early childhood experiences in preschool, day care, or at home focus on play and creativity, kindergarten is the first truly academic experience for children. Educators want children entering kindergarten to be ready to succeed socially, behaviorally, and academically.

Children with a phonological disorder might have a harder time with this adjustment for several reasons. First, because of speech-sound problems, these children may not have a history of successful communication, which can lead to social and behavioral difficulties. Second, because of the way in which phonology impacts literacy learning, these children may have underdeveloped early literacy skills, which can undermine their readiness for academic learning, including literacy, in the kindergarten classroom. Parents and professionals must pay special attention to helping children with phonological disorders to have a successful transition to kindergarten.

For Further Discussion

What are some specific ways parents might prepare their children for the transition to kindergarten? What are some factors in a child's life that may impede or promote successful kindergarten transition?

To answer these questions online, go to the Ecological Contexts module in chapter 5 of the Companion Website.

loss is commonly associated with Down syndrome. Cleft palate, which describes a genetic anomaly of the development of the palate, often results in problems with articulation of specific sounds. Possibly because of these difficulties with articulation, children with cleft palate are prone to delays in phonological development (Broen & Moller, 1993).

Motor Speech Disorders. This subtype describes disorders of speech production that result from an underlying problem with the motor or muscular processes associated with speech-sound production. Apraxia of speech is a disorder of speech production that accounts for 3% to 5% of cases of childhood speech disorders (Shriberg, 1997). Apraxia of speech is not a phonological impairment per se; rather, it is an impairment of the motor system that plans and sequences the delivery of speech sounds (see Chapter 6). **Myofunctional disorders** describe a type of speech production problem resulting from inaccurate or unusual learned movements of the articulators. For instance, tongue thrust is a myofunctional disorder in which the tongue is pushed forward through the teeth for alveolar speech sounds, resulting in a type of lisp; therefore, /s/ is produced more like *th*. Tongue thrust, like apraxia of speech, is not a phonological disorder, as the underlying phonological system is intact.

Discussion Point: *Consider the case of Emily in Box 5-1. Which of the subtypes in the SDCS best describes Emily's condition?*

Psychosocial Involvement. An estimated 7% of cases of speech delay result from psychological or social causes (Shriberg, 1997). Potential contributors may include maturity, personality, temperament, attention, and behavior. These types of speech-sound problems do not result from a faulty phonological system.

What Are the Defining Characteristics of Phonological Disorders?

The SDCS describes three subtypes of phonological disorders: unknown origin, otitis media with effusion, and special populations. This section discusses the defining characteristics, causes, and risk factors for each subtype.

Phonological Disorder of Unknown Origin

Defining Characteristics

Children with a phonological disorder of unknown origin exhibit delayed development of the phonological system for reasons that cannot be unequivocally identified. This disorder affects more boys than girls, with a ratio of about 1.5 boys to 1 girl (Shriberg et al., 1999). Overall, about 4% of preschool-to-kindergarten-age children experience this disorder.

The defining characteristic of phonological disorders of unknown origin is a significant delay in development of the phonological system, which affects a child's speech-sound production and intelligibility. Four characteristics of the delay in speech development include

1. *Small phonemic inventory:* The child with a phonological disorder has a smaller set of phonemes and phonemic contrasts compared to other children. For instance, a 2-year-old child with a phonological disorder might use only four consonant sounds consistently at the beginning of words, whereas same-age peers would be using 10 sounds in this position.
2. *Phoneme collapse:* Phoneme collapse occurs when several phonemes are represented by only a single phoneme, common for children with a small phonemic inventory (Williams, 2000). For instance, a child may collapse seven phonemes into a single phoneme, as illustrated in Figure 5-6. In this figure, seven phonemes are represented by a child as the phoneme /d/, significantly affecting the child's intelligibility.
3. *Persisting errors:* Although all children go through a period when they simplify their phonology (e.g., saying "tuck" for *truck* and "dun" for *fun*), for children with phonological disorders these errors persist past the time they are usually suppressed.
4. *Reduced intelligibility:* A smaller phonemic inventory, phoneme collapses, and persisting errors combine to make the final characteristic of phonological disorders—reduced intelligibility. **Unintelligibility** refers to the degree to which a child's speech is understood by a naive or unfamiliar listener, and it ranges from mild to severe (Fudala & Reynolds, 2000):
   - Mild: speech is understood but contains noticeable errors
   - Moderate: speech is difficult to understand
   - Severe: speech cannot be understood at all

FIGURE 5-6 Collapse of seven phonemes into one phoneme.

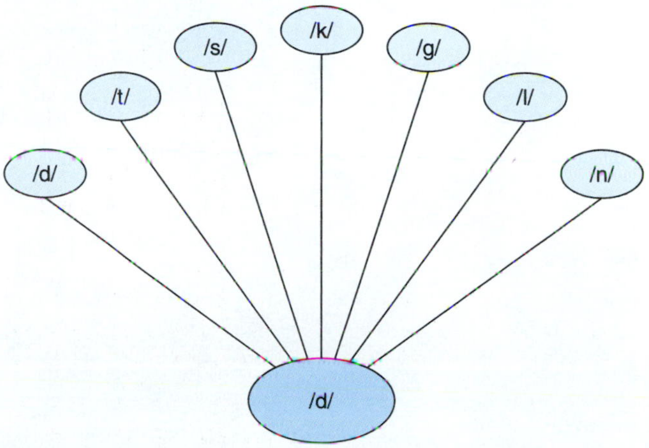

Source: Williams, L. (1993).

Usually, unintelligibility relates to the number of errors a child makes in producing sounds, with more errors resulting in greater unintelligibility. About one-third of children with phonological disorders have severe unintelligibility (Shriberg & Kwiatkowski, 1994).

About 30% of children with a speech delay also have a significant language impairment that affects vocabulary, grammar development, or both (Shriberg et al., 1999). Children who experience language disorders concomitant with speech delay experience more significant problems with social and academic performance compared to children with only phonological disorders.

Causes and Risk Factors

Discussion Point: *Adults with severe reading problems may have a weak underlying phonological system. Consider the case of Barcley in Box 5-1. Why would Barcley's underlying problem with phonology not have been previously identified?*

The cause of this subtype of phonological disorders, as the name suggests, is unknown. In general, difficulties with motor skills, intelligence, and home environment do not serve as specific risk factors in the development of phonological disorders (Bernthal & Bankson, 2004). There is, however, a tendency for phonological disorders to run in families, suggesting that most children experience phonological impairment as a result of a specific inherited weakness of the phonological system (Felsenfeld et al., 1995). This same underlying weakness is also implicated in **dyslexia**, which is a significant disability in learning how to decode words using the alphabetic principle. Children with a weak phonological system, including those with phonological disorders, seem particularly vulnerable for developing dyslexia.

Phonological Disorder: Otitis Media with Effusion

Defining Characteristics

The defining characteristics of a phonological disorder resulting from otitis media with effusion (OME) are the same as those of the unknown subtype: (1) small phonemic inventory, (2) phonemic collapse, (3) persisting errors, and (4) reduced intelligibility. As with the other subtype, these characteristics stem from poorly established phonological representations within the child's language system. In the case of OME, however, the problems with the development of phonological representations result from periods of **auditory deprivation**—a lack of input to the auditory system that occurs when a child has fluid in the middle ear for a sustained period of time. The risk for problems with phonological development is heightened when OME recurs repeatedly; OME is considered recurrent when children experience at least six episodes in the first 3 years of life (Shriberg, 1997).

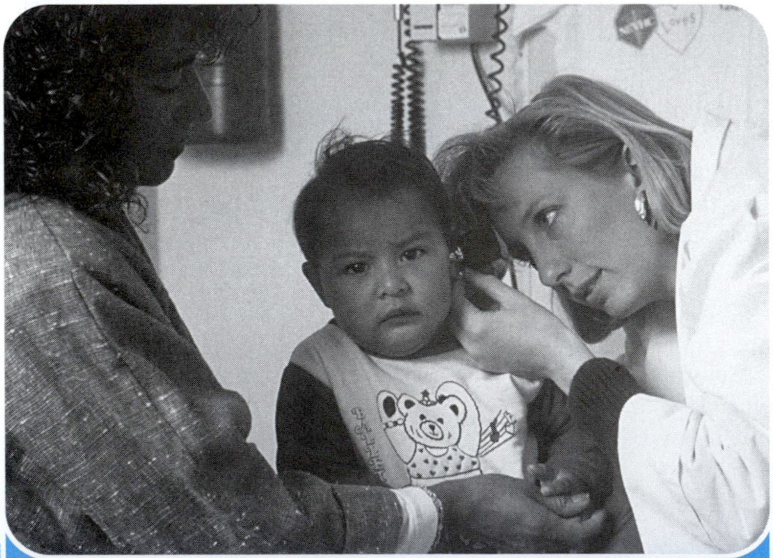

Although many children are resiliant to the impact of ear infections on the phonological system, some children are not.

Research on children with recurrent OME suggest specific markers of this type of phonological disorder, which include (1) delayed onset of babbling during the first year of life, (2) delayed onset of the use of meaningful speech, (3) reduced intelligibility compared to children with phonological disorders of unknown origin, (4) problems with specific classes of sounds (like *s* and *sh*), and (5) use of nonnatural sound changes (errors that are not expected with the child's native language) (Churchill, Hodson, Jones, & Novak, 1988; Miccio et al., 2002; Shriberg, 1997; Shriberg, Kent, et al., 2003).

Causes and Risk Factors

Any child can experience otitis media, although it is most common in children who are under 3 years old. This infection of the middle-ear cavity is caused by a bacterial or viral infection or allergens. These microorganisms reach the middle-ear space through the Eustachian tube and affect hearing in the following ways. First, the middle-ear space, typically filled with air, may fill with a thick fluid, which inhibits the processing of auditory information from the outer ear to the auditory centers of the brain. Second, the microorganisms can degrade and perforate the eardrum, which also negatively affects the processing and relay of auditory information.

Discussion Point: *Otitis media seems to be an equal opportunity disorder in that it knows no geographic or economic boundaries in whom it affects. Survey your friends to find out how many of them were affected by this disorder. Did it have an impact on their development?*

Many children experience these passing challenges to the health of the middle-ear cavity with few obvious negative effects. Perhaps someone you know had chronic ear infections during early childhood and appears none the worse for the experience. In such cases, the individual was resilient to the potential negative repercussions of this illness. On the other hand, some individuals are not resilient, and the experience of chronic OME tips the scale toward the negative impact of this disease. Many variables can affect the risk and resilience related to OME, such as poverty, language quality in the home or other caregiving environment, genetic predisposition for language disorders, and other health problems. For children who are not resilient, chronic OME can have a negative impact on phonological development, particularly when infections are recurrent, resistant to treatment, and/or incompletely treated (Katz, 1994).

Special Populations

Down Syndrome

Down syndrome is a congenital developmental disability that affects about 1 of 700 children (Bishop, Huether, Torfs, Lorey, & Deddens, 1997). Common characteristics associated with Down syndrome include mental retardation, small stature, heart defects, hearing loss, small oral cavity, and language delays. Phonological disorders are also prevalent among children with Down syndrome. These children often show delays in early phonological development of a variety of speech sounds, including a limited inventory of phonemes, delayed development of phonological representations, and poor phonological memory (Laws & Bishop, 2003). These basic deficits in phonology may be further compounded by the increased risk for hearing loss and articulation difficulties resulting from dental and oral cavity anomalies among children with Down syndrome.

Causes and Risk Factors. Down syndrome (also known as trisomy 21) results from a chromosomal abnormality and is associated with higher maternal age (Bishop et al., 1997). The majority of cases result from a defect in the 21st pair of chromosomes. Early intervention is important for promoting the positive development of children with Down syndrome and can help enhance phonological and communication development.

Hearing Loss

Defining Characteristics. For children to develop phonological representations of their native language, they must have access to the phonological code of that language via exposure.

This exposure need not be oral, as we know from research on children who are deaf who develop phonological representations through their exposure to a signed language (Luetke-Stahlman & Nielsen, 2003). As is explained in greater detail in Chapter 13, children who experience either transient or permanent impairment of their hearing are at significant risk for lack of adequate exposure to the phonology of their language. Inadequate exposure during the first 5 years of life is particularly detrimental as this is when phonological representations are rapidly being acquired and laying the foundation for reading ability.

Phonological disorders resulting from hearing loss tend to reflect the severity of the hearing loss and the extent to which the child receives intervention to ensure exposure to oral (speech) or manual (sign) phonological representations. Characteristics of phonological development for children with hearing loss are similar to those of children with unknown or other subtypes of phonological disorders and include limited inventory of phonemes and decreased intelligibility. Hearing loss commonly affects a large range of consonant types, including stridents (*s, sh, ch*), velars (*k, g*), nasals (*m, n*), and glides (*y, w*). Speech of affected children includes substitutions of sounds, omissions of sounds, and distortions of sounds (Hodson, 1997), which together can have a significant negative impact on effective and intelligible communication.

Causes and Risk Factors. Hearing loss occurs prenatally, perinatally, and postnatally. Prenatal causes of hearing loss include chromosomal abnormalities, maternal ingestion of toxins, and medications. Perinatal causes include birth trauma and anoxia, or loss of oxygen to the brain. Postnatal causes include bacterial infections, such as bacterial meningitis; trauma or accident; exposure to noise; and medications. The ear is a fragile and complex mechanism, and many things can impact its sensitivity to sound and its role in the development of phonology. Thus it is critically important to protect children's hearing. Adults who work with young children should watch for seven signs of possible hearing loss (Hall & Mueller, 1997): (1) ear pain or fullness, (2) discharge or bleeding from the ear, (3) sudden or progressive hearing loss, (4) unequal hearing by the ears, (5) hearing loss after an injury or loud sound, (6) slow speech and language development, and (7) balance disturbance. Chapter 13 provides a more detailed explanation of causes and risk factors in early childhood hearing impairment.

FIGURE 5-7 Unilateral cleft of the lip and palate.

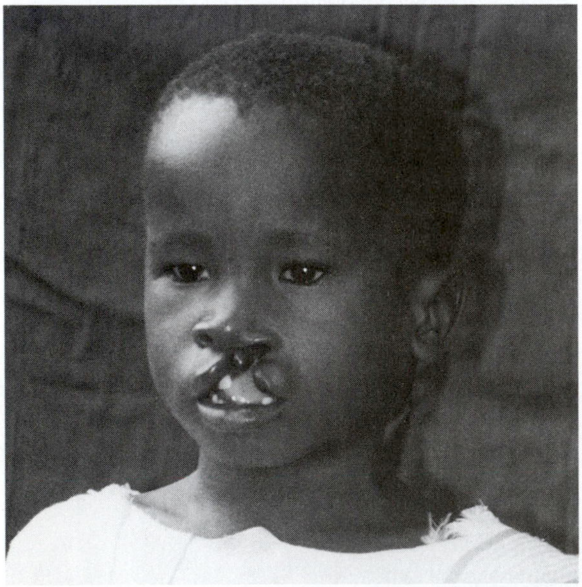

Cleft Palate

Defining Characteristics. Cleft palate is a congenital malformation of the palate, or roof of the mouth, that affects about 1 in 700 newborns (Bauman-Waengler, 2004). The name of the condition refers to the fissure or gap that is present in the roof of the mouth when the two sides of the palate do not fuse together during prenatal development. The fissure may affect only the soft palate or both the hard and soft palates, or it may extend to the lip; the latter is called cleft lip. The cleft may be unilateral (on one side) or bilateral (affecting both sides of the oral structures). Figure 5-7 illustrates a unilateral cleft of the lip and palate.

Surgery is typically performed to correct clefts within the first year of life, after which the cleft is considered repaired. The average age of children undergoing surgical repair for cleft palate is 12 months (Chapman, Hardin-Jones, & Halter, 2003). Prior to surgical repair, children with cleft palate have a range of articulation difficulties, including problems producing specific sounds, and considerable phonological delay. Also involved are problems with managing the valving of sounds and pressure between the nasal and oral cavities. Thus children with cleft palate have particular problems with consonants that require the building up of pressure in the oral cavity, such as the stops /p/ and /b/.

A child with cleft palate is prone to phonological delays both before and after repair that stem mainly from these challenges with the articulation of specific sounds. Children with cleft palate show preferences for production of certain sounds, such as nasals and glides, with only limited use of other sounds, including those requiring pressure in the oral cavity. During the months preceding repair, when children with cleft palate begin to babble and use a few words, they practice and receive reinforcement for using a small inventory of preferred sounds and do not practice or receive reinforcement for the use of other phonemes. Even after surgery, children with repaired clefts have a smaller consonant inventory compared to other children (Chapman et al., 2003). Several speech-sound patterns are observed for children with cleft palate:

- Consonant and vowel distortions due to nasal emissions and hypernasality (inappropriate valving of airflow into the nasal cavity during production of consonants and vowels)
- Consonant distortions due to misarticulation (inappropriate placing of articulators for production of specific consonant features)
- Consonant distortions due to lack of pressure in oral production, particularly /p/, /b/, /t/, /d/, /k/, and /g/

Causes and Risk Factors. The fusion of the palatal structures occurs between the 8th and 12th weeks of gestation (Siren, 2004). There are 400 different syndromes with which cleft palate is associated (Pore & Reed, 1999), including Van der Woude syndrome and Smith-Lemli-Opitz syndrome. Van der Woude syndrome is a chromosomal disorder commonly associated with cleft palate and phonological disorders, although it carries few other physical

BOX 5-4 Spotlight on Research

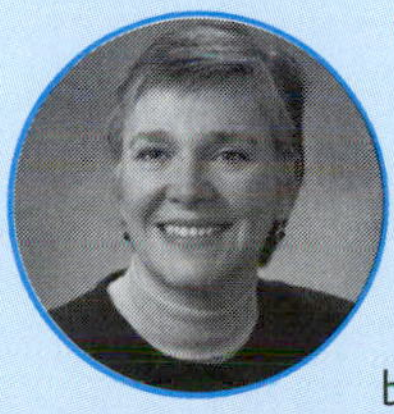

Lynn Williams, Ph.D.
Professor, East Tennessee State University

Lynn Williams is a professor and clinical researcher with an extensive background working with children who have severe speech disorders. At East Tennessee State University, Dr. Williams currently teaches courses on clinical phonology, supervises graduate students in the Phonological Intervention Program (PIP), and conducts intervention research with children who have speech disorders.

Dr. Williams's research program started in 1990 with the development and investigation of a new model of phonological intervention called *multiple oppositions.* Through PIP, she studies disordered sound systems to develop assessment approaches for children with speech disabilities. In this program, the child's entire sound system is described as an exotic native language of its own, utilizing methodologies and principles borrowed from linguistics. Then interventions based on the multiple oppositions approach are designed. A recent goal of her research is the development of a software program called Sound Contrasts in Phonology, or SCIP, supported by the National Institutes of Health and a collaboration with Thinking Publications. SCIP will ideally provide a "better, faster, cheaper" approach in the development of intervention materials to increase clinician access to recent innovations in phonological intervention, including multiple oppositions, minimal pair therapy, maximal oppositions, and treatment of the empty set. More details on Dr. Williams's work can be found in the following resources:

Williams, A. L. (2000). Multiple oppositions: Theoretical foundations for an alternative contrastive intervention approach. *American Journal of Speech-Language Pathology, 9,* 282–288.

Williams, A. L. (2000). Multiple oppositions: Case studies of variables in phonological intervention. *American Journal of Speech-Language Pathology, 9,* 289–299.

BOX 5-5 Spotlight on Practice

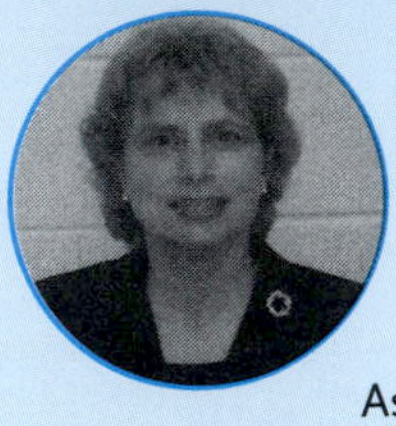

Patricia Ann Ritter, Ph.D.
Speech-Language Pathologist and Assistant Executive Director
The Treatment and Learning Centers, Rockville, MD

As the Assistant Executive Director of the Treatment and Learning Centers, I am responsible for the outpatient departments of Speech, Audiology, Occupational and Physical Therapy, Psycho-Educational Testing, Tutoring, and Vocational Services. I am a member of the management team, making decisions related to the Centers' mission, direction, and operations. My duties include budget, recruitment and retention, staff supervision, and program quality, as well as marketing and front-desk administration. During my 14 years of management, serving initially as the Director of Outpatient Speech, I have used the knowledge and skills gained from a variety of positions in speech-language pathology.

My jobs as a public school clinician fostered independence and resourcefulness. Early in my career I traveled to schools in Germany for the British and American military. The isolation from other clinicians required independent study and an efficient use of networking on my part. With no Internet, the link to others was travel by train for periodic meetings at various sites. I quickly learned sign language in order to communicate effectively as a speech-language pathologist with individuals with hearing impairments. Later, in Canada, I became a diagnostician, providing evaluations and consulting with school personnel regarding programming. Since there were no speech-language pathologists in many schools, it was essential to offer ideas that could be integrated into the classroom environment.

The school experience culminated in my most rewarding accomplishment, working with a colleague to start a school for children with learning disabilities. We created a philosophy, model, staffing pattern, and admission criteria, opening the school with approximately 35 children less than a year after the idea was proposed. Today, the Katherine Thomas School at the Treatment and Learning Centers has 11 classrooms with a capacity of 110 children.

My work with adults with neurological disorders in a hospital setting expanded my knowledge of other disciplines and fostered the teamwork needed to achieve outcomes. From compromise on scheduling to collaboration on goals, learning to be a member of a team became a necessity. It also was essential that I expand my understanding of the implications of a disability on other family members. Support and empathy were critical from initial communication of the problem, to ongoing evaluation of progress, to reintegration into home and community.

Being a speech-language pathologist has been a varied and rewarding career choice. I have developed professional and personal skills in a variety of job settings that have helped me to be successful in my current management position. Perhaps most important, speech-language pathology has allowed me to fulfill my personal goal of making a difference in the lives of others.

characteristics. Smith-Lemli-Opitz syndrome is a disorder linked to the X chromosome and thus affects only males. Cleft palate is one of many markers of Smith-Lemli-Opitz syndrome; others include mental retardation and learning disabilities (Siren, 2004).

How Are Phonological Disorders Identified?

Discussion Point: *A team approach is beneficial for truly representing a child's phonological capabilities. Consider the case of Octavio in Box 5-1. Who should be involved in the study of his phonological performance?*

Speech-language pathologists use a systematic and comprehensive process of assessment to identify phonological disorders in children. To ensure the accuracy of identification, the SLP typically consults with others to gather information about the child, including an audiologist for input on hearing, a pediatrician for input on general development and health history, a psychologist for input on the child's well-being and mental health, classroom teachers for input on the child's learning skills and classroom behaviors, reading specialists for input on reading development, and, most important, the parents for input on the child's communicative performance in the home and elsewhere. Information from all these constituents is crucial for developing an accurate profile of a child's phonological and more general communicative abilities and for understanding the contribution of specific factors of risk and resilience for the child.

The Assessment Process

Referral

Referral for phonological evaluation is typically made by a parent, a pediatrician, or an early childhood educator. All of these adults are in a good position to note that a child does not appear to be using speech sounds at a level that is age appropriate. For children who are under 2 years of age, signs of a possible phonological delay may include the following:

- Suspected hearing loss or chronic ear infections
- Known physical impairment, particularly of the oral-facial structures, such as cleft palate
- Known mental or cognitive impairment, such as Down syndrome or Prader-Willi syndrome

Specific vocal and verbal behaviors also serve as warning signs and suggest the need for referral:

- Delay in vocal play, babbling, appearance of the first word (expected around 1 year of age) and use of two-word combinations (expected between 18 and 24 months of age)
- Limited repertoire of phonemes (the child should use at least three or four different phonemes by 1 year, such as /b/, /m/, /p/, and /n/)
- Lack of intelligibility of early words for familiar caregivers
- Reliance on nonverbal communication to get needs met, such as gesturing, and inability to use verbal communication for functional purposes (e.g., to request, to reject)

Identifying phonological problems as early as possible may help prevent these problems from growing in severity. In the first few years of life, the difference in phonological skill between a child with a delay and a child without a delay might be quite small. However, over time, this gap grows, and the problems become much more difficult to remediate. To ensure that the gap stays narrow—or, in the best scenario, disappears—two things must happen for children with early phonological delays: (1) they must be identified and (2) they must receive early intervention services focused specifically on building phonological skills.

Most children are not identified as having phonological difficulties until they start using language as a primary means to communicate. In the second year of life, usually between 12 and 18 months, children shift to using spoken communication to get their needs met and to comment on the world around them. They use their slowly emerging vocabulary and phonology, saying such words as *no, night-night, Mommy,* and *milk.* It is normal for some of these productions to be unintelligible. By the time the child turns 2 years old, however, he or she should be intelligible a majority of the time (more than 50%) when communicating. At this age, children should not show persistent frustration when trying to communicate with others, nor should they rely on close caregivers to translate their words so that others can understand them. By 3 years of age, children should be intelligible 75% of the time when talking with a person unfamiliar to them (Vihman & Greenlee, 1987). Children who do not meet these guidelines should be referred to a professional.

Screening

Nearly all children show errors in their sound use during early development, such as omitting the final consonant in words or deleting a sound in consonant clusters. Children also only gradually acquire all of the phonemes of their language; some phonemes are not acquired until kindergarten or first grade. For these reasons, it is sometimes challenging to determine whether a child is showing a delay in phonological development or merely demonstrating phonological errors that are normal.

Screening is a way to take a quick look at a child's phonological development to determine whether a child's speech errors go beyond what is normal and warrant a more comprehensive assessment. It is not used to identify whether a child should receive treatment. Screening can be conducted using informal or formal measures. An informal measure might involve a screener engaging a child in play for a few minutes to observe communicative patterns during spontaneous speech. The screener might try to elicit specific sounds or processes that should have been mastered by a child of this age. The screener might also ask the child to imitate some specific sound targets, for example,

> ***I saw seashells on the seashore. I love lollipops and licorice. Rufus the rabbit is really tired.***

Some formal measures a screener might use as a quick check of phonological performance include the Denver Articulation Screening Test (Drumwright, 1971) and the Quick Screen of Phonology (Bankson & Bernthal, 1990), both of which take just a few minutes to administer. Regardless of whether an informal or a formal protocol is used, the screener should be familiar with the normal phonological characteristics of children at various stages of development in order to determine whether a child is showing improper phonological development.

Comprehensive Phonological Assessment

For children showing signs of a phonological disorder, a comprehensive assessment is needed. This assessment is administered by a specialist in phonological disorders, usually a speech-language pathologist. This individual must be skilled in administering a variety of assessment procedures, working with children, and phonetically transcribing phonological productions, and must have an arsenal of tools for eliciting the child's speech. A comprehensive assessment is designed to achieve six aims (Miccio, 2002):

1. To characterize the child's general developmental background, including family characteristics
2. To characterize the status of hearing and oral structures and functions
3. To characterize current phonological and language performance
4. To characterize the nature and severity of the phonological disorder
5. To determine the prognosis for phonological outcomes
6. To determine the course of treatment

These aims are met through an assessment lasting as long as 2 hours and including such activities as caregiver interview and case history, oral mechanism screening, hearing screening, language screening or evaluation,

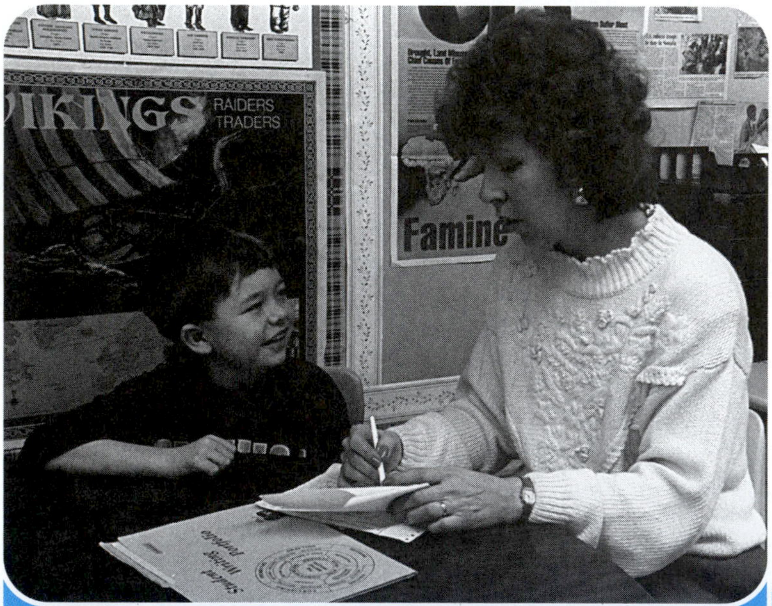

The phonological assessment is conducted by a clinician skilled at enticing children to use speech during informal and formal activities.

and phonological analysis. The assessment usually ends with the professional meeting with a caregiver to present the findings and make recommendations.

Caregiver Interview and Case History. An interview with a child's primary caregivers, which includes administering a case history, is needed to develop a broad understanding of the child's phonological, social, communicative, and health history. The caregiver interview helps the professional understand the child's communication challenges from the family's perspective (Miccio, 2002). The interview also enables the clinician to (1) recognize cultural factors that may influence the assessment, (2) create a familiarity with the family that can facilitate the assessment process, and (3) understand family variables that may complicate or complement the child's phonological development (Miccio, 2002). Table 5-5 details specific questions for an interview with caregivers. Sometimes these questions can be gathered in a telephone interview prior to assessment.

Oral Mechanism Screening. An **oral mechanism screening** carefully examines the structures and the functions of the systems that are needed for effective speech production. An examination of structures looks at the appearance of the articulators, including the lips,

TABLE 5-5 Questions for caregiver interview during phonological evaluation

General Topic	Specific Questions
Communication	When did the child first begin to babble regularly?
	When did the child first speak three different words? What were they?
	When did the child start saying two- and three-word sentences on a regular basis?
	When did the child begin to speak in sentences, even if some of the words in the sentences were missing?
Birth/Medical	Were there any complications during the pregnancy?
	Was the baby full-term?
	How much did the baby weigh?
	How long was the baby in the hospital after delivery?
	Did the baby have any diagnosed medical conditions?
	Does the child take any medications regularly?
	Has the child ever been hospitalized?
	Has the child ever had an ear infection?
	How is the child's present health?
Social	Who are the members of the child's family?
	Who are the main people with whom the child interacts?
Education	Has the child attended any type of day care or preschool? Did she/he receive any special services?
	Describe the child's current education program and any special services.

Source: From Bleile, K. (2002). Evaluating articulation and phonological disorders when the clock is running. *American Journal of Speech-Language Pathology, 11,* 243–249. Reprinted with permission.

teeth, tongue, jaw, hard palate, soft palate, and tonsils, for any deviations that may impact speech production. The clinical tools for this inspection include surgical gloves, a tongue depressor, cotton swabs, and a flashlight. After examining the structures, the clinician looks at how the speech system functions during speech and nonspeech activities. An example protocol is shown in Table 5-6. In this protocol, the clinician studies lip rounding, lip spreading, tongue movement, lip closure, and mandible movement and looks for possible neuromuscular abnormalities that may contribute to or cause phonological difficulties (Miccio, 2002).

Hearing Screening. A hearing screening is an essential part of phonological assessment to rule out the possibility that a hearing impairment is the cause of any phonological difficulties. The hearing screening is conducted at standard thresholds—typically a loudness of 20 decibels (dB) in each ear at four frequencies (500, 1000, 2000, and 4000 hertz). Careful questioning of caregivers for a history of hearing difficulties, including otitis media, is also

TABLE 5-6 Items for Oral Mechanism Screening

Prompt	Purpose
Show me a kiss	Lip rounding
Say /u/	Lip rounding
Smile	Lip spreading
Say /i/	Lip spreading
Say /i/-/u/	Forward-backward movement of tongue, lip rounding and spreading
Say /ki/-/ku/	Up-down movement of tongue dorsum
Close your lips tight and don't let me open them	Lip closure strength
Say /ib/-/ib/	Lip closure and adduction of vocal folds
Say /bi/-/bi/	Lip closure and adduction of folds
Slowly open your mouth as wide as you can and then close it	Nonspeech mandible lowering and raising
Say /pa/-/pa/	Lowering mandible
Say /ap/-/ap/	Raising mandible
Open your mouth wide	Structural appearance of oral cavity
Say /ab/	Raising the velum
Say /am/	Lowering the velum
Touch your teeth with your tongue	Forward-backward movement of tongue
Say "th"	Forward-backward movement of tongue, contact of teeth and tongue
Touch the tip of your tongue to the ridge behind your teeth	Upward-downward movement of tongue

Source: From Miccio, A. W. (2002). Clinical problem solving: Assessment of phonological disorders. *American Journal of Speech-Language Pathology, 11,* 221–229. Reprinted with permission.

important. If a child does not pass the screening, referral to an audiologist for a more comprehensive hearing evaluation is warranted.

Language Screening/Evaluation. Many children who exhibit a phonological disorder also have problems with language development, including grammar and vocabulary (Fey et al., 1994; Tyler, Lewis, Haskill, & Tolbert, 2002). Often, a child sees a speech-language pathologist because of poor speech intelligibility. Sometimes, however, the speech-sound problems are just the tip of the iceberg, and the child's phonological problems present a "warning that other linguistic systems need attention" (Khan, 2002, p. 250). For many children, a problem with speech-sound production reveals not only a disorder of phonology, but also a more extensive problem with the language system. Thus, including measures of receptive and expressive language is an important part of phonological assessment. Clinicians often collect measures of spontaneous language use during play and conversation, supplemented by a formal evaluation with a standardized assessment (Williams, 2002).

Phonological Analysis. The heart of the phonological assessment is a careful examination of the child's phonological system to determine whether it is disordered. Clinicians use a variety of tools to identify errors in the phonological system, to identify patterns and consistencies in these errors, and to determine the stimulability of certain sounds and patterns. **Stimulability** refers to the extent to which a child can produce a new sound or pattern when given some sort of assistance. The main tools used in phonological analysis include (1) standardized testing, (2) spontaneous speech sampling, and (3) probing.

Standardized testing is used to gather a summary of a child's use of specific sounds and patterns and compare it to similar information for children of the same age. Typically, a child is shown a series of pictures and is asked to name each one. The stimuli are designed to elicit the full range of English phonemes in a variety of different word positions. One popular test is the Goldman-Fristoe Test of Articulation–2 (GFTA; Goldman & Fristoe, 2000), in which the child produces 53 words (e.g., *duck, yellow, finger*) and production errors are recorded on a score sheet. The total number of errors the child makes are summed and translated into a percentile rank, which indicates a child's standing in speech production compared with children of the same age. When a child's percentile rank is sufficiently low (e.g., 10th percentile or lower), a delay or disorder may be indicated.

Standardized testing is also used to examine other aspects of the phonological system, such as phonological awareness and phonological memory. The Phonological Awareness Test (PAT; Robertson & Salter, 1995) is a standardized test that asks children to make rhymes ("What rhymes with *cat*?"), identify the beginning sounds in words ("What is the first sound in *dog*?"), and identify the number of syllables in words ("How many parts are in *pizza*?"), among other tasks. These tasks tap the child's ability to reflect on the phonological structure of language. Phonological memory is tested in the standardized Comprehensive Test of Phonological Processing (CTOPP; Wagner, Torgesen, & Rashotte, 1999). On one task, for instance, children listen to spoken strings of increasing length and must repeat them to an examiner. Tests such as these are useful for comparing a child's phonological capabilities with age-based normative references.

Spontaneous speech sampling is a second critical tool for phonological analysis. By collecting a sample of a child's phonological production across a variety of activities, clinicians can observe the child's phonological strengths and weaknesses in everyday conversational activities. Sometimes children perform very well producing sounds during the structured tasks of standardized tests, but cannot communicate intelligibly during naturalistic activities. Experienced clinicians are quite skilled at eliciting children's use of specific sounds during play activities and making sense of patterns observed and how the context influences those patterns.

When collecting spontaneous speech samples to evaluate phonology, clinicians can determine a child's overall intelligibility by calculating the Percentage of Consonants Correct (**PCC**) metric (Shriberg, Austin, Lewis, McSweeney, & Wilson, 1997a). The PCC is the ratio of the number of consonants produced correctly to the total number of consonants:

$$\frac{\text{Total number of correct consonants produced}}{\text{Total number of consonants produced}} \times 100$$

Thus, a child who produced 500 consonants in a conversation but produced only 288 of them correctly has a PCC of 57.6%, meaning that only about 58 of 100 consonants are produced correctly. The PCC is used to characterize a child's conversational intelligibility as (Shriberg et al., 1997a):

>90%	mild unintelligibility
65–85%	mild to moderate unintelligibility
50–65%	moderate to severe unintelligibility
<50%	severe unintelligibility

For the child in our example, whose PCC is about 58%, intelligibility is moderately to severely compromised.

Probing is a third important tool clinicians use for conducting phonological analysis and complements standardized testing and conversational speech sampling. The clinician uses probing to look at how the child performs on specific sounds or patterns. For instance, based on observations during testing and conversation, the clinician may suspect that a child has not developed representations of final consonant sounds. The clinician therefore develops probes to study the child's ability to differentiate words on the basis of final consonants (e.g., *hoe* versus *hope; bow* versus *bone, pop* versus *pod*) and also asks the child to produce a series of real and nonsense words differing only on final consonants (e.g., /pIk/, /pIm/, /pIt/, /pIn/).

***Discussion Point:** What is the added benefit of using probing? Why wouldn't a clinician rely solely on standardized testing to study a child's phonology?*

Probing is also used to determine stimulability. Once a child is shown *not* to have a particular sound or pattern, such as final consonant sounds, the clinician studies how much and what type of support is needed for the child to produce that sound or pattern. This is called stimulability testing, and it helps a clinician select sounds and patterns for therapy and identify specific techniques that may be useful for bringing about change.

Diagnosis

Diagnosis of a phonological disorder is made by considering the cumulative evidence from the comprehensive evaluation. A phonological disorder is present if the child's phonological system is developing at a rate sufficiently different from age-based expectations; if the phonological differences are not accounted for by cultural or linguistic factors, such as dialect; and if the phonological difference has an impact on the child's ability to effectively communicate for social or academic purposes. The extent of the disorder can range from mild to severe. Children with a mild disorder make only a few distortions of sounds, which do not affect intelligibility, such as saying *f* for *th.* This type of problem is sometimes seen in adolescents who as children had severe phonological problems but who now have mild residual errors. Children with a moderate disorder show some sound substitutions and sound omissions, with an occasional impact on intelligibility. Children with a severe disorder also use substitutions and omissions, and intelligibility is often compromised. Children with a profound disorder are unable to effectively communicate their needs because sound substitutions and omissions are extensive, and they have few speech sounds to use (Hodson & Paden, 1991).

***Discussion Point:** Consider the case of Emily in Box 5-1. Her difficulties are probably consistent with a mild impairment. In what ways might a mild impairment affect a child's educational performance?*

How Are Phonological Disorders Treated?

Treatment Paradigms

This chapter has emphasized the phonological basis for the majority of cases of speech delay in young children, which represents a paradigm shift in speech-language pathology. Since the 1990s, treatment paradigms have moved away from therapies emphasizing the child's learning of better articulatory movements toward phonologically oriented therapies, which emphasize the child's achievement of distinct, underlying representations for each phoneme. The more traditional motor- and articulatory-oriented therapies emphasized the child's gradual learning of improved ways to produce specific sounds, typically one at a time. In the traditional approach, the clinician would select a sound and help the child to improve production of it over time through a series of highly controlled drill-like activities. In a given session, the client might produce the target sound in isolation ten times with reinforcement, then produce the sound in different contexts (e.g., at the beginning of words, at the end of words) multiple times, and perhaps complete some motor exercises with a mirror to study how the tongue moves during production of the sound.

Clinicians are gradually shifting from these traditional techniques to more phonologically oriented approaches, which seem more effective for many children (Klein, 1996). Some of the governing principles of phonologically oriented approaches follow (Bauman-Waengler, 2004):

1. *Phonological processes or rules are treated, rather than the individual sounds themselves.* The clinician identifies patterns or processes that explain the child's errors. For instance, the child who leaves out the /s/ at the beginning of such words as *star, skunk,* and *spot* is using the process of cluster reduction. Rather than training the child to use the /s/ sound, the clinician remediates the underlying pattern of cluster reduction.
2. *The contrasts between phonemes are emphasized.* Therapy emphasizes the child's development of an awareness of how phonemes signal changes in meaning, as with the minimal pairs *swipe* and *wipe,* in which the inclusion of the /s/ in the first word signals a difference in meaning from the second. Accordingly, in phonologically based therapies, words, phrases, and sentences are used to train children to recognize contrasts between phonemes; a focus on training children to produce individual sounds accurately in isolation is rare.
3. *Efforts to enhance language and communication are included.* Many children with phonological disorders also have impairments in other domains of language, including morphology, syntax, and vocabulary. Children with phonological disorders are also at risk for problems developing important literacy skills, such as phonological awareness and reading abilities. Phonologically oriented therapies emphasize the role of phonology in communication and move away from drill-like activities focused on sounds in isolation that do not feature authentic communication. Phonologically oriented therapies also often incorporate attention to other linguistic targets, such as improved morphology and the child's development of phonological awareness (Tyler, Lewis, Haskill, & Tolbert, 2003).

The following sections provide a brief overview of four common approaches to phonological intervention: minimal opposition contrast therapy, multiple oppositions therapy, cycles therapy, and phonological awareness therapy.

Minimal Opposition Contrast Therapy

Minimal opposition contrast therapy trains children to recognize and produce the phonemic contrasts between words that differ by only a single phoneme (Bauman-Waengler, 2004). The word *minimal* in the name of this approach emphasizes the focus on helping children become aware of minimal differences among words that are marked by phonemes,

Discussion Point: *For a child whose intelligibility is compromised by consonant cluster reduction, what are some minimal pairs that might be used in treatment to build use of consonant clusters?*

and *opposition contrast* emphasizes the focus on teaching through contrasts. The purpose of this therapy is to help children develop representations of phonemes or phonological rules that are not yet present in their underlying phonology. It does so by training children to be conceptually aware of the phonemic differences among words that differ by only a single contrast. For instance, when a child does not represent final consonants in words—known as final consonant deletion—a clinician trains this pattern by teaching the child to sort words into those that have a final consonant and those that do not (e.g., *bow, bone, boat*).

Multiple Oppositions Therapy

Multiple oppositions therapy is also based on the principle of teaching children to focus on the contrasts, or oppositions, between words (Williams, 2000). This therapy builds contrasts within a phonemic collapse. Recall from earlier in this chapter that a phonemic collapse is when a number of phonemes are represented by a single phoneme. To build up the child's phonology, multiple oppositions therapy focuses on each contrast that is collapsed. Thus, for a child who collapses /t/, /k/, /g/, and /z/ into /d/, training will build contrasts between /d/ and /t/, /d/ and /k/, /d/ and /g/, and /d/ and /z/.

Cycles Therapy

Cycles therapy is a popular phonologically based approach that tries to stimulate children's use of certain phonemes or patterns by treating them in cycles. A cycle is a period of therapy, usually about 2 to 6 hours over several weeks, in which a small set of phonemes or patterns are exclusively targeted (Hodson & Paden, 1991). At the end of the cycle, the therapist selects a new set of phonemes or patterns to target. Phonemes and patterns that are not resolved within a cycle are recycled and addressed in a future cycle. For a child with severe unintelligibility who uses many different processes, cycle 1 might focus on final consonant deletion, cycle 2 might focus on consonant cluster reduction, cycle 3 might recycle final consonant deletion in addition to focusing on weak syllable deletion, and so forth. The principle of cycles training is to stimulate the emergence of a particular phoneme or pattern rather than targeting it until mastery is reached. By cycling through many different targets, children's speech skills may improve more quickly than they would using approaches that focus on several targets at once over a lengthy period of time.

Phonological Awareness Therapy

The significant challenges faced by many children with phonological disorders in the area of phonological awareness argue the need to integrate phonological awareness therapy into phonological interventions. The goal of phonological awareness therapy is to develop the child's sensitivities to the sound structure of language. For children who are under 5 years old, phonological awareness therapy helps develop an awareness of (1) words as sentence units (word awareness), (2) syllables as word units (syllable awareness), and (3) intersyllabic units, such as beginning sounds (e.g., *s* in *sit*) and rhyme patterns (e.g., *og* in *bog* and *hog*). As important as these early sensitivities are, what is most crucial is that children come to recognize the phonemic structure of language, or that words and syllables are made up of phonemes. One program that helps children develop this awareness is the Gillon Phonological Awareness Training Program, described in Gillon (2004). In this program, children participate in a range of activities to help them focus on the phonemic elements of words, including blending activities, in which children identify words that are presented as broken segments (e.g., "What word is this: /b/ . . . /I/ . . . /g/?") and segmenting activities, in which children identify the phonemes in a word ("Tell me all the sounds in the word *big*."). One useful activity for helping children develop these phonemic sensitivities is moving blocks that represent sounds, which makes the phonemes more concrete for children. For instance, given a red block to represent the /I/ sound and a blue block to represent the /z/ sound, the clinician might instruct the child to arrange the blocks to make /Iz/ and then rearrange them to make /zI/.

Goals and Targets in Phonological Therapy

Phonological therapy may last for months or years, depending on the age of the child, the severity of the disorder, and the type of treatment used for remediation (Klein, 1996). The time taken for resolution of problems is also related to the goals of therapy and the targets selected for therapy.

A therapy goal is an objective to be reached and may be a short-term or a long-term goal. A short-term goal focuses on more immediate change, whereas a long-term goal identifies the end goal of treatment. Effective short-term goals concentrate on eliminating broad patterns rather than on training specific sounds. For instance, a child who never uses /k/ in the final position of words might be using a pattern of final consonant deletion whereby all final consonants in words are omitted. A short-term goal might read something like "Johnny will suppress final consonant deletion in 80% of opportunities during spontaneous speech." When setting short- and long-term goals in phonological therapy, it is important to keep in mind the end of improving children's ability to communicate more effectively in social and academic situations.

A target is the phoneme or error that is addressed in a given therapy session. Many children who receive phonological therapy have multiple errors in their speech-sound production and have widespread gaps in their underlying phonological knowledge. Some children may be highly unintelligible when they first begin therapy and may not even be able to communicate their most basic needs and interests. These children (and their family members) might be frustrated and even angry about how hard it is to communicate. Clinicians must select the specific speech-sound targets that will bring about the greatest amount of change in the shortest possible time for these children. In general, five approaches are preferred by practicing therapists in selecting targets:

1. *Target errors or patterns that most affect intelligibility.* Typically, errors that occur more than 40% of the time affect children's intelligibility.
2. *Target sounds or patterns that are stimulable.* Children show greater progress during therapy on stimulable sounds and patterns than on those that are not stimulable (Rvachew, Rafaat, & Martin, 1999). Some clinicians prefer to target stimulable sounds during therapy to achieve immediate and observable success.
3. *Target sounds or patterns that are not stimulable.* Some clinicians target sounds and patterns that are not stimulable for the child based on the view that a child will likely resolve stimulable sounds without assistance or therapy, whereas sounds that are not stimulable require help through therapy (Rvachew et al., 1999). Thus, therapists following this paradigm target sounds and patterns with which the child has the greatest difficulty.
4. *Follow developmental norms and select early-acquired sounds and patterns.* Many clinicians select phonological targets using developmental norms for the order in which children attain phonemes and the order in which certain error patterns are suppressed. In this paradigm, clinicians select targets according to the pattern of normal phonological development based on the assumption that mastery of earlier-developing phonemes will be easier for children than later-developing phonemes (Gierut, Morrisette, Hughes, & Rowland, 1996).

5. *Follow developmental norms but select later-acquired sounds and patterns.* Just as some clinicians might select early-acquired sounds and patterns, other clinicians take the opposite approach and select later-acquired sounds and patterns based on developmental norms. The rationale for selecting later-developing sounds is to bring about greater phonological change than will be realized using early-developing sounds (Gierut et al., 1996).

Discharge

Children are generally discharged from therapy when their speech skills have normalized, usually defined as producing more than 85% of consonants correctly in spontaneous speech and being adultlike in speech production (Gruber, 1999). For children who are in school, it is also important that their speech skills do not interfere with educational progress. Some children experience **short-term normalization**, meaning that they achieve articulate and intelligible speech prior to 6 years of age, whereas others experience **long-term normalization**, in which articulate speech is achieved after age 6 (Shriberg, Gruber, & Kwiatkowski, 1994). For children who do not normalize by age 6, problems persist primarily with the *s* sounds (*s, z, sh*), with *r*-influenced vowels (*or, ar, ir*), and with the liquids (*l, r*) (Shriberg, Gruber, & Kwiatkowski, 1994). These sorts of residual errors are most common in children with a history of moderate to severe phonological problems during early childhood (Shriberg, Gruber, & Kwiatkowski, 1994).

As a final note, some children may normalize in their speech production and have intelligible, adultlike speech but continue to have phonological problems in areas associated with literacy. These include difficulties with phonological awareness and with applying this awareness to phonics instruction. Although the child's speech production skills have normalized, the history of phonological weakness may have set the child back in important ways that influence literacy and reading development (Gillon, 2004). Intervention may be needed to promote the child's application of phonological skills to literacy activities.

Case Study and Clinical Problem Solving

Carpenter Speech-Language Therapy Associates
2276 Oak Avenue
Springfield, Michigan

QUARTERLY PROGRESS REPORT

Client Name: Kayley Hart
Diagnosis: Phonological disorder
Date of Birth: 3/7/98
Age: 5; 6
Dates of Therapy: 6/8/03–9/12/03
Date of Report: 9/15/03

Background Information

At the referral of Dr. Arriana Lonigan, ENT, Kayley has received speech-language therapy for treatment of a phonological disorder at the Carpenter Center since 6/8/03. Her therapy program has consisted of one-hour small-group sessions and one-hour individual sessions two times a week for 12 weeks. Goals at the Carpenter Center were aligned with objectives on Kayley's Individualized Education Plan (IEP). In addition, the group sessions emphasized literacy-based activities and promoted phonological awareness and effective communicative skills with peers.

Pretherapy Assessment

Kayley's performance on standardized speech and language tests, including the Goldman-Fristoe Test of Articulation–2 and the Preschool Language Scale–3, were below the expected range for her age. The GFTA assessed Kayley's speech-sound performance and demonstrated a need to remediate the production of classes of sounds, including fricatives, and the suppression of a number of processes. Deletion of nasals and use of final consonant deletion and cluster reduction affected most Kayley's intelligibility. These goals were emphasized in this 3-month period of therapy. The PLS–3 showed that Kayley's performance in auditory comprehension tasks and expressive language skills fell below the normal limits.

Taking into account Kayley's test results, school recommendations, and observations, the following goals were established for the 12-week period discussed in this report:

Short-term goals and performance levels included:

Focus Area No. 1: Intervention to improve phonology/articulation
Kayley will:

1. Represent all sounds in consonant clusters in the initial position of single-syllable words when first modeled by clinician with at least 85% accuracy across all sessions.
   Results of treatment: Kayley achieved this goal during the final three individual sessions.
2. Suppress final consonant deletion for a range of sounds when first modeled by clinician with at least 85% accuracy across all sessions.
   Results of treatment: Accomplished for final position /t/ and /k/.
3. Use nasals in word-initial positions when first modeled by the clinician with at least 90% accuracy across all sessions.
   Results of treatment: Initial performance was 15%, and performance at final session was 92%, with an average performance of 74%.

Focus Area No. 2: Intervention to improve receptive and expressive language
Kayley will:

1. Use appropriate grammatical markers to mark plurals and possessives when first modeled by the clinician with at least 85% accuracy across all sessions.
   Results of treatment: Kayley used plurals with approximately 74% accuracy across sessions. Due to Kayley's difficulty in producing the /s/ sound, the measuring of the plural marker *s* at the end of a word (e.g., cats) was not an easy task. If she produced the *th* sound instead of the /s/ sound at the end of a plural word, it was assessed as correct.
2. Use novel words—nouns, verbs, object complements—upon introduction in therapy during communicative interactions.
   Results of treatment: Kayley consistently used novel words following their introduction in interactions with her therapist. Novel words used in the final session included, for instance, *trapeze, tiptoe, carefully, circus, giant,* and *stilts*.
3. Initiate with her peers to request and to question three or more times within group sessions.
   Kayley was prompted to initiate with her peers during group activities using prompted initiations in which she was given phrases to use to request and question her peers. In the final four sessions, Kayley averaged 6 initiations with her peers per session, with >80% successful.

Therapy Schedule was as follows (two days per week):

9:00 A.M. to 10:00 A.M.	Individual therapy session
10:00 A.M. to 11:00 A.M.	Group therapy session

Techniques included:

In the group therapy sessions:

- Activities that involved letter and sound correspondence and identification of the names of pictures and their initial sounds (with the sounds *b, t, l, g, m,* and *s*)

- Rhyme discrimination and rhyme matching activities (with the endings *-ell*, *-ock*, and *-op*)
- Sorting through various letters to correctly spell her name
- Promoting listening skills with specific directions for the activities and story time.

In the individual therapy sessions:

- Games were built on the use of flashcards to elicit the production of targeted sounds and patterns.
- Mirror work was introduced to promote awareness of oral motor movements in sound production.
- Minimal pairs were used to heighten awareness of contrasts between words (e.g., *star* vs. *tar*)
- Structured play with dolls and dollhouses was used to elicit expressive language. Clinician recast and expanded on Kayley's verbalizations to elicit the targeted goals and provide language modeling.

Summary

Kayley was always very cooperative, talkative, and willing to work. A number of phonological and language goals were achieved during this therapy period. Her Percentage of Consonants Correct (PCC) increased from 61% in June 2003 to 72% at present. Kayley also showed increases in self-confidence concerning communication. However, Kayley's mother reported that Kayley has also shown increases in frustration regarding her difficulties with effectively communicating, particularly at home. Continued speech-language intervention is recommended to promote age-appropriate language, speech, and literacy skills.

If you have any questions about this report, please do not hesitate to contact us.

Sincerely,

Kindra Osling, CCC-SLP
Speech-Language Pathologist

CLINICAL PROBLEM SOLVING

1. Kayley's therapy plan included both group and one-on-one sessions. What are some reasons for including both types of sessions in a child's therapy?
2. The report indicated that Kayley's PCC had increased over the 3 months of therapy. What is PCC? What does it measure?
3. The report indicated that Kayley's group sessions targeted phonological awareness and other literacy skills. Why would these be included as goals in speech-language intervention?
4. In your opinion, given that Kayley received approximately 24 hours of therapy during the report period, was her progress slow, moderate, or good? What kind of factors might contribute to a child' rate of progress during therapy?

CHAPTER SUMMARY

The term *phonological disorder* describes a condition in which an individual's phonological system is impaired. Children with phonological disorders develop their phonological system slowly and have deficient or immature phonological representations. This condition affects the production of speech sounds and is most serious when the child's intelligibility is severely compromised, making communication difficult.

The four primary symptoms of phonological disorders are difficulties with expressive phonology, phonological awareness, verbal working memory, and word learning and word retrieval. Expressive phonology refers to the production of specific speech sounds and patterns and is the hallmark of a phonological disorder. Phonological awareness describes an individual's awareness of the segmental aspects of spoken language, such as words, syllables, and phonemes. Many children with phonological disorders have problems with phonological awareness, which is a necessary skill for early reading development. Verbal working memory describes an individual's capacity to hold verbal information in storage for processing. Verbal working memory is important for language comprehension and is commonly weak in children with phonological disorders. Word learning and word retrieval describe the ability to learn new words and to retrieve words from the mental lexicon; this area, too, is weak in people who have a phonological disorder. Not all children have all four symptoms, but children with a poor underlying phonological system are at risk for difficulties in each area.

Five subtypes of speech delays include three varieties of phonological disorder—phonological disorder–unknown origin, phonological disorder–otitis media with effusion, and phonological disorder–special populations. Additional subtypes of speech delays include motor speech disorders and psychosocial involvement. For most cases of phonological disorders, the cause is unknown.

Treatment of phonological disorders requires early identification. With referral, a child who shows signs of a phonological disorder receives a comprehensive assessment by a specialist that involves case history, parent interview, articulation testing, speech sampling, and language assessment. The specialist identifies whether the phonological system is underdeveloped or disordered and develops a treatment plan for remediation. Phonologically oriented therapies focus on developing the underlying representations of phonology while simultaneously improving the child's intelligibility. Common approaches include minimal opposition contrast therapy, multiple oppositions therapy, and cycles therapy.

KEY TERMS

allophone, p. 148
alphabetic code, p. 154
articulation disorder, p. 146
articulatory phonetics, p. 149
assimilation, p. 154
auditory deprivation, p. 162
coarticulation, p. 154
cognates, p. 146
consonant, p. 149
cycles therapy, p. 174
dyslexia, p. 162
expressive phonology, p. 156
grapheme-phoneme correspondence, p. 154
IPA, p. 149
long-term normalization, p. 176
manner of articulation, p. 151
minimal opposition contrast therapy, p. 173
multiple oppositions therapy, p. 174
myofunctional disorders, p. 160
oral mechanism screening, p. 169
PCC, p. 172
phonics, p. 154
phonological awareness, p. 155
phonological disorder, p. 146
place of articulation, p. 149
residual errors, p. 159
short-term normalization, p. 176
speech delay, p. 143
stimulability, p. 171
surface representation, p. 147
underlying representation, p. 147
unintelligibility, p. 161
verbal working memory, p. 155
voicing, p. 151
vowel, p. 149

ON THE WEB

Check out the Companion Website at http://www.prenhall.com/justice! On it, you will find:

- suggested readings
- reflection questions
- a self-study quiz
- links to additional online resources, including information about current technologies in communication sciences and disorders

Motor Speech Disorders

Apraxia and Dysarthria

Edwin Maas and Donald A. Robin

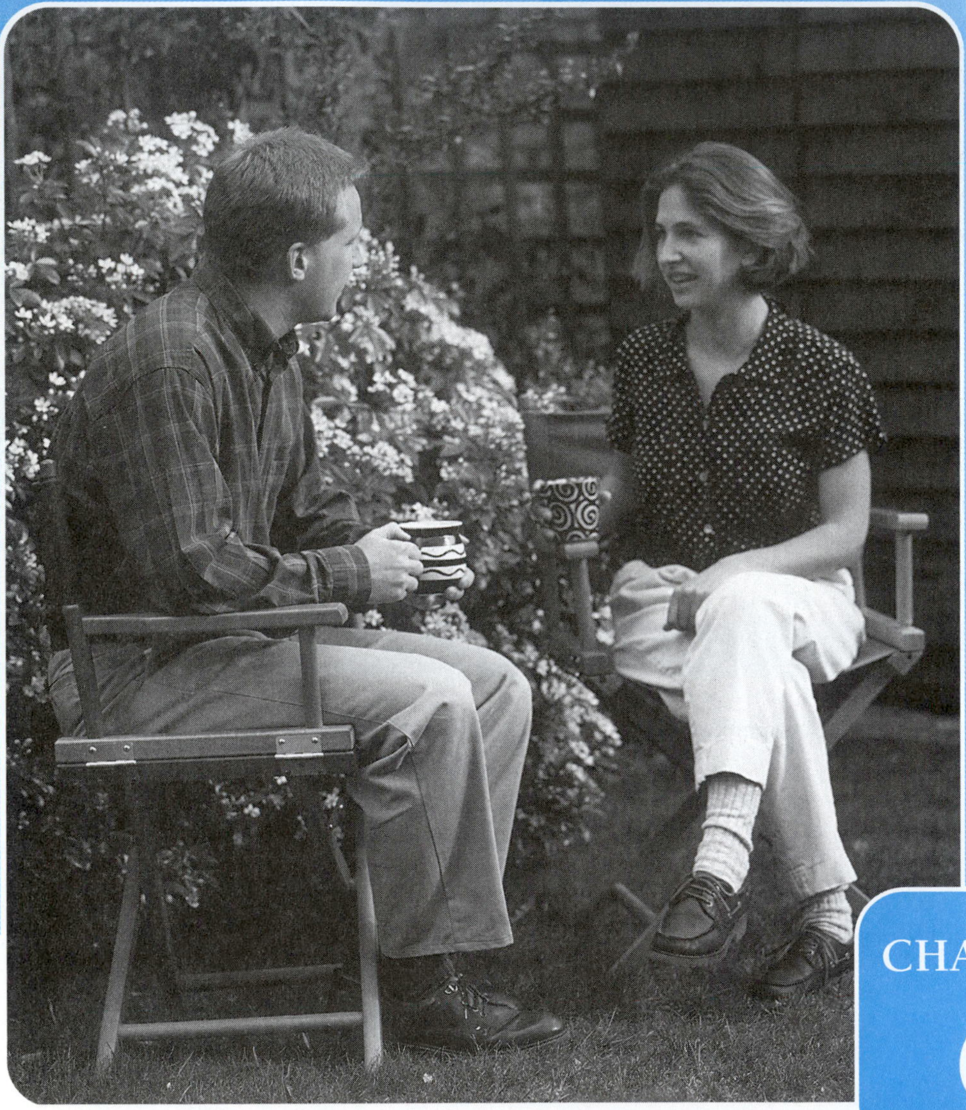

CHAPTER 6

FOCUS QUESTIONS

This chapter answers the following questions:

1. What is a motor speech disorder?
2. How are motor speech disorders classified?
3. What are the defining characteristics of prevalent types of motor speech disorders?
4. How are motor speech disorders identified?
5. How are motor speech disorders treated?

INTRODUCTION

Speech production is the most effective way to communicate. It is also one of the most impressive motor skills possessed by the human species. Speech production involves the rapid and fine-tuned coordination of many muscles and muscle groups in a fluent, continuous manner. A difference in the onset of muscle contractions of as little as 40 to 50 milliseconds can mean the difference between two sounds (e.g., /b/ vs. /p/); thus accuracy in motor production is critical for effective communication. The fact that speakers can reliably produce such small differences in timing indicates the degree of control speakers must and can exert over the coordination of muscle contractions. An individual's control over the muscular coordination involved with producing speech is called **speech motor control.**

Speech motor control follows a course of development that begins at birth and continues to about age 12. During these years, children's speech movements are less accurate and show greater variability compared to those of adult speakers (Clark, Robin, McCullagh, & Schmidt, 2001; Maner, Smith, & Grayson, 2000; Moore & Ruark, 1996; Smith & Goffman, 1998; Wohlert & Smith, 2002). By adolescence, most children exhibit adultlike speech motor control.

Some children, however, have great difficulty acquiring the degree of speech motor control seen in adult speakers or other typically developing children. These children have difficulty articulating the stream of speech needed to accurately and consistently produce speech for conversation. Although in many cases the exact cause of children's problems with the motor control of speech is unknown, most experts agree that such problems are related to neurological difficulties. Adults also can experience difficulty with motor control of speech, particularly after injuries or illnesses that affect the brain regions linked to speech motor control. This chapter discusses these disorders of communication, called motor speech disorders, from a lifespan perspective. The two major categories of motor speech disorders are apraxia of speech and dysarthria, both of which can affect children and adults.

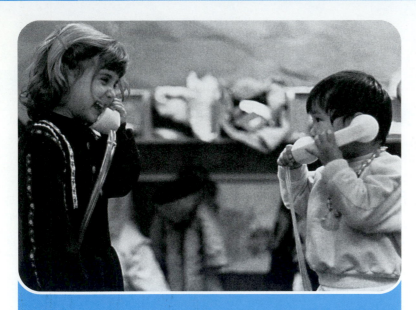

A difference in the onset of muscle contractions of just milliseconds means the difference between a /b/ and a /p/.

What Is a Motor Speech Disorder?

Definition

A **motor speech disorder** is an impairment of speech production caused by defects of the neuromuscular system, the motor control system, or both (Clark, Stierwalt, & Robin, 2000). With a motor speech disorder, defects in these underlying systems involved with planning, programming, and executing speech result in significant difficulties producing fluent, intelligible speech. A motor speech disorder does not result from and cannot be explained by other disorders, such as language impairment or phonological disorders, although these types of communication disorders may co-occur with a motor speech disorder. People with motor speech disorders may also exhibit difficulties with other functions that involve oral movements aside from speech, such as chewing and smiling, since the impairment affects the motor system.

Terminology

This section presents the concepts and terminology required to understand breakdowns in the control of motor speech. The first section describes four systems involved with speech production—the respiratory, phonatory, resonatory, and articulatory systems—and offers a review of concepts presented in chapter 3. The second section describes key concepts for understanding motor control, including motor units; motor planning, programming, and execution; and motor learning.

Systems of Speech Production

Speech production involves the coordination in space and time of muscles and muscle groups from four major systems. The four systems are the respiratory, phonatory, resonatory, and articulatory systems (see Table 6-1). Three of these systems (respiration, phonation, and

TABLE 6-1 The four systems of speech production

System	Key Structures	Muscles and Articulators Involved
Respiratory	lungs	respiratory and postural muscles
Phonatory	larynx	vocal folds
Resonatory	velopharyngeal port, pharynx	velum, pharynx
Articulatory	oral cavity	jaw, lips, tongue

articulation) were described in chapter 1. The resonatory system is introduced here. Each system includes many muscles, which must be carefully coordinated temporally and spatially with other muscles within and across subsystems.

FIGURE 6-1 **Respiratory system.**

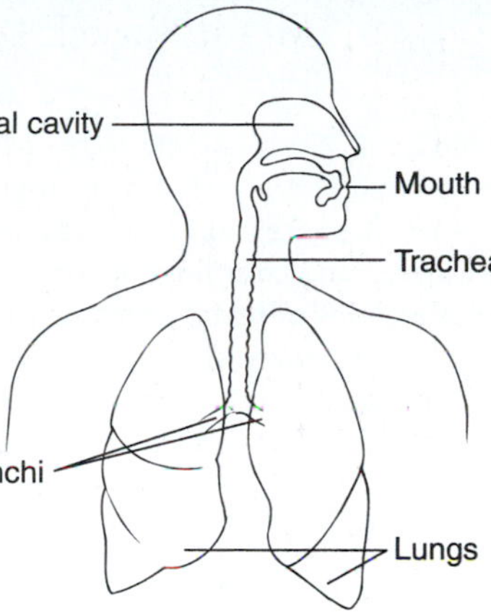

Respiratory System. Speech production requires airflow to produce sound. The airflow for speech may be ingressive (going in) or egressive (going out), but most languages, including English, rely on egressive airflow for sound production (Ladefoged, 2001). The most important mechanism for producing airflow is the pulmonary mechanism, including the lungs, which produces airflow by pushing air out of the lungs through the trachea, or windpipe, using various muscle groups (see Figure 6-1). The pulmonary mechanism is a major structure in the **respiratory system**, which regulates the inhalation/exhalation cycle for passive breathing and for producing speech.

To produce fluent speech, an individual must carefully control the exhalation cycle so that it extends the length of an utterance in a controlled and coordinated manner. In passive breathing, the duration of inhalation versus exhalation corresponds to a ratio of approximately 1:1, but in speech production this ratio ranges from about 1:6 to 1:9 (Yorkston, Beukelman, Strand, & Bell, 1999). When speaking, speakers inhale briefly, typically at clause boundaries (Winkworth, Davis, Adams, & Ellis, 1995), and extend the exhalation period to the end of the utterance (Kent, 1997; Robin, Solomon, Moon, & Folkins, 1997; Winkworth et al., 1995). For instance, to produce a brief narrative such as that presented below, the speaker pauses at clauses (marked here with a #) to inhale for continued airflow:

> When we received the letter in the mail# we immediately contacted our insurance agent# to let them know about our concerns# they didn't seem too worried# so we didn't pursue the matter . . .

To further complicate speech production, utterances require stress assignment on some syllables and words. For instance, in the example presented here, the words *we, letter,* and *mail* in the first utterance are emphasized relative to the other words. This means that the exhalation cycle not only needs to be extended in time for speech production, but also must be manipulated to produce stress. In short, breath support is crucial for oxygen intake as well as for speech production.

FIGURE 6-2 **Phonatory system.**

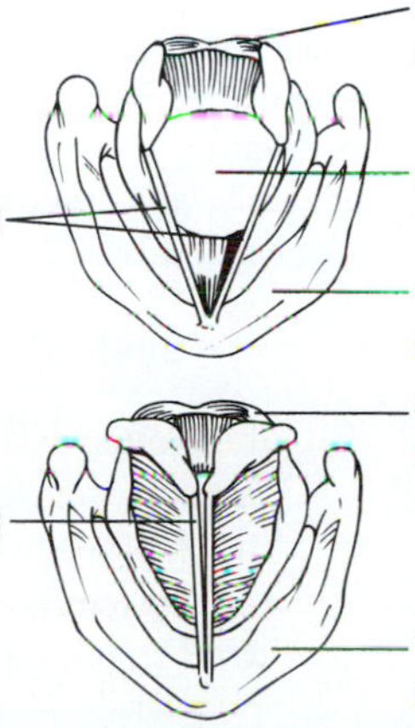

Phonatory System. Humans produce speech sounds by modulating or changing the airflow in various ways and at various points along the vocal tract. One major source of sound production is the vibration of the vocal folds that sit within the larynx, as discussed in Chapter 3 and shown in Figure 6-2.

The various muscles and structures in the larynx, including the vocal folds, form the phonatory system of speech production. The **phonatory system** regulates the production of voice and the prosodic or intonational aspects of speech. To produce many of the consonant sounds (e.g., /m/, /b/, /z/) and all the vowel sounds, the vocal folds are brought close together (adduction) by various muscle groups so that the airflow causes them to vibrate. The vocal folds are stretched lengthwise to manipulate the frequency or pitch of the voice, which carries both linguistic and nonlinguistic information. The opening between the vocal folds is

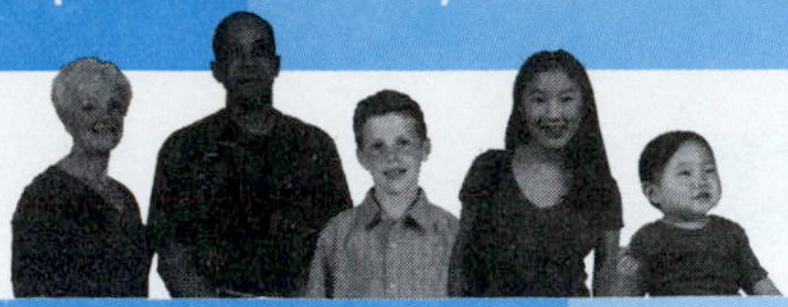

BOX 6-1 Motor Speech Disorders Across the Lifespan: Case Examples

Bob is a 42-year-old bank vice president in the Midwest. He is married, with four children, and is bilingual, speaking both English and Spanish fluently. He travels regularly to visit family in Mexico, California, and Texas. Until recently, Bob coached a children's soccer team and was involved in church and town activities. In 2003, however, Bob began to have difficulty walking and coordinating arm movements. When he finally saw a neurologist for an assessment, the neurologist ordered a series of tests, which revealed a tumor in the cerebellum. Surgery was performed within the week, and the tumor was removed successfully. Despite the removal of the tumor, Bob is now ataxic, showing serious difficulty in coordinating voluntary movements, and he has a severe tremor. He requires a wheelchair to get around and has moderately to severely impaired speech, with estimates of about 30% intelligibility by those close to him.

Internet research

1. According to current estimates, how many Spanish-English bilingual speakers live in the United States?
2. What percentage of speech-language pathologists are fluent in both Spanish and English?
3. What is the incidence and prevalence of brain tumors in the United States?

Brainstorm and discussion

1. What are some ways in which Bob's current motor difficulties affect his participation in life at home and in the community?
2. What types of strategies might you suggest to improve Bob's participation in life?

Walter is a 60-year-old man who lives with his second wife in the Pacific Northwest. His two daughters from his first marriage live close by and visit with him almost every week. In his spare time, Walter likes to read, play tennis, improve the house, and play the piano. Walter holds a doctorate in business administration and is a professor in the Business Administration Department at a local university.

At age 59, Walter suffered a left-hemisphere stroke, which resulted in weakness on the right side of his body and almost complete loss of speech production abilities. In the months following his stroke, Walter's speech improved slowly, but it currently remains slow, effortful, and inconsistently distorted, with about 75% intelligibility. His language comprehension and language production skills are largely intact, with the exception of occasional word-finding problems. The right-sided weakness remains, which also affects the oral structures (tongue, lips). Walter currently uses a cane to walk, and he writes with his nondominant left hand. Walter was diagnosed by his speech-language pathologist as having mild aphasia and a mild apraxia of speech, characterized by slow and effortful speech with inconsistent distortions and prosody impairments.

Internet research

1. What are the incidence and prevalence of stroke in the United States? How do these figures vary as a function of educational attainment?
2. What is the average duration of hospitalization for a person who has had a stroke?
3. What percentage of people who experience a stroke return to live independently at home?

the glottis, and the buildup of sufficient air pressure below the glottis, called subglottal air pressure, sets the vocal folds into cycles of vibration. The phonatory system coordinates with the respiratory system, which provides the airflow needed for phonation. In short, the phonatory system is essential for producing both voiced and voiceless sounds and for modifying word stress, intonation, and other aspects of prosody.

Brainstorm and discussion

1. Walter has improved his speech intelligibility from total unintelligibility to 75% intelligibility. What are some factors influencing his recovery?
2. How likely is it that Walter will teach again? What strategies could be used to promote his communication in the classroom?

Hikaru is a 5-year-old boy who came to the United States from Japan with his family when he was 2. Hikaru attends an English-only public school because that is the only option in his state. Expressively, he is primarily an English user, but receptively, he also understands Japanese because it is used at home. He was referred for a speech and language evaluation by his mother because of concerns about articulation difficulties. His mother reported that Hikaru was slow to talk and has always drooled a lot while talking. During the evaluation, the clinician observed that Hikaru had social skills appropriate for the North American culture and interacted well with the clinician. Hikaru's communication strategies included the use of gestures, facial expressions, changes in prosody, and verbal expression using both English and Japanese words. Hikaru exhibited severe delays in expressive language, in particular, in syntax (reduced utterance length) and phonology (sound substitutions and deletions). His speech production was imprecise and appeared weak, consistent with flaccid dysarthria. Based on the evaluation, these motor difficulties seemed largely restricted to the articulatory system. Hikaru's mother is concerned about his speech difficulties and is considering delaying Hikaru's entry into first grade by a year.

Internet research

1. How many states have adopted legislation that mandate public schools to provide English-only education?
2. What proportion of children in the United States are bilingual?

Brainstorm and discussion

1. What are some possible reasons Hikaru's parents did not pursue an evaluation earlier in light of Hikaru's history of speech problems (e.g., drooling)?
2. The Japanese language does not have consonant clusters and syllable-final consonants (as in *truck*). How relevant is this to the speech evaluation? What other differences between Japanese and English might be relevant for fully understanding Hikaru's problems?
3. In your opinion, will holding Hikaru back from first grade be an advantage or a detriment to his development? After stating your opinion, investigate research on the topic to see what researchers say about the advantages and detriments of grade retention.

Resonatory System. The **resonatory system** regulates the resonation or vibration of the airflow as it moves from the pharynx into the oral and/or nasal cavities. Resonance refers to the effect of the shape and size of the vocal tract on sound quality, and an important aspect of vocal resonance is whether the nasal cavity is used as a vibrating chamber. This is determined by the state of the **velopharyngeal port**, which is the opening between the velum

FIGURE 6-3 Resonatory and articulatory systems.

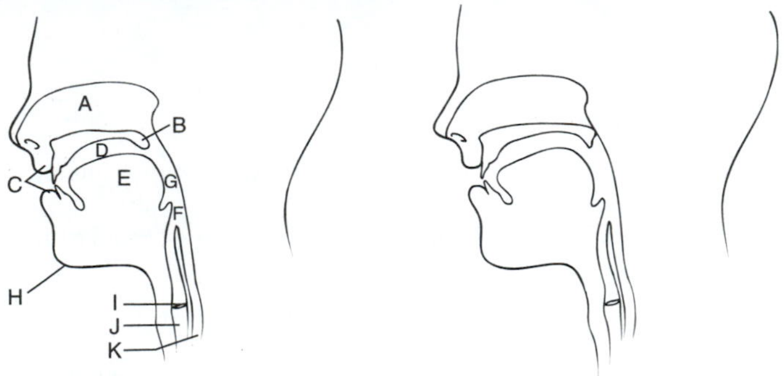

In the left panel the velum (B) is lowered, opening the velopharyngeal port (G) to produce a nasal sound; in the right panel, the velum is raised and the velopharyngeal port closed, to produce an oral sound. A = nasal cavity; B = velum; C = upper and lower lips; D = oral cavity; E = tongue; F = pharynx; G = velopharyngeal port; H = jaw; I = larynx; J = trachea; K = esophagus.

(soft palate) and the back of the pharynx wall (see Figure 6-3). When the velum is raised, the velopharyngeal port is closed (the velum touches the back wall of the pharynx), and air flows out through and resonates within only the oral cavity. When the velum is lowered, the velopharyngeal port is open, and air flows out through both the oral and nasal cavities, affecting the quality of the sound (nasality). Regulation of the velopharyngeal port is important for producing the difference between oral and nasal sounds (e.g., /b/ and /m/) and for ensuring a normal sound quality. The resonatory system must be carefully timed and coordinated with the respiratory and phonatory systems for fluent speech production.

Articulatory System. The fourth system of speech is the **articulatory system**, which regulates the control of the articulators within the oral cavity to manipulate the outgoing airflow in different ways, usually at very high speeds. The major structures involved in articulation are the lower jaw and lips for opening and closing movements and creating constrictions at the end of the oral cavity. The tongue also is an important structure for creating constrictions and obstructions within the oral cavity (see Figure 6-3). In fact, the tongue is probably the most important articulator because of its flexibility and capacity for high-speed motion. The tongue is a muscular hydrostat, which means that it does not contain bone or cartilage and that it maintains its volume regardless of muscle contractions (Kent, 1997). The tongue comprises many muscles and muscle groups, and these are categorized as intrinsic muscles, which originate within the tongue, and extrinsic muscles, which originate outside the tongue. The intrinsic muscles regulate the more fine-tuned movements of the tongue. The extrinsic muscles regulate coarser movements, such as tongue protrusion, tongue retraction, tongue elevation, and tongue depression (Kent, 1997). Contractions of these muscle groups create constrictions of varying degrees and locations within the oral cavity. The tongue is sometimes divided into four sections: the apex (tip of the tongue), the lamina or blade (front of tongue), the center (middle part of tongue), and the dorsum (back of tongue). These sections are shown in Figure 6-4.

Changes in the positions and shapes of the tongue and other articulators result in different speech sounds. At a very general level, speech sounds are divided into consonants and vowels, as discussed in Chapter 5. To review, *consonants* are a group of speech sounds that involve a constriction in the vocal tract; *vowels* are a group of speech sounds that

FIGURE 6-4 **Subdivisions of the tongue. A = tip or apex; B = blade or front; C = center; D = dorsum or back.**

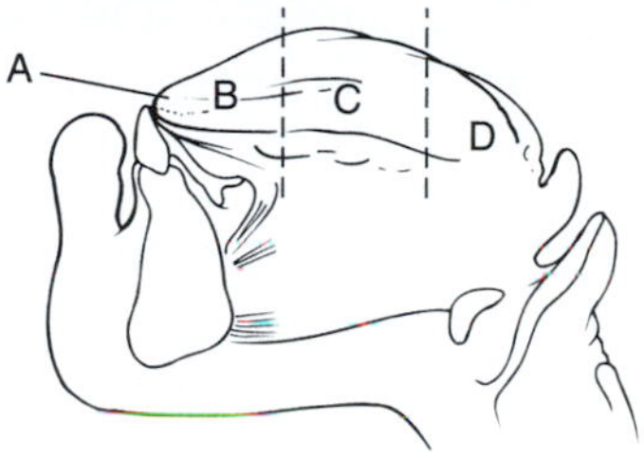

involve relatively little or no constriction of the vocal tract but a modulation of the shape of the oral cavity by the tongue, lips, and/or jaw.

For consonants, the constriction may be a complete obstruction of airflow, as in the case of stop consonants, such as /p/ (obstruction at lips), /d/ (obstruction at tongue tip), and /k/ (obstruction at tongue dorsum), and nasal consonants, such as /m/ (obstruction at lips), /n/ (obstruction at tongue tip), and /ŋ/ (obstruction at tongue dorsum). Some consonants involve a partial constriction, such as /f/, /z/, and /ð/, for which a narrow constriction is created to push a turbulent airflow through the constriction location. For some sounds, such as /w/, /r/, and /l/, the constriction is wider, so that the airflow is smoother and continuous rather than turbulent.

For vowels (at least for the English vowels), the airflow is never turbulent, and the continuous airflow is manipulated by the tongue in the oral cavity to create the varying vowel sounds. Diphthongs are an interesting variety of vowels that involve a gliding movement in the production of the sound, as in *oy*.

In producing the consonants and vowels, the actions of the tongue and the articulatory system must work seamlessly with the other systems—respiratory, phonatory, and resonatory—to produce well-articulated and fluent speech that unfolds over time.

This brief overview of the motor systems involved in speech production demonstrates the complexity of speech as a motor skill and the requirement for fine-tuned and rapid coordination of the four systems involved with speech production. Given this complexity, it is not surprising that both children and adults may experience failures in motor speech coordination. Sometimes the four individual systems are poorly coordinated, resulting in breakdowns in the larger motor speech production system. Or, deficits in the coordination of the muscles and muscle groups within a specific system may cause the entire system to break down because of the complex interrelationships among the four systems.

Speech Motor Control

Production of fluent speech requires the rapid coordination of muscle activity across a wide range of muscle groups within the four systems. To maintain speed and fluency when speaking as well as accuracy of movements, the sequences of movements are programmed together as a single movement unit. If we consider the vast number of muscles and muscle groups involved in fluent articulation, and thus the large number of degrees of freedom (the number of elements, such as muscles, that can be independently controlled), the magnitude of the challenge facing the speaker becomes apparent. One way to contend with the challenge of controlling all these different muscles in a coordinated and fluent manner is to reduce the number of degrees of freedom by organizing motor actions into motor units (Kent, Adams, & Turner, 1996). A motor unit is a single control mechanism that controls more than one degree of freedom.

Motor Units. A **motor unit**, sometimes called a **motor program** or muscle synergy, is "a piece of behavior that can be utilized repeatedly in various actions, producing essentially the same movements (but scaled to the environment) each time" (Schmidt & Lee, 1999, p. 208). Motor units are those aspects of a movement that remain constant over repeated productions in different contexts and therefore seem to be planned and executed as a whole, although timing and force can vary across executions.

Consider the following as an example. In order to kick a ball, you have to swing your leg backward, using muscles in the back of your thigh, and then reverse to swing your leg forward, using muscles in the front of your thigh. The timing and force of these two aspects of the movement are closely related, so that when your leg swings backward, it must also swing forward at least the same distance to hit the ball. The relative force and timing of the muscle contractions with respect to each other are organized as a whole. The actual absolute force produced by these muscles depends on other factors, such as the distance between kicker and ball, the size and weight of the ball, and how far the ball is to be kicked. The basic pattern of the movement components remains constant, however, while more specific aspects of the movements (e.g., muscle contractions) are influenced by the specific circumstances.

Speech production is even more complicated than kicking a ball. When producing speech, an individual is producing linguistic units—phrases, words, syllables, and phonemes—and is simultaneously producing acoustic events—pitch and loudness variations—that map onto the linguistic units. It is not clear whether the motor units produced during speech correspond to the linguistic units or the acoustic events (Ballard, Granier, & Robin, 2000; Folkins, 1985; Folkins & Bleile, 1990; Knock, Ballard, Robin, & Schmidt, 2000; Smith & Goffman, 1998). What this means is that the relationship between the linguistic and motor systems involved with speech production is not completely understood (Kent et al., 1996). However, experts generally agree that the linguistic system provides input to the motor system in speech production, as discussed in the model of speech production presented in Chapter 1 (Browman & Goldstein, 1990, 1997; Gracco, 1997; Levelt, Roelofs, & Meyer, 1999; Van der Merwe, 1997). It is also clear that speech motor control involves a tight integration and coordination of various muscle groups and systems (Abbs, Gracco, & Cole, 1984; Gracco & Abbs, 1987; Kelso, Tuller, Bateson, & Fowler, 1984). This coordination involves programming particular configurations of muscle activity into single motor units to ensure accurate and fluent articulation.

Motor Planning, Programming, and Execution. Planning and programming a motor unit are different from executing a motor act (Schmidt & Lee, 1999). Motor planning and programming are aspects of motor control that occur *before* initiation of movement, whereas execution occurs *at* or *after* initiation. For example, when a person produces a sentence, intonation typically shows a decline across the sentence so that the sentence ends at a lower pitch than it began. This change occurs in part because of the decreasing breath support at the end of the exhalation phase as the speaker runs out of breath. We might consider that this loss of pitch at the end of a sentence relates solely to motor execution or the actual delivery of speech. However, this would not be quite accurate. Speakers usually start at a higher pitch when they have to produce a longer sentence than they do when they have to produce a shorter sentence. This phenomenon provides evidence that speakers prepare how they will modulate intonation over a whole sentence. In other words, speakers spread out the exhalation across the entire utterance so they do not have to pause for inhalation. The higher pitch at the beginning of longer utterances is actually a phenomenon of motor planning (Cooper & Klouda, 1987; Manjula & Patil, 2004).

Discussion Point: *Ask a peer to tell you about something he or she did recently, such as going on a trip. Examine how pitch changes over utterances, and consider how many of these changes were planned in advance.*

Motor planning and programming—which happen prior to execution of a movement—are important aspects of motor behavior that professionals must consider when they work with individuals experiencing motor problems. Professionals must determine whether a breakdown in motor performance occurs in the planning and programming or in the execution of the motor act. The exact nature of the processes involved in motor planning and programming are not totally understood (McNeil, Doyle, & Wambaugh, 2000), but experts do recognize that aspects of a movement are planned, or preprogrammed, based on central processes and without any external feedback since the movement has yet to be executed (e.g., Abbs et al., 1984; Guenther & Perkell, 2004; Klapp, 1995; McNeil et al., 2000; Perkell et al., 2000; Schmidt & Lee, 1999; Shea, Lai, Wright, Immink, & Black, 2001).

On the basis of this background, the remainder of this chapter will use the following terminology to describe motor speech control:

- **Motor planning** refers to the processes that define and sequence articulatory goals (e.g., lip closure, onset of voicing) prior to their occurrence.
- **Motor programming** refers to the processes responsible for establishing and preparing the flow of motor information across muscles for speech production and specifying the timing and force required for the movements.
- **Motor execution** refers to the processes responsible for activating relevant muscles during the movements used in speech production. (Van der Merwe, 1997)

It is sometimes difficult for experts to tease apart motor planning and motor programming; therefore, motor planning and programming will be considered together throughout this chapter.

Motor Learning. The ability to effectively plan and program speech movements requires extensive practice to achieve the stability and flexibility that characterizes skilled speech production. Extensive practice using speech is needed to learn and develop motor control through motor learning. **Motor learning** is the way in which "practice or experience leads to relatively permanent changes in the capability for movement" (Schmidt & Lee, 1999), and it is an important concept for understanding normal and disordered speech motor control.

When considering normal and abnormal development of speech motor control, an important question is how the motor speech system learns to form the appropriate units to ensure fluent and accurate execution of movements during speech. One concept to describe this learning, called schema theory, suggests that individuals develop **schemas**—memory representations of relationships between various sources of information (Schmidt, 1976, 2003; Schmidt & Lee, 1999). These schemas represent the motor specifications needed to reach a desired outcome, including the initial state of the muscles or structures as well as the actual outcome of the movement. A schema becomes stronger with experience because information about the movements and muscle configurations is stored after every movement. For future movements, the person can then use the stored schema to produce the corresponding motor specifications that will lead to the desired outcome.

The stored schemas of people who produce motor speech movements that are well planned and executed, resulting in precise and intelligible speech, provide a solid representation of speech production processes. The schemas of people who have motor speech disorders provide representations of motor planning, programming, and execution that are flawed. The stored schemas specifying these behaviors need to be unlearned and replaced with schemas that specify improved motor control.

Prevalence and Incidence

Reliable estimates of prevalence and incidence for specific motor speech disorders are rare. For adults who exhibit communication disorders due to trauma or illness (e.g., stroke), one estimate comes from a study of 3,417 patients seen in the Mayo Clinic for acquired neurogenic communication disorders. This study found that motor speech disorders accounted for more than 50% of these communication disorders; 46.3% were diagnosed with dysarthria and 4.6% with apraxia of speech (Duffy, 1995). At least at the Mayo Clinic, the prevalence of motor speech disorders among those who seek treatment for acquired neurogenic communication disorders is quite high.

Among children, estimates of prevalence for motor speech disorders are also hard to come by. Speech delays affect about 4% of children (Shriberg, Tomblin, & McSweeney, 1999). However, what number of these children exhibit speech delays because of a motor speech disorder is not clear. Experts contend that these children represent a very small subsection of the larger population of children with speech delays, with some estimates suggesting that about 5% of cases of childhood speech delays occur because of motor speech problems (Kwiatkowski & Shriberg, 1993). However, these are rough estimates. No comprehensive investigation of incidence or prevalence of motor speech disorders among children is available at present, primarily because of difficulties identifying specific motor speech disorders and long-standing debates over the tools and criteria used to identify motor speech problems in children.

How Are Motor Speech Disorders Classified?

Discussion Point: *Consider each of the cases in Box 6-1. Characterize each motor speech disorder in terms of acquired versus developmental and identify the cause of each.*

Etiology

Motor speech disorders may be acquired or developmental. Acquired motor speech disorders result from damage to a previously intact nervous system, most often caused by cerebrovascular accidents (CVAs) or strokes, degenerative diseases such as Parkinson disease and amyolateral sclerosis, brain tumors, and traumatic brain injury.

Developmental motor speech disorders result from abnormal development of the nervous system or from damage to the nervous system in its early development (Thompson & Robin, 1993). Abnormal development may result from various congenital diseases, including cerebral palsy and a variety of genetic syndromes such as fragile-X and Down syndrome. Damage to the developing nervous system may be caused by traumatic brain injury, brain tumors, and CVAs.

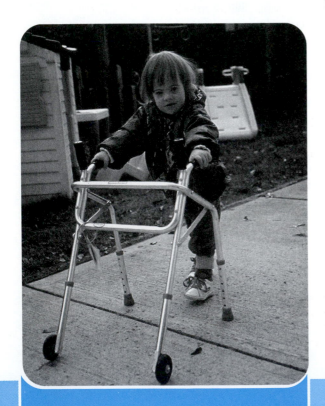

Children with cerebral palsy, because of its impact on neuromuscular functioning, often exhibit motor speech disorders.

Manifestation

Motor speech disorders are divided into impairments of motor planning and programming and impairments of motor execution. For fluent, articulate speech, the individual systems and muscles of speech production as well as the coordination of muscle contractions within and among systems must be intact. Breakdowns at all levels of the motor speech system are possible.

Sometimes breakdowns occur at the level of execution, as with disruptions of muscle physiology. For example, paralysis of the tongue will seriously impede speech production, regardless of whether speech is planned and programmed normally or not. Similarly, speech production will be affected by involuntary movements (e.g., tremors) of muscles and by reductions in range, speed, and consistency of movement. In such cases, the speech motor problem results from difficulties or impairment with execution of speech.

Breakdowns can also occur at the level of planning and programming. In such cases, muscle physiology and movement abilities (e.g., range, speed, and direction of movement) are intact, but the coordination of the relevant muscles and muscle groups (within and among systems) for a given speech target is disrupted. For instance, the individual may not experience paralysis of the tongue, but may have difficulty moving the tongue in the right way at the right moment in time for a given speech target. This situation would be consistent with a disruption at a level of processing prior to execution, namely, at the motor planning and programming levels.

Severity

Motor speech disorders, whether developmental or acquired, or affecting children or adults, range from mild to severe. The degree of severity is determined not only by the symptoms, but also, and more importantly, by how the disorder affects the person's participation in life. An individual person may have a motor speech disorder that profoundly affects speech intelligibility but does not have any impact on daily living activities. What is most critical to consider when determining a disorder's severity is the distinction between different levels of disorder, as detailed by the World Health Organization (WHO). The WHO distinguishes between three aspects of a disorder, namely, disease, activity, and participation in life (WHO, 2001).

- The **disease** is the underlying physiological condition that impedes performance. Disease also refers to the psychological cause of a disorder. For motor speech disorders, the disease is the neurological deficit impacting speech production and its systems.
- The **activity** level refers to the actual behavioral or performance deficits that result from the disease. In motor speech disorders, the most important indices of activity are speech intelligibility and fluency or naturalness.
- **Participation in life** considers how the disease impacts the quality of life of the individual, that is, how it affects the person's ability to live a happy and productive life as defined by that person (Clark et al., 2000). For motor speech disorders, this factor refers to how the speech impairment impacts an individual's performance at home, at school, at work, and in the community.

Professionals who work with individuals with motor speech disorders must consider the severity of the disorder on all three aspects: disease, activity, and participation in life. A person may have severe symptoms of the disease but be relatively unaffected in terms of activity and participation. On the other hand, the disease and its symptoms may appear relatively mild, but they may have a great impact on the person's activity and participation. By considering severity using the WHO scales, professionals are able to focus more holistically on motor speech disorders, taking into account the symptoms as well as how those symptoms affect an individual's life at home, at school, at work, and in the community.

Discussion Point: *Consider the case of Walter in Box 6-1. In what ways has his impairment impacted his life? Have these impacts been serious or mild?*

Characterizing Individual Differences

As is the case with many abilities and disorders, a range of individual differences occur for motor speech disorders. The effects of a neurological disease on an individual differ from person to person, even if the cause and severity of the disease are similar. Individuals differ in their

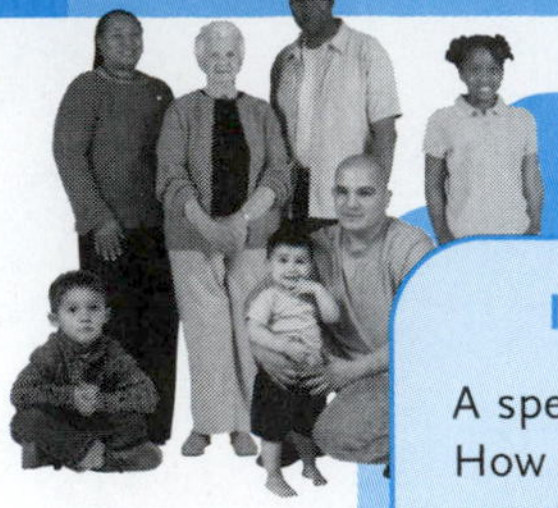

BOX 6-2 Multicultural Focus

Issues for Motor Speech Disorders

A speech sound is never produced exactly the same way twice, even by the same speaker. How a speech sound is produced depends on many factors, including the surrounding speech sounds (e.g., the *k* sound at the beginning of *cook* involves lip rounding, but the *k* sound at the beginning of *kit* does not), speech rate and loudness, the emotional state of the speaker, and the particular dialect and language of the speaker. Differences between speakers in how they produce speech sounds exist even for people who speak the same language and dialect, but these differences are greatest for speakers with different language or dialect backgrounds. Such differences are important to consider in the assessment and treatment of motor speech disorders.

The distinction between a language and a dialect is based on the principle of mutual intelligibility. If two speakers can understand each other they are considered to be speaking the same language (they are mutually intelligible). A dialect refers to variation in a language's syntax, vocabulary, phonology, and pronunciation (e.g., Garn-Nunn & Lynn, 2004) and may vary along geographical, social, economical, religious, or political boundaries. For example, most speakers of American English produce the *th* sound (in *teeth*) by sticking their tongue tip between their teeth, whereas most speakers of British English place the tip of their tongue behind their upper front teeth (Ladefoged, 2001). Moreover, even within American English there are differences. For instance, speakers of the dialect African American English may not produce the *th* sound at all since it is not part of their dialect, substituting *d* (as in "dat" for *that*) or *f* (as in "bof" for *both*). These are considered dialect differences between speakers of the same language. As another example, the production of the sound *r* differs greatly among speakers, even speakers of the same general dialect. In American English, there are two broad ways to produce *r*, one with the tongue tip behind the teeth and the other with the tongue bunched up toward the palate (e.g., Guenther, Hampson, & Johnson, 1998); they are perceptually indistinguishable.

Given that dialects are important for a sense of belonging to a particular community, treatment targets must be appropriate for each individual to ensure consideration of the speech community or communities to which the person belongs. In addition, an awareness of other possible ways to produce a sound may help in identifying useful compensatory pronunciations, especially when the resulting sound is perceptually indistinguishable, as with the *r* example.

When planning assessment and treatment, consideration of factors such as the individual's community and language background and associated variations in pronunciation are perhaps even more important when working with individuals who speak multiple languages (and dialects thereof) or for whom English is not a native language. For example, an impairment of the phonatory system resulting from dysarthria may be more obvious during assessment of a speaker of Mandarin Chinese, a tonal language, than during assessment of a speaker who does not speak a tonal language. Such an impairment may also be much more devastating for a speaker of Mandarin Chinese, since subtle tone variations can lead to quite different meanings, which is not the case for a language like English.

For Discussion

What are some specific ways that the dialect of a client might affect the assessment process? How would you go about finding an interpreter for a client whose language you do not speak? What are some potential problems that might arise when working with an interpreter?

Companion Website

To answer these questions online, go to the Multicultural Focus module in chapter 6 of the Companion Website.

ability to compensate for a motor or muscle physiology problem, their ability to use unimpaired systems to take over for the loss of the impaired system, and their general life response to major medical problems. In addition, treatment of motor speech disorders produces widely varying results as a function of several factors, including the person's perceptions of disability, family support systems, adherence to intervention activities, and desire to improve, among others.

What Are the Defining Characteristics of Prevalent Types of Motor Speech Disorders?

Motor speech disorders are divided into disorders of motor planning and programming and disorders of motor execution (Darley, Aronson, & Brown, 1975; McNeil, Robin, & Schmidt, 1997; Van der Merwe, 1997). Motor planning and programming disorders are caused by an inability to group and sequence the relevant muscles with respect to one another in order to plan or program a movement. **Motor execution disorders** are caused by deficits or inefficiencies in basic physiological or movement characteristics of the musculature, such as muscle tone, movement speed, and movement range. Motor speech disorders also affect other oral motor behaviors, such as smiling (e.g., Folkins, Moon, Luschei, Robin, Tye-Murray, & Moll, 1995; Robin et al., 1997).

The following sections first discuss disorders of speech motor programming and planning, including acquired apraxia of speech (AOS) and developmental or childhood apraxia of speech (CAS). They then describe speech execution disorders, namely, acquired and developmental dysarthria. An overview of important characteristics of these motor speech disorders and how they affect speech production is provided in Table 6-2.

Motor Programming and Planning Disorders and Acquired Apraxia of Speech (AOS)

Defining Characteristics

Apraxia of speech (AOS) is an impairment of motor programming and planning that involves an inability to transform a linguistic representation into the appropriate coordinated movements of the articulators (Clark et al., 2000). Thus, a child may have the linguistic representation of the word *cup* well formed in the language systems of the brain but be unable to transform this representation into fluent and well-articulated motor sequences. AOS is not the result of a language disturbance or an impairment of the neuromuscular system (e.g., muscle weakness, spasticity, abnormal reflexes), but rather is an impairment of the ability to plan and program the relevant articulator movements. The location of the impairment is in the articulatory system of speech production, and the resonatory, phonatory, and respiratory systems are relatively intact (McNeil et al., 1997; Wertz, LaPointe, & Rosenbek, 1984).

The speech of individuals with AOS is marked by certain salient characteristics:

- Effortful, slow speech with increased pauses between syllables and sounds
- Prolonged durations of speech sounds
- Distortions of speech sounds
- Reduced prosody, including a reduction of differences in pitch, duration, and loudness between stressed and unstressed syllables
- Errors that are consistent in type and location *within* an utterance although the actual error may vary across utterances or productions. (McNeil et al., 1997, 2000; Shuster & Wambaugh, 2003)

TABLE 6-2 Characteristics of various motor speech disorders

	Apraxia of Speech	Spastic Dysarthria	Flaccid Dysarthria	Hypokinetic Dysarthria	Hyperkinetic Dysarthria	Ataxic Dysarthria	Unilateral Upper Motor Neuron Dysarthria
Impairment	motor planning for speech, groping and posturing of the articulators	low muscle tone, muscular weakness	weakness, atrophy, low muscle tone	slow movement, rigidity, tremors	variable muscle tone, involuntary movements	incoordination, tremors, overshooting and undershooting movements	unilateral facial or tongue weakness
Respiration	typically normal	reduced respiratory support and control for speech	reduced respiratory support for speech	shallow breaths, reduced breath support	sudden and irregular respiratory patterns	irregular respiratory patterns	typically normal
Phonation	typically normal, some irregular changes in pitch or loudness	strained and strangled voice quality, reduced pitch, reduced variations of loudness	breathiness, monoloud-ness, monopitch	reduced loudness	sudden changes in pitch, loudness, and voice quality	hoarse or breathy voice quality, irregular pitch, loudness changes	harsh voice quality, reduced loudness
Resonation	typically normal	hypernasal	hypernasal	typically normal	typically normal	typically normal	typically normal
Articulation	sound distortions, substitutions, omissions, and additions; groping of the articulators	reduced precision of articulators	reduced precision of articulators	reduced precision of articulators, reduced range of motion	sudden, irregular breakdowns in precision of articulators	reduced and irregular precision of articulators	reduced precision of articulators, irregular motion rates
Prosody	slow rate, irregular prolongations and pauses, reduction in stress difference between stressed and unstressed syllables (dysprosody)	excess stress and/or equal stress, short phrases	short phrases	rapid bursts of speech, long pauses	rapid bursts of speech, inappropriate phrasing	irregular pitch and loudness changes, irregular speech rhythm	typically normal

Source: Clark, H. M., Stierwalt, J. A. G., & Robin, D. A. (2000). Motor speech disorders. In J. B. Tomblin, H. L. Morris, & D. C. Spriestersbach (Eds.), *Diagnosis in speech-language pathology* (2nd ed., pp. 337–352). Reprinted with permission of Delmar Learning, a division of Thomson Learning: www.thomsonrights.com. Fax 800 730-2215.

FIGURE 6-5 Location of brain damage in apraxia of speech.

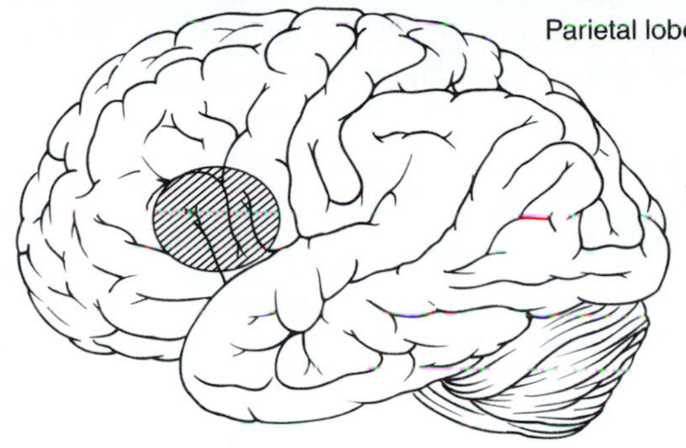

Additional characteristics of AOS that may occur include difficulties with initiating speech and groping of the articulators when producing speech (Ballard, 2001; Kent & Rosenbek, 1983; McNeil et al., 1997, 2000). For example, a patient may be unable to say the phrase "Bless you" when explicitly asked to do so in a structured assessment task, but the same patient may spontaneously and without error produce the phrase in response to the assessor's sneeze.

Causes and Risk Factors

Acquired apraxia of speech occurs as a result of neurological damage. The specific site of the brain lesions are typically in the left frontal cortex in the area surrounding Broca's area, as shown in Figure 6-5 (e.g., McNeil et al., 1997, 2000). Common causes include stroke, in which the loss of oxygen to the brain causes tissue damage or death, brain injuries, and illness and infections.

Childhood Apraxia of Speech (CAS)

Defining Characteristics

Childhood apraxia of speech (CAS) is a phonetic-motoric disorder of speech production. Children with COS are unable to translate linguistic or phonetic information concerning speech production to accurate motor behaviors or are unable to learn the motor behaviors to execute planned speech. The symptoms of COS are the same as those of AOS, including effortful and slow speech, prolonged durations of speech sounds, speech-sound distortions, reduced prosody, and errors that vary across utterances or productions. Children with CAS often show considerable delays in their development of speech production and have a limited sound inventory when producing syllables and words. They also typically have severe unintelligibility and progress slowly in speech therapy.

Causes and Risk Factors

The causes of CAS are not well understood. Experts recognize that some children have enormous difficulty in planning, programming, and executing speech movements and that these difficulties stem from a motor disorder rather than a phonological disorder (discussed in Chapter 7). Although the incidence of CAS is relatively low, children with CAS struggle

Discussion Point: *Hikaru, described in Box 6-1, has a motor speech disorder. What were some early indicators of this disability?*

greatly with speech production, highlighting the need for experts to better understand what causes this disorder. Some research shows a hereditary component to the developmental form of CAS (Duffy, 2002), but for many cases of CAS, there is no evidence of specific neurological damage to the brain (Hall, Jordan, & Robin, 1993). For some cases, CAS results from stroke or traumatic brain injury damaging the brain.

Acquired Dysarthria

Defining Characteristics

Dysarthria is a cluster of speech disorders caused by disturbances of neuromuscular control of the speech production systems (Darley, Aronson, & Brown, 1969; see also Clark et al., 2000; Duffy, 1995). In contrast to apraxia of speech, dysarthria is not an impairment of planning and programming of speech movements, but rather is a disruption in the execution of speech movements. Dysarthria results from underlying neuromuscular disturbances to muscle tone, reflexes, and kinematic aspects of movement, such as speed, range, accuracy, and steadiness (Duffy, 1995; McNeil et al., 1997). Any or all of the systems of speech production may be affected (Wertz et al., 1984). As with AOS, dysarthria is complicated by a relatively high co-occurrence of language disturbances.

Dysarthria is characterized by speech that sounds slow, slurred, overly harsh or overly quiet, or uneven, depending on the type of dysarthria (Clark et al., 2000). In addition, individuals with dysarthria may have problems initiating speech, and they may grope with the articulators when producing speech. Dysarthric speech is generally more consistent in types of errors and amount of intelligibility compared to apraxic speech.

Three concepts are important for understanding dysarthria and neuromuscular impairments: (1) spasticity, (2) dyskinesia, and (3) ataxia (Bauman-Waengler, 2004). These describe ways in which the muscles and motor functions are affected. Spasticity is a common symptom of neuromuscular impairment and refers to increased deep tendon reflexes, hypertonic muscles, and underdevelopment of limbs (Pore & Reed, 1999). Dyskinesia refers to "slow, writhing, involuntary movements" due to disturbances in muscle tone (Pore & Reed, 1999, p. 15). Ataxia refers to weakness, tremors, and lack of coordination. These terms are often used to describe the different types of dysarthria (e.g. Duffy, 1995; Thompson & Robin, 1993), as described next (see also Table 6-2). These types of acquired dysarthria result from neuromuscular damage caused by a progressive disease, such as Parkinson disease, or because of trauma, as in serious brain injuries.

Spastic Dysarthria. Spastic dysarthria is characterized by abnormal muscle tone (hypertonicity and weakness) and a state of hyper reflexes (hyperreflexia). Spastic dysarthric speech is characterized by reduced speech rate, distorted consonants and vowels, reduced or exaggerated stress, reduced pitch and loudness variation, breathy, harsh or strained-strangled voice quality, and hypernasality (Clark et al., 2000; Murdoch, Thompson, & Theodoros, 1997).

Flaccid Dysarthria. Flaccid dysarthria involves muscle weakness, atrophy, and hypotonicity. The speech associated with flaccid dysarthria is characterized by reduced breath support, breathy voice quality, monoloudness and monopitch, hypernasality, reduced articulatory precision, and reduced utterance length (Clark et al., 2000; Duffy, 1995).

Hypokinetic Dysarthria. Symptoms of hypokinetic dysarthria include bradykinesia (slowness of movement), rigidity, and static tremor (Adams, 1997; Clark et al., 2000; Duffy, 1995). Speech characteristics include reduced breath support, reduced loudness, reduced articulatory precision, often with limited range of motion, and rapid bursts of speech and long pauses (Clark et al., 2000; Duffy, 1995). Hypokinetic dysarthria is most often observed with Parkinson disease.

Hyperkinetic Dysarthria. Hyperkinetic dysarthria is characterized by variable muscle tone and (slow or fast) involuntary movements. Speech characteristics include sudden, irregular breathing patterns, sudden changes in pitch, loudness, and quality, sudden breakdowns in articulatory precision, and rapid bursts of speech and inappropriate phrasing (Clark et al., 2000).

Ataxic Dysarthria. Ataxic dysarthria results from damage to the cerebellum, causing incoordination, dysmetria (undershooting or overshooting when reaching for a target), and tremors (Cannito & Marquardt, 1997; Clark et al., 2000; Duffy, 1995). Speech characteristics include irregular breathing patterns, hoarse or breathy voice quality, irregular pitch and changes in loudness, reduced and irregular articulatory precision, and irregular speech rhythm (Clark et al., 2000; Duffy, 1995).

Unilateral Upper Motor Neuron Dysarthria. Unilateral upper motor neuron (UUMN) dysarthria involves weakness of the lower face or tongue on one side (Duffy, 1995). Breathing for speech is usually normal, but there may be a harsh voice quality, reduced loudness, reduced articulatory precision, and irregular alternating motion rates (Clark et al., 2000; Duffy, 1995).

Discussion Point: *Consider the case of Walter in Box 6-1. Which symptoms might lead you to suspect the presence of dysarthria, even though he is diagnosed with AOS?*

Developmental Dysarthria

Defining Characteristics

Developmental dysarthrias are present at birth and usually accompany a known disturbance to neuromuscular functioning, as might occur with anoxia (loss of oxygen to the brain) during birth. The most common types of developmental dysarthria are spastic dysarthria and dyskinetic dysarthria, although other types and mixed spastic-dyskinetic dysarthrias may occur as well (Hardy, 1983; Thompson & Robin, 1993). Cerebral palsy, a neuromuscular disorder that varies considerably in severity, is a frequent result of anoxia and is also often accompanied by dysarthria.

Spastic Dysarthria. Spastic dysarthria is characterized by hypertonicity (increased muscle tone) and hyperreflexia (increased sensitivity of reflexes). There is considerable variability among children with respect to severity and the systems affected. Many children with spastic dysarthria also have spasticity of upper or lower limbs or both. As with the acquired version, spastic dysarthric speech has a slow speech rate, distorted consonants and vowels, reduced or exaggerated stress, reduced pitch and loudness variation, a breathy, harsh, or strained-strangled voice quality, and hypernasality (Clark et al., 2000; Murdoch et al., 1997). Children with spastic dysarthria may have inadequate breath support for producing speech and may produce speech in short phrases.

Dyskinetic Dysarthria. Dyskinetic dysarthria is characterized by impaired coordination of muscles and involuntary movements, including chorea (sudden fast, flailing, jerking movements) and athetosis (slow, writhing movements). In most children with dyskinetic dysarthria, all four limbs are also affected. As with spastic dysarthria, a great deal of variability exists across children. Children with dyskinetic dysarthria may have a hard time producing speech, and speech may be strained, harsh, and low. Child may make abnormally large jaw movements when producing speech, resulting in imprecise and unintelligible speech (Bauman-Waengler, 2004).

Discussion Point: *Differentiating among the dysarthrias can be difficult for students of communication disorders. Think of a strategy for knowing the major characteristics of each type.*

Causes and Risk Factors

Developmental dysarthria results from pre-, peri- or postnatal damage to the nervous system. Prenatal factors that may lead to abnormal development of the motor system include genetic factors (e.g., blood incompatibilities between mother and child, metabolic disturbances), deficient oxygen supply to the fetus, maternal infections, exposure to chemicals, and other problems occuring during early pregnancy. Perinatal factors that may disrupt normal development of the neuromotor system include head trauma in difficult deliveries, premature and rapid deliveries, and respiratory problems during and following birth. Postnatal causes of developmental dysarthria include infections (meningitis, encephalitis), brain abscesses, tumors, head injuries, and strokes. Neurological developmental disorders affecting the motor system are often labeled cerebral palsy in the case of pre- and perinatal factors, but less often in the case of postnatal causes (Thompson & Robin, 1993).

How Are Motor Speech Disorders Identified?

The Assessment Process

Professionals use a variety of methods of measurement to evaluate motor speech disorders. They examine how the disorder affects the individual's activities and participation in life to determine the most appropriate course for treatment. Although speech may be the most affected motor skill and the reason for the referral, assessment of motor speech disorders should include measures of nonspeech oral motor performance so that the underlying impairment may be isolated from the overall behavior. Each of the four systems (respiration, phonation, resonation, articulation) may be impaired to different degrees, influencing speech production in different ways. Since in production of speech all systems interact to carry out communicative demands, observations of speech alone may obscure these differential contributions of the systems or their coordination on speech production. Thus, assessment of nonspeech oral motor performance designed to isolate a particular system or function is invaluable in determining the underlying impairment.

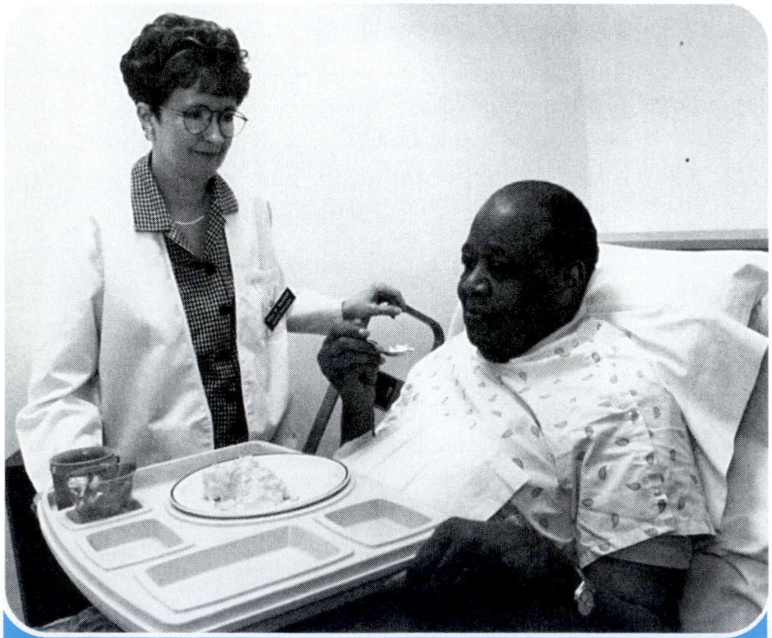

Clinicians rely on perceptual observations to study an individual's motor speech performance in a variety of informal and formal tasks.

Measurement Methods

Professionals use perceptual measures, acoustic measures, and physiological measures to document motor speech disorders.

Perceptual measures are the most common tools used and typically involve perceptual judgments of intelligibility, accuracy, and speed in an individual's speech production. The clinician listens and watches the individual during a variety of speech and nonspeech motor tasks. Perceptual measures help the professional characterize the impact of the disorder on various aspects of speech (e.g., loudness, pitch, breath support) and are also crucial for differentiating motor speech disorders. For instance, the professional can likely differentiate spastic dysarthria from flaccid dysarthria through perceptual observations alone.

Acoustic measures involve a visual representation of the speech sound wave (e.g., a spectrogram) and allow for more detailed examination of speech abnormalities that may not be perceptible to the eye and ear of the professional. Several computer programs are available that transform the auditory signal into a visual form and include various analysis options, thus providing a relatively accessible measurement method (e.g., PRAAT; see Boersma & Weenink, 2004).

Physiological measures involve measurement of physiological aspects of the speech motor system, such as muscle strength, endurance, and airflow.

Complimenting these tools are other measures used to examine language performance, as disorders of language frequently co-occur with motor speech disorders. In addition, memory, attention, vision, hearing, and mental health should also be examined to determine an individual's ability to process task instructions and perform and learn speech tasks both inside and outside the therapeutic setting. These assessments may be conducted by the speech-language pathologist or other team members, such as a neuropsychologist.

Discussion Point: *Consider the case of Hikaru in Box 6-1. The speech evaluation provided detailed information on many aspects of Hikaru's speech and language skills. Consider each finding and whether it was obtained from perceptual, acoustic, physiological, or other measures.*

Referral

Patients are generally referred for a motor speech assessment by health care professionals, typically a pediatrician for children or a family physician for adults. In cases of acute injuries, such as traumatic brain injury, speech-language pathologists are often part of an inpatient hospital team that evaluates the patient for the presence of motor speech and other communicative impairments. In cases of developmental disabilities that occur at or after birth, such as cerebral palsy, speech-language pathologists are often part of early intervention teams that provide multidisciplinary assessments of all critical areas of development. Some children, however, show signs of CAS only after they begin talking and have no other impairment. These children are often referred through their pediatrician at the request of their parents.

Screening

Screening of general motor speech performance is an important first step when people with suspected motor speech disorders are seen by a professional. The nature of the possible disorder is determined based on interviews with the client and the family. In addition, the person's medical history is obtained to determine the cause, or etiology, of the disorder and factors relevant to its prognosis (e.g., presence of strong social support system, smoking habit, history of depression, hypertension, progressive disease process). For adolescents and adults, it is important to interview both the client and the family, since they may have different perceptions of the disorder (Clark et al., 2000). For instance, an adolescent with suspected dysarthria following a traumatic brain injury may view his or her speech difficulties as mild or insignificant, whereas family members may see the difficulties as severely detrimental to academic and social performance.

Comprehensive Motor Speech Evaluation

Assessment should include motor control tasks that involve speech and nonspeech movements (Clark et al., 2000; Folkins et al., 1995; Robin et al., 1997). This practice is important to determine how much the language and motor systems contribute to observed speech difficulties. Often, a language impairment may be present simultaneously with a motor speech disorder, and the effect of the language impairment on speech production

Discussion Point: *Consider the cases presented in Box 6-1 of Bob, Walter, and Hikaru. Which of these individuals likely exhibit a language impairment in addition to a motor speech disorder? What evidence is available to support your view?*

should be identified so that the impairments resulting from motor speech deficits can be identified separately. By definition, motor speech disorders involve an impairment of the motor system and thus cannot be explained by a language impairment. The examination of motor speech tasks that do not involve language (e.g., pursing the lips, smiling, clucking the tongue) should exhibit some degradations of motor control when a motor speech disorder is present, even if these degradations are subtle.

The professional assesses an individual's problems at each of level of functioning—disease, activity, and participation in life—to determine the impact on daily life and to formulate appropriate therapy goals and strategies. Assessment of participation in life is difficult and typically depends on detailed interviews with the patient and his or her family. The effects of the speech disorder on daily life may also be observed in real-life situations (e.g., interactions with family, work situation).

A comprehensive motor speech evaluation should include assessments of each of the speech systems separately to determine the contribution of each system to the overall speech disturbance. An overview of the types of tasks that may be used in evaluations for each system is provided in Table 6-3.

Respiration. Motor speech disorders rarely result from isolated impairment of the respiratory system; however, when combined with impairments of the other speech production systems, respiratory difficulties can undermine speech. Symptoms might include short phrasings, reduced syllable repetitions, decreased speech rate, and uncontrolled phonation (Hardy, 1983; Thompson & Robin, 1993). Breathing may be irregular, shallow, or noisy, which may affect the rhythm, loudness, and rate of speech. The motor speech assessment encompasses tasks to examine the respiratory system, including both perceptual measures, such as examining how long the individual can sustain a breath, and physiological measures, such as examining an individual's vital capacity. Vital capacity is the total amount of air that can be inspired into the lungs after emptying them fully.

Phonation. The motor speech system assessment also involves careful study of the phonatory system. For some people with motor speech disorders, phonation is directly impaired because there is abnormal strength or control of the muscles in the larynx. Or, phonation may be impaired due to deficits in the other speech production systems, particularly respiration. A variety of phonatory problems may be observed in motor speech disorders, including reduced loudness, variable loudness, sudden changes in pitch or reduction in pitch range, and breathy or harsh voice quality (Davis, 1982; Thompson & Robin, 1993). The motor speech assessment examines the phonatory system using perceptual, acoustic, and physiological measures, as described in Table 6-3.

Resonation. Individuals with motor speech disorders may exhibit an impairment of the functioning of the velum, the pharynx, or both. Either structure may exhibit a decreased range or speed of motion, changes in muscle tone, and abnormal reflexes (Thompson & Robin, 1993). In addition, patients may compensate for slowed movements of the velum by reducing their speech rate. These deficits in functioning typically affect resonatory characteristics, such as hypernasality. The motor speech assessment examines resonatory characteristics using perceptual tasks, such as watching the velum functioning during a sustained "aah" and studying for nasal emissions during production of oral sounds. The assessment may also use physiological measures, such as nasendoscopy, which examines the functioning of the velopharyngeal port when producing speech sounds.

Articulation. Motor speech disorders often result in abnormal articulation. Abnormal articulation can arise from impairments of the other systems, such as the respiratory system. Reduced capacity for breath support, as occurs in some cases of dysarthria, may lead to reduced pressure in the oral cavity necessary for production of stop sounds, for instance.

TABLE 6-3 Tasks used to assess motor speech function

Subsystem	Method	Task
Respiration	Perceptual	Observe an inhalation-exhalation cycle for a deep breath Observe breathing during rest and conversation Count words per exhalation during counting Observe a prolonged vowel "ah" Observe counting from one to ten
	Physiological	Determine vital capacity Study body posture during speech Determine respiratory pressure and flow during speaking tasks
Phonation	Perceptual	Study voice quality during conversation Compare voiced consonant-vowel repetitions (ba-ba) to unvoiced consonant-vowel repetitions (pa-pa) Study ability to vary pitch and loudness during conversation Examine ability to vary pitch and loudness from minimum to maximum on vowel sound
	Acoustic	Determine pitch and intensity range during conversation Determine fundamental frequency for sustained vowel sounds
	Physiological	Study laryngeal resistance during vowel production Study the vibration patterns of vocal folds during vocalization
Resonation	Perceptual	Observe production of prolonged /s/ Observe counting from one to ten Examine for nasal emissions during counting using a dental mirror under the nose
	Physiological	Use nasendoscopy to study palatal movement for sustained vowel sound Use videoflouroscopy to study velopharyngeal functioning during conversation
Articulation	Perceptual	Conduct oral mechanism assessment to include all structures and functions Examine ability to repeat multisyllable words and sentences of varying complexity Examine performance during automatic speech tasks like counting and reciting days of the week
	Physiological	Conduct EMG to study timing of articulatory gestures of lip, jaw, and tongue for different syllables

Sources: Barlow (1999); Clark, Stierwalt, & Robin (2000); Love (1992).

However, articulatory abnormalities may also result from impairment of the articulatory system itself. For example, reduced muscle strength of the tongue will impede the ability to produce lingual sounds, including all the vowels and most of the consonants. Depending on the particular muscles involved and the extent of the neuromuscular deficits, a variety of articulatory problems may be observed, including speech-sound substitutions and distortions and reduced speech rate.

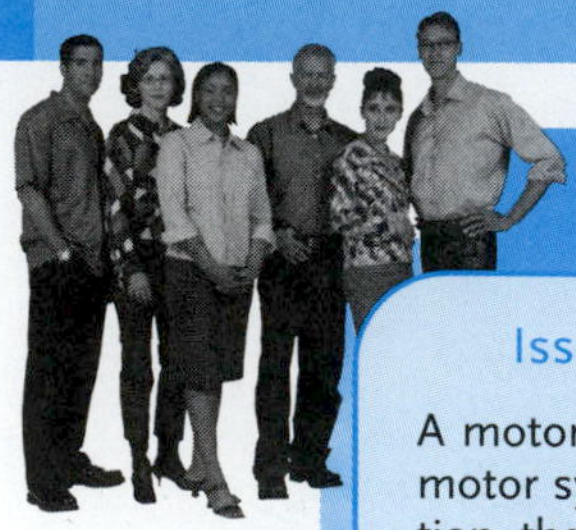

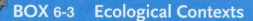

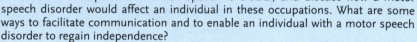

BOX 6-3 Ecological Contexts

Issues for Motor Speech Disorders

A motor speech disorder seldom occurs in isolation. For example, impairment of the oral motor system often also affects vital functions such as swallowing and respiration. In addition, there may be other cognitive impairments present, such as a language disorder. However, a motor speech disorder even by itself can severely impact the quality of life. Speech is the main means of communication, and an impairment of speech production limits the ability to convey thoughts, needs, and questions and affects a person's social, personal, and professional life.

The impact of a motor speech disorder on participation in life differs from person to person, depending not only on the severity but also on the importance of speech production in the person's life. For example, certain occupations rely more on the ability to produce fluent speech than others (e.g., a newscaster vs. a columnist), and people differ in terms of the importance of social interactions to their lives. However, since speech is one of the defining features of human beings and permeates virtually every aspect of life, the effects of a motor speech disorder on the life of any patient and his or her communication partners cannot be underestimated.

For Further Discussion

What are some differences between an acquired and a developmental motor speech disorder in terms of the impact on an individual's participation in life and well-being? Consider some specific situations or occupations in which speech is crucial, and discuss how a motor speech disorder would affect an individual in these occupations. What are some ways to facilitate communication and to enable an individual with a motor speech disorder to regain independence?

Companion Website

To answer these questions online, go to the Ecological Contexts module in chapter 6 of the Companion Website.

When examining the articulatory system, the clinician studies the stability of speech errors under different circumstances. If a motor speech disorder is the result of a basic physiological malfunction of the articulatory system, as in muscle paralysis in some dysarthrias, speech errors are likely to be consistent across repetitions, contexts, and tasks (e.g., in repetition, reading, and spontaneous speech). In contrast, if the motor speech disorder results from a malfunction in the coordination or planning and programming of speech (as in apraxia of speech), errors may be more variable across repetitions, contexts, and tasks. The individual may produce a given sound clearly and accurately in one word but not in another, and performance may vary depending on the context in which the sound is elicited. For instance, a phrase may be produced accurately in an automatic or reflexive response, such as greeting someone entering a room, but the phrase may be degraded in its sounds and intelligibility in a volitional task, as with a greeting that is elicited (e.g., "Say this: 'Hello, Mr. Green, I am happy to see you today.'")

The motor speech assessment involves a variety of perceptual, acoustic, and physiological tasks for assessing the articulatory system. Of great importance is the professional's ability to closely study the individual's motor speech performance perceptually during a variety of structured and unstructured tasks. The professional will supplement these perceptual observations of motor speech performance with tools that document intensity and loudness in different speech tasks and that study how well the larynx functions.

Prosody. Although prosody is not generally considered a separate system of speech production, it is an important aspect of speech that characterizes a person's naturalness when speaking. The ability to produce normal prosody results from a complex interaction of all speech production systems and therefore is critical in understanding and treating motor speech disorders. Specifically, prosody requires the controlled exhalation of air divided across series of syllables (for assigning relative loudness and duration), coordinated with the phonatory system (for assigning relative pitch differences) and the articulatory system (for extending or shortening articulator movements relative to syllable duration). Disorders of prosody may help differentiate among impairments because by examining prosodic aspects of speech, the professional can determine what systems of speech production are most affected by the disorder.

Assessment of prosody examines the individual's prosodic variations as a function of different types of language use, such as producing a declarative versus an interrogative sentence, and for different emotional states (e.g., happy, angry, surprised) (Robin, Klouda, & Hug, 1991; Seddoh & Robin, 2001). In addition to perceptual observations of prosodic variations, professionals use acoustic measures to provide important information about which aspect of prosody is impaired (e.g., loudness, duration, pitch, rhythm).

Discussion Point: *In the case of Bob in Box 6-1, which aspects of prosody might be impaired? Describe some tasks that could be used to test his ability to vary prosody.*

Diagnosis

Following the motor speech assessment, the professional interprets findings to arrive at a speech diagnosis. Depending on the findings, a patient may receive a diagnosis of one of the various motor speech disorders discussed previously. A diagnosis that differentiates a person's disorder from other similar disorders, for example, spastic dysarthria from flaccid dysarthria, is called a differential diagnosis. It is important to note that a differential diagnosis of a motor speech disorder is based primarily on the perceptual findings and judgment of the clinical professional, which are derived from extensive experience. No one test can provide a differential diagnosis. Current research is investigating the use of acoustic and physiological measures in diagnosis (see Box 6-4), but as yet, this work is best categorized as research and has not become a routine part of clinical practice.

Differential diagnosis in motor speech disorders is important because the type of treatment depends on the nature of the disorder, and what may be effective for one disorder may not be effective for another. For example, a focus on improving posture and breathing may be useful for patients who have an impairment of the respiratory system, but may not lead to improved speech for patients with aphasia or patients with tongue paralysis.

How Are Motor Speech Disorders Treated?

Individuals with motor speech disorders often also have other clinical problems, such as aphasia, limb paralysis, hypertension, or a learning disability. Therefore, treatment options are typically explored and recommended by an interdisciplinary team consisting of physicians, physical therapists, occupational therapists, neuropsychologists, teachers, speech-language pathologists, and the client and family.

Treatment Goals

Treatment for the motor speech impairment itself is typically provided by the speech-language pathologist through inpatient or outpatient therapy. An important consideration in treatment is clear identification of therapy goals. In motor speech treatment, the goal of therapy is to *learn or relearn accurate production of speech* for improved speech intelligibility. In many treatment contexts, professionals face great pressure to achieve maximal progress with limited resources (time, money, staff). Earlier, we defined motor learning as "a set of processes associated with practice or experience leading to relatively *permanent* changes in the *capability* for movement" (Schmidt & Lee, 1999; italics added). Accordingly, a primary goal of treatment is that an individual not only learn a new skill, but also maintain that skill over time to show evidence of permanent changes. This is the principle of retention. Therapy differentiates treatment outcomes into temporary performance enhancements observed during treatment (acquisition) and lasting performance enhancements observed after treatment has ended (retention). Evidence from the motor learning literature strongly suggests that improvements during acquisition do not necessarily result in improvements during retention tests (e.g., Schmidt & Bjork, 1992; Schmidt & Lee, 1999). In fact, factors that enhance acquisition may have negative effects on retention (e.g., Schmidt & Bjork, 1992). This finding has important implications for evaluating the outcomes of motor speech treatment. In many settings progress is measured almost exclusively in terms of acquisition, yet the hope is that improvements observed during treatment will continue after treatment ends. Thus, measures of retention must be included to determine the effectiveness of the treatment for permanent improvements.

A second important goal of treatment relates to the principle of **generalization**, which refers to application or transfer of a skill to related but untrained movement patterns. According to this principle, an individual's underlying capability for movement should be facilitated by treatment so that untrained tasks also improve. Two types of generalizations are desirable (Ballard, 2001; Wambaugh, Kalinyak-Fliszar, West, & Doyle, 1998; Wambaugh, Martinez, McNeil, & Rogers, 1999; Wambaugh, West, & Doyle, 1998). Response generalization refers to improvements of untrained behaviors (e.g., speech sounds), whereas stimulus generalization refers to improvement of targeted behaviors in different contexts, tasks, or settings (e.g., in conversational speech vs. repetition tasks).

Discussion Point: *For multilingual speakers such as Bob and Hikaru, described in Box 6-1, in what language should intervention be provided?*

Goals in the treatment of motor speech disorders must thus consider improvements and treatment effectiveness according to the principles of retention and generalization and not simply measure temporary performance enhancements observed during acquisition.

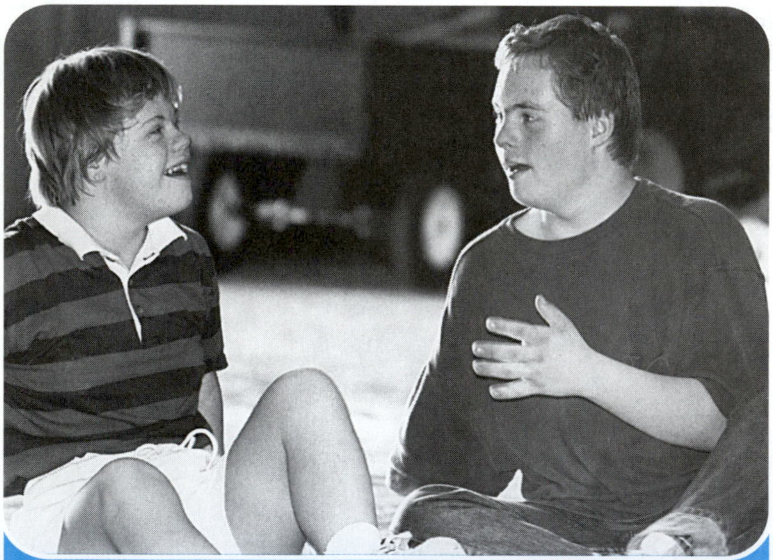

The principle of generalization refers to how motor speech goals achieved in the therapy context apply to other contexts of communication.

Targets and Strategies

Treatment Targets

Clinical professionals carefully select treatment targets based on the nature of an individual's speech difficulties and the impact of the speech disorder on daily living function. When deciding on targets for treatment programs, clinicians must answer several questions, including: Should we target speech or nonspeech motor tasks? Should we target simple speech tasks or complex speech tasks? A brief summary of these important questions follows.

Speech and Nonspeech Tasks. Some clinicians select both speech and nonspeech treatment targets. For instance, a clinician may target improved intelligibility of certain speech sounds or words for a given client while also targeting improved tongue strength and range of motion. The latter types of activities are called oral motor exercises. The tongue strength and range of motion targets are selected based on the notion that certain basic physiological components (such as muscle strength or endurance) must be strengthened in isolation in order to be functional in speech production. However, it is important to note that increasing nonspeech motor movements, in this case for a patient with tongue muscle weakness, will not likely improve speech intelligibility. In fact, evidence suggests that practicing oral motor exercises will not result in improved speech production (e.g. Campbell, 2003; Lof, 2004). Since presumably the goal of speech therapy is to improve speech production, it seems reasonable to target speech as an integrated behavior with an emphasis on intelligibility and using speech to communicate functionally.

Some patients may be unable to produce speech in early stages of treatment, particularly after an acute incident, such as stroke. In such cases, targeting isolated speech sounds or articulatory movements may be justified. For instance, an individual may not be able to produce any speech sounds, and the clinician may select specific speech sounds to target (e.g., /b/, /m/). However, given that the goal of speech treatment is to improve speech production, speech targets should be included as early as possible.

Simple and Complex Tasks. The selection of treatment targets should take into account the complexity or difficulty level of the target behavior. For instance, producing sounds intelligibly in a phrase (e.g., "I want some milk.") is clearly more complex than producing sounds in isolation (e.g., *m-m-m*). Some experts contend that focusing on more complex targets results in greater learning than does focusing on simpler targets (e.g., Ballard & Thompson, 1999; Gierut, 1998, 2001; Kiran & Thompson, 2003; Maas, Barlow, Robin, & Shapiro, 2002; Thompson, Ballard, & Shapiro, 1998). Targeting complex sounds, syllables, and sentences leads to improvements in these targeted items as well as improvements in simpler but untrained items. In contrast, when clinicians target simpler items in therapy, these items improve but more complex items do not. These recent findings from clinical research show that when a patient is unable to produce either a simple or a complex item, targeting the complex item will improve both simple and complex items, whereas targeting the simple item improves only that simple item. This finding is important clinically because it suggests that the simpler items do not need to be specifically targeted, which can make treatment more efficient. It is important to note, however, that these recent research findings go against a common approach in clinical treatment that involves beginning with simple items and working up to more complex items.

Treatment Strategies

The goal of speech treatments for motor speech disorders is generally to improve the accuracy, stability, and intelligibility of speech and the naturalness or fluency of speech. The two primary therapeutic strategies are to (1) improve the impaired system(s) and (2) teach compensatory strategies.

Improvement of individual systems involves focusing on specific functions in relevant speech tasks, for example, by emphasizing the modification of speech breathing patterns, the use of intonation in utterances, or words with specific speech sounds that are difficult. More specific approaches for each system are presented in the next sections.

In addition to directly targeting impaired abilities, teaching compensatory strategies may also be useful. Compensatory strategies may focus on the individual with a motor speech disorder or on the environment and communication partners. Compensatory strategies may include slowing down the rate of speech and using gestures, writing, or

***Discussion Point:** For a college professor with a motor speech disorder, such as Bob in Box 6-1, what are some compensatory strategies that may facilitate teaching in the classroom?*

alternative and augmentative communication devices such as communication books and handheld computers (e.g., Van de Sandt-Koenderman, Wielaert, & Wiegers, 2003). Clinicians also need to treat the WHO level of participation in life by working with family members and other communication partners as well as by making environmental adaptations. Compensatory strategies in this regard may involve environmental modifications (e.g., noise reduction) and communication partner training. For example, communication partners may be instructed to ask more effective yes/no questions.

Pretreatment Considerations. Treatment is most effective when the clinician pays careful attention to what the client brings to the therapy context. The most influential client characteristics for motor speech treatment include memory, attention, motivation, goal setting, and correctness reference. Descriptions of these considerations are drawn from Yorkston, Beukelman, Strand, and Bell (1999).

> *Memory*. Since learning involves storage of information in long-term memory, it is important to determine whether any memory impairments are present in addition to the motor speech disorder. A memory impairment may impede learning and the potential benefits of therapy.
>
> *Attention*. If a client has limited capacity to focus and sustain attention, learning may be impeded as well; therapy sessions may be structured in such a way as to maximize attention (e.g., by providing frequent breaks).
>
> *Motivation*. The client's motivation is important to learning. Understanding the relevance of the therapy task for the goal of improving speech production may help motivate the patient to perform the therapy task.
>
> *Goal Setting*. Setting specific goals, such as "request the newspaper effectively," will be more effective than asking patients simply to "do the best you can" (McNeil et al., 1997, p. 333).
>
> *Correctness Reference*. The client needs a reference of correctness to know which productions are considered normal or acceptable and which are not. This reference enables the learner to develop internal error-detection mechanisms.

***Discussion Point:** Consider the case of Walter in Box 6-1. What indicators are available to suggest that treatment may or may not be effective?*

Treatment of the Respiratory System. Treatment of the respiratory system may focus on improving respiratory support, modifying inspiration and exhalation and their interrelationship, increasing respiratory flexibility, or a combination of these goals, depending on the nature of the motor speech problem. To improve respiratory support, the clinician works with the client to improve and control the buildup of subglottic airpressure, adjust and improve posture for improved breath support, and if needed, provide a respiratory prostheses, such as a paddle or board to push against.

Activities to modify inspiration and exhalation may include increasing the duration of air intake and using various ways of monitoring the duration (e.g., tactile, visual, auditory, torso monitoring). Increasing the inhaled lung volume will also assist exhalation through elastic recoil of the diaphragm. Modifying exhalation can begin with vowel prolongation and counting, followed by production of larger units of speech (phrases, sentences). Since speech breathing involves rapid inhalations with protracted exhalations, it is important to establish or improve the appropriate relationship between these two parts of the respiratory cycle. For example, the clinician can train brief inhalations followed by controlled, slow exhalations in using vowels and then consonants. Furthermore, speakers may be taught where to take inhalations relative to breath groups and to hold their breath until exhalation and speech can begin. In addition, the clinician should teach the patient where to terminate exhalation and how to plan utterances in advance. Maladaptive respiratory patterns should be eliminated if possible.

BOX 6-4 Spotlight on Research

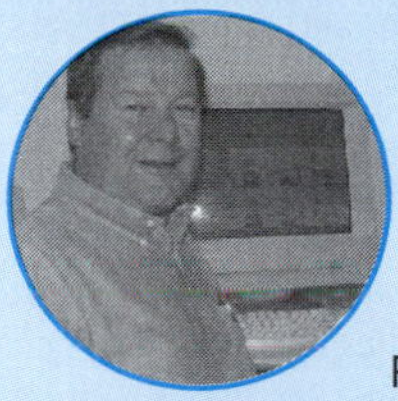

Raymond D. Kent, Ph.D.
Professor,
Waisman Center
University of Wisconsin at Madison

Ray Kent received his Ph.D. from the Department of Speech Pathology and Audiology at the University of Iowa and has been at the Waisman Center at the University of Wisconsin-Madison since 1975. He is widely acknowledged as one of the leading scholars in the field of motor speech disorders, has received numerous honors for his work in this area, and currently serves as Vice President for Research and Technology for the American Speech-Language-Hearing Association.

Ray has an active research lab focusing on neurogenic motor speech disorders in children and adults. His work examines how specific impairments of motor and sensory processes affect various communicative aspects (such as speech intelligibility) and how such impairments relate to neural lesions. Through studies of a wide variety of motor speech disorders resulting from different types of neurological damage (e.g., cerebral palsy, stroke, neurodegenerative disease), his work also aims to contribute to a more complete understanding of brain-behavior relationships with respect to speech motor control.

Throughout his career, Ray has consistently contributed to refinement of descriptions of various motor speech disorders, to increasing our understanding of typical and atypical speech motor control both in terms of behavior and in terms of the neural basis of speech, and to methodological improvements. His recent work also includes the application of a neural network model to understanding speech motor development. In addition to being at the forefront in the field in both basic and applied research, Ray has written many reviews of relevant literature, with important directions to help guide future research. More details on Ray's work can be found in the following papers:

Kent, R. D., & Kim, Y. J. (2003). Toward an acoustic typology of motor speech disorders. *Clinical Linguistics and Phonetics*, 17(6), 427–445.

Kent, R. D., Duffy, J. R., Slama, A., Kent, J. F., & Clift, A. (2001). Clinicoanatomic studies in dysarthria: A review, critique, and directions for research. *Journal of Speech, Language, and Hearing Research*, 44, 535–551.

Callan, D. E., Kent, R. D., Guenther, F. H., & Vorperian, H. K. (2000). An auditory-feedback based neural network model of speech production that is robust to developmental changes in the size and shape of the articulatory system. *Journal of Speech, Language, and Hearing Research*, 43, 721–736.

Treatment of the Phonatory System. Treatment of the phonatory system may focus on improving voice quality or on control over the vocal folds to enhance production of prosodic aspects of speech and thereby enhance the naturalness of speech. Treatment approaches to improving voice quality are described in Chapter 11 and may include postural adjustments and training to increase effort when producing voice. Treatments to improve prosody are discussed later in this chapter.

Treatment of the Resonatory System. Treatment of the strength and control of the velopharyngeal port may involve having the patient view nasal airflow in the form of biofeedback or by practicing nasal versus oral airflow patterns (negative practice). The use of a palatal lift, a device that helps raise the velum, should be considered when resonatory difficulties severely impact intelligibility.

Treatment of the Articulatory System. Generally, the use of nonspeech tasks, such as oral motor exercises, have little if any effect on speech production; therefore, the goal of improving speech production requires the use of authentic speech tasks. Exceptions may involve patients whose impairment is so severe as to preclude production of even the simplest speech sounds or utterances. Articulatory treatment should focus the patient's attention on the accuracy, range, and direction of movement during speech. The clinician provides feedback, including modeling the correct positioning or using a diagram with the correct articulatory configuration, to guide improved articulation.

BOX 6-5 Spotlight on Practice

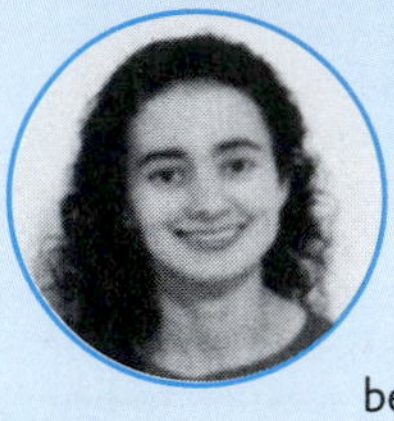

Cindy Trujillo-Hale, CCC-SLP
San Diego City School District
Childhood Apraxia of Speech Resource Center

What a versatile and rewarding field to be in! These two attributes drew me to the field of speech and language disorders, and the profession has certainly been what I anticipated. I graduated with my M.A. in Speech-Language Pathology from San Diego State University, where I focused on the assessment and treatment of motor speech disorders and disorders in bilingual-multicultural populations. I obtained a bilingual-multicultural certificate in speech-language disorders.

I am currently working for San Diego city schools, a large district that provides numerous professional growth opportunities for its speech-language pathologists. As a district employee I have two assignments: I work as an elementary school clinician and as the coordinator for the Childhood Apraxia of Speech Resource Center; in addition, I work in conjunction with a former professor, mentor, and now colleague in private practice.

The Childhood Apraxia of Speech Resource Center was created as a staff development opportunity for speech-language pathologists in San Diego city schools. Our mission through the Childhood Apraxia of Speech Resource Center is to change common misconceptions about childhood apraxia and improve the efficacy of treatment programs. The center provides opportunities for speech-language pathologists to receive assistance with planning and implementing research-based interventions for students who have or are suspected of having apraxia of speech. I assist speech-language pathologists in developing stimuli, activities, and treatment goals for their students. Consultation is also provided to guide the selection of an appropriate assessment battery as well as to assist in the interpretation and differential diagnosis of speech assessments. Multiple opportunities for speech practice are necessary for children with apraxia to correctly program speech patterns; as a result, I train school support staff on ways to support students' speech production growth. I work closely with a licensed speech-language pathology assistant who provides additional speech practice to children in need of more intense speech practice and makes resources related to apraxia of speech available to speech-language pathologists and families.

The Childhood Apraxia of Speech Center has allowed me to collaborate with many speech-language pathologists throughout the district as well as professors from San Diego State University. By combining knowledge from clinicians and researchers we have been able to improve the current apraxia treatment within San Diego city schools. I have had the opportunity to work with and learn from children with varying disorders and severities throughout the district as well as through private practice. I enjoy what I do, knowing that I can make a positive change in the lives of many children and their families. I also like knowing that I have many choices available in terms of the settings and populations I can work with and that there are numerous disorders in which I can choose to specialize. Versatile and rewarding, most definitely!

Treatment of Prosody and Rate Control. Prosody is essential for producing natural-sounding speech. Prosody involves manipulation of three factors: loudness, pitch, and duration. Impairments of prosody may result from reductions in the range of any one of these factors. Treatment should include exercises geared toward increasing the range of the affected factors. For example, the professional may lead the client through contrastive stress drills, such as producing sets of words or phrases that differ only in stress pattern (e.g., *differ* and *defer* or *a project* and *to project*) and asking questions that elicit differential stress or intonation patterns (e.g., "Is the ball in the red *bag*?" "No, the ball is in the red *box*.").

Speech rate contributes significantly to intelligibility, and it may be helpful to reduce the rate of speech, even if the rate is already slower than normal. There are two types of techniques to improve speech rate, rigid control techniques and nonrigid control techniques (Yorkston et al., 1999). Examples of rigid control techniques include pacing boards and alphabet boards. Examples of nonrigid control techniques include rhythmic cueing (in which the clinician points to words in a text at a given rate) and computerized cueing (words are presented on the screen one at a time at a given rate, or words in a text are highlighted at a given rate, and the speaker produces only those words). Nonrigid control techniques are less disruptive to prosody than are rigid techniques.

Case Study and Clinical Problem Solving

TREATMENT RECOMMENDATIONS REPORT

Los Angeles Pediatrics, Inc.

Client: Sharon Richardson
Evaluation date: 5-12-2004
Date of report: 5-14-2004
Date of birth: 7-6-1995
Age: 8 years, 10 months
Referred by: Mother, teacher

Overview

Sharon was referred to the Pediatrics Clinic for evaluation of her communication skills. Sharon stayed on task for the entire 2½ hour evaluation on May 12, 2004. She cooperated with the examiners and demonstrated appropriate pragmatic and social skills, such as turn taking and eye contact. We believe the results of the evaluation are an excellent reflection of her current level of speech and language abilities.

Background

Based on previous reports, Sharon, an adopted child, was the product of "an unremarkable pregnancy." There were no complications during labor or delivery, except for low amniotic fluid during the last trimester. Sharon suffered from chronic ear infections and allergies for the first 12 months. Parent report indicates that Sharon was a late talker. She did not babble and spoke her first word ("moo") at 18 months of age. Sharon was reported to have a limited sound repertoire, and the mother summarized Sharon's speech development as "she was a quiet baby." Sharon would produce a sound or a word "for a while" only to lose it approximately 2 weeks later. By age 3, Sharon only had 5 "semblances of words" but she appeared to understand what was said to her. Sharon was diagnosed with apraxia of speech in kindergarten. A report from a private consultant for the school concluded later that there was no "motor programming or planning problem" and changed the diagnosis to phonological disorder. Sharon is currently receiving speech services from a private speech-language pathologist in addition to minimal services provided by the school district. Sharon attends the second grade in the Los Angeles school district. With the exception of speech and mathematics, the mother reported that Sharon is doing well. She has friends and appears to be able to handle the current academic curriculum. She is receiving occupational therapy on a pull-out basis to improve visual-motor skills. The mother estimated that strangers can understand Sharon's speech about 50% of the time. When she is not understood she may repeat or use gestures to enhance communication.

Motor Speech Findings

Sharon's speech production indicated mild to moderate apraxia of speech. Her speech production errors were primarily characterized by sound distortions and sound substitutions, errors that were consistent in type and location on repeated trials (but that varied in the exact error on different productions), intonation abnormalities, and slow rate of speech. We also saw trial-and-error groping during speech, the loss of speech sounds and words in early development (from parental report), the history of a limited sound repertoire, increased errors with increased utterance length, limited early sound play, intact receptive language skills compared to reduced expressive language abilities, imitative skills superior to spontaneous speech, and sound sequencing difficulties.

With the correct therapy program, there is a positive prognosis for improved speech production skills. Sharon has strong social skills. She is a friendly girl who enjoys communicating with people. Her speech production difficulties do not appear to affect her willingness to communicate at this time. Sharon's age-appropriate receptive language skills and age-appropriate academic level also support a positive prognosis.

A critical issue in the remediation program for children with apraxia of speech is the need for intense speech and language therapy services. Intensive services should provide the most efficacious means of improving her speech production and expressive language and prevent future possibilities of social, emotional, and academic problems associated with her apraxia of speech and expressive language delays.

Recommendations

To treat Sharon's apraxia and expressive language delays, the following steps are recommended:

1. Sharon should receive intensive speech therapy (5 days a week, 45-minute sessions, and an

additional group session) to improve her intelligibility and expressive language skills. To minimize the disruption of taking a child out of the classroom, it is often optimal to provide these services before or after school.

2. Because it is important to maximize the amount of speech practice, a speech-language assistant can provide extra speech practice under the guidance of a qualified speech-language pathologist.
3. It is imperative that parent training be provided to maximize the effects of therapy. This means allowing parental visitation during therapy, videotaping of sessions, and a home program developed for practice outside of therapy.
4. The speech-language pathologist working with Sharon should receive training in working with children who have apraxia of speech in order to enhance the outcome of therapy.

TREATMENT PLAN

Client: Sharon Richardson
Plan date: 5-19-2004

Objectives: Expressive Language

1. Sharon will use free and bound morphemes such as plural endings and verb tense markers (e.g., *-ed*) functionally 10 times per session.
2. Sharon will formulate complete sentences 80% of the time during each session.

Objectives: Speech Production and Prosody

1. Sharon will accurately produce multisyllabic words without syllable segmentation and with appropriate stress assignment 90% of the time.
2. Sharon will accurately produce the sounds *t, g, s, z, r, sh, j,* and *ch* in initial, medial, and final word position in single words with 90% accuracy.
3. Sharon will produce the sounds *t, g, s, z, r, sh, j,* and *ch* accurately in conversational speech 75% of the time.
4. Sharon will produce appropriate prosodic components (pitch, loudness, duration, pause, tempo, intonation, stress, and rhythm) at the sentence level to indicate contrastive stress and emotional state 90% of the time.
5. Sharon will learn strategies to prevent and repair communication breakdown.

Plan of Activities

1. Sharon will receive speech therapy 5 days a week for 45 minutes and an additional group session at her school. Treatment will take place before and after classes so as to not interrupt the regular academic curriculum.
2. The above objectives will be addressed in the context of conversational speech and targeted tasks such as role-playing games, storytelling, voicing and devoicing drills, and sentence construction with target words containing difficult sounds.
3. Activities will be alternated, and presentation of items will be randomized. Feedback about accuracy will be provided on approximately 60% of attempts to encourage self-monitoring skills and will be provided after 3–4 seconds so as not to interfere with internal evaluation processes.
4. Parent training will be provided, including parental visitation during therapy, videotaping of sessions, and a home program for practice outside of therapy.

If you have any questions about this report, please do not hesitate to contact me.

Sincerely,

River Reynolds, M.Ed., CCC-SLP

CLINICAL PROBLEM SOLVING

1. This report recommended group therapy for Sharon. What might group therapy provide that one-on-one therapy would not?
2. In the background section of this report, it was noted that Sharon's diagnosis had changed from apraxia of speech to phonological disorder. Why are these disorders confusable?
3. This report recommended parental involvement in Sharon's treatment. Why involve Sharon's parents? What can they offer that the professional cannot?

CHAPTER SUMMARY

Speech production involves the coordination in space and time of four separate systems of speech production: the respiratory, phonatory, resonatory, and articulatory subsystems. Each of these systems may be impaired independently and to different degrees. These systems exhibit impairments due to deficits at the level of motor planning and preprogramming or at the level of execution.

There are two categories of motor speech disorders, both of which are caused by a neurological impairment of the motor systems involved with speech production. Apraxia of speech results from a disruption of motor planning or programming, whereas dysarthria results from a disruption of basic aspects of the motor system (e.g., muscle weakness, abnormal reflexes). Both dysarthria and apraxia of speech have acquired and developmental variants, the former describing disorders that result from injury, disease, or illness to the neurological systems and the latter describing disorders present at birth.

Assessment examines motor performance in both nonspeech and speech activities. Assessment of nonspeech oral motor performance is essential to determine the relative contribution of the respiratory, phonatory, articulatory, and resonatory systems to the speech impairment. The functioning of each system and their collective involvement in efficient and intelligible speech is considered at the levels of disease, activity, and participation in life, and assessment may involve perceptual, acoustic, and physiological measures.

The goal of treatment for motor speech disorders is to improve the accuracy, stability, and intelligibility of speech and the naturalness of speech. Treatment aims to maximize learning to ensure that effects are maintained over time and show generalization to other, untrained tasks. Treatment targets should primarily include speech, and the clinician should take into account the complexity of targets as there is evidence suggesting that more complex targets may lead to better learning. Specific approaches are used to treat impairments of the respiratory, phonatory, articulatory, and resonatory systems.

KEY TERMS

apraxia of speech, p. 193
activity, p. 191
articulatory system, p. 186
disease, p. 191
dysarthria, p. 196
generalization, p. 204
motor execution, p. 189
motor execution disorders, p. 193
motor learning, p. 189
motor planning, p. 189
motor programming, p. 189
motor speech disorder, p. 182
motor unit (motor program), p. 188
participation in life, p. 191
phonatory system, p. 183
resonatory system, p. 185
respiratory system, p. 183
schemas, p. 189
speech motor control, p. 181
velopharyngeal port, p. 185

ON THE WEB

Check out the Companion Website! On it, you will find:

- suggested readings
- reflection questions
- a self-study quiz
- links to additional online resources, including information about current technologies in communication sciences and disorders

Language Disorders in Early and Later Childhood

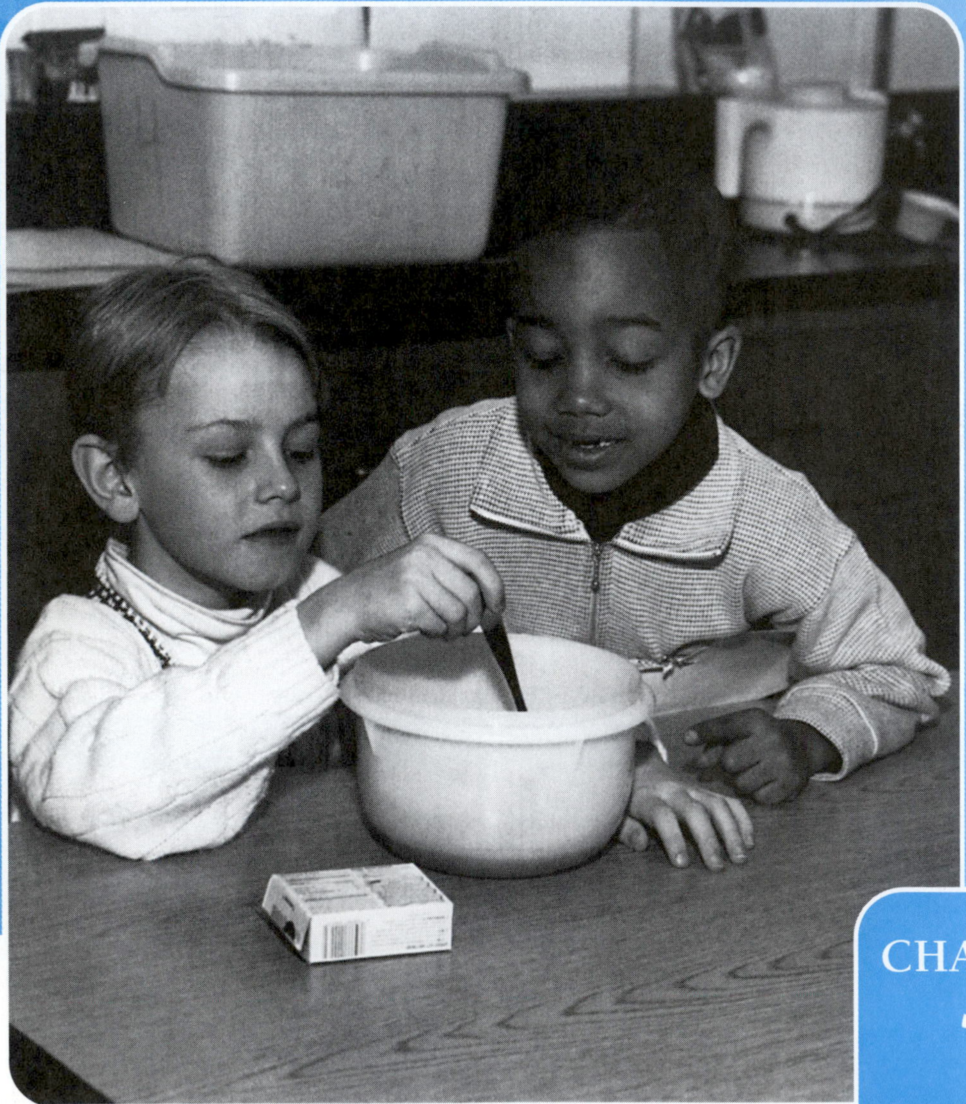

CHAPTER 7

FOCUS QUESTIONS

This chapter answers the following questions:

1. What is a language disorder?
2. How are language disorders classified?
3. What are the defining characteristics of prevalent types of language disorders?
4. How are language disorders identified?
5. How are language disorders treated?

INTRODUCTION

For many children, the development of language follows a predictable pathway in both the rate and the type of accomplishments. Recall from chapter 2 that most children say their first word at around 1 year, begin to combine words to form two-word sentences at about 18 months, are able to produce three-word sentences by 24 months, and so forth. In fact, one of the remarkable features of language is that it is *species uniform* (see chapter 1), meaning that regardless of where a child is born and reared—whether in Antarctica, Laos, or Zimbabwe—critical language accomplishments adhere to a strikingly similar pathway.

However, for reasons that are sometimes never known, a small but consequential portion of young children have considerable problems with the development of language. These children have a **language disorder**. They typically show delays in obtaining critical language precursors, such as babbling and gesturing, in the first year of life. In the toddler and preschool years, they are slow to achieve important early language milestones, such as speaking the first word, combining words into sentences, and initiating conversation with adults or peers. During the school-age years, these children often struggle with academic skills that rely on language proficiency, including reading and writing. They also are likely to have problems with complex language tasks, such as using and understanding figurative (e.g., idioms, proverbs) and abstract language. As adults, persons with language disorders face ongoing challenges in living and working in a culture that places enormous value on language proficiency.

What Is a Language Disorder?

Definition

A language disorder refers to

> impaired comprehension and/or use of a spoken, written, and/or other symbol system. The disorder may involve (1) the *form* of language (phonology, morphology, and syntax),

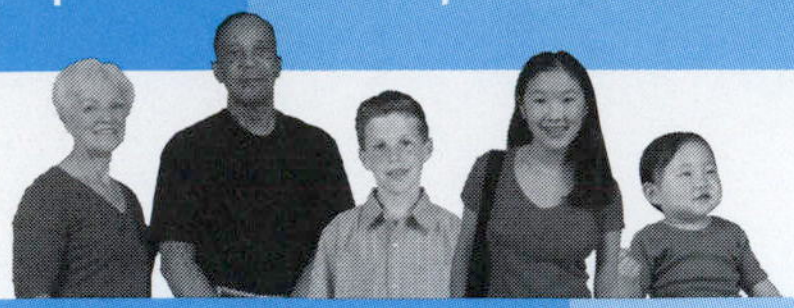

BOX 7-1 Language Disorders in Early and Later Childhood: Case Examples

Alejandro is a 6-year-old student in Mr. Allen's kindergarten classroom in a small elementary school in rural Washington. Alejandro is the youngest child in a migrant Spanish-speaking family that travels annually from Texas to Washington state for the pear and apple harvest. Like many other migrant families, Alejandro's family is living in a small tent in a state-run temporary housing camp. Mr. Allen, a monolingual English speaker, has difficulty communicating with Alejandro, who speaks very little English. Mr. Allen recognizes that there is a language mismatch, which explains much of the difficulty in their effective communication with one another, but he is concerned that Alejandro may also have a communication disorder. Mr. Allen has noted that Alejandro does not interact well with his peers—for instance, he uses communication cues inappropriately (e.g., talks too loud, refuses eye contact) and is very clumsy and defensive in social interactions. Mr. Allen has asked the speech-language pathologist to come and observe Alejandro in the classroom and to consider the need for a comprehensive speech-language evaluation.

Internet research

1. Is Alejandro's circumstance common in the United States?
2. What educational resources are available for children like Alejandro?
3. What challenges face migrant families?

Brainstorm and discussion

1. What strategies can be used to identify whether Alejandro's suspected communicative difficulties are the result of a language difference or a language disorder?
2. What are some strategies Mr. Allen might use in the classroom to promote Alejandro's success when communicating with classmates?

Natasha is a 28-month-old child adopted 4 months ago from Ukraine by Mr. and Mrs. Scarbrough. The adoption agency reported that Natasha had been abandoned by her parents at 3 months of age because of her severe lactose intolerance. From 3 months to 2 years of age, Natasha lived in an orphanage outside Kiev with 120 other children. Although the adoption agency indicated that Natasha had received a full developmental screening and showed no developmental delays or medical problems (aside from lactose intolerance), Mr. and Mrs. Scarbrough are very concerned about Natasha's communication development. When Natasha was adopted, she was not talking at all. Currently, she uses only about four English words (*mama*, *dada*, *wawa*, *car*) and understands several more. She rarely initiates communication with her parents, does not consistently respond to their initiations, and seems more content sitting and looking at storybooks than interacting with others. Mr. and Mrs. Scarbrough have heard friends talk about institutional delays in children adopted from foreign countries and are concerned that Natasha will have ongoing problems with speech and language, given her apparent late start. They have arranged for a comprehensive speech-language evaluation at the local foreign-birth adoption clinic and are eager for suggestions to help Natasha at home.

Internet research

1. Approximately how many children are adopted each year through international adoption agencies?
2. What community resources are available to families adopting children from overseas?
3. What is the developmental prognosis for children who have been institutionalized for long periods of time?

Brainstorm and discussion

1. What information concerning Natasha's first 2 years of life would be helpful for understanding her current communicative abilities?

> (2) the *content* of language (semantics), and/or (3) the *function* of language in communication (pragmatics) in any combination. (American Speech-Language-Hearing Association [ASHA], 1993, p. 40; emphasis added)

A disorder is present if a child's language skills in these areas—form, content, or use—are not consistent with what is typically seen in children of a similar age and a similar cultural and

2. To develop a comprehensive understanding of Natasha's current communicative patterns in the home environment, what questions would you ask her adoptive parents?

Savannah Wasserstrom is a 10-year-old student in a suburban middle school in Ohio. She lives with her mother and is an only child. Savannah struggled with speech and language development when she was little; she did not start talking until she was nearly 3, and even then she was very hard to understand. Savannah had nearly constant ear infections as a young child and received speech-language therapy at Head Start for 2 years, until she entered kindergarten. Now a fourth-grade student, Savannah continues to have a few minor speech problems (like saying "w" for *l* and *r*), difficulties with some aspects of language (e.g., understanding jokes), problems following classroom directions, challenges in participating in conversations with other children, and serious struggles in learning to read. However, she has not received any special help since preschool.

Savannah's teachers view her as a late bloomer whose problems with communicating with others are due to shyness and embarrassment over her mild speech difficulties. Lately, however, Savannah's mother, Mrs. Wasserstrom, has become more concerned about her communication problems and reading difficulties. Savannah struggles with reading at home and at school and never wants to look at books or talk about her reading problems. She seems unable to carry on conversations with other children and has few friends. Mrs. Wasserstrom is wondering if Savannah's reading problems are related to her communication problems and is concerned that she will not be able to pass the state reading tests scheduled for the end of the year. If Savannah does not pass, she will probably be held back, and Mrs. Wasserstrom absolutely does not want her to be held back, as her self-esteem already seems so fragile. Mrs. Wasserstrom has requested that the school provide a speech-language and reading evaluation for Savannah, but school personnel have rejected her request, noting that her Savannah's problems are too mild for an evaluation to be necessary.

Internet research

1. How many states have mandated fourth grade reading tests? Do children with disabilities have to take these tests?
2. What does the 2001 No Child Left Behind Act say about mandated testing for young children?

Brainstorm and discussion

1. Why might a school district reject a request for a speech-language evaluation?
2. A comprehensive language evaluation involves investigation of classroom curriculum-based performance. What types of classroom artifacts of Savannah's should be examined?
3. Savannah has difficulty following classroom directions and conversing with peers. This may be the result of a communication disorder or could be attributed to other circumstances. What are some of these other circumstances, and how might these be ruled out?

linguistic background (Paul, 2002). A language disorder may impact all three areas—whereby a child has difficulties with phonology, morphology, syntax, semantics, and pragmatics—or it may impact only one area. In addition, a language disorder can affect spoken or oral language as well as written language (e.g., reading, spelling) or another system of symbolic communication, such as sign language.

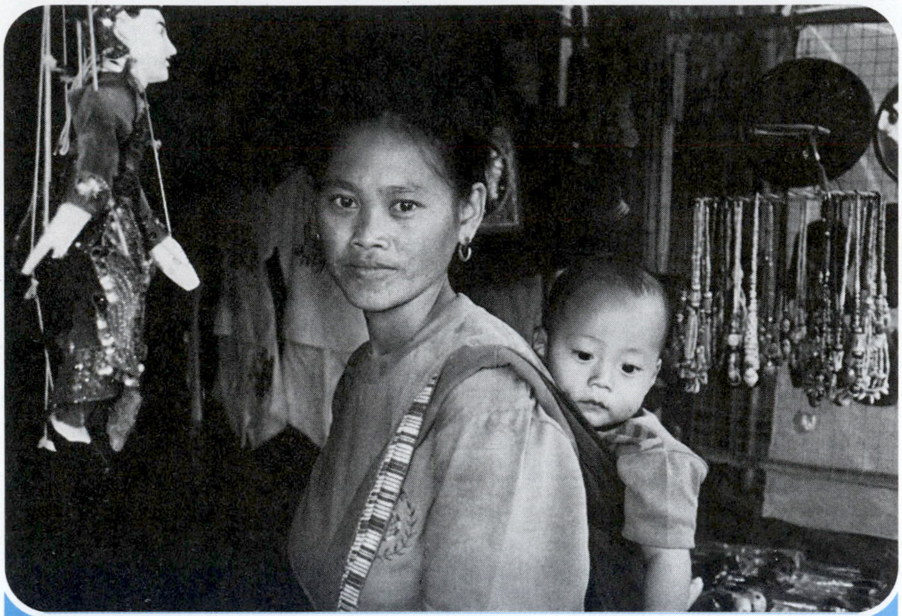

Across the communities of the world, children develop language along a predictable pathway.

Additional Considerations in Defining Language Disorders

This definition of a language disorder is a theoretical definition, and applying it to everyday clinical and educational work with children suspected of having language disorders is, as Fey (1986) has written, "not simple at all" (p. 31). Theoretical definitions must be refined for work with children by (1) considering the extent to which observed or suspected language problems have adverse social, psychological, and educational impact upon the children, (2) differentiating between language disorders and language differences, and (3) deciding when language problems are significant enough to be classified as disordered.

Discussion Point: Functional consequences *refers to the impact of a disorder on an individual's ability to perform daily living activities and to be a full member of a community. What aspects of daily living would you expect to be most affected by a language disorder? In thinking about this question, consider the case of Savannah in Box 7-1.*

Social, Psychological, and Educational Impact. If a child exhibits difficulty with language but the difficulty does not adversely affect the child socially, psychologically, or educationally, it could be argued that what appears to be a disorder is not a disorder at all (Fey, 1986). Emphasizing the social, psychological, and educational impact of language skills focuses attention on *functional consequences:* Does a child's language performance have a negative impact on the child's ability to function in society? (Fey, 1986). Some experts argue that a language disorder can exist only "when that person is at some risk for disvalue in one or more domains of life function because of the person's current or projected language abilities" (Tomblin, 1983, as cited in Fey, 1986).

Language Disorder Versus Language Difference. An accurate definition of *language disorder* must also take into consideration the cultural contexts in which a child is reared and is expected to perform. Consider, for instance, the case of Alejandro in Box 7-1. Alejandro's communication difficulties may be the result of a language disorder or a **language difference**. A language impairment should be evident when examining a child's language skills against both norm-referenced expectations and cultural expectations (see Figure 7-1; Fey, 1986; Paul, 2002).

Discussion Point: *What are some ways in which a child's culture may affect her language development?*

Norm-referenced expectations are based on a child's peer group. For instance, to determine whether a boy who is 3 years, 6 months of age is experiencing impaired language development, his language skills would be compared to the language skills typically seen in boys of the same age. This is a normative reference. On the other hand, cultural expectations are based on the cultural contexts in which a particular child is raised. One would expect slightly different language patterns when comparing the oral language skills of a 3-year-6-month-old European-American child reared in inner-city Boston and an African American child of the same age reared in an Appalachian region of southeast Ohio. Thus, definitions of language disorder should refer to language expectations based on normative references, as well as the expectations of a child's cultural group and the language-learning environment.

FIGURE 7-1 Determining a language disorder.

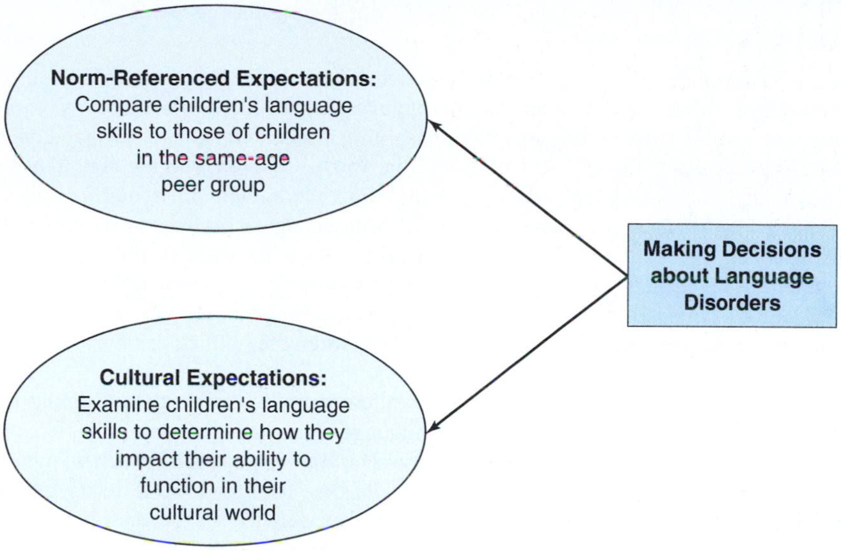

The Meaning of Significant. A definition of language disorder also must specify the difference between language difficulties that are not serious enough to be classified as disordered and those that are. By many accounts, a language disorder is present if *significant* problems are present (see Paul, 2002). However, it is difficult to determine when a child's language problems are serious enough to be called significant.

Because of the challenges in determining the presence or absence of significant difficulties, speech-language pathologists and other professionals who diagnose language disorders tend to rely on the use of tests and their outcomes. However, even scores from norm-referenced tests are not always absolute when considering the meaning of *significant*. For instance, a child may receive a standard score of 81 on a standardized test of language development. (Recall from chapter 4 that a standard score is a type of derived score from a norm-referenced test.) In many clinical or educational settings, this score of 81 would be interpreted as showing a significant problem with language development because a score of 85 is used as a cut-off; that is, a score of 86 or over is not disordered, whereas a score of 85 or below is disordered. However, in other clinical settings a score of 81 would not be considered disordered, or significantly different from normal. It is important to realize that these cut-off scores are arbitrary; there is currently no universally accepted test score that differentiates significant from nonsignificant problems with language (Aram, Morris, & Hall, 1993).

Obviously, this particular issue has serious implications for clinical practice and has often been the subject of serious debate among speech-language researchers and clinicians. In reality, decisions about the meaning of *significant* are often made at the level of the service provider (e.g., school district, health agency, private practice). These organizations set guidelines for speech-language pathologists and other professionals to follow in clinical decision making.

Discussion Point: *In the case of Alejandro in Box 7-1, how would a professional charged with completing a speech-language evaluation find out about speech-language expectations of Alejandro's cultural group and language-learning environment?*

Discussion Point: *In the case of Savannah in Box 7-1, school personnel do not feel that Savannah's difficulties are severe enough to be considered significant. What does* significant *mean to you?*

Terminology

Many terms are used to describe language disorders in children, including *language delay, language impairment, language disability,* and *language-learning disability*. The terms *childhood aphasia* and *language deviance* are outdated and inaccurate classifications of this condition

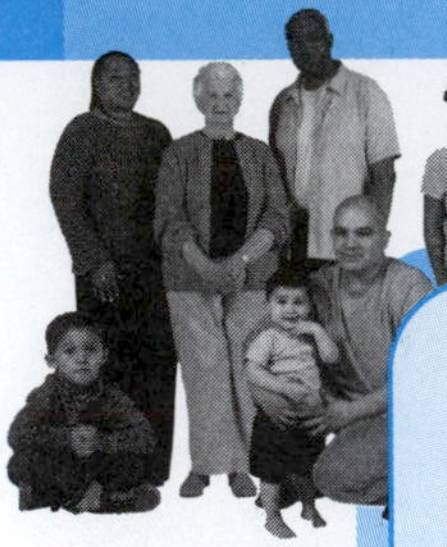

BOX 7-2 Multicultural Focus

Dual Language Learners

Children who are under 5 years of age and are acquiring two languages simultaneously (e.g., English and Spanish) are described as *simultaneous bilinguals;* children who are over 5 years of age and who have a native (home) language but are learning a second language, such as English, are described as *sequential bilinguals* (August & Hakuta, 1997). Children who are simultaneous and sequential bilinguals develop language differently from children who are acquiring only English and are native English speakers. Some children with limited English proficiency (LEP, also referred to as English language learners, or ELLs) may appear to have a language disability but, in fact, are simply going through the normal stages of learning a new language. These differences must not be mistaken for a language disorder; federal law legislates that children who are struggling academically should not be identified as having a disability when their difficulties are associated with limited proficiency in English.

Learning two or more languages—either simultaneously or sequentially—should have no negative impact on a child's ability to acquire language. Fears that learning multiple languages can confuse children are derived from flawed research in the early 1900s in which bilingual immigrant children in the United States were given intelligence tests and found to have lower test scores than monolingual children had. These early studies were flawed for many reasons, including the fact that many more of the immigrant children studied were from low socioeconomic households, whereas the monolingual children were from more advantaged homes. More recent and well-conducted studies have shown bilingualism to have an overwhelmingly positive impact on children's cognitive and linguistic development, once the effects of socioeconomic status are accounted for (August & Hakuta, 1997).

Large numbers of children who are learning English as a second or foreign language are being educated in American schools. In the 2000–2001 school year, more than 300,000 children were receiving LEP services in California's Los Angeles Unified School District; in Florida's Dade County School District, more than 60,000 LEP children were served; and in Texas's Houston Independent School District, more than 50,000 children were served (National Center for Education Statistics, 2003). About 10% of these children can be expected to exhibit a primary or secondary language disorder on the basis of epidemiological estimates of the prevalence of language impairment in young children. For some groups of children within the broader population of LEP students, the incidence may be slightly higher, particularly among children who are being reared in poverty conditions or whose families have had limited access to health care. In such cases, however, language disorders are not arising from limited English proficiency or second/foreign language acquisition, but rather from socioeconomic and broader cultural influences that have impacted the children's language-learning conditions.

When providing language services to ELL children, accurate assessments of needs and strengths are critical for "differentiating linguistic and cultural differences from learning difficulties,

and are therefore no longer used. The term **language delay** carries the connotation that children exhibiting problems with language achievements are having a late start with language development and can be expected to catch up with their peers (Leonard, 2000). However, as can be seen in Figure 7-2, many children with language disorders do not catch up with their peers over time; rather, the gap in language skill between children with normal development and those with language disorders tends to widen. In addition, for some children with language disorders, their language skills plateau at a point of arrested development. Therefore, the term *language delay* is not really an accurate characterization. There are some children, termed **late talkers**, who do show delays in the earliest stages of language development; approximately half of these children will catch up with their peers by and developing an appropriate educational program that addresses students' linguistic, cultural and experiential backgrounds" (Salend & Salinas, 2003, p. 37). Salend and Salinas (2003) provide six recommendations for individuals working with ELL students:

1. *Work as a multidisciplinary team.* Team members should include educators with training in working with ELL students (e.g., migrant educators, bilingual educators), as well as community members, parents, and professionals who speak the child's language.
2. *Study children's performance in both their native language and English.* Assessment data from both languages will detail the student's language proficiency in both languages and will document language dominance, language preference, and the extent to which language difficulties in one language are present in the other language.
3. *Know the factors associated with second language learning.* Team members need to understand that second language acquisition is a complex process and should understand factors that influence the rate and type of accomplishments.
4. *Use assessment alternatives.* A variety of assessment strategies should be used, including curriculum-based measures, dynamic assessment, observation, and analysis of classroom artifacts and curriculum participation.
5. *Examine diverse life experiences of the child that may influence learning.* These include length of time in the United States, school attendance patterns, attitude toward school, home language and dialect, and health and developmental history.
6. *Analyze the data.* Data analysis for ELL students includes examining diverse life experiences that may have influenced learning and determining the extent to which any language difficulties are present in the native or preferred language. Data analysis also includes determining whether any biases were present in the assessment process (p. 37).

For Discussion

In what ways might being reared bilingually have a positive impact on children's language development?

What are some factors that might influence the rate of language acquisition for children learning English as a second language?

There is currently grave concern over the possibility of misdiagnosing a child with a language difference as having a language disorder. Why is this a concern? What are some solutions to the problem of misdiagnosis?

Companion Website

To answer these questions online, go to the Multicultural Focus module in chapter 7 of the Companion Website.

3 or 4 years of age (Girolametto, Wiigs, Smyth, Weitzman, & Pearce, 2001; Rescorla, Roberts, & Dahlsgaard, 1997), whereas the other half will continue to show ongoing difficulties with language development.

The terms *language disorder* and *language impairment* provide the most accurate representation and are currently preferred for describing children experiencing significant challenges in language development relative to other children (Paul, 2002). The term *language disability* may also be used to suggest that children's language difficulties are exerting a significant, negative impact on their daily-living activities or functions (Paul, 2002). The term *language-learning disability* often describes older children with language disorders who experience difficulties with academic achievement in areas associated with language, such as

FIGURE 7-2 Normal and disordered language development over time.

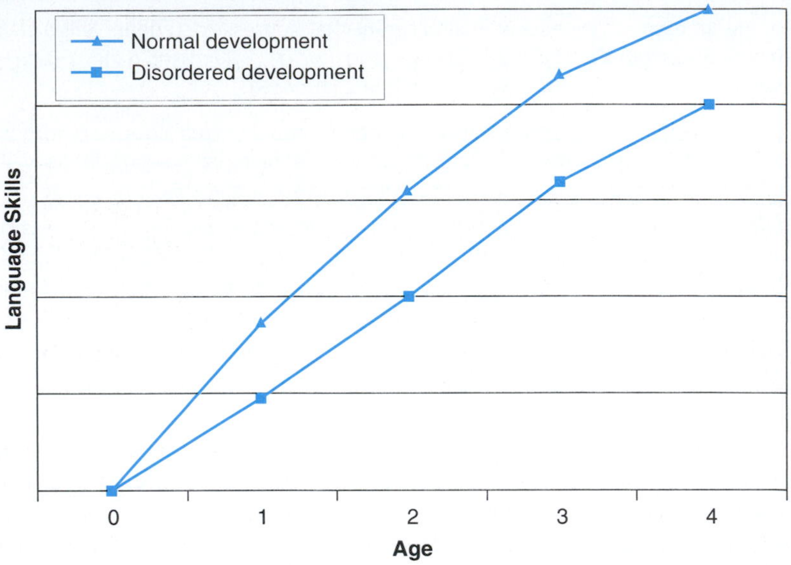

Source: From *Children with Specific Language Impairment* by L. Leonard, 2000, Cambridge, MA: MIT Press. Copyright 2000 by MIT Press. Adapted with permission.

reading, writing, and spelling (Heward, 2003). Finally, federal legislation (U.S. Congress, 1997) uses *specific learning disability* to describe children having substantial problems "in one or more of the basic psychological processes involved in understanding or in using language, spoken or written, which . . . may manifest itself in imperfect ability to listen, think, speak, read, write, spell, or do mathematical calculations" (p. 13).

Prevalence and Incidence

Language disorders are the most common type of communication impairment affecting children. They represent the most frequent cause for early intervention and special education services for children from toddlerhood through the elementary grades. About 15% of toddlers are late talkers (Rescorla, Hadicke-Wiley, & Escarce, 1993), and some of these youngsters will go on to receive a diagnosis of primary language impairment in the later preschool years (Rescorla & Schwartz, 1990). **Primary language impairment** describes a significant impairment of language in the absence of any other developmental difficulty (e.g., mental retardation, brain injury); it affects about 7–10% of children over the age of 5 years (Beitchman et al., 1989; Tomblin et al., 1997). Many of these children will continue to experience significant problems with language skills into middle and later adolescence (Catts, Fey, Zhang, & Tomblin, 2001; Catts, Fey, Tomblin, & Zhang, 2002; Johnson et al., 1999). Well over 1 million children receive special education services in American schools because of speech or language impairments (U.S. Department of Education, 2001).

A **secondary language impairment** is the result of other developmental disorders (e.g., mental retardation) or is acquired by a brain injury; it is more difficult to estimate in terms of prevalence. About 1 in 1,000 children exhibit mild to severe mental retardation (Fujiura & Yamaki, 1997), and about 1 in 500 children exhibit autism or an autism spectrum disorder (Autism Society of America, 2000; Ehlers & Gillberg, 1993). In addition, approximately 2% of children experience significant head injuries each year (U.S. Department of Health and Human Services, 1999). Annually, these percentages translate into about 600,000 school children receiving services for mental retardation, 65,000 children receiving services for autism, and 14,000 children receiving services for brain injuries (U.S. Department of Education, 2001). Many of these children will experience significant challenges with language and will need special communication supports.

How Are Language Disorders Classified?

Every child with a language disorder has an individual profile of language strengths and weaknesses. To capture these differences among children, language disorders are usually classified according to etiology, manifestation, and severity.

Etiology

Primary and Secondary Disorders

Etiology refers to cause. Language disorders result from many diverse causes, although in some cases cause can never be determined. Language disorders are often differentiated as having primary versus secondary etiologies (Schuele & Hadley, 1999). As was mentioned earlier, a primary language impairment occurs in the absence of any other disability that can clearly be held accountable for the disordered pattern of language development. A secondary language impairment occurs as a consequence of another disorder. For instance, mental retardation, hearing loss, and brain injury are primary conditions that often result in a secondary language disorder. So, a child with a severe congenital hearing loss may receive a diagnosis of having a language disorder secondary to hearing loss. Similarly, language disorders resulting from such conditions as prenatal or postnatal exposure to toxins (e.g., fetal alcohol syndrome, lead ingestion) or child abuse (e.g., shaken baby syndrome) may also be considered secondary language impairments.

Discussion Point: *Consider the case of Natasha in Box 7-1. Natasha clearly is showing some delays in acquiring the English language. If she is found to have a language impairment, would you consider it primary or secondary in etiology?*

Developmental and Acquired Disorders

Language disorders also are often classified as developmental language disorders or acquired language disorders. A **developmental language disorder** is present from birth; it can describe a primary language impairment that has no obvious cause or an impairment that is secondary to another congenital disability, such as Down syndrome, which results in mental retardation. An **acquired language disorder** is acquired sometime after birth, typically as the result of some type of insult or injury to the developing child (e.g., a car accident).

Manifestation

Language disorders are also classified according to which aspects of language are affected or how the disorder is manifested. Does the disorder impact comprehension, expression, or both? Does the disorder affect form, content, and use, or just one or two of these domains?

Comprehension and Expression

Some children exhibit significant problems with comprehending language but have normal expressive language skills—a language comprehension disorder (Beitchman et al., 1989). Other children have problems only with expressive language—an expressive language disorder (American Psychiatric Association [APA], 1994). This is also referred to as a **specific expressive language disorder (SELD)**. Children who show impairments in both comprehension and expression have a **mixed receptive-expressive disorder** (APA, 1994).

Form, Content, and Use

Children with language disorders differ in the area of language affected. Recall from chapter 2 that language form refers to the structure of language (i.e., morphology, syntax, and phonology), content refers to the meaning expressed through language (i.e., semantics), and use describes how language is used in social contexts (i.e., pragmatics). Some children may have problems only with syntax and morphology—a language disorder of form. Children who have a disorder of phonology also have a form problem. Some children may have difficulties only with aspects of word meaning; word finding problems, difficulties with abstract language, and slow vocabulary development would characterize a content problem. Some children have problems only with use, or pragmatics. These children may have problems initiating conversations with peers, engaging in extended discourse, or using a wide range of communicative behaviors (e.g., questions, requests, comments, greetings).

Although some children have a problem specific to one area or domain, a great number of children have difficulties in two or all three areas. A disorder affecting only one domain is a **focal disorder**, whereas a disorder affecting multiple domains is a **diffuse**, or widespread, **disorder**. Typically, a disorder that is diffuse is less likely to resolve and is viewed as more serious than a focal impairment (Bishop & Edmundson, 1987).

Severity

The severity of language disorders ranges from mild to profound, as shown in Figure 7-3. Mild impairments may be perceptible only to a child, parent, or professional and may have little impact on a child's ability to function at home or school. In contrast, children with a profound impairment may have no language skill at all and therefore may be severely limited in their ability to participate in many home, school, or community functions (Paul, 2002).

Characterizing Individual Differences

Interchild Differences

These classifications represent the variation among children in the cause, manifestation, and severity of language disorders. For instance, a 7-year-old child may have a severe acquired language disorder, secondary to traumatic brain injury and impacting comprehension and

FIGURE 7-3 Variations in severity of language disorders.

Mild	Has some impact on child's ability to perform in social or academic situations but does not preclude participation in normal, age-appropriate activities in school or community
Moderate	Involves a significant degree of impairment that necessitates some special accommodations for the child to participate in mainstream community and academic settings
Severe	Usually makes it very difficult for a child to function in community and educational activities without extensive supports
Profound	Implies that the child has little or no ability to use language to communicate and is unable to function in community and educational activities

Source: From *Language Disorders from Infancy Through Adolescence* by R. Paul. Copyright 2002. Reprinted with permission from Elsevier.

FIGURE 7-4 Symptom variations of language disorders over time.

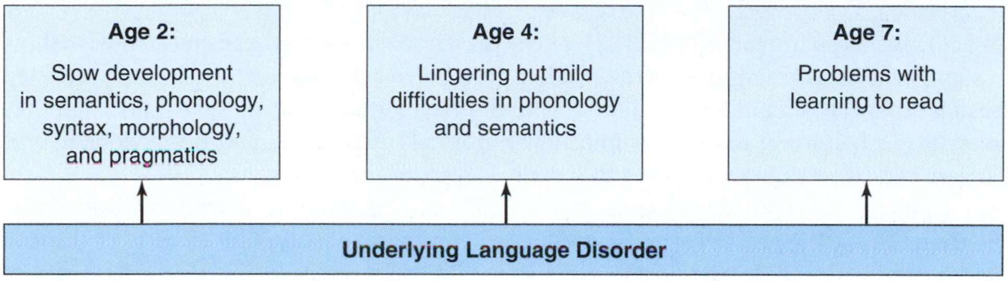

Source: Based on Scarborough, H. S., (2000).

expression in the areas of content and use. Professionals must be sensitive to this appreciable diversity among children, which has important implications for accurate assessment and treatment. Clearly, there can be no one-size-fits-all approach when working with children with language disorders.

Intrachild Differences

There are also important **intrachild differences** in how a language disorder is manifested. The symptoms and severity of a language disorder may change dramatically over time as a result of developmental maturation, treatments, and educational opportunities. Many young children with specific language impairment, which is discussed later in this chapter, show significant difficulties across the full range of language domains during the early preschool years. By the time these children enter school, however, as many as half of them will have completely resolved their language difficulties (Rescorla & Schwartz, 1990). For the other half with more persistent problems, some will have only lingering difficulties in one or two domains, whereas others will continue to show widespread challenges affecting multiple areas of language (Bishop & Edmundson, 1987).

However, even those children whose language difficulties are resolved by the time they enter school face a general vulnerability to once again exhibit a language disorder. This is particularly true when educational experiences make significant requirements of the underlying language system, as is the case when children begin to learn to read (Bashir & Scavuzzo, 1992; Menyuk et al., 1991); the process of learning to read may once again reveal an underlying language problem. One way of describing this phenomenon, whereby children manifest different language problems at different points in time, is presented in Figure 7-4. This figure shows how a child's language symptoms may vary across time; a language disorder may be a lasting condition that persists across the lifespan (Botting, Faragher, Simkin, Knox, & Conti-Ramsden, 2001; Girolametto et al., 2001; Johnson et al., 1999).

What Are the Defining Characteristics of Prevalent Types of Language Disorders?

Four types of language disorders are particularly prevalent among young children. **Specific language impairment** is a primary, developmental language impairment with no known cause. **Autism spectrum disorder** and mental retardation are two types of developmental disabilities that often result in secondary language impairments. Traumatic brain injury is an acquired disorder that also often results in a secondary language impairment.

Specific Language Impairment

Defining Characteristics

Specific language impairment (SLI) describes preschool and school-age children who show a significant impairment of expressive and/or receptive language that cannot be attributed to any other causal condition. Children with SLI have typical hearing skills (although they may have a history of middle ear infections), normal intelligence, and no obvious neurological, motor, or sensory disturbances, such as seizures or brain injury.

Children are typically diagnosed with SLI after their third birthday (Rescorla & Schwartz, 1990). Although signs of language difficulty may be present as early as the first and second years of life, toddlers who are slow to talk are typically classified as late talkers rather than language impaired. Because at least 35% and as many as 60% of late talkers outgrow their language problems by 3 years of age (Rescorla et al., 1997; Thal & Tobias, 1992), the diagnosis of SLI is usually not made until age 3 or later, when it is clear that a child is exhibiting a true disorder of language rather than a late start.

Discussion Point: *What are some benefits of early diagnosis of SLI? Can you think of any drawbacks of early diagnosis?*

The language profile of children with SLI is difficult to capture, because these children are a very diverse group. Some children with SLI have problems in only one area of language, whereas others have problems that transcend all areas of language performance. Some children have difficulties with expressive language only (SELD), while others have problems with both expression and comprehension (a mixed disorder).

An overview of language challenges for children with SLI from toddlerhood through adolescence is presented in Table 7-1. Hallmark characteristics include these:

1. Inconsistent skills across different domains; for instance, a child might have a strength in phonology and a weakness in syntax and morphology.

TABLE 7-1 Language difficulties associated with SLI

Age	Language Difficulties
Infancy and toddlerhood	Late appearance of first word (average age of 23 months); delayed use of present progressive (*-ing*), plural (*s*), and possessive (*'s*); late use of two-word combinations (average age of 37 months); less frequent use of verbs and less variety in verbs; slow development of pronouns; longer reliance on gestures for getting needs met; difficulty initiating with peers; difficulty sustaining turns in conversation
Preschool	Use of grammar that resembles that of younger children (e.g., pronoun errors, as in *me want dolly*); late use of verb markers (e.g., third person singular *is* as an auxiliary); frequent errors of omission (e.g., leaving out key elements of syntax); shorter sentence length; problems forming questions with inverted auxiliaries; difficulty with accurate use of *be* as an auxiliary or copular verb form; slow development of pronouns; requests similar to those of younger children; difficulty with group conversations (i.e., conversing with more than one child); difficulty with verbal resolution of conflict
Early and later elementary	Word-finding problems accompanied by circumlocutions and pauses; naming errors (e.g., *shoes* for *pants*); slower processing speed; use of earlier developing pronoun forms; low sensitivity to the speech of others (e.g., difficulty responding to indirect requests); difficulty maintaining topics; difficulty recognizing need for conversational repair
Adolescence	Difficulty expressing ideas about language; inappropriate responses to questions and comments; poor social language; insufficient information for listeners; redundancy; inadequate sense of limits or boundaries; difficulty expressing needs and ideas; difficulty initiating conversations with peers; immature conversational participation

Sources: Based on Conti-Ramsden and Jones (1997); Leonard (2000); McGregor and Leonard (1995); Ratner and Harris (1994); Watkins, Rice, and Molz (1993).

2. A history of slow vocabulary development: on average children with SLI produce their first words at about 2 years of age and continue to struggle with learning new words through the elementary years (see Leonard, 2000).
3. A tendency toward **word finding problems**, that is, difficulties in coming up with the right words at the right time (Oetting, Rice, & Swank, 1995). Word finding problems are usually accompanied by frequent pauses, filler words (e.g., *um, uh*), a reliance on nonspecific and general words (e.g., *thing, stuff*), and naming errors (e.g., calling a plate a glass; McGregor, 1997).
4. Considerable difficulty with grammatical production and comprehension that begins during toddlerhood and continues through school age (Conti-Ramsden & Jones, 1997). This problem is particularly evident with verbs. Children with SLI use verbs less frequently than do their same-age peers, use fewer types of verbs, and show delayed development of verb morphology (Conti-Ramsden & Jones, 1997; Rice, 1996; Watkins & Rice, 1994). Leonard (2000) has written that verb use is an "extraordinary problem" for children with SLI (p. 61).
5. A tendency toward problems in social skills, behavior, and attention (e.g., problems making friends or initiating with peers; Fujiki, Brinton, Morgan, & Hart, 1999; Fujicki, Brinton, & Todd, 1996; Redmond & Rice, 1998).
6. The likelihood of language difficulties persisting over time. Well over 50% of children who exhibit SLI at kindergarten age continue to show language weaknesses in adolescence and adulthood (Johnson et al., 1999; Stothard, Snowling, Bishop, Chipchase, & Kaplan, 1998).

Causes and Risk Factors

There is currently no known cause for SLI, a fact that is frustrating for both parents and professionals. Recent advances in brain imaging and epidemiological investigations suggest a strong biological and genetic component to this disorder (Gauer, Lombardino, & Leonard, 1997). The current theoretical view is that biological or genetic factors predispose a child to SLI. For instance, children who have immediate family members with language impairment are more likely than other children to develop SLI (Ellis Weismer, Murray-Branch, & Miller, 1994; Rice, Haney, & Wexler, 1998; Tomblin, 1989; Van Der Lely & Stollwerck, 1996). About 20–40% of children with SLI have a sibling or a parent with a language disorder.

Whether a biological or genetic predisposition to SLI is eventually manifested as a disorder is linked to a child's exposure to additional risk factors. Not all children who are genetically or biologically predisposed to SLI

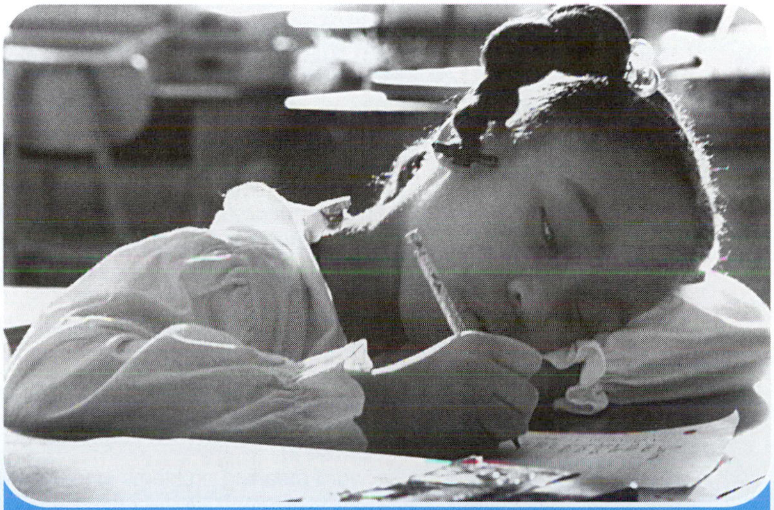

More than 50% of kindergarteners with language impairment will continue to have language problems in adolescence.

Discussion Point: *Survey your classmates to find out how many had chronic middle ear infections as children. Chronic middle ear infections can increase a child's risk for language difficulties, although the connection has been difficult for researchers to establish. Why would it be difficult to study ear infections in young children?*

will experience SLI. Specifically, it appears that sensory deprivation due to environmental factors (e.g., limited language input) or biological factors (e.g., chronic middle ear infections) contributes to a developmental fragility that increases the risk for SLI, as can physical health challenges resulting from adverse perinatal influences (e.g., low birth weight, prematurity) and postnatal influences (e.g., exposure to toxins, undernutrition).

Autism Spectrum Disorder

Defining Characteristics

Autism spectrum disorder (ASD) is an umbrella term describing a variety of developmental conditions that are characterized by significant difficulties in social relationships, communication, repetitive behaviors, and overly restricted interests (Lord & Risi, 2000). While the prognosis for autism has historically been poor (Heflin & Simpson, 1998) and few individuals have been able to live and work independently, recent advances in early identification and intervention provide increasing promise for individuals with autism and their families.

The term *autism spectrum disorder* includes four types of disabilities: autism, childhood disintegrative disorder, Asperger's syndrome, and pervasive developmental disorder–not otherwise specified (PDD). These four conditions are childhood disabilities that together impact about 1 in 500 children (Autism Society of America, 2000). There is a higher rate of these disorders in children with family members who are also affected, indicating a strong genetic component. The prevalence of autism across the genders is markedly uneven: with the exception of childhood disintegrative disorder, boys are about four times as likely as girls to be affected (APA, 1994). However, when girls are affected, they tend to have more severe symptoms than boys.

Children with any one of the autism spectrum disorders usually will exhibit a mild to severe or profound secondary language impairment. The language characteristics of children with ASD are presented in Figure 7-5.

Autism. Autism is a severe developmental disability with symptoms that are present before a child's third birthday. Diagnostic criteria from the most recent *Diagnostic and Statistical Manual of Mental Disorders* (*DSM;* APA, 1994) are presented in Table 7-2. The

FIGURE 7-5 Language characteristics of children with ASD.

1. Delays in language development are often the first warning sign for this disorder.
2. Approximately 50% of children with ASD never develop functional language.
3. The language of children with ASD shows a prevalence of
   - echolalia (functional or nonfunctional repetition of phrases heard elsewhere)
   - pronominal confusions (referral to self using third-person pronouns or proper name)
   - self-stimulatory speech (use of same sounds or phrases repeatedly without communicative intent)
   - dysprosody (use of inappropriate or unusual pitch, rhythm, pace, or articulation)
   - paralinguistic difficulties (difficulty with eye gaze, proximity, gestures, and body contact)
   - word meaning problems (difficulty with nonliteral language and abstract concepts)
   - context-bound usage (inability to use language to refer to events away from the here and now)

Source: From *Childhood Language Disorders in Context* (2nd ed.) by Nickola Wolf Nelson. Published by Allyn & Bacon, Boston, MA. Copyright 2004 by Pearson Education. Adapted by permission of the publisher.

TABLE 7-2 Diagnostic criteria for ASD

Disorder	Onset	Hallmark Characteristics
Autism	Prior to 3 years	Abnormal functioning in social interaction, communication, and behavior, with at least six specific areas of deficit from the following (at least two must be in social interaction, and at least one in the other two categories): 1. Social interaction a. Marked impairment in using multiple nonverbal behaviors (eye-to-eye gaze, facial expression, body posture, gestures) b. Failure to develop peer relationships appropriately c. Lack of spontaneous seeking to share enjoyment, interests, or achievements with others d. Lack of social or emotional reciprocity 2. Communication a. Delay in or total lack of development of spoken language b. Marked impairment in ability to sustain conversation with others c. Stereotyped and repetitive use of language or idiosyncratic language d. Lack of varied, spontaneous or make-believe play or social imitative play 3. Behavior a. Preoccupation with one or more stereotyped patterns of interest that are abnormal in intensity or focus b. Inflexible adherence to specific nonfunctional routines or rituals c. Repetitive motor movements d. Persistent preoccupation with parts of objects
Childhood disintegrative disorder	Between 2 and 10 years	Normal development for at least first 2 years, significant loss of skills in two or more of the following: language, social skills or adaptive behavior, bowel or bladder control, play, and motor skills. Significant impairment must also be observed in at least two of the following: 1. Social interaction, including impaired nonverbal behaviors, failure to develop peer relationships, and lack of emotional reciprocity 2. Communication, including lack of spoken language, inability to sustain or initiate conversation, and repetitive use of language 3. Behavior, including restrictive, repetitive, or stereotyped patterns of behavior and interests
Asperger's syndrome	Onset before or after 3 years	No clinically significant delay in language, cognitive, self-help, and adaptive behavioral skills, but significant impairment in two or more areas of the following: 1. Social interaction a. Impairment in use of nonverbal behaviors b. Failure to develop peer relationships c. Lack of spontaneous seeking to share enjoyment, interests, or achievements with others d. Lack of social or emotional reciprocity 2. Behavior a. Preoccupation with one or more stereotyped patterns of interest that are abnormal in intensity or focus b. Inflexible adherence to specific nonfunctional routines or rituals c. Repetitive motor movements d. Persistent preoccupation with parts of objects
Pervasive developmental disorder	Onset before or after 3 years	A severe and pervasive impairment in social interaction, communication, and/or behavior without meeting criteria for diagnosis of autistic disorder, childhood disintegrative disorder, or Asperger's syndrome

Source: From *Diagnostic and Statistical Manual of Mental Disorders* (4th ed.) by American Psychiatric Association, 1994, Washington, DC: APA. Copyright 1994 by APA. Adapted with permission.

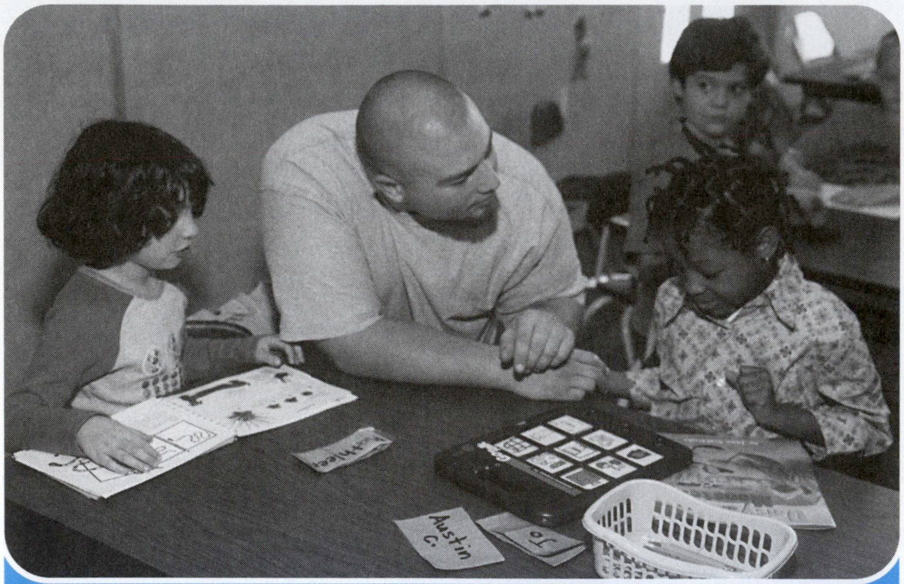

Autism results from a neurological disturbance, but the exact cause of the disorder remains unknown.

three hallmark characteristics of autism are difficulties with social interactions with others, severe impairment of communication skill, and restricted and stereotypical behaviors and interests.

Children with autism show significant difficulties in interacting and relating with others. This includes impaired nonverbal behaviors (e.g., eye contact, posture, facial expressions), an inability or lack of interest in developing relationships with peers and participating in social games or routines, and little awareness of the feelings or needs of others (APA, 1994). Children with autism also have severely impaired communication skills. Some children with autism never develop any functional oral language skills; the language of those who do develop language is often characterized by idiosyncratic, repetitive language (e.g., **echolalia**, stereotypical repetitions of specific words or phrases) and an inability to initiate or reciprocate in communicative interactions with others.

In addition, children with autism also show "restricted, repetitive, and stereotyped patterns of behaviors, interests, and activities" (APA, 1994, p. 67). These children may have very few interests and are overly preoccupied with certain objects or activities. For instance, a child may be preoccupied with a set of plastic dinosaurs and may spend hours each day lining up the dinosaurs along the edge of a table in a particular order. **Stereotypical behaviors** are also common, such as rocking back and forth, humming, or flapping the arms.

Childhood Disintegrative Disorder. **Childhood disintegrative disorder** describes children under 10 years of age who appear to be developing normally until at least their second birthday but then display a significant loss or regression of skills in two or more of the following areas: language, social skills, bowel control, play, or motor skills (APA, 1994). Like children with autism, children with disintegrative disorder display significant problems in their social interactions and communication skills and also show restricted and repetitive behaviors and interests.

Asperger's Syndrome. Children with **Asperger's syndrome** are often referred to as "higher functioning" children with autism. Like children with other autism spectrum disorders, children with Asperger's have substantial problems with social interaction and show restricted and idiosyncratic behavioral patterns and interests. The language skills of children with Asperger's tend to be relatively well developed and are not viewed as clinically disordered. However, because of their challenges with social relationships, children with Asperger's often have considerable difficulty using language as a social tool and a means of developing and maintaining social relationships. They may, for instance, have difficulty initiating conversations with peers and may use language that is situationally inappropriate.

Pervasive Developmental Disorder (PDD). PDD describes children who have severe problems with social interactions and communication and who display repetitive behaviors and overly restricted interests but do not otherwise meet the criteria for autism, childhood disintegrative disorder, or Asperger's syndrome.

Discussion Point: *Even though children with Asperger's syndrome tend to have well-developed language skills, they still benefit from language intervention to enhance their pragmatic skills, such as conversational participation and initiating with peers. Can you think of some ways these skills might be targeted in a therapy session?*

Causes and Risk Factors

Autism spectrum disorders are currently viewed as neurobiological disorders resulting from an organic brain abnormality (Lord & Risi, 2000). Several risk factors may contribute to the likelihood of a child's developing an autism spectrum disorder. Prenatal and perinatal complications, particularly maternal rubella and **anoxia** (i.e., lack of oxygen to the brain), have been associated with increased risk for autism (APA, 1994). The presence of other developmental or physical disabilities, such as encephalitis (an inflammation of the brain) and fragile X syndrome (a genetic disorder that results in mental retardation), also can contribute to the occurrence of autism. Seizure disorder is seen in 25% of children with autism (APA, 1994). Severe sensory deprivation, as seen in severe cases of neglect and child abuse, can have profound impact on communication and social development and in extreme cases may result in patterns of development similar to that of autism spectrum disorders (Kenneally, Bruck, Frank, & Nalty, 1998).

Some professionals and parents believe there is a link between childhood vaccinations and autism, particularly the MMR (measles, mumps, rubella) vaccine. However, the most extensive study to date examining the evidence for the autism-vaccination connection found no link between this vaccine and the risk for developing autism. Published in 2002 in the *New England Journal of Medicine* (Madsen et al., 2002), this study examined the incidence of autism in 537,303 children in Denmark, of whom 440,655 had received the MMR vaccine. The study showed the rate of autism to be no higher for children who had received the vaccine than for children who had not received the vaccine. Research focused on determining the cause of autism, including further study of the vaccine-autism link, is currently underway in the United States.

Mental Retardation

Defining Characteristics

Mental retardation, according to the American Association on Mental Retardation (AAMR, 2002), is a "condition of arrested or incomplete development of the mind, which is especially characterized by impairment of skills manifested during the developmental period" (p. 103). About 1% of children in American schools have a diagnosis of mental retardation, reflecting about 10% of children receiving special education services (U.S. Department of Education, 2002). The diagnosis of mental retardation is made in children under the age of 18 years who experience "significant limitations both in intellectual functioning and in adaptive behavior as expressed in conceptual, social, and practical adaptive skills" (AAMR, 2002, p. 1).

In accordance with this definition, an accurate diagnosis of mental retardation is made on the basis of two key considerations (AAMR, 2002):

1. Limitations in intelligence, to include difficulties with reasoning, planning, problem solving, abstract thinking, comprehending abstract and complex concepts, and learning skills

2. Limitations in **adaptive behavior** and the activities of daily living, including difficulties in conceptual skills (communication, functional academics, self-direction, health and safety), social skills (social relationships, leisure), and/or practical skills (self-care, home living, community participation, work)

Consideration of limitations in both intelligence and adaptive behavior is made in reference to the broader context of an individual's peers and community and must include the impact of linguistic and cultural diversity (AAMR, 2002). In other words, the unique contexts in which an individual is reared—referring to the "conditions within which people live their everyday lives"—must be closely examined for any determination of mental retardation to occur (AAMR, 2002, p. 15). Examination of context should include an individual's *microsystem* (close family), *mesosystem* (neighborhood and community), and *macrosystem* (society).

Mental retardation can affect an individual only minimally, with an individual exhibiting mild learning difficulties but able to participate fully in society and develop strong social relationships, or it can affect an individual profoundly. People with profound mental retardation may be unable to care for themselves, communicate, or participate in any community or employment activities. Four levels of mental retardation, ranging from mild to profound, are presented in Table 7-3 and can be determined by considering both intellectual limitations and adaptive behavior limitations. Of the four levels presented in Table 7-3, mild and moderate levels are much more prevalent (about 95% of persons with mental retardation) than severe and profound levels of retardation (only about 5% of cases; AAMR, 2002).

TABLE 7-3 Categories of mental retardation

Classification	IQ Range	Adaptive Skills
Mild (85% of MR)	50–69	Mild learning difficulties; able to work, maintain good social relationships, and make contributions to society. Can acquire academic skills up to about a sixth-grade level. By adulthood usually achieve social and vocabulary skills adequate for minimum self-support; apt to need supervision and assistance. Usually live successfully in community, either independently or in supervised settings.
Moderate (10% of MR)	35–49	Marked developmental delays in childhood; able to develop some degree of independence in self-care and acquire adequate communication and academic skills. As adolescents may have problems with peer relationships because of difficulties with social conventions. Can benefit from vocational training. Need varying degrees of support to live and work in community but are able to perform unskilled or semiskilled work with supervision. Adapt well to community life, usually in supervised settings.
Severe (3–4% of MR)	20–34	Significant developmental delays; acquire little or no speech and language skill in preschool years but may later develop minimal communication skills. Can master some preacademic skills (sight reading of important words). Need continuous levels of support to care for self and participate in community activities but can adapt well to community life with close supervision.
Profound (1–2% of MR)	<20	Severe limitations in self-care, continence, communication, and mobility; usually identified with a neurological condition that accounts for mental retardation. Need constant aid and supervision; may perform simple tasks with much support.

Source: From *Diagnostic and Statistical Manual of Mental Disorders* (4th ed.) by American Psychiatric Association, 1994, Washington, DC: APA. Copyright 1994 by APA. Adapted with permission.

The language skills of a person with mental retardation usually approximate the degree of cognitive impairment. In general, children with mental retardation show delays in early communicative behaviors (e.g., pointing in order to request, commenting vocally) and are slow to use their first words and to produce multiword combinations (Rosenberg & Abbeduto, 1993). The path of language acquisition tends to follow the same path as that of children who are developing typically, albeit at a slower rate.

Children with mild forms of mental retardation may have well-developed oral language skills, particularly in vocabulary, with minor difficulties with abstract concepts, figurative language, complex syntax, conversational participation, and communicative repairs (Ezell & Goldstein, 1991; Kuder, 1997). For instance, children with mild mental retardation often have difficulty understanding abstract notions such as *liberty* or *cooperation*, understanding and using idiomatic expressions (e.g., *hit the books*), using conjunctions to temporally and causally sequence their thoughts, and recognizing when communication breakdowns have occurred. Despite these difficulties, many children with mild levels of mental retardation exhibit oral language skills that allow them to fully participate in the academic curriculum, communicate competently with peers and adults, and relay their needs and interests to others.

Comparatively, children with more severe forms of mental retardation display severe to profound levels of language disorder. Some individuals with mental retardation never learn to express themselves through verbal means. They may produce only a few words or sounds and few gestures. For some individuals, an augmentative and alternative communicative (AAC) device can facilitate their ability to express themselves. AAC devices and other means of enhancing the communicative abilities of individuals with severe communicative disabilities are described in chapter 15.

Historically, it was thought that individuals with mental retardation reached an early plateau in language development. Recent research has shown, however, that new language skills continue to emerge well into adolescence for persons with mental retardation. Chapman and colleagues' research on persons with Down syndrome, which is a fairly prevalent cause of mental retardation, show significant gains in syntax and vocabulary development through later childhood and adolescence (Chapman, Seung, Schwartz, & Kay-Raining Bird, 1998). For instance, children who are 5 to 8 years of age produce utterances that average about two words in length, compared to utterances of about 4.5 words in length for older adolescents. Although continuing to develop over time, the language skills of children and adolescents with Down syndrome tend to be characterized by short sentences (about three words in length), a fairly small expressive vocabulary, a slowed rate of speech, and often compromised intelligibility. Function words, such as copular and auxiliary verbs (e.g., *is, were, does*), may be frequently omitted, as are pronouns, conjunctions, and articles. Language comprehension tends to be better than language expression.

Causes and Risk Factors

Mental retardation can occur for many reasons, although in about 30–40% of cases the cause cannot be identified (APA, 1994). For the other 60–70% of cases, prenatal damage to the developing fetus due to chromosomal abnormalities or maternal ingestion of toxins accounts for the majority of cases (about 30% overall). Environmental influences and other mental conditions, such as sensory deprivation (e.g., neglect) or the presence of autism, account for about 15–20% of all cases. Pregnancy and perinatal problems—such as fetal malnutrition, prematurity, anoxia (lack of oxygen to the child's brain before, during, or following birth), and viral infections—account for an additional 10% of cases. Medical conditions such as trauma, infection, and poisoning cause about 5% of cases of mental retardation, and heredity alone accounts for 5% of cases.

Brain Injury

Defining Characteristics

Brain injury refers to damage or insult to an individual's brain. Although brain injuries can occur in utero (before birth) and perinatally (during the birthing process), this chapter focuses on *acquired* brain injuries. Brain injuries sustained before or near the time of birth that result in significant intellectual challenges are usually viewed as cases of mental retardation. Acquired brain injuries are the leading cause of death and disability among young children, and the majority of these injuries result from transportation-related accidents (U.S. Department of Health and Human Services, 1999).

Acquired injuries occur sometime after birth as a result of an incident that inflicts damage on the brain matter. Brain injuries affect approximately 1.5 million persons each year, the majority of whom do survive but often with significant, lasting neurological damage. Young children, adolescent males, and the elderly are at greatest risk, and males are affected twice as often as females. The impact of a brain injury on children and their families can be enormous; about 60% of those affected by a brain injury have lifelong serious impairments that negatively impact daily living activities (Beukelman & Yorkston, 1991). The financial costs of brain injuries are substantial. Many families directly impacted by a brain injury deplete all or most of their financial resources to care for the injured person, and the annual economic burden to the United States is billions of dollars (U.S. Department of Health and Human Services, 1999).

The severity of a brain injury is often associated with the amount of unconsciousness resulting from the injury. Mild injuries, characterized by a concussion and loss of consciousness for 30 minutes or less, are the most common type of brain injury and are associated with less serious repercussions. A severe injury is accompanied by a coma of 6 hours or more (Russell, 1993). Serious brain injuries can result from infection (e.g., meningitis), disease (e.g., brain tumor), and physical trauma. Brain damage resulting from physical trauma, particularly blunt trauma to the head, is referred to as traumatic brain injury, or TBI. Causes of TBI in children include abuse (e.g., shaken baby syndrome), intentional harm (e.g., being hit or shot in the head), accidental poisoning through ingestion of toxic substances (e.g., prescription medications, pesticides), car accidents, and falling.

The most common type of TBI is a closed-head injury (CHI), in which brain matter is not exposed or penetrated. CHI is frequently associated with rapid acceleration and deceleration, as in a car, in which people may hit their heads on the dashboard or steering wheel. Among children CHI may result from child abuse, sports injuries, falls, and pedestrian-vehicle accidents (National Institute on Deafness and Other Communication Disorders [NIDCD], 2003). In contrast, in open-head injuries (OHI) brain matter is exposed through penetration.

Injuries may be diffuse, affecting large areas of the brain, or they may be focal, affecting only one specific brain region. The frontal and temporal lobes of the brain, which house the centers for much of our executive functions (e.g., reasoning, planning, hypothesizing) and our language functions, are often damaged in head injuries, as they sit more anterior in the brain where damage is most likely to occur (e.g., during a car accident) [NIDCD, 2003]. CHI tends to be associated with diffuse damage to the brain, whereas OHI, such as injury from a gunshot wound, usually results in a focal injury.

The immediate injury to the brain, whether diffuse or focal, may also be accompanied by secondary brain injuries that result from the primary trauma. For instance, an injury to the brain may result in edema, a swelling of the brain due to increased fluid. This swelling can cause brain damage beyond what was sustained in the original injury. Loss of blood, decreased blood pressure, or airway obstruction accompanying a brain injury can cause anoxia, which can cause additional brain damage (Brooke, Uomoto, McLean, & Fraser, 1991).

Most children with an acquired brain injury have a history of normal language skills. Language disorders resulting from brain injury are influenced by the severity of the injury, the *site* of the damage, and the characteristics of the child before the injury occurred (Chapman, 1997). Children with more severe injuries have less of a chance for full language recovery. Contrary to popular thought, the brains of young children are not better able to withstand and heal from injury than those of older children. Infants, toddlers, and preschoolers show long-lasting cognitive and language impairments following TBI (Aram, 1988). However, some young children may have a delayed onset of impairment; that is, problems sustained during a brain injury may not be evident until later years when damaged areas of the brain are applied to certain skills and activities (Goodman & Yude, 1996).

***Discussion Point:** Contrary to historical belief, infants, toddlers, and preschoolers show long-lasting cognitive and language impairments following a TBI. A prevalent cause of TBI in children is shaken baby syndrome. What are other causes of TBI in children? What are some ways to decrease the occurrence of TBI in children?*

In many cases of CHI, the brain injury affects the frontal lobe of the brain, resulting in difficulties associated with language use and cognitive, executive, and self-regulatory functions. About 75% of children with severe CHI have language use problems in the area of discourse (Chapman, 1997). Major language difficulties commonly associated with brain injury are presented in Figure 7-6 and include giving less information in discourse, producing language that is fragmented and difficult to follow, and having difficulties with word retrieval (Chapman, 1997; Russell, 1993).

Brain injury can also impact a child's cognitive, executive, and behavioral skills (Russell, 1993; Taylor, 2001). These include difficulties with sustained and selective attention (e.g., maintaining attention during an ongoing activity, when distractions might be present), storing new information, retrieving known information, planning and goal setting, organizational skills, reasoning and problem-solving, self-awareness, and behavioral monitoring (Taylor, 2001). Children and adolescents with brain injury may be more likely to exhibit aggression, irritability, depression, and anxiety. Because the prevalent long-term repercussions of brain injury are more subtle than obvious physical manifestations, brain injury is often referred to as an invisible epidemic (U.S. Department of Health and Human Services, 1999).

Causes and Risk Factors

The most common causes of brain injuries are automobile accidents, falls, and sports injuries (Beukelman & Yorkston, 1991). For children, recreational and sports injuries—such as bicycling, football, and horseback riding—are common causes of brain injury. Risk factors

FIGURE 7-6 **Language problems associated with brain injury.**

- Language comprehension difficulties, affected by decreased attention and decreased speed in processing information
- Difficulty with abstract information, such as identifying a main idea and understanding abstract concepts
- Disruption of newly learned language information (e.g., new vocabulary) due to long-term memory deficits
- Problems organizing complex or main ideas and information in verbal and written language
- Difficulties in word retrieval and rapid naming
- Ineffective, tangential, or socially inappropriate discourse
- Impaired coherence in discourse: fragmented, irrelevant, and lengthy utterances

Source: Based on Russell (1993).

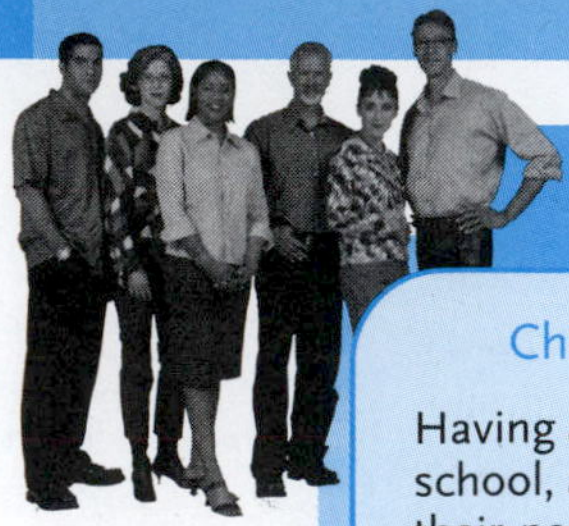

BOX 7-3 Ecological Contexts

Children with Language Disorders in Home, School, and Community

Having a language impairment can have a profound influence on children's lives at home, at school, and in the community. Language skills are the means by which children interact with their parents, siblings, and friends and the principal way in which children get their needs met and tell others how they are feeling. Children who have language disorders may be unable to effectively ask for needed actions, such as help going to the restroom, to request desired objects, such as a favorite toy or something to eat, or to comment on what they like or don't like. These challenges can have serious consequences on children's motivation to communicate; continually unsuccessful efforts can cause children to give up trying to tell others what they want or feel. Such situations can also cause frustration for the children's conversational partners, particularly parents and siblings.

For Discussion

What are some specific ways that a language disorder might impact a child at school, at home, and in the community?

How can language treatments be structured to improve children's functioning in broad ecological contexts?

Companion Website

To answer these questions online, go to the Ecological Contents module in chapter 7 of the Companion Website.

include participating in contact sports or other recreational activities that may result in a fall or a collision and using drugs or alcohol during these activities or when driving or riding in vehicles. Adolescents who are new drivers are at increased risk for brain injury as well.

The potential for experiencing a brain injury has no social or economic boundaries. For example, skiing, which is a sport associated with affluence, places an individual at an increased risk for brain injury. Brain injuries occurred at a rate of about 0.77 per 100,000 ski visits to Colorado resorts from 1994 through 1997 (Diamond, Gale, & Denkhaus, 2001). Males were more likely to be injured than females, and children and older adults were also at increased risk. Of injured skiers 24% experienced a skull fracture, and 79% experienced amnesia; their average hospital stay was 4.3 days.

How Are Language Disorders Identified?

The Assessment Process

Discussion Point: *Referral is a critical first step in beginning the assessment process. What are some barriers to referral? Consider the case of Savannah in Box 7-1 in answering this question.*

Identifying children who exhibit language disorders is a multistage process that often involves many team members working together at each stage of the process; team members often include speech-language pathologists, special and general educators, audiologists, pediatricians, psychologists, and parents. Referral and screening are the first steps in the process, followed by a comprehensive language evaluation to gather evidence concerning the extent of linguistic strengths and weaknesses. On the basis of this evidence, a diagnosis is made.

Referral

For children under 5 years of age, referral for language assessment is usually made by pediatricians in consultation with the children's parents. Generally, referrals are made because children exhibit a developmental or acquired disorder, such as Down syndrome or traumatic brain injury, that places them at increased risk for language problems or because warning signs signal the presence of a language disorder. By the time children are 12 months of age, they should be babbling often with a variety of consonants, using some gestures (e.g., pointing and showing), showing pleasure and excitement toward others, comprehending several common words (e.g., *daddy, mommy, bye-bye, up*), engaging in periods of joint sustained attention with others, and participating in vocal routines (Rossetti, 2001). For children between 1 and 5 years of age, delayed attainment of key language milestones is usually viewed as a warning sign of a possible language disorder and the need for referral.

Table 7-4 provides a checklist that can be used to determine whether infants, toddlers, and preschoolers are meeting milestones according to expectations. Children who

TABLE 7-4 Key milestones in early language development: a parent checklist

Age	Does Your Child . . .?
0–3 months	__ startle to loud sounds? __ smile when spoken to? __ seem to recognize your voice and quiet if crying? __ increase or decrease sucking behavior in response to sound? __ make pleasure sounds (cooing, booing)? __ cry differently for different needs? __ smile when seeing you?
4–6 months	__ move eyes in direction of sounds? __ respond to changes in tone of your voice? __ notice toys that make sounds? __ pay attention to music? __ produce babble that sounds more speechlike with many different sounds, including *p, b,* and *m*? __ vocalize excitement and displeasure? __ make gurgling sounds when left alone and when playing with you?
6 months–1 year	__ enjoy games like peekaboo and pat-a-cake? __ turn and look in direction of sounds? __ listen when spoken to? __ recognize words for common items like *cup, shoe, juice*? __ respond to some requests? __ produce babble that has both long and short groups of sounds such as "tata upup bibibibi"? __ use speech or noncrying sounds to get and keep attention? __ imitate different speech sounds? __ have 1 or 2 words (*bye-bye, dada, mama, no*) although they may not be clear?
1–2 years	__ point to pictures in a book when named? __ point to a few body parts when asked? __ follow simple commands and understand simple questions ("Roll the ball," "Kiss the baby," "Where's your shoe?")? __ listen to simple stories, songs, and rhymes? __ say more words every month? __ use some 1–2-word questions ("Where kitty?" "Go bye-bye?" "What's that?")? __ put 2 words together ("more cookie," "no juice," "mommy book")? __ use many different consonant sounds at the beginning of words?

(*continued*)

TABLE 7-4 *(continued)*

Age	Does Your Child . . .?
2–3 years	__ understand differences in meaning (*go/stop, in/on, big/little, up/down*)? __ follow two requests ("Get the book and put it on the table")? __ have a word for almost everything? __ use 2–3-word sentences to talk about and ask for things? __ produce speech that is understood by familiar listeners most of the time? __ often ask for or direct attention to objects by naming them?
3–4 years	__ hear you when you call from another room? __ hear television or radio at the same loudness level as other family members? __ understand simple who, what, where questions? __ talk about activities at school or at friends' homes? __ usually talk easily without repeating syllables or words? __ produce speech that people outside the family are able to understand? __ use a lot of sentences that have 4 or more words?
4–5 years	__ pay attention to a short story and answer simple questions about it? __ hear and understand most of what is said at home and in school? __ use sentences that give lots of details (e.g., "I like to read my books.")? __ tell stories that stick to a topic? __ communicate easily with other children and adults? __ say most sounds correctly except a few like *l, s, r, z, j, ch, sh, th?* __ use adultlike grammar?

Source: From "How Does Your Child Hear and Talk?" Retrieved October 1, 2004, from http://www. asha.org/ Copyright 2004 by American Speech-Language-Hearing Association. Reprinted with permission.

Discussion Point: *Infants can be screened for early indicators of language disorder (e.g., slow start in babbling, few gestures, and limited periods of joint attention). What are some other possible indicators? If you were speaking with Alejandro's parents (Box 7-1) about his early communication development, what questions would you ask them?*

are not displaying particular behaviors should be seen by their pediatricians to determine whether a referral for a comprehensive speech-language evaluation is needed. Although some pediatricians prefer to take a wait-and-see approach, children who show delays in attaining early communication milestones should always be referred for further evaluation by a speech-language specialist, particularly children who have a history of abuse or neglect, medical problems, developmental disability, trauma, hearing loss, exposure to drugs or other poisons, or any other significant risk factor (Paul, 1996). There is no good reason to wait and see when the topic is a young child's health and development.

Once children enter school, referrals for language evaluation are usually made by classroom teachers or by other school personnel. Language disorders are not always readily recognizable, however. Speech-language pathologists and other knowledgeable specialists can provide in-service workshops and develop referral checklists (see Figure 7-7) to help teachers recognize signs of possible language difficulties (Paul, 2002).

Screening

Screening should follow referral to determine the need for a comprehensive language assessment. After the referral, a speech-language pathologist, a special educator, or another trained professional may administer a screening tool that is specially designed to

FIGURE 7-7 Example of a referral checklist for teachers of older students.

Does the student's language or communication exhibit:

__ 1. Insufficient information: Student does not provide the amount or type of information needed by listener.

__ 2. Nonspecific vocabulary: Student uses pronouns, proper nouns, and possessives without supplying appropriate referents. Student overuses generic terms like *thing* and *stuff.*

__ 3. Informational redundancy: Student continues to stress a point or relate a fact even when the listener has acknowledged its reception.

__ 4. Need for repetition: Student requires repetition of material for accurate comprehension even though material is not difficult.

__ 5. Poor topic maintenance: Student makes rapid and inappropriate changes in topic without providing transitional cues to listener.

__ 6. Inappropriate response: Student makes responses that are radically unpredictable interpretations of meaning.

__ 7. Failure to ask relevant questions: Student does not seek clarification of material that is unclear.

__ 8. Situational inappropriateness: Student produces utterances that are irrelevant to the discourse and the situation.

__ 9. Linguistic nonfluency: Student's language use is disrupted by frequent repetitions, pauses, and hesitations.

__ 10. Frequent revision: Student speaks with many false starts and self-interruptions.

__ 11. Delay in responding: Student responds to utterances following pauses of inordinate length.

__ 12. Turn-taking difficulty: Student does not attend to cues indicating the appropriate exchange of conversational turns.

__ 13. Failure to structure discourse: Students speech lacks forethought and organizational planning.

__ 14. Inappropriate intonation: Student uses inappropriate vocal intensity, pitch levels, and inflectional contours.

Source: From "Clinical Discourse Analysis: A Functional Approach to Language Assessment" by J. S. Damico, 1991, in C. S. Simon, *Communication Skills and Classroom Success,* Eau Claire, WI: Thinking Publications. Copyright 1991 by Thinking Publications. Reprinted with permission.

efficiently and effectively determine whether a child has difficulties using or understanding language (Paul, 2002). Some formal tests, such as the *Early Screening Profiles* (Harrison et al., 1990) and the *Denver II* (Frankenburg et al., 1990) are available for this purpose and can be administered in about 10 or 15 minutes.

If a child does not pass a benchmark score on such screening tests, then a full evaluation is conducted to determine whether a language disorder is present and, if so, what the nature and type of language difficulty is. If the child passes the screening test, a full evaluation is not conducted. Obviously, then, the quality of a screening test is important. Children who pass a screening test but show minor communication difficulties or exhibit significant developmental risk factors should be continually monitored, with screening repeated every 3 to 6 months for children under 3 years and every 6 to 12 months for children between 3 and 5 years (Paul, 1996).

Many preschools and kindergarten programs regularly conduct language screening when children enter these programs. In such cases all children in a particular program are administered a brief language screening; children who do not pass the screening are referred for a more comprehensive language evaluation. However, because language screening programs are uncommon after kindergarten, it is important that classroom teachers are well aware of warning signs for possible language difficulties.

Comprehensive Language Evaluation

A comprehensive assessment determines whether a language disorder is indeed present. The language evaluation develops a profile of linguistic strengths and weaknesses and identifies needed supports for improving language form, content, and/or use. A comprehensive language evaluation includes a case history, interview, comprehensive analysis of language skills and communicative behaviors, and evaluation of collateral areas of performance.

Case History. The case history involves a questionnaire administered to parents by an examiner or completed on their own. Older children can also provide information, but parents are always important to document children's history of early and later language skills. The questionnaire examines a child's developmental history and gathers information about general health, medical conditions and allergies, family size and resources, the child's language and communicative history, current skills, interests, and behaviors, and the parents' and the child's perceptions of suspected problems.

Discussion Point: *When interviewing older students, it is important that students are fully informed of the reason for the interview. Students should be guided through a self-assessment that allows them to identify areas in which they excel, areas in which they do fine, and areas in which they need help. Why is this important?*

Interview. Personal interviews are an important part of the evaluation process. For infants, toddlers, and preschoolers, a parent interview follows the case history to focus on particular issues identified in the case history, to further explore parental perceptions of the child's language difficulties, and to determine parental goals for the evaluation. For older children, interviews with teachers and the child are critical for developing an accurate profile of the child's language abilities.

Comprehensive Language Analysis. To be comprehensive, a language evaluation must be broad-based and functional and use multiple methods of inquiry.

A **broad-based assessment** examines all domains of language (form, content, use) in both comprehension and production. For younger children who are not yet talking, a broad-based evaluation can examine the development of critical language precursors, including babbling, gesturing, affect and expression, participation in early communicative routines, and periods of joint attention. For older children, a broad-based assessment examines both oral and written language skills—including reading, writing, and spelling—and performance on classroom and curriculum-based tasks.

A **functional assessment** characterizes the extent to which children's language skills impact their ability to function in home, school, and community environments. For young children, the assessment must examine their ability to use language skills to get their needs met through various communicative functions, including requesting objects and actions; expressing feelings of interest, pleasure, and excitement; responding to the questions, requests, and comments of others; and using social behaviors, such as greeting (Halliday, 1975). For older children, the language assessment must examine the extent to which their language skills impact their ability to participate in the school curriculum and to interact effectively with friends, teachers, and parents.

An assessment that uses multiple methods of inquiry involves a variety of assessment tools, including criterion-referenced and norm-referenced tests, dynamic assessment, and observational measures. Criterion-referenced tasks examine the level of performance on a particular type of language task against a standard, or criterion, such as the percentage of one-step directions the child can correctly follow. Norm-referenced tasks examine the level of language performance against a national sample of same-age peers. Dynamic assessment examines children's performance with different types of assistance, providing valuable information about what kinds of supports are needed to optimize children's language performance. Observational measures examine children's language form, content, and use in naturalistic activities with peers or parents. Particularly important is an examination of children's conversational skills—the ability to initiate conversation, to take turns, to maintain topics, to identify breakdowns in conversation, and to attend to listener needs.

For older children, language assessment must also include curriculum-based assessment, which examines their strengths and weaknesses in participating in the academic curriculum. Methods of curriculum-based assessment include classroom observations of children's ability to work independently, work collaboratively with peers, complete assignments, and gain information from lectures and other assignments. Curriculum-based assessment also involves close examination of curriculum artifacts, including assignments and tests.

Discussion Point: *Curriculum-based assessment examines students' linguistic strengths and weaknesses when performing authentic academic tasks in the classroom. What are some examples of authentic academic tasks?*

Evaluation of Collateral Areas. To determine whether other difficulties may be present that impact a child's development of language, the language evaluation should screen cognitive skills, oral-motor structure and function, and hearing. If any of these areas are not developing appropriately, a more comprehensive evaluation by a specialist or other team member may be warranted.

Cognitive abilities can be estimated by examining play development for younger children; play and cognitive achievements are highly interrelated. Table 7-5 provides an overview of the major milestones in early play development that may guide the screening process. For older children, a formal cognitive screening may be administered, such as the *Kaufman Brief Intelligence Test* (Kaufman & Kaufman, 1990). Oral-motor structures are screened by examining the structures of the lips, teeth, and oral cavity (e.g., hard and soft palate), whereas oral-motor function involves children's ability to use the oral structures for different purposes. Screening of function might involve asking children to purse their lips, blow a bubble, lick a lollipop, and repeat the sound sequence puh-puh-puh, among other tasks. A hearing screening is a quick check of hearing acuity.

Diagnosis

How does one determine whether a language disorder is indeed present? The answer to this million dollar question comes through careful consideration of the evidence gained through the case history, interviews, comprehensive evaluation of all areas of language performance, and screening of collateral areas. An evaluation of the evidence indicates whether observed problems are serious enough to be considered significantly different from normal and ensures that observed problems are not the result of cultural or linguistic factors. Once the decision is made that a language disorder is present, the diagnosis usually designates the type of impairment (primary, secondary), impacted domains (form, content, and/or use; comprehension and/or production), and the severity (mild, moderate, severe, profound). Additionally, diagnosis may include a prognosis statement; a good prognosis states that a disorder is likely to resolve, whereas a poor prognosis states that a disorder is unlikely to resolve. In some cases professionals withhold a statement of prognosis, pending further information from other specialists or a period of observing how children respond to treatment.

In addition, diagnosis is usually accompanied with a recommended course of treatment, which typically describes the targets of treatment, the professionals who will provide the treatment, and the frequency of treatment. For instance, a recommendation might state:

> Language therapy is recommended to develop semantic and syntactic skills in comprehension and production to help Johnny participate in home and school activities. Therapy should be provided three times weekly in small-group sessions by a speech-language pathologist, who will work closely with Johnny's preschool teacher and parents. Given Johnny's strong support system at home and school, the prognosis is good.

Discussion Point: *A prognosis statement might differ for children who make quick progress versus those who progress more slowly. What other factors might influence prognosis? Consider the case of Natasha in Box 7-1 in answering this question.*

TABLE 7-5 Milestones in early play development

Age Range	Play Behaviors
9–12 months	Is aware that objects exist when not seen Crawls or walks to get what is wanted Pulls string toys Does not bang or mouth all toys (some used appropriately)
12–17 months	Purposefully explores toys, discovers operation through trial and error Uses variety of motoric schemes Hands toy to adult if unable to operate Begins to use objects in appropriate ways Places objects into containers
17–19 months	Uses early symbolic/pretend play (pretends to go to sleep or drink from cup) Uses most common objects and toys appropriately
19–22 months	Extends symbolic play beyond self (brushes doll's hair, feeds doll) Performs pretend activities on more than one object (feeds self, doll, and stuffed bear) Combines two toys in pretend manner (pours from pot to cup)
22–24 months	Represents daily experiences through play (play house or school) Includes short and isolated events without true sequences Stacks up and knocks down blocks
24–30 months	Represents events less frequently observed, including traumatic events (doctor and sick child)
30–36 months	Continues pretend activities; begins to incorporate sequence (mix cake, bake cake, serve cake) Reenacts play events with different outcomes
36–42 months	Carries out play activities of previous stages with miniature representations (toy house, barn with animals) Uses blocks and sandbox for imaginative play Uses objects to represent other objects (block for a phone) Uses dolls and puppets as participants in play
42–48 months	Begins to problem-solve and hypothesize through play (what would happen if . . .) Uses dollars and puppets to act out scenes Builds 3-dimensional structures with blocks
48–60 months	Plans a sequence of pretend events and organizes what is needed Is highly imaginative; sets the scene without realistic props Fully cooperates in play with other children

Source: From "Assessment of Cognitive and Language Abilities Through Play", by C. Westby, 1980, *Language, Speech, and Hearing Services in Schools, 11,* pp. 155–168. Copyright 1980 by ASHA. Reprinted with permission.

The Importance of Accurate Diagnosis

The importance of accurately determining whether a child has a language disorder cannot be overemphasized. Of two possible scenarios for inaccurate diagnosis, one is that of a **false-positive**, meaning that a child who does not have a language disorder is diagnosed as having a language disorder. The other scenario is a **false-negative**, whereby a child who has a language disorder is not accurately identified as having one.

Misdiagnoses happen for a variety of reasons. False-positives can occur because of poorly constructed tests or tests that are biased in cultural or linguistic factors. In addition, children may perform poorly during a language evaluation because of illness, fatigue, or shyness or because they have another condition (e.g., behavioral problem, attention deficit disorder) that shares characteristics with language disorders (e.g., difficulty following directions). There is also the alarming tendency of professionals to misdiagnose language differences as language disorders. Children who speak a nonstandard dialect of English or who are learning English as a second language may be diagnosed as language disordered when, in fact, their underlying language capabilities are culturally, linguistically, and age appropriate. This problem is at least partly to blame for the overrepresentation of children from diverse linguistic, racial, and/or ethnic backgrounds in special education (U. S. Congress, 1997).

What are the implications of a false-positive? First, children receive a label that is inappropriate and that may have serious and practical consequences, including the possibility that the children will be stigmatized by their peers or that educators may hold low expectations for these children (Heward, 2003). Second, children inaccurately diagnosed with a language impairment are likely to receive speech-language services to remediate their perceived language problems. Treatment for a language disorder is an expensive and time-consuming process on the part of the health and educational professionals involved, as well as the children and their families. And providing services to children who do not need them may keep those services away from children and families who really do need the help.

False-negatives happen for many of the same reasons that false-positives occur, including the use of poorly constructed tests or tests that are inappropriate for children of a particular cultural, ethnic, or language group. In addition, for children who have other disorders (e.g., mental retardation, attention deficit disorder), a clinician may mistakenly view poor language performance as a result of that disorder rather than as evidence of a language disorder.

The implications of a false-negative are also of serious consequence to the child and family affected. Children with a language disorder that is not identified do not receive the services to which they are entitled by federal law. Thus, these children are denied the services that might help them overcome or at least better cope with their disorders.

Discussion Point: *A false-negative occurs when a child with a language disorder is identified as developing typically in language. What are some reasons this might occur?*

How Are Language Disorders Treated?

The nature of a child's language impairment drives the treatment. In other words, difficulty with language form requires a treatment approach focused on developing form; if problems are severe, the treatment approach will be more intensive than it will be if problems are mild. A child whose language disorder is secondary to autism will receive a treatment approach distinct from that of a child whose language disorder is secondary to traumatic brain injury. Treatment approaches are tailored to the unique needs of individual children in terms of treatment targets, strategies, and contexts.

Targets, Strategies, and Contexts

Treatment Targets

Treatment targets are the elements of language that are addressed during intervention. For instance, a treatment target for a 2-year-old child might be to produce two-word utterances to communicate needs, whereas a treatment target for an adolescent might be to comprehend figurative language (e.g., jokes heard on the playground). A treatment target for a young child with autism might be to communicate nonverbally for a variety of purposes

BOX 7-4 Spotlight on Research

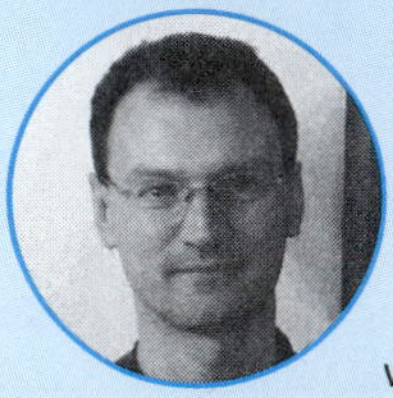

Luigi Girolametto, Ph.D., CCC/SLP
Associate Professor, University of Toronto

Luigi Girolametto is a speech-language pathologist and researcher who has worked in two agencies in Toronto, Canada, with children who have language disorders—the Hanen Centre (a language intervention program that trains parents) and the Hospital for Sick Children. He received his training in speech-language pathology at McGill University and his doctorate in early childhood special education at the University of Toronto. He is an associate professor in the graduate department of speech-language pathology at the University of Toronto, where he teaches child language development, disorders, and intervention.

Luigi has an active research lab where he and his colleagues ask questions about the efficacy of language intervention with young children with language disorders. One branch of his research focuses on the efficacy of a parent training program to provide language intervention for preschool children—*It Takes Two to Talk: The Hanen Program® for Parents*. His intervention studies have shown that parents successfully learn to apply language intervention strategies during everyday, naturally occurring situations in the home. Specifically, parents learn to use intervention strategies that are child centered (e.g., wait and listen, respond to your child's focus), promote interaction (e.g., take one turn and wait, ask questions to encourage turns), and model language at the child's level (e.g., label, expand). In addition, parents learn to use a focused stimulation strategy that involves repetitive modeling of a language goal without prompting the child to respond.

This parent-training program has been enormously successful with late-talking toddlers and young children with Down syndrome. Following intervention, children talk more, use a larger vocabulary, use more mature sentence forms, and acquire more speech sounds than do children in control groups that do not receive intervention. More details on Dr. Girolametto's work can be found in these two articles:

Girolametto, L., Verbey, M., & Tannock, R. (1994). Improving joint engagement in parent-child interaction: An intervention study. *Journal of Early Intervention, 18*, 155–167.

Girolametto, L., Pearce, P. S., & Weitzman, E. (1996). Interactive focused stimulation for toddlers with expressive vocabulary delays. *Journal of Speech and Hearing Research, 39*, 1274–1283.

BOX 7-5 Spotlight on Practice

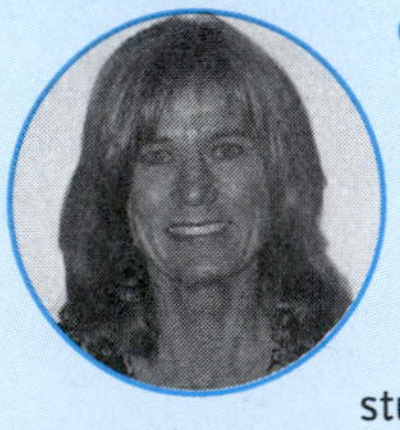

Claudia Dunaway, M.Ed., CCC-SLP
Speech-Language Pathologist
San Diego Unified School District

I never dreamed when I began my studies in anthropology that I would become a speech-language pathologist. In retrospect, 30 years later, the seemingly erratic roads that I traveled all fit neatly together. My fascination with social change, ethnography, and linguistics, tempered by the necessity to support myself, resulted in a challenging and fulfilling career in communication disorders. From my parents I inherited a strong commitment to community service. I am fortunate that each day, as a speech-language pathologist, I have a chance to make a difference.

Currently, I am the lead for a staff of 180 speech-language pathologists in San Diego City Schools. I took the long road to get here, accepting every opportunity that came my way to learn something new. I thrive on challenge, and this field offers an abundance of opportunities. Over the years, I have worked in many different settings and with individuals of every age and disorder. These experiences broadened my worldview as well as my clinical expertise. Today, I enjoy sharing these experiences by mentoring and coaching younger speech therapists, although I also continue to provide direct services to children with specific language impairment. I rank the establishment of an intensive program for these students in San Diego as one of my finest accomplishments. My biggest challenge is finding the time to make sure that my clinical work is informed by current research. It is tempting to use a method that seems effective without understanding its theoretical basis. By disciplining myself to always look for the connection, I have constructed a detailed mental map of both normal and disordered language development. This blueprint allows me to solve even the most perplexing communication problems.

As for the future, I am working with a team to effect district change by deepening our knowledge of descriptive, performance-based assessment and curriculum-based intervention. For anyone considering a clinical career, I suggest that you study with as many mentors as possible. There is no substitute for hands-on experience and immediate feedback.

(e.g., to request, reject, comment), whereas a treatment target for a first grader with traumatic brain injury might be to answer questions with appropriate, on-topic responses. Some professionals may emphasize only one or two targets at a time, whereas others may target many goals at once.

Treatment Strategies

Treatment strategies describe the manner in which treatment targets are addressed. **Child-centered approaches** are those in which the child is "in the driver's seat" (Paul, 1995, p. 68). The child sets the pace and chooses the materials, and the professional seeks ways to facilitate language form, content, or use in the context of child-selected activities. One example of a child-centered treatment approach is *focused stimulation* (Cleave & Fey, 1997; Fey, Cleave, Long, & Hughes, 1993; Girolametto, Pearce, & Weitzman, 1996). With focused stimulation, the adult provides multiple and highly salient models of language targets that are goals for the child. For instance, if a child is not able to request using the word *want,* the clinician would set up communication temptations in the context of play-based interactions to entice the child to use the word *want.* The clinician would also model use of this word repeatedly ("I want the cookie," "The boy wants candy," "The dog wants the bone"). To make the word stand out, the clinician might say it loudly, slowly, or with dramatic pitch changes (Fey, Long, & Finestack, 2003). During focused stimulation, the child is not required to respond at all; however, the parent or professional arranges the environment and uses verbal techniques to *entice* the child's verbal participation and use of language targets. Focused stimulation and other child-centered strategies are often used with young children (infants and preschoolers) and can be implemented by parents in the home following training by a professional (Girolametto et al., 1996).

Clinician-directed approaches are those in which the adult (i.e., therapist, teacher, parent) is in the driver's seat. The adult selects the activities and materials and sets the pace of instruction. Rather than waiting for opportunities to occur that address a particular treatment target, the clinician deliberately structures a therapy session for frequent, ongoing opportunities for the child to experience and practice a form, content, or use target. Clinician-directed approaches are useful for older children in particular and can be used to target skills that arise infrequently in naturalistic communications. These approaches are also used to teach children with language disorders how to apply strategies to compensate for underlying challenges with language comprehension and production.

A strategy is the way an individual approaches a task; it includes both cognitive and behavioral components—that is, how one thinks and acts when doing something. Strategy training can be an effective way to improve children's abilities with diverse language tasks, such as understanding jokes, initiating conversation with friends or adults, or deciphering unknown words when reading. Strategy instruction focuses on teaching students specific ways to approach a linguistic task. The steps in strategy instruction include (1) pretesting the child on strategy knowledge, (2) describing the strategy, (3) modeling the strategy, (4) having the child discuss and rehearse the strategy, (5) having the child practice the strategy with feedback until acquisition occurs, and (6) having the child use the strategy in other settings (Mercer, 1997). Figure 7-8 shows the typical sequence of strategy instruction and ways to maximize its success.

Treatment Contexts

Treatment contexts describe the settings in which treatment targets and strategies are used. Treatment contexts should include as many settings as possible to promote generalization of skills learned in treatment—that is, the application of skills to many diverse settings. For instance, children may experience treatment targets and strategies at home with their parents, in the classroom with their teachers, and in the clinic with their speech-language

FIGURE 7-8 **Stages in strategy instruction.**

Stage 1: Pretest and make commitments

- Give rationale and overview, administer pretest, describe the strategy, discuss results others have achieved, ask for a commitment to learn the new strategy

Stage 2: Describe the strategy

- Describe situations in which the strategy can be used, describe the overall strategic process, set goals for learning the strategy, discuss self-instruction

Stage 3: Model the strategy

- Review previous learning, state expectations, present the strategy using think-aloud and self-monitoring, perform task while student observes, check student understanding

Stage 4: Verbal elaboration and rehearsal

- Have student describe intent of strategy and the process involved, have student describe each step and what it is designed to do, work until student is automatic in describing each step

Stage 5: Controlled practice and feedback

- Review the strategy steps, prompt reports of strategy use and errors, prompt student completion of steps as teacher models, prompt increasing student responsibility, provide peer-mediated practice opportunities

Stage 6: Advanced practice and feedback

- Repeat last stage with grade-appropriate materials, fade prompts and cues for use and evaluation

Stage 7: Confirmation of acquisition and generalization commitments

- Congratulate student on meeting mastery, discuss achievements, explain goals of generalization, prompt commitment to generalize

Stage 8: Generalization

- Identify settings for strategy use, discuss how to remember to use strategy, prompt and monitor application to other settings, help other teachers cue use of strategy, help student set goals for long-term use

Source: From *Students with Learning Disabilities (5th ed)* by Cecil D. Mercer, © 1997. Adapted by permission of Pearson Education, Inc., Upper Saddle River, NJ.

Discussion Point: *Home-based interventions are also useful for observing the quality of parent-child interactions, including maternal and child affect, mood, proximity, and initiations and responses to one another. What would this information tell us? If you were conducting a home visit to document Alejandro's interactions with his parents (Box 7-1), what would you look for?*

pathologists. Clearly, collaboration among parents, teachers, speech-language pathologists, and other professionals is critical for ensuring that treatment occurs in many contexts.

For many young children receiving language intervention, treatment is provided in the home environment, allowing parents to directly observe and even implement treatment targets and strategies. Home-based interventions are particularly prevalent for children under the age of 3 years who receive language therapy. The professional providing intervention comes to the child's house and collaborates with the child's parent(s) and possibly other professionals (e.g., a physical therapist). For older children, treatment is usually provided in the school setting—preschool, elementary, middle, or high school—although parental involvement remains important and should be pursued at all opportunities. Some children also receive language treatment in outpatient hospital clinics or private centers.

In the school setting, treatment contexts can vary. Although historically children have received language intervention in a pull-out model, in which language therapy was provided in a speech room, this model is less common today. Frequently, children receive language intervention through collaborative classroom-based models, with teachers and speech-language pathologists working together to target language goals within the classroom environment (Farber & Klein, 1999). Speech-language pathologists may work individually with children during small-group or center times, may team-teach particular lessons with teachers, or may train teachers to integrate special language enhancement techniques into their classroom instruction (DiMeo, Merritt, & Culatta, 1998).

The Treatment Plan

A treatment plan is the guide to a particular child's treatment targets, strategies, and contexts. A treatment plan is established following a comprehensive language evaluation and is updated periodically as children progress. For children who are served through public agencies governed by the federal IDEA—such as early intervention programs, public preschools, and elementary schools—the treatment plan can appear in two forms. An individualized family service plan (IFSP) is required to provide any early intervention services to infants and toddlers with disabilities. The IFSP states the frequency, intensity, method, location, and expected duration of services; it must be reviewed every 6 months and updated annually. An individualized education program (IEP) is used to provide special services to preschoolers and school-age children with disabilities. The IEP includes a series of measurable annual goals and short-term objectives and describes the services, programs, and aids the child will be provided to meet those objectives and goals. An annual goal for language might state that "by the end of the academic year, Juan will improve his receptive and expressive vocabulary skills to levels consistent with his chronological age."

Intervention Principles

Researchers are continually seeking more effective and efficient strategies for reducing or ameliorating the consequences of language disorders. This chapter presents 10 key research-based principles for providing effective treatments to children with language disorders: five principles focus on working with younger children (infants, toddlers, and preschoolers), and five focus on working with older children.

Intervention Principles for Infants, Toddlers, and Preschoolers

Key principles for providing language intervention to infants, toddlers and preschoolers include early intervention, parental involvement, naturalistic environments, social interaction, and functional outcomes.

Early Intervention. Early intervention refers to therapeutic interventions for children 3 years of age and under. Children receiving early intervention may have a developmental disorder, such as Down syndrome, an acquired disorder, such as a brain injury, or may be vulnerable for developing a disorder because of various risk factors. Early intervention is a primary prevention strategy aimed at keeping a disorder from developing at all or at least reducing the severity of a disorder. Early intervention services, when applied in a timely and rigorous manner, can be very effective in both regards (Guralnick, 1997).

Critical to such efforts is identifying children with established disorders and those at risk for developing disorders as early as possible and enabling them to access needed therapeutic interventions. For some types of language disorders, such as SLI and autism, there may be a tendency to ignore early warning signs that can signal a possible problem with language development. Professionals and parents may be overly optimistic about the likelihood of problem resolution (Schuele & Hadley, 1999), or there may be a lack of information concerning early indicators of possible problems. Regardless, scientific evidence shows that early intervention is an effective route for reducing the negative outcomes associated with early language difficulties (Maclean & Cripe, 1997).

The key, however, is *early* detection and treatment; once a language disorder manifests itself, reversal of competence to normal levels of functioning is highly unlikely. Epidemiological data show that 73% of children clinically identified as language impaired in kindergarten maintain that diagnosis at age 20, even in the context of ongoing interventions (Johnson et al., 1999).

Discussion Point: *Hart and Risley's book* Meaningful Differences *(1995) shows that the differences in language experienced by children can be large; for instance, in a given year, some children will hear about 11,000,000 words, whereas others will hear only 3,000,000 words. How important are these differences? Consider the case of Natasha in Box 7-1. What do you think the first 2 years of her life were like?*

Parental Involvement. Parental involvement is important for a variety of reasons when working with young children. First, it is absolutely true that parents are children's first teachers. The interactions between children and their primary caretakers are critical to developing firm language foundations (Landry, Miller-Loncar, Smith, & Swank, 1997; Tamis-LeMonda, Bornstein, & Baumwell, 2001). For instance, the number of words children experience in their interactions with family members contributes to how fast those children learn new words and what types of words they learn (Hart & Risley, 1995).

Second, parental involvement respects the role of parents in their children's lives. Involving parents in interventions helps professionals understand the values and beliefs of the families with whom they work. Third, parents can play key roles in language intervention programs (e.g., Fey et al., 1993; Girolametto et al., 1996). Parents can be trained to use certain techniques when they interact with their children to stimulate development of important language skills. This is a cost-effective and family-centered way to provide early intervention treatments.

Naturalistic Environments. The provision of services in children's most natural environments is an important part of working with young children. For many children receiving early intervention, therapists and special educators come to the home to provide treatment, and parents are hands-on partners. Working in the child's most natural environment promotes the child's sense of control and comfort and allows treatment to involve familiar activities and objects, thereby increasing the generalization of intervention to other situations of use. Working in the child's home also helps parents to learn specific language stimulation strategies. For example, a home-based interventionist might observe a mother and child eating lunch together and afterwards suggest ways the mother can structure the mealtime routine to encourage the child's use of

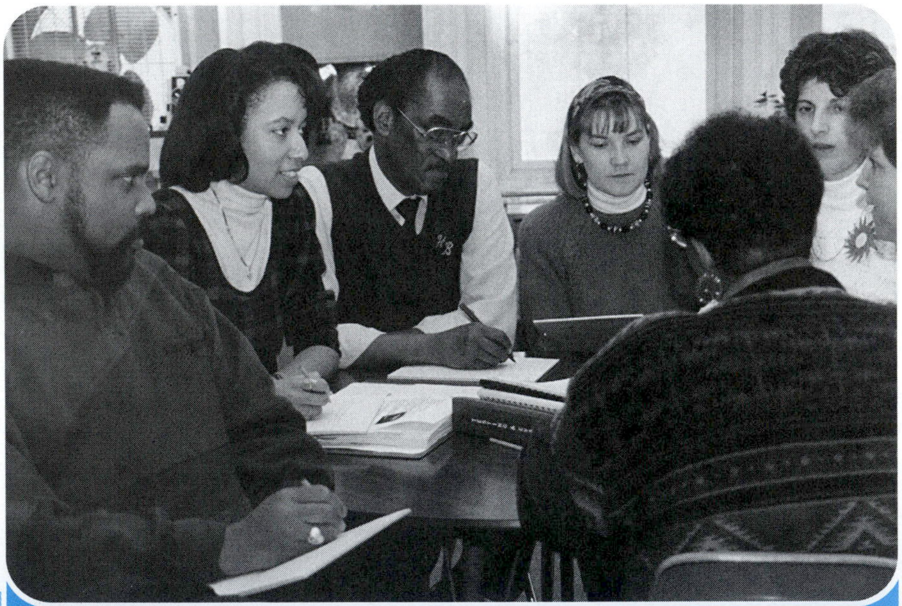

Parental involvement is not only required by law when providing early intervention services, but also respects the roles of parents as their children's first teachers.

requesting behaviors. For medically fragile children, providing services in the home can also offer protection for their health (Rossetti, 2001).

Social Interaction. A social interactionist account of language acquisition argues that language is learned through children's meaningful interactions with others. Social interaction creates opportunities for children to apply new language forms, content, and use. An important part of social interactionist perspectives is that therapies should embrace the communicative value of language; children need to be engaged in meaningful social interactions during which their use of emerging forms and functions is recognized as having communicative value. Social interactionist approaches would not value a speech-language pathologist or early childhood educator showing a young child a series of pictures and having the child repeat the name of each picture. Rather, engaging children in meaningful, authentic opportunities to communicate (e.g., asking for a real toy) is an integral part of therapies that embrace social interactionist accounts of language development (Kaderavek & Justice, 2002).

Functional Outcomes. Language interventions for young children must target language outcomes that have real value—outcomes that improve children's ability to be valued members of home, school, and community. All language goals should apply directly to improving children's ability to communicate with others. For example, for a child struggling with grammatical development, a language goal that targets repetition of 10 noun phrases (*the* + *noun*) per therapy session has little direct functional value. The goal must have a functional aim that adds value to the contexts in which the child lives. For this child the goal might be to use complex noun phrases to accurately specify the child's wants during mealtime routines.

Intervention Principles for School-Age Children

The goals and techniques of language intervention with older children differ somewhat from those used with younger children. First of all, enlisting the support and commitment of older children is critical to the intervention process; children who are unmotivated or who do not want to participate in therapeutic activities make it hard to achieve positive outcomes. Second, intervention goals shift for older children from primary prevention (i.e., keeping a disorder from manifesting itself) to secondary and tertiary prevention (i.e., helping children compensate for a disorder that is already present). Third, intervention for older children must be linked directly to the academic curriculum. Because children with language impairment are likely to struggle academically, improved academic performance should be a principal goal of intervention. And fourth, intervention with older children tends to move at a much slower pace than intervention with younger children. The rate of language acquisition slows as children age, and the types of skills that are targeted in later intervention are usually quite complex, requiring considerable time for learning to take place.

Five key principles for providing language intervention to older children include metalinguistic awareness, functional flexibility, discourse-level skills, literacy achievement, and least restrictive environment.

Metalinguistic Awareness. Metalinguistic awareness refers to the ability to focus on language as an object of scrutiny. When a teacher asks a child, "Is the word *caterpillar* a long word or a short word?" or tells the child to "circle all the nouns in this passage," these are metalinguistic tasks that require conscious reflection on language as an object of thought (Chaney, 1998; Justice & Ezell, 2001). Being able to scrutinize language is a highly abstract activity, one that does not come easily for children with language impairment. However, because metalinguistic awareness is so highly integrated into the academic curriculum at all levels, providing frequent opportunities for children with language disorders to engage in metalinguistic tasks—with support and guidance—is an important aspect of language intervention for school-age children.

Discussion Point: *Just the act of thinking about the meaning of the term* metalinguistic awareness *is itself a metalinguistic activity. Think of a metalinguistic activity that might take place in a preschool classroom, a first-grade classroom, and a third-grade classroom. Which children in the classroom would struggle with these activities?*

Functional Flexibility. Children need to be able to use language to communicate in a variety of situations and to readily assume the listener and speaker roles in any communicative interaction (Simon, 1991). Establishing functional flexibility means that children are helped to develop skills that allow them to accurately portray all thoughts, feelings, and needs within any communicative interaction. For school-age children this means acquiring five key communicative functions: (1) control (e.g., command, suggest, permit, warn, refuse, argue), (2) feel (e.g., exclaim, express, disagree, reject), (3) inform (e.g., question, answer, justify, demonstrate, explain), (4) ritualize (e.g., greet, recite, take turns, joke, pray), and (5) imagine (e.g., role-play, fantasize, speculate, dramatize, theorize; Simon, 1991). Being able to use language for diverse purposes should be an integral goal of language intervention for school-age children.

Discourse-Level Skills. Language intervention for school-age children requires an intensive focus on discourse-level skills. Discourse refers to the stream of language that occurs when a person produces a series of sentences, as in relating a personal event or a fictional story (narrative) or participating in a conversation. Too often, language intervention focuses on smaller units of language—such as the word, the sound, or a part of speech—rather than on the child's ability to use language for narrative and conversational purposes.

Discourse is the unit of language used in the curriculum; *instructional discourse* refers to the exchanges that occur in the classroom between teachers and students. The goal of instructional discourse is to teach—to give new information and to teach new skills (Merritt, Barton, & Culatta, 1998). However, instructional discourse can be very challenging to children with language disorders, because it requires the integration of form, content, and use—all of which may be areas of weakness. Typically, classroom discourse is decontextualized, meaning that it is not accompanied by cues to help with meaning interpretation. Children must rely solely on their linguistic skills to interpret what is being relayed through the discourse.

Language intervention for school-age children, rather than focusing on discrete subcomponents of language, needs to engage children at the level of instructional discourse (Damico, 1991). Indeed, intervention should provide them with ample opportunities to participate in discourse at various levels of complexity—conversation, narrative, and instructional discourse—with the interventionist providing supports to maximize the children's ability to participate and learn (Merritt et al., 1998).

Literacy Achievement. Children with language disorders are more likely to struggle with reading and spelling. Language intervention should therefore help children develop skills that are critically linked to success in these areas. One area of particular difficulty for children with language impairment is phonological awareness (PA; Justice & Schuele, 2004). *Phonological awareness* is the ability to attend to the units of sound that make up running speech. A sentence, for instance, can be broken into a series of smaller sound units, including words, syllables, and phonemes. The phoneme is the smallest unit of sound, and in the English alphabetic system, the mapping between phonemes and graphemes (i.e., sounds and letters) is the key to unlocking the alphabetic system.

Children with language impairment tend to have problems with phonological awareness; during the preschool years they are slower than other children to begin to play phonological awareness games (e.g., making rhymes; Magnusson & Naucler, 1993), and in the early elementary grades they have difficulty identifying the number of phonemes in words. Figure 7-9 provides an overview of key developments in phonological awareness. Timely attainment of these skills helps children become successful readers (Chaney, 1998).

Problems with phonological awareness contribute to the problems with reading and spelling that are prevalent among children with language disorders (Catts et al.,

FIGURE 7-9 Development of phonological awareness.

Stage I: Recognition that running speech can be broken into words (word awareness)

- Child can identify how many words are in a sentence.
- Child can clap with each word in a sentence.

Stage II: Recognition that multisyllabic words are made up of syllables (syllable awareness)

- Child can identify how many syllables are in a word.
- Child can delete the first or last syllable in a multisyllabic word.

Stage III: Recognition that syllables and one-syllable words can be divided into onset and rime* units

- Child can identify the first sound in a word.
- Child can match or produce words that rhyme.
- Child can segment the first sound from the rest of a syllable.

Stage IV: Recognition that syllables and words can be divided into a series of phonemes

- Child can identify how many sounds are in a word.
- Child can segment a word into all of its phonemes.
- Child can blend a series of phonemes into a syllable.

Sources: Based on Justice and Kaderavek (2004); Justice and Schuele (2004).

*Rime is a linguistic term. It is the part of a syllable that remains when the initial consonant(s) are removed (e.g., the rime of dog is og, and the rime of pay is ay).

2001, 2002). Integrating literacy goals into language intervention is becoming increasingly important for school-age children with language disorders. For instance, when working on specific speech targets, children can be prompted to think about the phonological composition of words (e.g., the word *wasp* has four sounds, and the word *wasps* has five sounds). Addressing literacy and language simultaneously can maximize the overall effectiveness of language interventions to promote children's academic success.

Least Restrictive Environment. Providing language intervention to children in the least restrictive environment (LRE) is federal law (IDEA 94-142). The law stipulates that children with disabilities are to be educated with their peers "to the maximum extent possible" (20 U.S.C 1412 [a][5]). Many children with language disorders receive their general education within regular classrooms but receive language intervention through pull-out therapies provided in a speech-language laboratory or resource room. This model has garnered a lot of criticism in recent years because pull-out therapies remove children from the very context in which they need to learn to perform (Bashir, Conte, & Heerde, 1998).

The premise behind LRE, in contrast, is that children need to "learn, practice, and apply skills with their classmates in the communicative context of the classroom" (DiMeo et al., 1998, p. 39). Alternative models of language intervention are therefore receiving increased attention. These include providing therapy to children directly in their classrooms and using a consultant or collaborative model in which speech-language pathologists and teachers address children's language goals together. The teacher and speech-language pathologist may team-teach lessons in which language and academic goals are targeted simultaneously (DiMeo et al., 1998).

Case Study and Clinical Problem Solving

DIAGNOSTIC REPORT: SUMMARY

Client: Evan Hartley
Evaluation Date: 09-30-05
Date of Report: 10-01-05
Date of Birth: 06-02-02
Age: 3 years, 4 months
Referral Source: Mother, day care personnel

Overview

Evan was referred to the Piedmont Child Development Center for evaluation of language skills because of parental concerns regarding possible slow expressive and receptive language development. Mother reports that Evan demonstrates some frustration with his inability to communicate. Personnel at PDI Learning Center, Evan's day care, have voiced concerns regarding Evan's language performance in comparison to that of the other children. Diagnostic information was attained via an assessment session with Evan at PDI Learning Center, supplemented by information attained in a parent interview conducted via phone on 09-27-05.

Pertinent History

Mrs. Hartley reported an unremarkable pregnancy with no pre-, peri-, or postnatal complications. Delivery was natural with epidural. Labor was 2 hours. Birth weight was 7 lbs, 14 oz; no unusual conditions were noted. Mrs. Hartley reported that Evan's general development has been slow. For example, Evan did not walk unassisted until 20 months. Delays also have been apparent in Evan's communicative skills: babbling occurred at approximately 16 months, first word occurred at approximately 22 months, and two-word combinations occurred at 33 months. At age 2 years, Evan spoke approximately 3 words. Evan has a positive history of otitis media and has had approximately seven occurrences of OM. Mrs. Hartley has never observed any hearing deficits. Evan's health is currently considered good. No feeding or swallowing difficulties have been observed, but Evan drools constantly. There is no family history of language problems. Evan currently attends a private day care 40 hours weekly and has three older siblings. Evan enjoys day care and gets along well with the other children. His parents both work full-time. His parents were unable to schedule an interview or home-based assessment with the examiner. Mrs. Hartley reported that Evan's day care providers are very interested in working with her and Evan's siblings and parents to help Evan develop better communication skills.

Test Results and Observations

Oral-Motor Screening

General and informal observations of Evan's oral-motor structure and function were conducted. All structure and function were unremarkable and appeared within normal limits. Dentition and alignment appeared normal. Tongue movement was excellent for imitative tasks. Evan was able to imitate lip rounding, lip spreading, mouth opening/mouth closing, and tongue protrusion. Constant and excessive drooling was observed throughout the assessment session.

Peripheral Screening

Evan resisted a hearing screening. Observation of play skills indicated symbolic skills that were age appropriate. Evan was observed to play appropriately with a barn with animals and to symbolically manipulate the horse to eat hay.

Language

Assessment of language skills was conducted via informal observations and administration of the following: Peabody Picture Vocabulary Test-III (PPVT-III) and the Preschool Language Scale-3 (PLS-3). The PPVT examines children's understanding of single-word vocabulary words through a picture-pointing task (e.g., given four pictures of various items, Evan was asked to point to a drum). The PLS examines children's expression and comprehension skills in diverse language areas, including grammar and vocabulary. Evan was very cooperative during testing, although he occasionally needed redirection to continue test tasks. In addition, much of the testing occurred in Evan's day care environment, within the context of much noise and activity. This may have influenced performance.

Standard scores for each test are reported below. [Standard scores represent a child's score on a scale where 100 is average (i.e., the mean) and a standard deviation is 15 points. Thus, a score of 85 or below is considered significantly below average. Percentile ranks present a child's standing in a group of 100 children. Thus, a percentile rank that is higher than 10 is generally considered within normal limits; scores lower than the 10th percentile suggest a significant problem.]

Expressive Language. Assessment of Evan's expressive vocabulary skill was difficult because of limited verbal output. He produced little spontaneous conversation. Results of the expressive communication portion of the PLS-3 showed an overall expressive language score of 79 (percentile rank = 8%). This standard score is more than one standard deviation below the mean, suggesting the presence of a disorder in expressive language skills. [The percentile rank of 8% means that out of 100 children, 92 children would have scored better than Evan.] Evan's expressive language consisted primarily of one- and two-word utterances, such as "get ball," "want book" and "me Evan." Evan uses spoken words to get his needs met and will persist to clarify but relies primarily on gestures to communicate. Overall, the results suggest a mild to moderate impairment in expressive language.

Receptive Language. Evan's single-word receptive vocabulary was examined via the PPVT-III. A standard score of 80 indicated difficulty in receptive vocabulary. Results of the auditory comprehension portion of the PLS-3 resulted in a standard score of 79. Evan performed well on a number of comprehension tasks, including demonstrating his knowledge of body parts (e.g., hair, eye, nose, foot, ear) and following directions requiring comprehension of locatives (e.g., put the block on the table; put the block in the box). He was unable to follow more complicated directions (e.g., put the yellow block in the box). Overall, receptive language performance suggests a mild to moderate impairment.

Conclusions

Evan is a social and cooperative child. He demonstrates age-appropriate play skills, suggesting no cognitive difficulties. His verbal output is limited to primarily single words and several multiword combinations. Both expressive and receptive vocabulary knowledge are below age-level expectations. Mild problems with oral-motor skills, primarily drooling, were observed. Communication is assisted via verbal persistence (i.e., repeating) and gestures. Evan has a strong support network in terms of family and caregivers at his daycare. Evan's parents and his day care providers are very interested in having specific suggestions to help Evan throughout the day.

Recommendations

Based on the initial language evaluation, Evan currently presents with a mild to moderate receptive/expressive specific language impairment. The following are recommendations for further evaluation:

1. Evan should be enrolled for language intervention at a private clinic or through public programming. One to two 50-minute sessions per week are recommended.
2. Evan should receive a comprehensive hearing evaluation, given his history of otitis media and present demonstration of language impairment.
3. Evan's parents should be provided with materials and training to implement a language stimulation program within the home environment. Information and language goals will also be provided to Evan's day care provider so that stimulation can occur consistently across home and day care environments.

Prognosis: Good

Ima Young, CCC/SLP
Speech-Language Pathologist
VA License 34-973

CLINICAL PROBLEM-SOLVING

1. What might a home-based observation of Evan have revealed? What would be the purpose of a home-based observation?
2. The clinician concluded that Evan had a mild to moderate receptive/expressive specific language impairment. What does this mean?

How should this information be communicated to Evan's parents?
3. What is the purpose of the audiological referral?
4. The clinician indicated a good prognosis for Evan. What factors likely led her to this judgment? What other information would be useful for making a prognostic statement about Evan's language difficulties?

CHAPTER SUMMARY

A language disorder refers to significant difficulties in the content, form, or use of spoken, written, or other symbol systems used for the purpose of communication. For a language disorder to be present, it must adversely impact an individual socially, psychologically, or educationally.

Language disorders are classified by etiology, manifestation, and severity. A primary language disorder describes an impairment attributable to no other cause, whereas a secondary impairment is caused by another primary source, such as hearing loss. Developmental disorders of language are present from birth; acquired disorders result from an insult or injury sometime after birth. Language disorders can affect comprehension, expression, or both. Disorders can affect all three domains of language (form, content, and use) or only one. These are described as diffuse and focal disorders, respectively.

Four of the most prevalent language disorders are specific language impairment (SLI), autism spectrum disorder (ASD), mental retardation, and traumatic brain injury (TBI). SLI is a primary language impairment in which children show significant challenges with language development in the absence of any other known developmental difficulty. ASD is an umbrella term that encompasses four neurologically based developmental disorders characterized by disordered communication, repetitive behaviors, difficulties with social relationships, and restricted interests. Mental retardation is a developmental disability associated with language disorders ranging from mild to profound. Language disorders resulting from TBI are typically characterized by discourse problems and additional executive difficulties.

A multistep assessment process includes referral, screening, comprehensive language evaluation, and diagnosis. Treatment principles for infants, toddlers, and preschoolers include early intervention, parental involvement, naturalistic environments, social interaction, and functional outcomes. Treatment principles for older children include metalinguistic awareness, functional flexibility, discourse-level skills, literacy achievement, and least restrictive environment.

KEY TERMS

acquired language disorder, p. 221
adaptive behavior, p. 230
anoxia, p. 229
Asperger's syndrome, p. 228
autism spectrum disorder, p. 223
broad-based assessment, p. 238
child-centered approaches, p. 243
childhood disintegrative disorder, p. 228
clinician-directed approaches, p. 243
developmental language disorder, p. 221
diffuse disorder, p. 222
echolalia, p. 228
false-negative, p. 241
false-positive, p. 240
focal disorder, p. 222
functional assessment, p. 238
intrachild differences, p. 223
language delay, p. 218
language difference, p. 216
language disorder, p. 213
late talkers, p. 218
mixed receptive-expressive disorder, p. 221
primary language impairment, p. 220
screening, p. 236
secondary language impairment, p. 220

specific expressive language disorder (SELD), p. 221

specific language impairment, p. 223

stereotypical behaviors, p. 228

word finding problems, p. 225

ON THE WEB

Check out the Companion Website! On it you will find

- suggested readings
- reflection questions
- a self-study quiz
- links to additional online resources, including current technologies in communication sciences and disorders

Adult Aphasia and Other Cognitive-Based Dysfunctions

Cynthia R. O'Donoghue

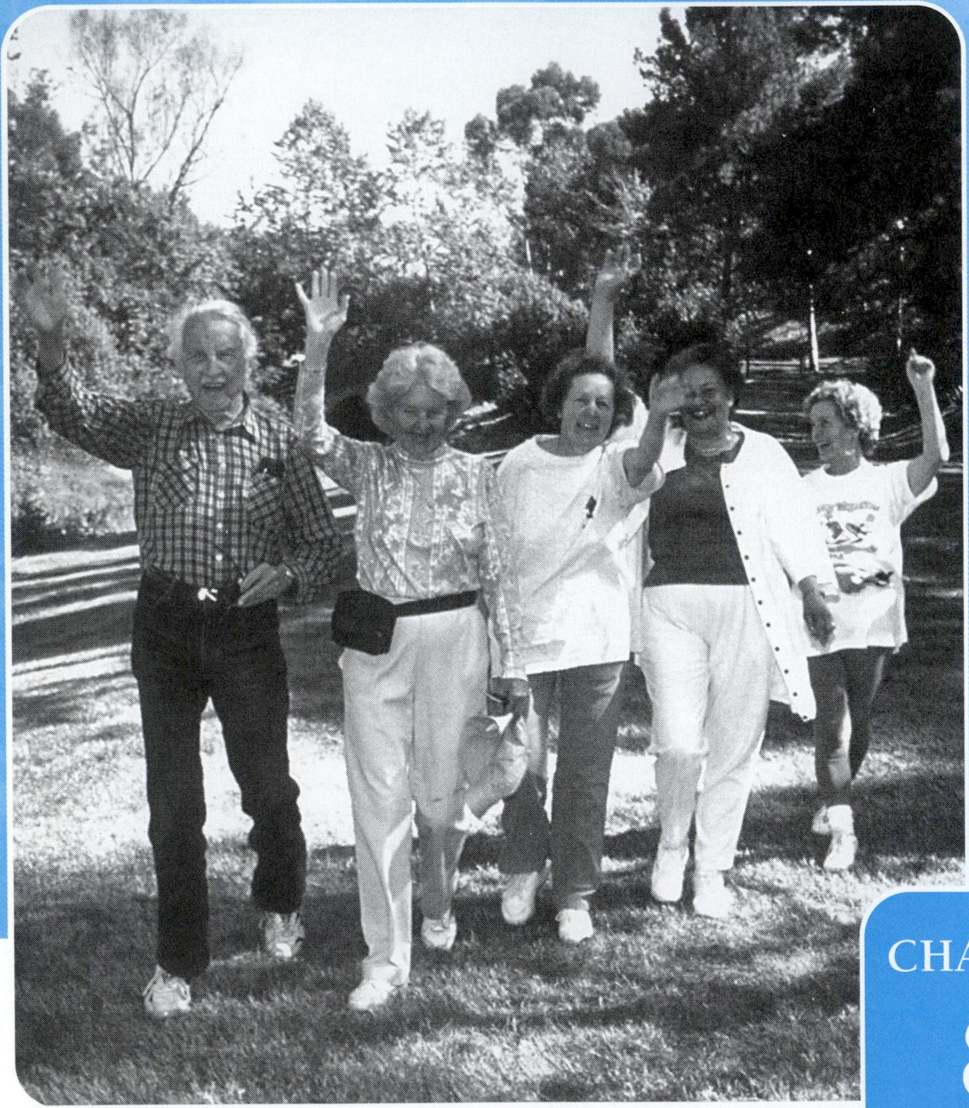

CHAPTER 8

FOCUS QUESTIONS

This chapter answers the following questions:

1. What is aphasia?
2. How is aphasia classified?
3. What are the defining characteristics of aphasia syndromes?
4. How is aphasia identified and treated?
5. What are right hemisphere dysfunction, traumatic brain injury, and dementia?

INTRODUCTION

When stroke, progressive neurological disease, or tumors damage the tissues of the brain, one's ability to effectively accomplish everyday tasks—like watching a movie, reading the newspaper, and conversing with friends—is often compromised. This chapter describes language and cognitive disorders associated with acquired neurological injury, specifically aphasia, right hemisphere damage, traumatic brain injury, and dementia.

Aphasia is an acquired disorder of language that typically results from injury to the left cerebral hemisphere, most often due to a stroke. Difficulties in expressing, understanding, reading, and/or writing oral and written language are some characteristics of aphasia. *Right hemisphere damage* (RHD) is an acquired cognitive disorder associated with damage to the right cerebral hemisphere. Like aphasia, RHD can result from stroke, and typical symptoms of this disorder include memory impairment, attention and impulsivity problems, and visual dysfunction. These problems are often accompanied by a lack of insight into or awareness of these problems. *Traumatic brain injury* (TBI) is another type of acquired neurological injury, which can result from car accidents, severe falls, and acts of violence. A variety of cognitive and linguistic difficulties can arise from TBI, with the symptoms varying based on the site and severity of the injury. *Dementia* describes a loss of linguistic and cognitive ability due to a progressive brain disease, such as Alzheimer's Disease (AD). The linguistic and cognitive abilities of persons with dementia become increasingly affected as the disease progresses.

The language and cognitive-based problems associated with acquired neurological injury can have far-reaching consequences on a person's ability to live life in a full and meaningful way. This chapter provides an overview of adult communication problems following neurological injury that causes impairment of language or cognitive-based processes. The chapter first focuses on aphasia, which is primarily a disorder of language resulting from damage to the left hemisphere. The chapter then focuses on disorders of cognitive-based functions that affect communication, including RHD, TBI, and dementia.

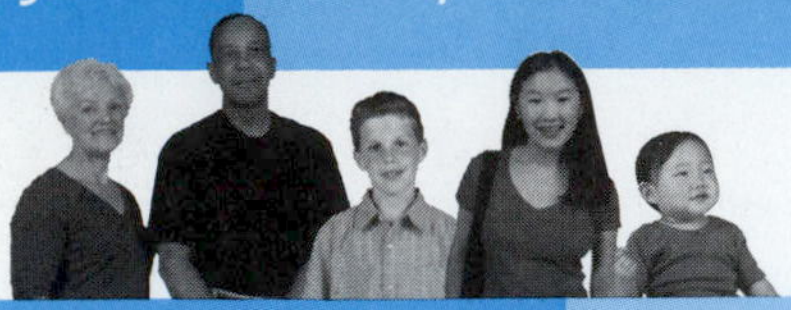

BOX 8-1 Adult Language and Cognitive-Based Dysfunction: Case Examples

Joe Gordon is a 48-year-old male who suffered a stroke 2 weeks ago and is now an inpatient on the acute rehabilitation unit of St. Patrick's Hospital. Joe understands others' speech and can communicate, although his speech is labored. He has weakness on his right side, affecting his face, hand, and leg. Prior to this incident Joe was employed as a carpenter and was the primary wage earner for his family. He did not complete high school but was literate and good with numbers. Joe has been happily married to Sarah for 29 years. They have three children, aged 17, 22, and 27. His wife works part-time as a housekeeper. Joe and Sarah have been told by Dr. Rather, the neurologist, that Joe suffered a moderate-sized stroke in the left frontal lobe, mostly affecting the superior portion. Dr. Rather has emphasized to Joe and Sarah that Joe's medical history of coronary artery disease and high-blood pressure coupled with his one pack per day of cigarettes puts him at risk for another stroke. Joe fears that he will be unable to return to work and that his family will be in financial difficulty. He is afraid that he now may not be able to afford to send his youngest child, the first college-bound Gordon, to college.

Internet research

1. What age group of the population is most at risk for experiencing a stroke?
2. How often do persons with strokes return to their jobs?
3. What information is available about leave of absence from gainful employment following a stroke?

Brainstorm and discussion

1. What psychological and social issues need to be considered by the rehabilitation team working with Joe?
2. What factors in Joe's life support his recovery and ultimate return to work?

Maria Garcia is a 68-year-old female who emigrated from Mexico to Odessa, Texas, in the early 1990s to be closer to her son and his family. Maria has lived with her son's family since coming to the United States. She speaks English competently, as do her other family members, although Spanish is the language spoken in the home. Maria cares for her four grandchildren after school while her son and daughter-in-law are working. She drives the children to after-school activities and prepares the evening meals for the family. Three weeks ago, Maria suffered a stroke in her right hemisphere and now has difficulty with her vision, experiences weakness in her left arm and leg (although she is walking safely with a walker), and has difficulty retrieving the words she wants to use. She finds that she has more problems retrieving words in English and so frequently switches to or inserts Spanish into her English, even in interactions with friends who do not speak Spanish. Maria has no insurance and thus is resisting consulting a speech-language pathologist for rehabilitation therapy.

Internet research

1. Of American adults, what percentage currently have health insurance?
2. Are there tests of language disorders for adults that are standardized in Spanish?

What Is Aphasia?

Definition

Aphasia is a disorder of language that is acquired sometime after an individual has developed language competence. Aphasia results from injury to the language functions of the brain. For most people these language functions are contained in the left hemisphere, although for a small percentage of the population the right hemisphere is the language-dominant hemisphere. The more common causes of neurological injury to the language-dominant hemisphere include stroke, infectious diseases such as meningitis or encephalitis, tumors, exposure to toxins or poisons, hydrocephalus, and nutritional or metabolic disorders. Of these, stroke is the neurological disorder that produces most aphasias. Stroke, also called a

3. Approximately what percentage of speech-language pathologists are bilingual with Spanish as one of their languages?

Brainstorm and discussion

1. Other than a lack of insurance, what are some reasons that might be preventing Maria from seeking therapy?
2. In your opinion, if therapy is provided, should it be conducted in English, Spanish, or both? Why?

Mable Green is a 72-year-old widow who lives alone in a single-level condominium in Sarasota, Florida. Mable is the mother of two adult children, Alice and Peter, who both reside within a 15-minute drive of Mable's home. Mable appears to have increasing periods of forgetfulness, which concerns Alice. Three weeks ago, Mable locked herself out of the house in her nightgown when going to retrieve the morning paper. Just last week, Alice received a call from her mother that she had gone to have her hair done at her usual beauty salon but then got lost on Independence Avenue and needed Alice to come and get her. Peter feels that his mother is fine and that her spells of confusion are expected at her age. Alice's concern is mounting. She wants her mother to see her family physician as soon as possible. Mable tells Alice to stop worrying: "I'm just fine and you know I always did have difficulty with directions. That's why your father always drove."

Internet research

1. Are these memory changes typical of individuals over 70 years of age?
2. What percentage of the current population in the United States is considered geriatric (over 65 years)?
3. What are some common warning signs of dementia?

Brainstorm and discussion

1. What are some reasons for Mable to resist a physician visit?
2. How might the family dynamics in this scenario influence Mable's outcome?
3. Should Mable be found to have dementia, what are some options for her caregiving?

cerebrovascular accident (CVA), occurs when the blood supply providing nutrients and oxygen to the brain is interrupted by a blood clot or other clogging material in an artery serving the brain. When this interruption affects the language areas of the brain, aphasia results from the damage to the brain tissue (see Figure 8-1).

Aphasia literally means "the absence of language," or "without language." Although this suggests that the individual with aphasia has no language abilities, people with aphasia exhibit a broad range of language difficulties, from only mild deficits to the most severe, in which an individual has few or no language functions. A classic definition follows:

> A disturbance of one or more aspects of the complex process of comprehending and formulating verbal messages that results from newly acquired disease of the central nervous system (A. Damasio, 1981, p. 51)

FIGURE 8-1 Damage to the brain due to stroke.

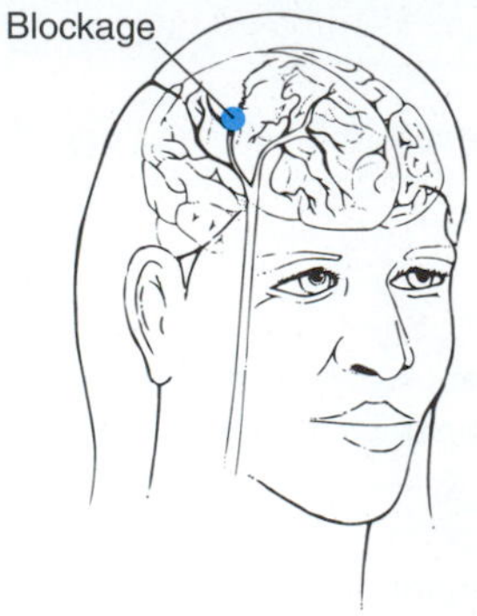

Discussion Point: *What other premorbid factors might affect the way aphasia affects a person? Consider the case of Joe, in Box 8-1, in your answer.*

This early definition by Damasio is used frequently in the aphasia literature (Rao, 1994; Rosenbek, La Pointe, & Wertz, 1989). However, it does not clearly address two very important facts about aphasia. First, aphasia is not limited solely to problems of spoken language; it also encompasses disturbances in written language skills, including reading and writing. Second, the damage to the central nervous system can be more specifically defined; it interrupts the language-dominant hemisphere of the brain (Brookshire, 2003).

Therefore, a more comprehensive definition of aphasia includes these points:

1. Aphasia is a disturbance in the language system *after* language has been established or learned.
2. Aphasia results from neurological injury to the language-dominant hemisphere of the brain.
3. Aphasia includes disturbances of receptive and/or expressive abilities for spoken and/or written language.

It is important that aphasia be differentiated from other types of communication disorders, such as developmental disorders of language, psychiatric problems, and motor speech disorders. First, aphasia is not a developmental disorder. Rather, it is an acquired disruption in the language system following neurological injury. It most often affects adults who have experienced a stroke and thus is often considered an adult language disorder, although it can also affect children and adolescents who experience a stroke. Because aphasia is acquired later in life for most people, its symptoms vary widely across those affected as a function of premorbid factors, which are characteristics of a person before an illness, in this case the neurological injury. The way aphasia affects a person is influenced by such factors as health, emotional well-being, occupational and educational attainment, and language abilities.

Second, aphasia is not a psychiatric problem. This fact requires mention because aphasia has sometimes been misdiagnosed as a psychological disturbance (Palmer, 1979; Sambunaris & Hyde, 1994). Some psychological disorders—such as psychosis, schizophrenia, or delirium—may yield a bizarreness in language (H. Damasio, 2001) that can also occur with aphasia. For example, some language oddities, such as difficulty coming up with the names of objects, may be the residual effects of a stroke after other functions have returned but might be confused with signs of a psychological

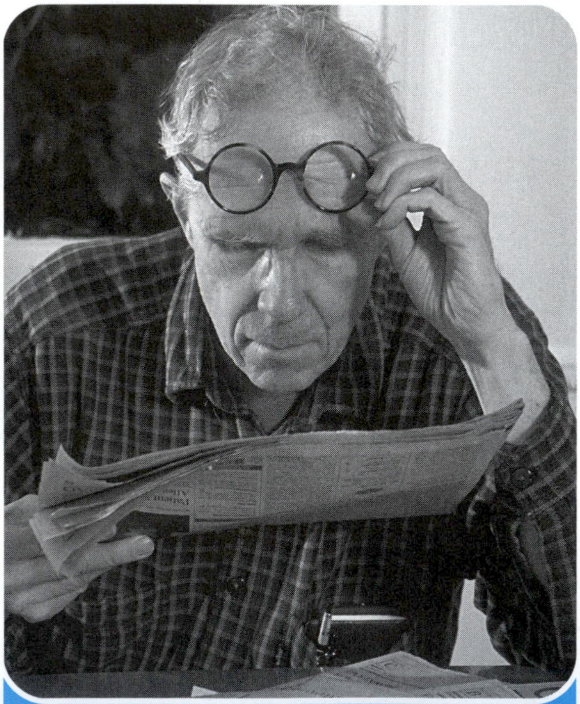

Aphasia includes impairment not only of spoken language but also of writing and reading.

disturbance. A language deficit is not the same as a psychological disturbance, even though the symptoms of both may, at times, appear similar. Thus, it is important that the language weaknesses of persons with aphasia are not mistaken for a more general psychological disturbance.

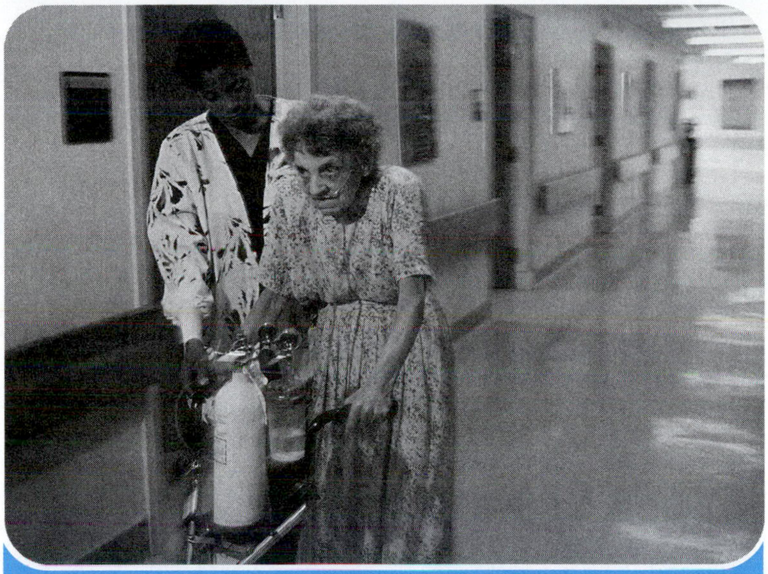

The symptoms of aphasia can be confused with symptoms of psychological disturbance.

Third, aphasia is not a motor speech disorder. Motor speech disorders, as discussed in chapter 6, refer to an inability to plan, program, and/or execute the motor movements required for efficient, intelligible speech production as a result of neurological deficits. **Dysarthria** is a motor speech disorder characterized by disruption in the range, speed, direction, timing, and strength of movements in the respiratory, phonatory, articulatory, and/or resonatory components of speech. **Apraxia**, another motor speech disturbance, is a difficulty in planning and executing the volitional movements of speech. Aphasia is a language-based dysfunction, not a motor-based dysfunction, but the symptoms of dysarthria, apraxia, and aphasia can appear similar in their impact on a person's ability to communicate effectively. Additionally, motor speech disturbances often coexist with aphasia, thus challenging professionals to identify which aspects of an individual's communication are undermined by motor speech problems and which by aphasia.

Discussion Point: *Motor speech disorders often coexist with aphasia. Using Box 8-1 and Joe's case, what information suggests that a motor speech disorder may be present as well as aphasia?*

Prevalence and Incidence

Stroke, or CVA, is the cause of most aphasias. The National Stroke Association reports that a stroke occurs every 45 seconds in the United States; approximately 750,000 citizens suffer strokes each year. The estimate of the total number of surviving stroke victims is 4 million in the United States alone. The associated health care costs are staggering, consuming about $30 billion annually.

Risk Factors

Risk factors for stroke, and subsequent aphasia, include both uncontrollable factors (those beyond the control of the individual) and modifiable factors (those that can be controlled). Uncontrollable risk factors include age, gender, racial or ethnic background, and family history. With increased age, the risk for stroke increases. In fact, for each decade over 55 years, the risk for stroke doubles. African Americans are twice as likely to suffer a stroke as are European Americans, and males are at greater risk than females. These are not factors a person can change.

Controllable, or modifiable, risk factors include hypertension (i.e., high blood pressure), diabetes, tobacco smoking, and alcohol use. With behavioral changes these factors can decrease the likelihood of a stroke occurring. For example, lifestyle changes, such as improving eating habits and exercise, as well as pharmaceutical intervention, can often improve symptoms of hypertension. And diabetes, although incurable, can be managed so that blood sugar levels remain within more normal ranges. Alleviating or reducing tobacco and alcohol use also decreases the risk of stroke. The National Stroke

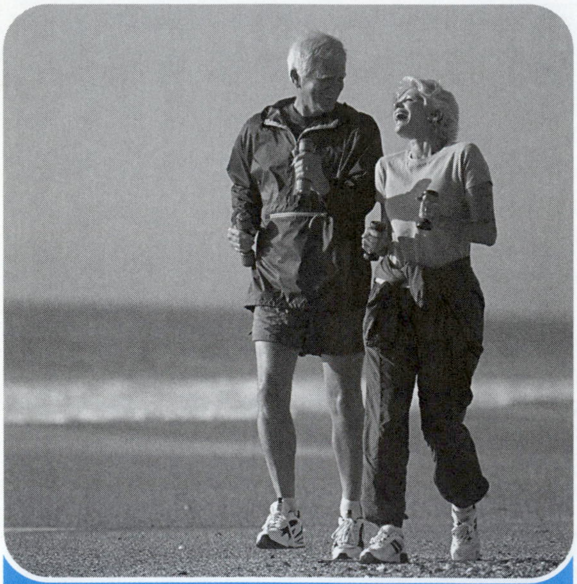

Lifestyle changes, such as ensuring regular exercise and eating a healthy diet, can decrease one's risk for stroke.

Association (NSA), the National Aphasia Association (NAA), and the National Institute on Neurological Disorders and Stroke (NINDS) are just a few of the many organizations working diligently on issues of stroke prevention, assessment, and treatment.

How Is Aphasia Classified?

Aphasia is a global term used to describe language disorders following neurological injury. The way in which language is affected varies widely based on the location of the damage to the brain. Thus, aphasia is differentiated into different types according to the location of the damage and the language-disorder symptoms that occur. This classification system for the aphasias is known as **taxonomy**; it draws upon those characteristics of aphasia that most differentiate disorders from one another and is similar to the way we might classify automobiles. Although automobiles might be grouped by year and color, the most useful taxonomy would use the factors that best differentiate one car from another. For example, saying, "I have a red car made in 1965" tells us much less than "I have a 1965 red Mustang convertible." Similarly, to differentiate aphasias, we need to describe each profile by using the most important factors.

Discussion Point: *Consider Joe's case in Box 8-1. What are his controllable and uncontrollable risk factors?*

Historically, there has been great debate over the best taxonomy by which to characterize aphasia. Some experts have advocated using the "locus of the lesion and the set of behavioral characteristics" (Rosenbek et al., 1989, p. 40) to differentiate aphasias. In this approach aphasia would be categorized by the cause and location of the brain damage, also called the site of the lesion. Based on this taxonomy, we would describe Joe in Box 8-1 as having an aphasia resulting from an infarct (i.e., damage) affecting the superior portion of the frontal lobe. The illustration in Figure 8-2 contrasts the effects of anterior and posterior sites of injury, which result in different kinds of aphasia symptoms.

Other experts prefer taxonomies based on the language skills, both strengths and weaknesses, evident in the aphasia (Goodglass & Kaplan, 1983). Such a taxonomy categorizes the aphasia by the most prominent language characteristics. For instance, this system might differentiate aphasias into those that result in nonfluent speech (i.e., short, choppy utterances) and those that result in fluent speech (i.e., long, flowing utterances that are devoid of content).

FIGURE 8-2 Aphasia types based on the site of injury.

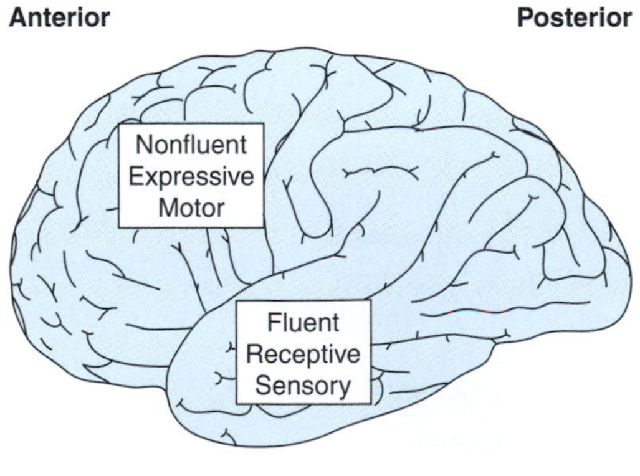

Needless to say, both of these approaches carry advantages and disadvantages. The most discriminating taxonomy differentiates aphasias by both the behavioral symptoms and the site of the lesion, and knowledgeable clinicians use all relevant factors when assessing and treating their patients with aphasia.

Behavioral Symptoms

A person with aphasia has an impairment of language. With this noted, it might be the only thing that two people with aphasia have in common. Indeed, the way acquired impairments of language are expressed varies widely across individuals. Some persons with aphasia are unable to initiate speech at all; others can initiate speech well but produce extended, flowery monologues that seem void of content and contain odd names for things. Still others with aphasia show relatively few symptoms of language impairment but can't seem to retrieve the names of common objects in the environment.

In general, the language deficits seen in aphasia are differentiated by their impact on fluency, motor output, comprehension, repetition, naming, and reading and writing. Problems in these areas, and the terminology used to identify them, are listed and described in Table 8-1.

Fluency

Fluency is a qualitative aspect of communication and speech that is used to describe its forward flow, including its phrasing, intonation, and rate. Fluent speech is easy, smooth, and well paced. Some people with aphasia exhibit a significant lack of fluency due to impairments in formulating and producing verbal output. This type of aphasia is called nonfluent and has these features:

- Short, choppy phrases
- Slow, labored production of speech

TABLE 8-1 Common speech-language problems seen in aphasia syndromes

Problem	Definition	Syndrome
Agrammatism	Leaving out grammatical markers in sentences and phrases, including verb inflections, articles, and prepositions (e.g., "He go store")	Broca's aphasia, transcortical motor aphasia
Word-finding problems (anomia)	Inability to come up with words or names of items in spontaneous conversation or in structured naming tasks	Broca's aphasia, transcortical motor aphasia, global aphasia, Wernicke's aphasia, conduction aphasia, transcortical sensory aphasia, anomic aphasia
Telegraphic speech	Phrases and sentences made up of mostly content words (nouns and verbs) with function words omitted (e.g., "Tom go store")	Broca's aphasia, transcortical motor aphasia
Paraphasias	Substitution of one word for another (e.g., *table* for *desk*)	Transcortical motor aphasia, Wernicke's aphasia, transcortical sensory aphasia
Jargon	Production of language that is meaningless and may run on and on	Wernicke's aphasia
Neologisms	Making up a new word (e.g., "The *bramble-thingie* is over there")	Wernicke's aphasia
Effortful articulation	Production of speech that seems physically laborious, often accompanied by reduced phases or sentence length; may grope with the articulators for positioning	Broca's aphasia, global aphasia
Initiation difficulties (adynamia)	Great difficulty or inability to initiate speech	Transcortical motor aphasia, global aphasia
Comprehension deficits	Compromised understanding or an inability to understand language	Wernicke's aphasia, transcortical sensory aphasia
Impaired repetition	Inability to repeat sounds, words, or phrases	Global aphasia, Wernicke's aphasia, conduction aphasia

Sources: Based on Rao (1994); Shipley and McAfee (1998).

- Grammatical errors
- Telegraphic quality

Discussion Point: *Fluency of speech output is a factor used in differentiating and classifying aphasia. In the case of Joe in Box 8-1, what information in his profile suggests that he is nonfluent?*

However, some aphasias are considered fluent; the speech flows well with adequate phrase length, although often the content of the language is affected. The extent to which a person with aphasia has fluent versus nonfluent speech gives insight into the location of the neurological injury. Generally, nonfluent aphasia correlates to injury anterior in the brain (i.e., the frontal lobe), whereas fluent aphasia correlates with posterior brain damage (i.e., the temporal-parietal regions).

Motor Output

For some people with aphasia, particularly those whose speech is nonfluent, motor systems involved with speech are compromised, resulting in a motor speech disorder. This occurs when the areas of the brain controlling motor planning and programming for speech are injured. These individuals may show slow and labored articulation of sounds, with some groping of the articulators as they seek accurate placement. In other types of aphasia the motor systems underlying speech are spared, but the comprehension of language is impacted.

Language Comprehension

Language comprehension, also called auditory comprehension, is the ability to understand spoken language; this is not acuity or the ability to hear the message, but the interpretation of what is heard. Most individuals with aphasia experience some degree of auditory comprehension deficit; some types of aphasia are characterized by significant problems with auditory comprehension, whereas other types of aphasia correlate with more mild difficulties. The extent of comprehension difficulties is useful for classifying the aphasias.

Aphasia characterized by comprehension problems is often referred to as receptive aphasia, to identify its impact on language reception. More posterior aphasias, particularly those affecting the temporal lobe, where language resides, tend to be coupled with more severe comprehension deficits. This contrasts with expressive aphasia, in which comprehension is relatively spared but expression is compromised. With anterior aphasias, which affect the frontal lobe, comprehension is relatively intact or only mildly to moderately affected.

Repetition

Repetition is the ability to accurately reproduce verbal stimuli on demand, as in the following tasks:

- Say /b/
- Say *cat*
- Say "My name is Billy"

Discussion Point: *Repetition ability is informative for classifying aphasia when compared to spontaneous speech and auditory comprehension skills. Why would an individual with aphasia be able to repeat better than he or she might speak spontaneously?*

The ability to repeat verbal stimuli is a major factor in differentiating among aphasias, and for many people with aphasia, it is an ability that is seriously compromised. In a repetition task, a person must receive and process the incoming stimulus, convey that information to regions of the brain that formulate and plan motor acts for speech, and then articulate to reproduce the initial stimulus. Repetition ability is most informative when considered in conjunction with performance in spontaneous speaking and in comprehending language; there are certain aphasia profiles in which repetition skills are preserved even though spontaneous expression or comprehension is severely impaired. Repetition abilities alone cannot differentiate between fluent and nonfluent or between receptive and expressive aphasia profiles. However, after these general groupings are established, an individual's repetition skills provide further details about the exact nature of the person's language impairment.

Naming

Naming, or word retrieval, is the ability to retrieve and produce a targeted word during conversation or more structured tasks. **Anomia** is the term used to describe word-finding problems or the inability to retrieve a word. *Anomia* literally means "no name." We have all experienced anomia at one time or another, perhaps when we were tired, ill, or simply stressed. Thus, it is a language difficulty with which we are all familiar. However, more serious deficits in word-finding are a typical symptom of aphasia, with nearly all persons with aphasia exhibiting some degree of difficulty with naming tasks (Best, Herbert, Hickin, Osborne, & Howard, 2002). Anomia is also one of the most persistent deficits in aphasia, meaning that word retrieval is the deficit most likely to remain even after recovery from aphasia (Basso, Marangolo, Piras, & Galluzzi, 2001; Cao, Vikingstad, George, Johnson, & Welch, 1999).

Discussion Point: *On the companion CD-Rom, Mr. Lamm shows difficulties with word-finding. How does he cope with anomia during normal conversations with others?*

Anomia patterns, or the type of word production errors seen in a person with aphasia, give insight into the type of aphasia. These patterns are called **paraphasias**, and they come in two varieties. A *phonemic paraphasia,* or literal paraphasia, occurs when there is a substitution or transposition of a sound. For example, looking at a picture of a sofa but producing "tofa" or "fosa" is a phonemic paraphasia. In "tofa" the /t/ is substituted for /s/. With "fosa" the /f/ and /s/ are transposed, or switched. In a *semantic paraphasia,* or verbal paraphasia, a word is substituted, often a word that is in the same category as the targeted word. Looking at a picture of a sofa but producing "chair" or "furniture" is a semantic paraphasia. Typically, phonemic paraphasias are more prevalent in nonfluent, expressive aphasias, whereas semantic paraphasias are associated with the fluent and receptive classifications.

Discussion Point: *Paraphasias are typically viewed as either phonemic or semantic. How would you characterize the paraphasias of Maria in Box 8-1?*

Reading and Writing

The language deficits of people with aphasia may extend to the domains of reading and writing, which involve the comprehension and expression of written language. Often, reading and writing deficits parallel the verbal language deficits. For example, persons who are nonfluent in spoken language frequently exhibit nonfluent oral reading. Likewise, persons who cannot understand sentence-length verbal messages often cannot comprehend sentence-level written information. It is unlikely that a person with mild to severe aphasia is unimpaired in reading and writing ability.

What Are the Defining Characteristics of Aphasia Syndromes?

Studying the language difficulties of people with aphasia provides information for classifying the types of aphasia into syndromes. We use the term *syndrome* to discuss aphasia because certain language difficulties tend to cluster for different aphasias.

The following discussion describes the seven major aphasia syndromes, based on the most prevalent clinical system (Rao, 1994). (Five of these categories are depicted in Figure 8-3 according to the most common site of the lesion.)

The discussion includes the most salient traits of all seven syndromes: Broca's, transcortical motor, global, Wernicke's, transcortical sensory, conduction, and anomic (Goodglass & Kaplan, 1983; Kertesz, 1982). Table 8-2 summarizes the description of each: the site of the lesion, the impact on speech fluency and expression, and the impact on language and auditory comprehension.

FIGURE 8-3 Aphasia syndromes and their lesion locations.

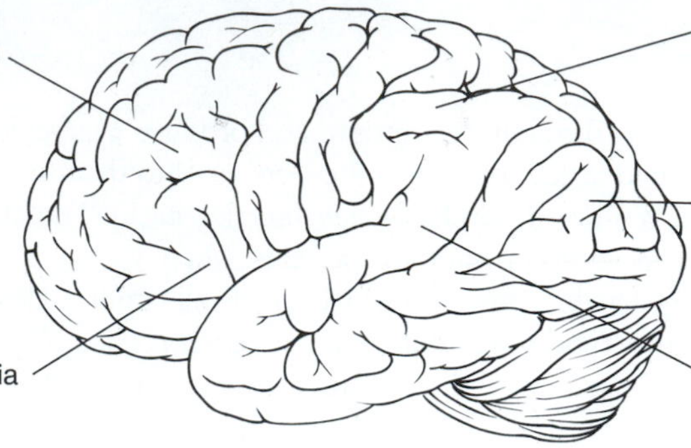

Source: From H. Damasio (1981). Cerebral localization of the aphasia. In M. T. Sarno (Ed.), *Acquired aphasia* (p. 29). New York: Academic Press. Copyright 1981, with permission from Elsevier.

Broca's Aphasia

Broca's aphasia results from damage to the frontal lobe of the brain, specifically Broca's area. This region, situated at the inferior portion of the premotor planning strip, plans and orchestrates the intricate motor movements for speech. In general, damage in Broca's area produces a nonfluent, expressive, motor aphasia profile.

Fluency and Motor Output. The individual with Broca's aphasia typically produces slowed, halting, and labored speech, yielding what some describe as a telegraphic or robotlike

TABLE 8-2 Defining characteristics of the aphasia syndromes

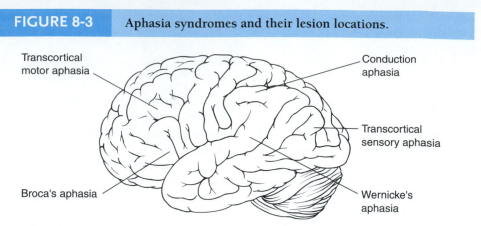

Aphasia Syndrome	Site of Lesion	Speech Fluency and Expression	Language and Auditory Comprehension
Broca's	Frontal lobe (posterior inferior region of left hemisphere)	Nonfluent, effortful articulation, telegraphic speech (mostly nouns and verbs), short phrases, impaired prosody, apraxia of speech	Fair to good
Transcortical motor	Prefrontal cortex (medial frontal region of left hemisphere)	Nonfluent, difficulty initiating speech, paraphasias, short utterances, good repetition	Good
Global	Multiple lobes and diffuse lesions	Nonfluent, delayed or no speech initiation and output, naming and word-finding problems	Poor
Wernicke's	Temporal lobe (posterior portion of left hemisphere)	Fluent, meaningless speech and jargon, paraphasias, naming difficulties	Poor
Transcortical sensory	Parieto-occipital region	Fluent, meaningless speech and jargon, paraphasias, naming difficulties	Poor
Conduction	Arcuate fasciculus	Fluent, imitation problems, naming difficulties, normal prosody and articulation	Fair to good
Anomic	Angular gyrus	Fluent, word-finding problems (loss of words)	Fair to good

Sources: Based on Brookshire (2003); Rao (1994).

quality. Additional characteristics include a decreased phrase length, typically no more than four to five words in an utterance. Because of the short phrasing, the melody of speech is affected. An additional characteristic is agrammatical speech, in which function words are omitted, such as articles, prepositions, and conjunctions. Missing or inaccurate tense markers (e.g., *-ed, -ing*) are also frequent. Yet despite these significant difficulties with expression, the individual with Broca's aphasia is likely to have intact self-monitoring abilities and an awareness of these spoken language difficulties, resulting in extreme frustration.

Language Comprehension. The person with Broca's aphasia exhibits mild to moderate auditory comprehension problems, particularly when messages increase in length and complexity or when contextual cues are removed. For instance, this individual may be able to follow simple directions, like "Point to the chair," but not more complicated directions with more complex language structures, such as "Point to the cat that is not white" or "Point to the chair and then to the table."

Repetition. People with Broca's aphasia are highly variable in their repetition abilities, ranging from mildly to severely impaired. In large part, these abilities reflect the extent of difficulty in verbal expression.

Naming. The individual with Broca's aphasia is likely to have mild to severe anomia, characterized typically by phonemic paraphasias.

Reading and Writing. Reading and writing are unlikely to be spared in Broca's aphasia. Typically, the impact of the neurological injury on reading and writing parallels its impact on verbal performance. Reading aloud is slow and laborious with misarticulations or distortions, and writing is effortful, characterized by oversized printing called **macrographia**. Misspellings are also common, with incorrect letter choices and letter transpositions.

Transcortical Motor Aphasia

Transcortical motor aphasia results from damage to the frontal lobe, typically the superior and anterior portions of the lobe. Like Broca's aphasia, this syndrome is characterized as nonfluent, expressive, and motor in its typology. The symptoms of transcortical motor aphasia are also similar to those of Broca's aphasia *except* that these individuals have repetition skills that are far better than their spontaneous speech. Thus, these individuals may have slow and labored expressive output on their own but are able to perform reasonably well on a repetition task. The relatively well-preserved repetition ability, in conjunction with the previously described language behaviors of Broca's aphasia, is the hallmark of transcortical motor aphasia. Most clients with this syndrome also demonstrate strong performance in oral reading.

Global Aphasia

Global aphasia occurs as a result of a large region of brain damage or multiple sites of brain injury in the language-dominant hemisphere. Because this aphasia syndrome results in deficits across all language modalities, a person is likely to be nonfluent *and* have poor comprehension of language. Such individuals experience severe problems communicating since they have difficulties receiving and sending messages. They are often nonverbal with limited gestures (e.g., head nods for yes or no, pointing to indicate a want). Likewise, understanding messages, even at the short-phrase or the single-word level, is usually impaired. And reading and writing abilities are similarly affected.

Wernicke's Aphasia

Wernicke's aphasia results from brain injury to the superior and posterior regions of the temporal lobe, possibly reaching to the parietal lobe of the language-dominant hemisphere. This area corresponds with auditory comprehension abilities. Wernicke's syndrome is a fluent, receptive, and sensory aphasia.

Fluency and Motor Output. The person with Wernicke's aphasia produces spontaneous speech that flows well with normal prosody. **Prosody** refers to the melody, intonation, and rhythm of speech. In addition, the length of utterances is not affected; utterances are typically at least five or more words in length. In fact, people with Wernicke's aphasia may appear verbose or may talk excessively, which is called **logorrhea**. However, the meaningful content of their utterances is limited, and they use frequent semantic paraphasias. These individuals are also prone to **neologisms**, the use of made-up words (e.g., *polyo* for *chair*), and **jargon**, the use of real words put together without any meaning (e.g., "days bone they could arms four kite"). Thus, although the spontaneous speech is quite fluent, the message is often empty or lost.

Unlike persons with Broca's aphasia, those with Wernicke's aphasia may have difficulty monitoring their own language production. Some people with Wernicke's aphasia may lack the insight that what they are attempting to say is not what they are actually saying. For this reason it can be difficult to treat these clients; they may think that the therapist is the one with the communication problem, not them!

Language Comprehension. Comprehension problems are the key disturbance in Wernicke's syndrome. Unfortunately, persons with this syndrome have great difficulty interpreting verbal and written messages. Even simple language can be difficult to comprehend, such as sentences like "Put your finger on the button." And when language becomes decontextualized to describe events away from the here and now or becomes more grammatically complex, such as "Put your finger on the button and then stand up and smile," the comprehension deficits become even more profound.

Repetition. Most persons with Wernicke's aphasia have difficulty with repetition. As discussed previously, repeating something spoken by another involves both comprehension and production of that message. For someone with this type of aphasia, the comprehension system is usually significantly impaired, which impacts the ability to repeat.

Naming. Moderate to severe naming difficulties are associated with the Wernicke's profile, along with frequent paraphasias of both the phonemic and the semantic variety.

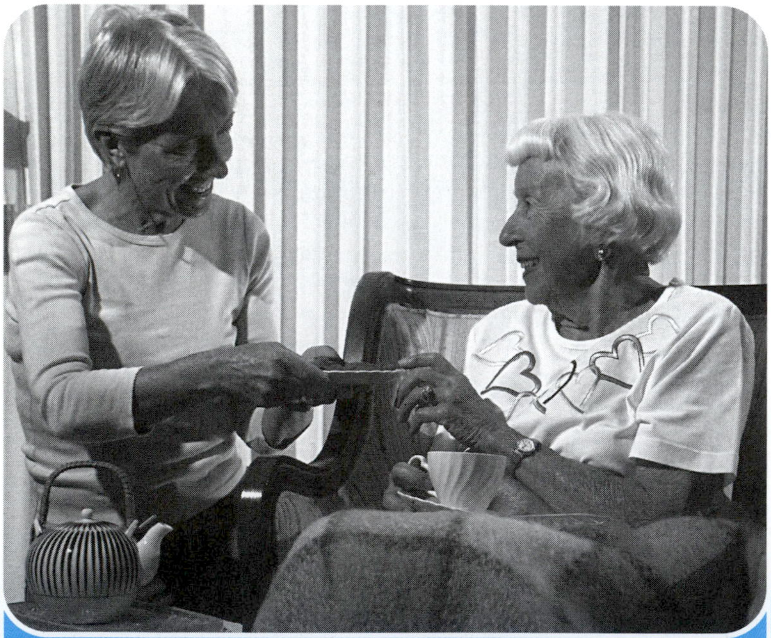

An individual with Wernicke's aphasia may be very fluent and talkative, but the speech lacks meaning and coherence.

In trying to describe a picture of a sailboat, for instance, an individual might say, "*Yep, that's a, uh, booty-dock, a nooty-dock, yep a nooty-boat, soap, it's a, uh, saily-boaty, taily-boaty.*"

The difficulties in coming up with the word *sailboat* result in not only paraphasias but also a behavior called **circumlocution**, which is, essentially, talking around a word that cannot be retrieved. A client trying to produce *refrigerator* might circumlocute and say, "That big box in the kitchen, it keeps food fresh, not spoiled, it is cold." These naming traits, coupled with the auditory comprehension deficits, contribute to the empty speech typical of Wernicke's aphasia.

Reading and Writing. With Wernicke's aphasia, reading may be intact, although comprehension of the text is likely to be degraded to the level of comprehension of spoken communication. Writing also parallels verbal expression. Although the writing is usually fluent and is in legible cursive with normal letter size, the message is unclear.

Transcortical Sensory Aphasia

Transcortical sensory aphasia results from injuries to the language-dominant hemisphere at the border of the temporal and occipital lobes (more inferior) or the superior region of the parietal lobe. Transcortical sensory aphasia is to Wernicke's aphasia as transcortical motor aphasia is to Broca's aphasia. These clients have the classic symptoms of a Wernicke's profile *except* they have stellar repetition skills. Further, they may also frequently repeat auditory stimuli called **echolalia**.

Conduction Aphasia

Conduction aphasia results from injury to the temporal-parietal region of the brain, typically to a connecting pathway called the *arcuate fasciculus*. This pathway provides communication between the speech production areas and the speech reception areas in the language-dominant hemisphere.

Fluency and Motor Output. The conduction profile is fluent, with only mild to moderate deficits in expressive output. Prosody and articulation tend to be normal.

Language Comprehension. Language comprehension in conduction aphasia also tends to be fair to good with relatively little impairment.

Repetition. Difficulties with repetition and reading aloud are the hallmark of conduction aphasia. These individuals receive and process the verbal or written stimuli to repeat or read aloud, respectively, but cannot transfer this input to the verbal output area (i.e., Broca's region) because of the impaired pathway between these processing centers. Therefore, they are unable to produce the target response despite intact comprehension. However, they are aware of their repetition and reading errors and will attempt to revise and improve their production, possibly numerous times and with considerable frustration.

Naming. Conduction aphasia, like all of the other syndromes, causes mild to moderate difficulties in naming and word retrieval.

Reading and Writing. An inability to read aloud is a hallmark characteristic of this disorder. Reading comprehension abilities are similar to those of auditory comprehension.

Anomic Aphasia

Anomic aphasia is not identified with a specific area of the brain or a site of lesion (i.e., injury). Anomic aphasia is fluent and expressive with relatively few deficits in language expression and comprehension with the exception of naming. Persons with anomic aphasia,

Discussion Point: *Consider Joe's case in Box 8-1. What aphasia syndrome might he have, based on the information supplied? What other information is needed to make this decision?*

as its name suggests, show significant impairment in word retrieval skills in both spoken and written language. This form of aphasia is the most pervasive type of chronic condition, even after treatment (Raymer, 2001), and it is the most common of aphasia profiles.

How Is Aphasia Identified and Treated?

The Assessment Process

For the individual who has sustained neurological damage, the interdisciplinary rehabilitation team includes physicians, nurses, physical therapists, occupational therapists, recreational therapists, social workers, respiratory therapists, registered dieticians, neuropsychologists, and of course, speech-language pathologists. These specialists work cooperatively to treat the client using a holistic approach, that is, attending to all problem areas as a whole picture, as opposed to focusing solely on isolated deficits. They may consult with still other disciplines, based on the client's individualized needs.

The speech-language pathologist's assessment of speech and language functioning provides insight for the entire rehabilitation team as they determine appropriate goals and treatment strategies. For example, if the client's aphasia impairs the ability to understand long phrases, it is important for the other team members to incorporate this finding into their treatment approaches. In this case the physical therapist should be using short phrases for instructions in treatment activities since multiple-step directions are beyond the client's ability (e.g., "Stand up straight" rather than "Lift up your head, straighten your back, and tuck your bottom in").

The speech-language pathologist evaluates the individual with suspected aphasia to answer a whole set of questions:

1. Is aphasia present?
2. If so, what type or syndrome of aphasia is indicated by the symptoms and the site of injury?
3. What treatment plan will be most beneficial?
4. What is the prognosis for recovery?
5. Are any referrals to other professionals needed?

It can be a challenge to gather all the needed information soon after a person sustains a neurological injury; the individual's medical condition may preclude extensive testing. If so, screening is recommended in the client's hospital room, often at the bedside.

A screening typically examines orientation and responsiveness, speaking ability, listening skills, and possibly reading and writing. The Aphasia Language Performance Scales (ALPS) (Keenan and Brassell, 1975), a standardized aphasia assessment tool, is a relatively brief aphasia battery that is often appropriate for clients at this stage. The Bedside Evaluation Screening Test (BEST) (Fitch-West & Sands, 1987) is also well suited for this purpose. Both of these instruments survey speech and language performance using a limited, yet informative, number of items; the testing takes about 30 minutes. Such informal bedside screening provides the starting point (i.e., baseline performance) for ongoing assessment and the start of a treatment plan.

As the neurological client becomes more medically stable, improved endurance will permit more extensive, comprehensive assessment. Most individuals will exhibit at least some level of recovery on their own, as part of the healing process. This **spontaneous recovery** is the natural, spontaneous healing of the brain without therapeutic interventions.

TABLE 8-3 Typical items included in aphasia batteries

Area of Testing	Typical Items
Spontaneous speech	• Answering questions • Describing a picture • Participating in informal or structured conversations
Auditory comprehension	• Answering yes/no questions • Pointing to objects or pictures as they are named • Following directions (single-step, multistep, and complex commands)
Repetition	• Repeating real words, phrases, and sentences • Repeating nonsense words and phrases
Naming	• Naming objects and pictures • Completing phrases • Naming items in a category • Providing names of general categories
Reading	• Reading words, phrases, sentences, and paragraphs
Writing	• Copying letters, words, and sentences • Writing from dictation • Writing about fictional or real experiences

When the client is able to participate for longer periods of time, standardized comprehensive aphasia batteries can be administered to evaluate levels of functioning and to develop a detailed plan for treatment. Numerous aphasia batteries are available from which the speech-language pathologist can choose. Often the choice of a test is influenced by clinician preference, test availability, guidelines of an organization, or unique client needs (e.g., a bilingual client or a client that speaks only Spanish). The areas assessed include language expression and motor output, language comprehension, repetition, naming, reading, and writing. Generally, test items have a hierarchical arrangement, moving from easier to more difficult tasks. Table 8-3 provides a sample of typical items included in an aphasia battery.

Discussion Point: *Consider the areas of testing presented in Table 8-3. For a person with conduction aphasia, which tasks would be more difficult? What about a person with Wernicke's aphasia?*

The speech-language pathologist also studies other variables that may affect communication. For example, a thorough examination of the oral structures and functions might reveal a coexisting dysarthria or apraxia. A hearing screening would indicate whether an audiologist should be consulted for further auditory and hearing assessment. A psychological screening could determine how any communication problems might be impacting the individual's psychological well-being, possibly warranting mental health counseling.

As the speech-language pathologist gathers input, findings are summarized in an evaluation report. This report provides the individual's history, current test findings, clinical impressions, and recommendations, as shown in Figure 8-4. This report then becomes part of the individual's medical file and is used to make treatment decisions.

It is important to recognize that assessment of aphasia is comprehensive and ongoing. As a function of treatment, time, and natural healing, persons with aphasia will show changes in their communicative status over time. Thus, the speech-language pathologist is constantly reevaluating an individual's performance and adjusting the treatment strategies accordingly.

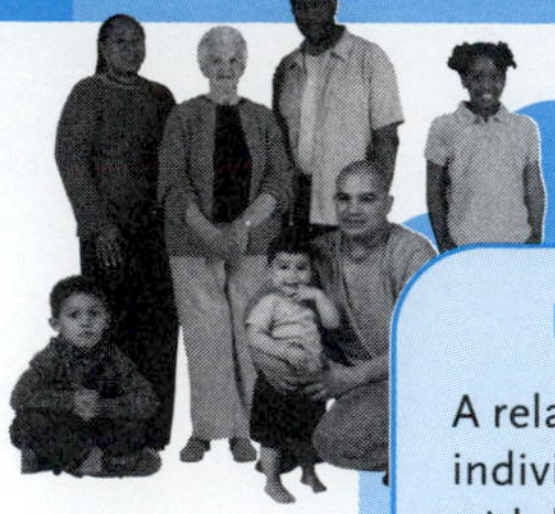

BOX 8-2 Multicultural Focus

Multilingualism and Language Disorders

A relatively new frontier of adult language rehabilitation is the evaluation and treatment of individuals who speak more than one language, that is, who are bilingual. Intervention with bilingual speakers requires the clinician to have knowledge of the languages spoken as well as the cultural backgrounds that influence language use. For individuals who speak multiple languages, optimal testing procedures will evaluate them in all spoken languages.

Although there are now tests that are standardized in multiple languages, therapists who are competent in multiple languages are scarce. Translators can be used to assist with this process, but they may miss subtle deficits in language or cognition. Further complicating matters are the multiple levels of bilingualism. For example, the individual who acquired both Spanish and English as a young child may have a different level of bilingual competency from that of the Spanish speaker who acquired English as a second language after moving to the United States at age 18.

Although there is still much to learn in this area of aphasia research, studies of bilingual persons with aphasia show several possible impacts (Roberts, 2001):

1. *Parallel impairment,* with both languages demonstrating similar strengths and weaknesses
2. *Differential impairment,* with one language showing greater impairment than another
3. *Differential aphasia,* with varying aphasia symptoms or profiles between languages
4. *Blended impairment,* with the individual appearing to mix features of the languages
5. *Selective aphasia,* with only one language revealing deficits and the other being preserved

These variations in aphasia profiles require much research. The rapidly expanding diversity in languages, dialects, and cultures in the United States necessitates better understanding of the most effective methods for evaluating and treating bilingual individuals (Niemeier, Burnett, & Whitaker, 2003).

For Discussion

What are some pros and cons involving an interpreter to assist in the assessment process?

What tests of adult language or cognitive-based disorders are available in Spanish? Arabic? French?

What language and cultural challenges might a therapist face in treating a bilingual individual with aphasia?

Companion Website

To answer these questions online, go to the Multicultural Focus module in chapter 8 of the Companion Website.

Prognostic Indicators

Determining treatment approaches and making prognostic judgments requires knowledge of those factors that predict which clients will benefit from what kind of therapy. **Prognostic indicators** are those variables that assist in predicting recovery: the site of the brain injury, the type and the size of the injury, the type and the severity of aphasia, handedness, age, preinjury health, and motivation for treatment (Robey, 1998b; Yamamoto & Magamonk, 2003). Often, prognostic indicators are used to specify treatment approaches, including the amount and the type of treatment. However, some clients do not respond as

FIGURE 8-4 Reporting format for the speech-language pathologist.

SPEECH-LANGUAGE PATHOLOGY EVALUATION REPORT

Client:
Date of birth/age:
Referral source:
Date of evaluation:

History

Include past medical, social, and educational information. Review current medical issues, presenting problems, and reason for referral.

Current Findings

Provide test results:

1. Oral motor examination
2. Swallowing status
3. Hearing screening
4. Articulation findings
5. Language findings
6. Voice findings
7. Fluency findings
8. Cognitive status

Clinical Impressions

Summarize the findings and provide the speech-language diagnosis (e.g., Broca's aphasia). Include a prognostic statement.

Recommendations

Include recommendations for therapy, if indicated; outline long- and short-term goals, as well as details on frequency and projected duration of treatment. List any referrals for other professional services.

Signature and credentials
State License Number

CC: List professionals receiving a copy of this report.

predicted. For this reason, a trial period of intervention is often worthwhile to evaluate an individual's responsiveness to the intensity and the approach.

Designing Treatment Plans

The goal of treatment for aphasia is to correct or compensate for speech and language deficits so that individuals can communicate functionally in their daily routines. Therapy should improve a client's communication skills beyond the level attributed to spontaneous recovery alone (Helm-Estabrooks & Albert, 1991). Since the time spent in treatment is positively associated with language improvements, a greater magnitude of change can be expected with a longer duration of treatment (Robey, 1998b). However, in the current health-care climate of cost monitoring and caps on services provided, there are often strict limits on the number of sessions allowed for aphasia treatment.

Treatment approaches focus on specific deficit areas identified in the evaluation and the underlying processes that produce these impairments. For example, consider a client with poor naming performance who consistently demonstrates phonemic paraphasias—a pictured flower is "tower." Rather than working specifically on improving the production of the word *flower,* the clinician wants to improve the underlying process that is impaired. Here, a motor planning or execution process is likely the cause of the naming error, because it appears that the client knows the correct label. The challenge is to produce gains in the therapy session that carry over or generalize into functional communication improvements. Designing a treatment regimen requires knowledge of **evidence-based practice**, those interventions that have been studied in a controlled manner and demonstrate improvement for a particular disorder.

Determining the Treatment Setting

Aphasia therapy is not limited to the speech-language pathologist and client working in a clinic or office setting. Therapy should encompass other environments to facilitate

BOX 8-3 Spotlight on Research

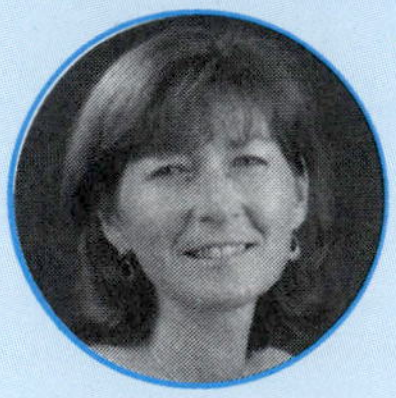

Anastasia Raymer, Ph.D., CCC-SLP
Associate Professor, Dept. of Early Childhood, Speech Pathology, & Special Education
Old Dominion University, Norfolk, Virginia

Dr. Anastasia (Stacie) Raymer is a speech-language pathologist, faculty member, and researcher who has worked with adults with acquired neurogenic communication disorders for the past 20 years. Her interests in adult neurogenic disorders were spurred during her master's studies at the University of Florida; she caught the research bug at the Gainesville Veteran's Administration (VA) Medical Center, where she completed her master's thesis under the guidance of Dr. Leonard LaPointe. It quickly became clear to her that every person with aphasia is a puzzle and that there are many unanswered questions about the effects of brain damage on language. This curiosity led her to complete her Ph.D. at the University of Florida and conduct postdoctoral research at the University of Maryland School of Medicine and the University of Florida Department of Neurology.

All of her research experiences prepared Dr. Raymer well to begin her faculty position at Old Dominion University, where she has remained for the past several years. She also has continued as an investigator in the Brain Rehabilitation Research Center at the Gainesville VA Medical Center. Spearheaded by Program Director Leslie Gonzalez Rothi, an interdisciplinary group of researchers there investigates novel, cutting-edge treatments for all types of acquired neurogenic communication disorders, supported by the National Institutes of Health.

Dr. Raymer's current research focuses on understanding the cognitive and neural underpinnings of disorders of word retrieval, reading, writing, and limb movement in individuals with stroke and Alzheimer's disease. She applies the knowledge gained to developing innovative interventions for acquired language disorders. Her specific interest is in treatments for word retrieval impairments in aphasia. Her recent studies demonstrate that treatments can lead to improvements in word retrieval but that generalization of improvements to functional communication is poor. Therefore, she is developing a new set of studies exploring treatment methods to promote generalized improvements.

One means Dr. Raymer uses to promote research is her role in ASHA Special Interest Division 2: Neurophysiology and Neurogenic Speech and Language Disorders. Division 2 affiliates are provided with the most recent and vital research findings related to neuroscience and clinical practice. With her colleagues in Division 2, Dr. Raymer encourages efforts to translate research into evidence-based clinical practice.

carryover and generalization of progress to different settings. For example, cotreatments with the occupational therapist are beneficial as the client works on activities of daily living (ADLs), such as grooming or dressing. This provides an opportunity for the speech-language pathologist to assess generalization of skills as the client interacts with the occupational therapist to sequence, follow directions, and communicate. Community reentry programs are also excellent simulations for carryover, with the client venturing out, accompanied by therapists, to practice therapy skills in real-world settings such as banks, restaurants, and grocery stores.

Discussion Point: *What are some additional specific ways that group therapy could benefit clients and their families? Consider Joe and Maria in Box 8-1.*

A group approach is another consideration for treating aphasia. Group therapy provides a functional setting for clients to practice communicating and an avenue for cooperative learning (Avent, 1997). At present, group treatment appears to be most beneficial for clients who have chronic or persistent aphasia (Bollinger, Musson, & Holland, 1993) and who also participate in individual treatment (Robey, 1998a). The group setting provides socialization and support for clients and their families.

Measuring Outcomes

Too often, language improvements for persons with aphasia are measured on the basis of standardized test scores, even though the gold standard for effective treatment is the carryover of test scores to *real-world* communication (Elman & Bernstein-Ellis, 1995). Real-world communication refers to communication used in functional and authentic conmmunication acts, and many third-party payers of communication therapy services

BOX 8-4 Spotlight on Practice

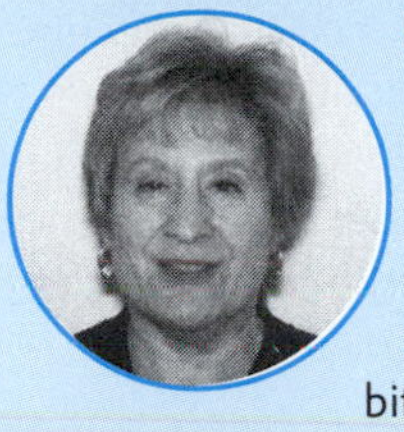

Fern Stillerman, M.Ed., CCC-SLP
Richmond Veteran's
Administration Hospital (retired)

During high school I was very involved with acting in the annual musical and drama production. I was bitten by the acting bug and thought I was Broadway bound. Eventually my father and I had "the talk" about what I was going to do with the rest of my life; he expressed his concerns regarding my career aspirations. In my senior year, I chose public speaking as my elective, little knowing how that class would impact my life. My teacher became my mentor as she discovered my love of communication—pubic speaking, debating, and oral interpretation of literature. One day, while driving home from a regional competition, we discussed my plans following graduation. She asked me whether I had heard of speech-language pathology; she had taken an introductory course in college on that topic and thought I might be interested. Soon after our discussion, she provided me with literature to read on this field. My interest was sparked and my career path established.

I have now been a speech-language pathologist for over 30 years. My first job after completing my master's degree was as a public school therapist. I loved working with the children. Then, during graduate school I had an opportunity to acquire clinical hours at a local VA medical center, working with adults with neurogenic communication disorders. When a position became available there, I applied and have been there ever since—I found my niche.

I have coordinated the speech-language pathology section of our service; developed protocols and procedures for new programs and equipment; lectured to medical students, medical residents, nurses, and other paraprofessionals; and supervised clinical graduate students from local universities. But most of all, I still enjoy clinical practice, working with patients and their families. It is such a thrill to see patients' progress.

One such patient I first evaluated 25 years ago. He was 21 years old and had suffered a left CVA due to occlusion of a carotid artery, resulting in a severe Broca's aphasia. When I first worked with him, he was aphonic, unable to produce any phonemes. Over time, he has progressed to a very mild Broca's aphasia with functional speech in conversation. He is also a computer wiz and has volunteered to fix wheelchairs at our medical center. I still see him periodically for reevaluation and am in awe of his cognitive-linguistic recovery.

Two areas have changed significantly during my career—technology and service delivery. Initially, technology consisted of a tape recorder and a language master. A CT scanner was purchased for my medical center soon after my arrival. The role of imaging in the diagnosis and treatment of cognitive-linguistic disorders has exploded with the advent of computerized tomography—the MRI and PET. As imaging techniques continue to improve, so will cognitive-linguistic diagnosis and treatment. Computer technology also affects how we document patient care, patient outcomes, and satisfaction with services. And speech-generating devices have expanded communication for those with no usable speech.

The second major area of change has been service delivery. When I started in the field, 90% of my inpatients and outpatients were seen for regularly scheduled diagnostic and therapy sessions *in my office* and were followed for several months. Today, many of my inpatients are initially screened or assessed at bedside, and I recommend where they will be best served—inpatient rehabilitation, outpatient rehabilitation, home health, or nursing home. The length of stay has decreased markedly; I may see them for only 3 days before they are transferred to another service. Then I may periodically reassess them for recertification of speech pathology services in the field. We also follow patients living at a distance from the medical center via computer programs and telemedicine. The challenge for speech pathologists today is to stay current with new technology, research, and outcomes measures in order to provide the best possible services to our clients.

emphasize the need for treatment to address real-world needs. For instance, Medicare guidelines focus on communicative interventions that enable individuals to "communicate basic physical needs and emotional states, and carry out communicative interactions in the community" (as cited in Busch, 1994). Thus, speech-language pathologists must consider how to measure treatment outcomes to document improvements such as these.

What is also important is tailoring functional goals to the specific needs of the individuals being treated. For some, a treatment goal might focus on establishing minimal communication functions, such as being able to say yes and no. For another, it might be to perform the communicative functions required of a trial attorney or a classroom teacher. Communication functions are as diverse as the clients we treat.

Tools that measure **functional outcomes**, or functional communication improvements, are considered an essential part of the speech-language pathologist's practice. The Communication Abilities of Daily Living (2nd ed.; Holland, Frattali, & Fromm, 1999), a standardized aphasia battery, is one example of a way to measure functional outcomes, as is the ASHA Functional Assessment of Communication Skills (Frattali, Thompson, Holland, Wohl, & Ferketic, 1995). These measures examine what individuals are able to do with independent and authentic communication tasks. Using such assessments to measure clinical effectiveness reminds speech-language pathologists of the importance of targeting real communication within therapeutic activities.

What Are Right Hemisphere Dysfunction, Traumatic Brain Injury, and Dementia?

Thus far, this chapter has focused on aphasia, one of the most common acquired communication disorders. However, there are other adult language disorders and cognitive-based dysfunctions that merit discussion. The rest of this chapter focuses on three additional acquired disorders of communication, namely right hemisphere dysfunction, traumatic brain injury, and dementia. Table 8-4 provides a summary of these disorders and their major impacts.

TABLE 8-4 Acquired disorders of language and cognition other than aphasia

Disorder	Description	Common Causes	Major Impacts
Right hemisphere dysfunction	Neurological damage to brain tissue in the right hemisphere due to loss of nutrients and oxygen to the brain	Stroke, illness, disease	Lack of attention to the left side of the body, including visual field Difficulty recognizing faces Compromised pragmatics (e.g., taking turns, reading others' cues) Wordy expression including tangents Lack of awareness of communicative and cognitive impairments Problems with higher level abstract thinking and language use Possible dysarthria and dysphagia
Traumatic brain injury	Neurological damage to brain tissue due to closed- or open-head injury	Motor vehicle accident, fall, recreational sports accident, act of violence	Possible significant personality changes Widespread language expression and comprehension problems, including expressing ideas, comprehending what others say, using and expressing humor, displaying and understanding emotions, and engaging in higher level abstract uses of language and cognition
Dementia	Gradual onset of declines in cognitive, language, and daily-living functions due to progressive central nervous system dysfunction	Neurological disease (Huntington's disease, Parkinson's disease, Pick's disease, Creutzfeldt-Jakob disease), multiple strokes	Memory impairment (both short- and long-term memory) Impairment in cognitive skills (abstract thought, judgment, and executive functions) Presence of aphasia, apraxia, or agnosia

Right Hemisphere Dysfunction

Right hemisphere dysfunction (RHD) results from neurological damage to the right cerebral hemisphere. When an individual experiences a stroke, the injury to the brain tissue can occur anywhere. Aphasia can result when the damage is to the left hemisphere; when damage affects the right hemisphere, language and cognition may be impacted, but the symptoms are quite different from those seen with aphasia. For most individuals, about 90% of the adult population, the left hemisphere is dominant for language. The right hemisphere is responsible for many nonlanguage functions, including comprehension of visual-spatial information and emotional expression. Because the two hemispheres do communicate, RHD may include a language disturbance, but cognitive, perceptual, and behavioral disruptions are the more consistent findings with this disorder. For this reason, RHD is commonly referred to as a cognitive-linguistic disorder.

Characteristics of RHD

There is currently no universally recognized taxonomy for RHD. However, there are behavioral symptoms that appear with relative consistency:

1. Lack of awareness of cognitive-linguistic deficits and possible denial of problem areas (Hartman-Maeir, Soroker, Oman, & Katz, 2003)
2. Lack of awareness, or complete neglect, of the left side of the body and external stimuli to the left side, including physical limitations, such as paralysis of the left leg or arm (*left hemiparesis*), and visual-spatial neglect, in which the individual does not process information in the left visual field and which can negatively impact reading and writing (Heilman, 2004)
3. Difficulty recognizing faces (*prosopagnosia*)
4. Compromised pragmatics, such as ability to "read" other people's cues, recognize others' communication interests, and use physical space and affect appropriately during communication
5. A tendency toward using wordy expression and providing tangential information
6. Difficulty understanding or using higher level cognitive-linguistic skills, such as problem solving or abstract thought
7. Dysarthria or dysphagia when neuromuscular systems are compromised

These characteristics vary in severity based on the size and the location of the injury; however, even mild cognitive-linguistic deficits can hinder functional abilities.

Identification of RHD

Like left hemisphere injury, right hemisphere damage requires a comprehensive speech-language assessment as part of an interdisciplinary team assessment. The speech-language pathologist should assess all aspects of communication, speech, and language performance, including those abilities examined in the aphasia battery (e.g., expression, motor control, auditory comprehension, naming, repetition, reading and writing). However, further testing is needed to determine the cognitive-linguistic profile to assess higher level language skills including predicting, reasoning, understanding humor and figurative language, and problem solving. Assessment should also study visual-perceptual performance and pragmatic appropriateness. And most individuals with RHD also benefit from comprehensive neuropsychological testing.

Specialized batteries are available specifically for the RHD population, such as the Mini Inventory of Right Brain Injury (MIRBI; Pimental & Kinsbury, 1989), the Right

Discussion Point: *Consider the case of Maria in Box 8-1. What characteristics in her profile are consistent with RHD?*

Hemisphere Language Battery (Bryan, 1989), and the Clinical Management of Right Hemisphere Dysfunction–Revised (Halper, Cherney, & Burn, 1996). Because evaluation of RHD is complex, it is best accomplished through an interdisciplinary team, whose collective findings can identify the strengths and weaknesses of cognitive, linguistic, and neuropsychological functioning that are pertinent to an individualized rehabilitation plan.

Treatment of RHD

Knowledge of treatments for RHD is more limited than that for left hemisphere damage and aphasia. Initial therapy for RHD targets the management of attention and visual disruptions, since these impact productive treatment activities. For instance, if the individual does not attend to visual stimuli in the left visual field, treatment materials in that space are not processed. Thus, improved attention to stimuli across both visual fields is a key factor in resolving reading and writing disturbances. A therapist can improve attention to the left visual field by placing a heavy, bright red marking, such as a line, on the left side of reading materials to direct the individual's attention to the left.

Therapy also targets higher level cognitive-linguistic tasks, such as thinking through functional problems (What would you do if you locked yourself out of the house? What are the steps to changing a flat tire?) and making inferences (If the alarm doesn't go off, what might happen?). Further, the pragmatics of communication interactions requires careful attention; improvements in facial expression, voice variation, turn taking, topic maintenance, and eye contact are frequent goals with RHD. Again, there is benefit to both individual and group settings for delivering intervention. Given the frequency of pragmatic issues, group treatment is especially helpful for building competence in functional interactions with others.

Traumatic Brain Injury

Traumatic brain injury (TBI) refers to neurological damage to the brain resulting from the impact of external forces. TBI most frequently occurs as a result of motor vehicle accidents (both cars and motorcycles), falls, or acts of violence. Incidence and prevalence statistics tend to vary because of difficulties in defining a TBI. For example, the mild concussion of a football player who briefly loses consciousness and memory of the incident may or may not be included in TBI numbers (Kaut, DePompei, Kerr, & Congeni, 2003).

Nonetheless, epidemiology studies show that TBI is a leading cause of death and disability in the United States. The yearly incidence of TBI in Americans is approximately 1.5 million with 50,000 deaths (Bruns & Hauser, 2003). Of those surviving TBI, 85,000 suffer long-term disabilities (Thurman, Alverson, Dunn, Guerrero, & Sniezek, 1999). Males are twice as likely to experience TBI as females, particularly males of lower socioeconomic backgrounds (Hanks et al., 2003). Certain age groups are also more prone to TBI; infants, adolescents, and senior citizens over 65 years of age have a greater incidence of TBI. Given the frequent long-term medical, vocational, and social needs of affected individuals, TBI represents a substantial health care issue in the United States.

Characteristics of TBI

Head injuries are grouped by the nature of the injury, whether open head or closed head. **Open-head injuries** occur when the skull and the meninges (i.e., the layers of tissue that encase the brain) have been penetrated. These injuries often stem from violent acts using guns, ice picks, and other sharp instruments. The injuries tend to be relatively localized (i.e., focal) with regard to the size and the extent of neurological damage.

One of the most famous cases of TBI was an open-head injury sustained by Phinneas Gage and described by Damasio (1995) in *Descartes' Error.* A railroad worker, Gage's brain was seriously damaged and his personality significantly changed when a metal rod went through his frontal lobe. The study of Gage's personality changes was important in advancing the field of psychology and explaining how traumatic brain injuries affect personality.

Closed-head injuries, by contrast, typically result from motor vehicle accidents, falls, physical assault, or abuse, such as shaken baby syndrome. Although the outer protection of the brain remains intact, the brain is jostled within the skull, yielding diffuse (i.e., nonfocal) neurological injury. The open or closed labeling is common in the clinical setting for diagnostic purposes.

The cognitive and linguistic impacts of TBI vary considerably across individuals and are often not the only aspects of well-being that are affected. As shown in Figure 8-5, TBI impacts the psychosocial realm as well, affecting emotions, temperament, motivation, and self-awareness. In fact, following a TBI, an individual's personality may seem totally changed. The combined impairments of cognition, language, and psychosocial functioning create significant difficulties with communication—expressing ideas, comprehending what others say, using and understanding humor, and displaying and comprehending emotions. As with other neurological injuries, there is often a correlation between the size, the location, and the overall severity of the injury and the impact on the individual's functioning. In short, there are numerous areas of impairment for most people following TBI. Consequently, comprehensive interdisciplinary testing by a team of professionals is imperative to determine baseline skills and target areas for rehabilitation.

Identification of TBI

The speech-language pathologist works as a member of an interdisciplinary rehabilitation team to assess an individual and plan for treatment following a TBI. Initially, many individuals

FIGURE 8-5 Impact of TBI on communication, cognitive, linguistic, and psychosocial realms.

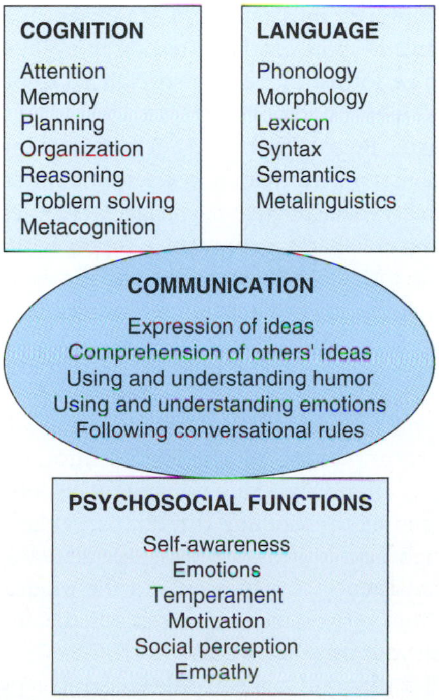

Source: From *Traumatic Brain Injury, Rehabilitation for Speech-Language Pathologists* by R. J. Gillis, 1996, Boston: Elsevier. Copyright 1996 by Elsevier, Inc. Adapted with permission.

TABLE 8-5 Rancho levels of cognitive functioning

Rancho Level	Behavior
I	No response to stimuli
II	Generalized response to stimuli
III	Localized response to stimuli
IV	Confused and agitated
V	Confused, not agitated, inappropriate
VI	Confused, not agitated, appropriate
VII	Automatic, appropriate
VIII	Purposeful, appropriate

Sources: Based on Hagen (1981); Malkus, Booth, and Kodimer (1980).

are comatose and require advanced medical support to survive. At this stage, testing for communication ability and potential relies on subjective, behavioral observations. Two instruments commonly used in the early phases of TBI recovery include the Glascow Coma Scale (Teasdale & Jennett, 1974) and the Rancho Los Amigos Levels of Cognitive Function (Hagen, 1981).

The Glascow Coma Scale (GCS) rates the best-observed response for eye opening, motor behavior, and verbal response to characterize an individual's functioning, from severe TBI (score of 3) to mild TBI (score of 15). The GCS is a predictor of eventual recovery. As an alternative estimate, the Rancho levels of the Rancho Los Amigos Levels of Cognitive Function (Hagen, 1981) use a subjective rating that outlines eight levels of cognitive functioning. These range from nonresponsiveness (Level I) to purposeful/appropriate behavior (Level VIII), as shown in Table 8-5. Since this scale reflects the entire continuum of TBI recovery, it applies throughout the rehabilitation process.

As the TBI client improves medically and stabilizes in functioning, the speech-language pathologist completes more extensive testing to evaluate the impact of the brain injury on communication performance. Several specialized tests are available, such as the Brief Test of Head Injury (Helm-Estabrooks & Hotz, 1991) and the Ross Information Processing Assessment (2nd ed.; Ross, 1996). These tests complement the additional testing that will examine both oral motor performance to determine whether dysarthria or apraxia is present and swallowing ability to ensure that dysphagia is not present. The speech-language pathologist then completes and shares a cumulative report with other rehabilitation team members. Because persons with TBI have many needs, the appropriate professionals collaboratively generate an interdisciplinary rehabilitation plan of care for the client.

Treatment of TBI

Treatment interventions will vary according to an individual's Rancho level. In the early stages of recovery, which correspond to Rancho levels I through III, stimulation treatment is common. Activities focus on arousing the individual's responses, such as being alert to the environment, and attending to incoming stimuli, particularly visual and auditory. For example, the therapist might use an irritating noise like an alarm clock or a bell to attract attention. Tracking the consistency of responses and the modes of stimuli yielding these responses is critical. At this early stage, responses will be inconsistent even for basic commands, such as "Blink your eyes" or "Make a fist."

Rancho levels IV to VI correspond to the middle phase of recovery. At this stage, tasks focus on establishing basic communication systems—whether verbal, gestural, or augmentative (i.e., alternative)—and enhancing the reliability of communication efforts. Initial communication systems may use a picture board, to which the client can point to indicate *bathroom, water,* or *food.* These clients need much structure and assistance from the therapist as they are still highly distractible and frequently are agitated or aggressive. Compensatory strategies, such as notebooks or schedule cards, can support orientation and memory and can improve goal-directed behavior. More structured therapy tasks are appropriate to improve memory, word retrieval, simple problem solving, and following directions as the client progresses.

Persons at Rancho levels VII and VIII are in the later phases of recovery. The focus at this stage is facilitating independence. Treatment stresses insight or judgment to solve problems encountered in daily activities. For example, a client might be helped to problem-solve the following scenario:

> You need to catch the bus and be at work by 9:00 AM. Look at the bus schedule and tell me which bus you should catch to get there on time.

Although much recovery has occurred prior to this stage, new or stressful situations are often difficult for the individual with TBI. Applying new communication and cognitive-linguistic skills to novel situations can cause anxiety and stress. Independence and safety issues should be addressed, using progressive community-based reintegration (e.g., planning a meal, making a grocery list, shopping at the store). Community outings can provide opportunities to apply treatment gains to real-world situations.

Treating clients with TBI requires great flexibility on the part of the therapist to meet their individualized needs as they progress through the Rancho stages. Many clients achieve an independent return to home, work, and society. Unfortunately, some clients do not and remain in early or middle Rancho stages. These individuals will require a structured, supervised, and supportive environment, such as a group home.

Dementia

Dementia is a chronic and progressive decline in memory, cognition, language, and personality resulting from central nervous system dysfunction (Bayles & Tomoeda, 1995). Diseases such as Alzheimer's disease, Huntington's disease, Parkinson's disease, Pick's disease, Creutzfeldt-Jakob disease, and multiple cerebral infarcts (i.e., strokes) can cause dementia. Alzheimer's is the most common cause, representing about 70% of all diagnosed cases (Brookshire, 2003). Dementia is most prevalent in the elderly, with as many as 35% of those 85 years or older exhibiting signs of dementia (Kart & Kinney, 2001). Because the geriatric population (i.e., those over age 65) represents the most rapidly growing demographic segment in the United States, dementia will continue to be a major health concern for this country.

The diagnostic criteria of the American Psychiatric Association (1994) identify three defining traits of dementia:

1. Memory impairment (both short- and long-term memory)
2. Impairment in cognitive skills (abstract thought, judgment, and executive functions)
3. Presence of aphasia, apraxia, or agnosia (i.e., inability to recognize objects, words, or sounds)

In addition, dementia must have a gradual onset with progressive functional decline over time. Dementia does not result from psychological disturbances such as psychosis, schizophrenia, or delirium, although these conditions may coexist in some cases. It is important to determine the cause of dementia since there are medical conditions that produce dementia-like profiles but are reversible, such as metabolic disturbances, infections, drug toxicity, vitamin deficiency, and thyroid disease.

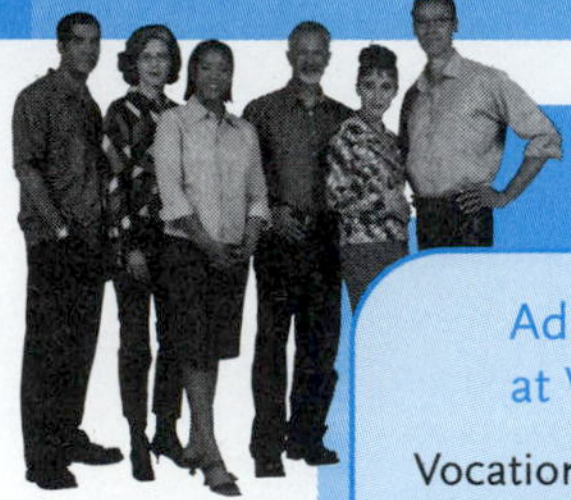

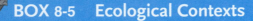

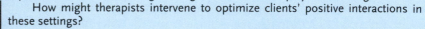

BOX 8-5 Ecological Contexts

Adults with Language and Cognitive-Based Dysfunction in the Home, at Work, and in the Community

Vocational challenges affect many adults with acquired language and cognitive impairments. Most jobs require the ability to communicate, problem-solve, and reason. Some estimates suggest that only about 10% of stroke survivors return to work without impaired performance (Rosenbek, LaPointe, & Wertz, 1989). With federal regulations such as the Family Medical Leave Act and the Americans with Disabilities Act, individuals now have greater potential to maintain their previous employment. These acts provide some degree of job protection and encourage reasonable accommodation for disabled employees.

However, even with these guidelines, gainful productive employment following a stroke can be challenging. Individuals may remain employed but may need to function in an altered capacity. And such changes may represent a change in status within the organization (i.e., a loss of responsibility), reduced wages because a 10-hour workday is now physically impossible, or job reconfiguration. Such modifications can result in work that is no longer professionally satisfying. Such factors likely contribute to the elevated incidence of depression following neurological injury (Bays, 2001).

For Discussion

What are some other ways a cognitive-linguistic impairment might impact an adult's experiences at work following re-integration into the employment setting?

How might therapists intervene to optimize clients' positive interactions in these settings?

Companion Website

To answer these questions online, go to the Ecological Contexts module in chapter 8 of the Companion Website.

Characteristics of Dementia

Since dementia is a progressive decline of skills, the characteristics of dementia are relative to how far the disease has progressed. People with dementia often progress from mild to moderate to severe deficits, with that progress ranging from a slow to a rapid decline.

Characteristics of Mild Dementia. Individuals with mild dementia exhibit forgetfulness, even of basic information or common routines. These memory problems appear as frequently losing or misplacing items, missing appointments, or forgetting a familiar phone number. Language skills at the mild dementia level show decreased vocabulary, reduced or verbose conversation, or anomia, in which the name of something cannot be retrieved. Typically, language comprehension is preserved even though information may not be remembered. Pragmatics and social skills are well preserved at this stage, and motor function is intact, so that the individual is walking, eating, and toileting without difficulty.

Characteristics of Moderate Dementia. The moderate dementia profile is the phase of most dramatic functional change. Here, the individual becomes increasingly disoriented in time and place, exhibits poor attention and memory, and also exhibits marked language difficulties. Deficits of language include significant anomia, difficulty repeating, problems understanding humor, and often empty conversations. At this stage, motor skills are still adequate for walking and eating, although restlessness and roaming are likely.

Characteristics of Severe Dementia. Extreme disorientation and minimal, if any, cognitive ability are defining characteristics of severe dementia. At this stage, language skills are profoundly compromised, with limited meaningful communication and frequent repetitions (i.e., parroting) and jargon. Comprehension skills are also severely impaired. Motor skills at this stage vary, although many individuals are wheelchair dependent and unable to control bladder and bowel functions.

***Discussion Point:** Speech-language treatment for dementia is determined largely by the severity of the disease progression. Consider the case of Mable in Box 8-1. What is the severity of her dementia?*

Identification of Dementia

A team of professionals evaluates suspected dementia to verify its presence, cause, and course of intervention. The speech-language pathologist assesses cognitive and linguistic skills in comparison to normal behaviors. Instruments commonly used to screen mental status include the Mini Mental State Examination (Folstein, Folstein, & McHugh, 1975) and the mental status subtest of the Arizona Battery for Communication Disorders of Dementia (Bayles & Tomoeda, 1993).

More comprehensive testing by the speech-language pathologist typically involves the complete Arizona Battery for Communication Disorders of Dementia (ABCD) (Bayles & Tomoeda, 1993). This standardized battery assesses and evaluates key areas of performance, including linguistic comprehension, linguistic expression, verbal memory, visuospatial skills, and mental status. Scores of the ABCD guide clinical judgments on the presence of dementia as well as the severity. Individualized intervention plans are then developed, based on these findings.

Treatment of Dementia

Speech-language treatment is determined largely by the severity of the dementia. In mild to even moderate cases, treatment can help to compensate for deficits (Bayles & Kim, 2003). Environmental changes to promote safety are imperative, and education for family members or caregivers is emphasized to provide specific training. Family members might be trained, for instance, to give verbal cueing for dressing or eating (e.g., "First you pick up the spoon"). Strategies to manage potential behavioral issues are important, as well as measures to minimize frustration for the client and the caregiver. Active support groups for care providers are encouraged. In cases of severe dementia, the speech-language pathologist and other professionals serve as consultants, providing management strategies. Unfortunately, the resources to provide care in many of these cases are beyond the physical, emotional, and financial capabilities of some families. At this point, long-term placement is necessary in a nursing home or supportive group environment where the client has professional caregivers.

Case Study and Clinical Problem Solving

SPEECH-LANGUAGE PATHOLOGY EVALUATION REPORT

Client: Thomas Driver
Date of Birth/Age: 18 May 1939, 66 years
Referral Source: Michael Demacio, M.D.
Date of Evaluation: 1 November 2005

History

Thomas Driver is a 66-year-old, right-handed Caucasian male, referred for a comprehensive speech-language evaluation following a left middle cerebral artery stroke on 26 October 2005. Mr. Driver's neurological status was initially stabilized on the acute medical floor at St. Patrick's Hospital, after which he was transferred to the acute rehabilitation unit on 31 October 2005.

Mr. Driver currently presents with right hemiparesis of the face, arm, and leg, right visual field deficits, and communication difficulties. His past medical history reveals hypertension, elevated cholesterol, and noninsulin-dependent diabetes (adult onset, Type II).

He was followed regularly by his family physician for these issues and was compliant in taking his prescribed medications. He is a smoker (reported at half a pack per day) and has limited alcohol intake (three drinks weekly, typically wine).

Mr. Driver is a retired architect who holds a master's degree. He resides with his wife of 40 years, Alice, in a single-level home that he designed for their retirement years. They have 4 adult children, 2 of whom reside in the area. Mr. Driver has enjoyed golfing and building model airplanes as hobbies. He has been very active in his church. The Drivers' goal is to return home and enjoy their retirement.

Current Findings

1. *Oral Motor Examination:* Mr. Driver's speech rates were slowed and labored. His right facial weakness was notable on appearance and in oral movement tasks (e.g., when he protruded his tongue, it deviated to the right). He showed some groping of articulators in repetition tasks.
2. *Swallowing Status:* Results from the videofluoroscopic modified barium study (VFMBS) conducted on 28 October 2005 showed a moderate oral phase dysphagia but no apparent aspiration. Please refer to the VFMBS report for a comprehensive review of findings.
3. *Hearing Screening:* Pure tone audiological screening was completed with passing performance.
4. *Articulation Findings:* Articulatory performance revealed slurring and slowed rate consistent with a mild dysarthria. His performance also suggested a coexisting mild verbal apraxia.
5. *Language Findings:* Mr. Driver was administered the Western Aphasia Battery to evaluate a suspected aphasia. He wore his prescribed reading glasses throughout the testing. He received an aphasia quotient of 56 of 100 possible points, suggesting a moderate to severe aphasia.
6. *Voice Findings:* No past medical history or new findings suggested a problem.
7. *Fluency Findings:* No past medical history or new findings suggested a problem.
8. *Cognitive Findings:* Results of this testing suggested no cognitive deficits. However, Mr. Driver is currently completing neuropsychological testing, which may be more sensitive to this area.

Clinical Impressions

Results of initial evaluation using the Western Aphasia Battery and behavioral observations show a moderate to severe Broca's aphasia with coexisting mild dysarthria and apraxia of speech. He has mild-moderate oral phase dysphagia, requiring an altered diet. His hearing, voice, fluency, and cognitive status seem normal. The prognosis for improvement in functional communication abilities is positive, given his short time postonset stroke, prestroke educational level, relatively young age, supportive family, and ability and efforts to actively participate in therapy.

Recommendations

Based on the information obtained through assessment, it is recommended that Mr. Driver participate in individual speech-language intervention for his aphasia for 2 30-min. sessions, 5 days per week. I also recommend participation in the Aphasia Communication Group twice weekly.

Arlyn Lucas, M.A., CCC/SLP

CLINICAL PROBLEM SOLVING

1. What aspects of Mr. Driver's background may have increased his risk of having a stroke?
2. The clinician indicated a positive prognosis for Mr. Driver. What are the reasons provided for this positive prognosis?
3. How likely is it that Mr. Driver will adhere to the treatment recommendations?

CHAPTER SUMMARY

Adult aphasia and other cognitive-based dysfunctions result from neurological injuries such as stroke, traumatic brain injury, or progressive diseases. These disorders occur after language and cognition are mature or established.

Aphasia occurs when the language-dominant hemisphere, typically the left hemisphere, is damaged. Stroke is the most common cause of aphasia. Aphasia is differentiated into several different syndromes based on analysis of fluency and motor output, language comprehension, repetition, and naming. The predominant aphasia syndromes include Broca's, Wernicke's, global, anomic, conduction, transcortical motor, and transcortical sensory.

Other acquired communication problems include right hemisphere dysfunction, traumatic brain injury, and dementia. Right hemisphere dysfunction (RHD) most often results from stroke, which damages regions of the right hemisphere. Characteristics of RHD may include difficulties with receptive and expressive language as well as significant problems in perception, behavior, and cognition. Traumatic brain injury (TBI) occurs with both open- and closed-head injuries. TBI is most frequently a result of motor vehicle accidents, falls, or acts of violence. Deficits following TBI are highly diverse but may include alterations in consciousness, cognition, language, and behavior. Dementia describes a progressive decline in functional skills, most notably cognitive abilities. There is variability across performance profiles of individuals with dementia, largely based on the disease progression or stage.

The adult communication disorders of aphasia, RHD, TBI, and dementia hinder an individual's ability to function in daily routines and responsibilities. Affected adults often face disruptions in their social, vocational, and psychological well-being. Family roles are also affected. An interdisciplinary team approach to prevention, evaluation, treatment, and education for these adults and their families is necessary. The speech-language pathologist plays a key role in the rehabilitation of aphasia and other cognitive-based disorders through comprehensive evaluation, efficacy-based and personalized treatments, and education.

KEY TERMS

anomia, p. 263
aphasia, p. 256
apraxia, p. 259
circumlocution, p. 267
closed-head injuries, p. 277
dementia, p. 279
dysarthria, p. 259
echolalia, p. 267
evidence-based practice, p. 271
functional outcomes, p. 274
jargon, p. 266
logorrhea, p. 266
macrographia, p. 265
neologisms, p. 266
open-head injuries, p. 276
paraphasias, p. 263
prognostic indicators, p. 270
prosody, p. 266
right hemisphere dysfunction, p. 275
spontaneous recovery, p. 268
taxonomy, p. 260
traumatic brain injury, p. 276

ON THE WEB

Check out the Companion Website! On it you will find

- suggested readings
- reflection questions
- a self-study quiz
- hot topics
- current technological innovations
- links to online resources

Pediatric Feeding and Swallowing Disorders

Mary C. Tarbell
Laura M. Justice

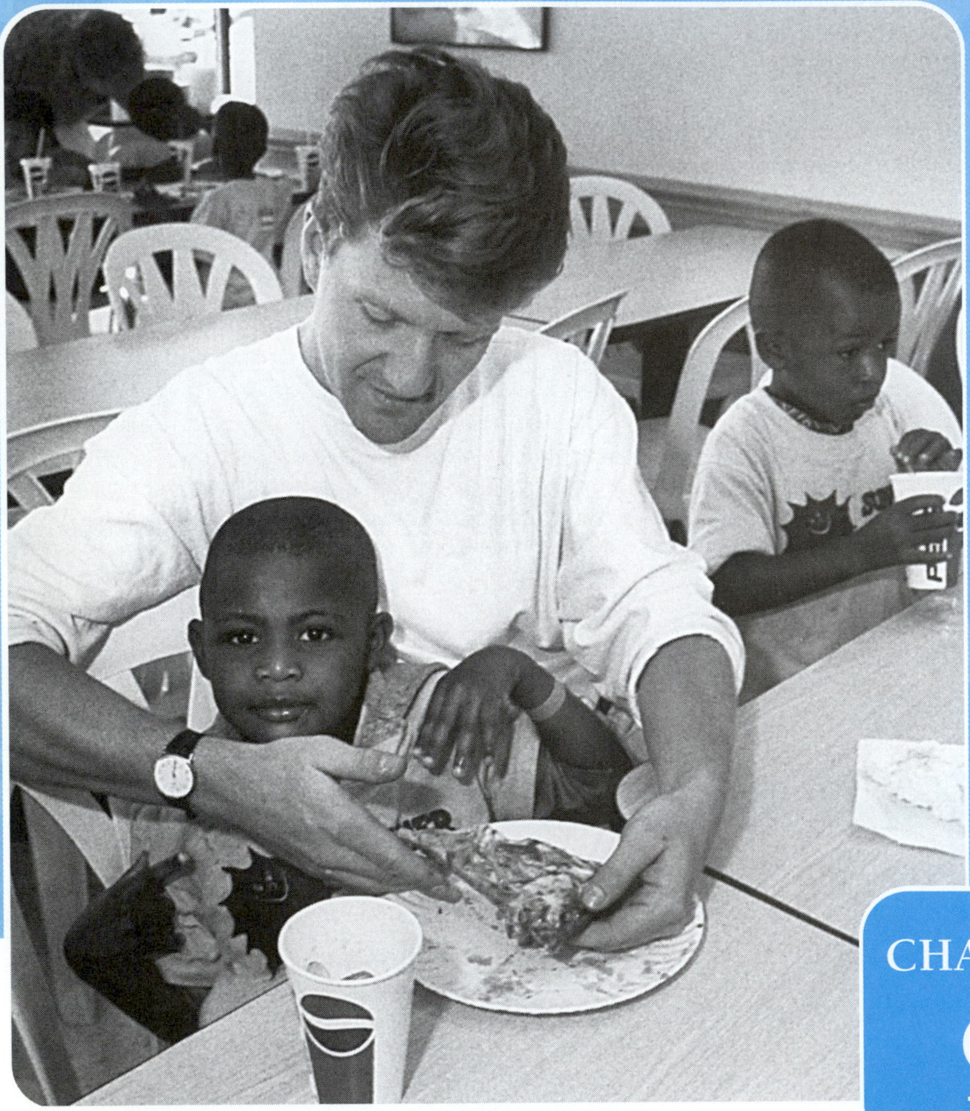

CHAPTER 9

FOCUS QUESTIONS

This chapter answers the following questions:

1. What are pediatric feeding and swallowing disorders?
2. How are pediatric feeding and swallowing disorders classified?
3. What are the defining characteristics of prevalent types of pediatric feeding and swallowing disorders?
4. How are pediatric feeding and swallowing disorders identified?
5. How are pediatric feeding and swallowing disorders treated?

INTRODUCTION

Children must eat to develop physically, cognitively, and psychologically. When eating does not happen regularly and effortlessly for young children, growth and development are compromised. Feeding in early childhood is also particularly important to communication development, as it promotes bonding and attachment between children and caregivers and the development of critical communicative routines, including turn-taking and joint attention. Thus, breakdowns in feeding can have serious nutritional consequences as well as a negative impact on the developing child's physical, cognitive, psychological, and communicative development.

This chapter provides a basic introduction to feeding and swallowing disorders in pediatric populations. You might wonder why a chapter on pediatric feeding and swallowing disorders is included in an introductory textbook on communication disorders. Good question! The assessment and treatment of feeding and swallowing disorders in young children involve many professionals because of the complexities of feeding and swallowing dysfunctions and the vital importance of feeding and swallowing to the child's short- and long-term growth and development. For both of these reasons, when children exhibit feeding and swallowing problems, many skilled professionals work together as a multidisciplinary team to share expertise. A number of disciplines offer a specialization in pediatric feeding and swallowing disorders, and each discipline brings unique and essential guidance—nutritionists, gastroenterologists, radiologists, feeding specialists, and more (see Table 9-1).

The speech-language pathologist who specializes in feeding and swallowing disorders in children serves as the **feeding specialist** and carries the responsibility of strengthening the child's oral-motor system and building the capacity for safe feeding and swallowing. The **oral-motor system** refers to the physical structures and neuromuscular functions involved with both eating and speaking. The feeding

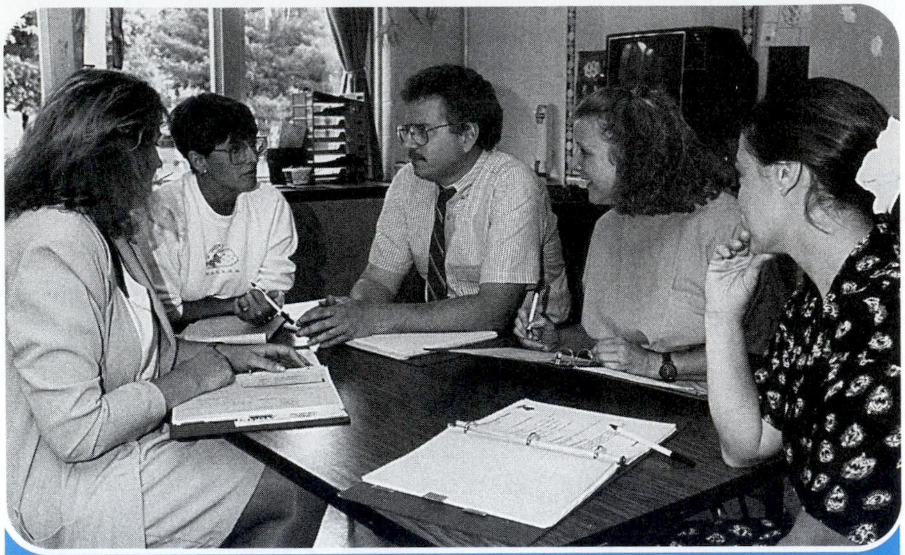

The last decades have seen considerable growth in research on how to rehabilitate swallowing functions.

specialist focuses on improving **oral-motor functions** (i.e., the strength and coordination of the articulators), **oral-motor muscular tone** (i.e., the tension and posture of the articulators), and **oral-motor sensation** (i.e., the sensitivity to taste, movement, and textures; Creskoff & Haas, 1999). This chapter provides basic information on pediatric feeding and swallowing disorders and the role of the feeding specialist in their management.

TABLE 9-1 Multidisciplinary team members involved with pediatric feeding and swallowing disorders

Professional	Role
Cardiologist	Evaluation and treatment of cardiac deficits
Cranio-facial surgeon	Evaluation and treatment of structural deficits such as cleft palate
Infant educator	Cognitive and developmental assessment
Nutritionist	Evaluation and treatment of growth and nutrition, including monitoring of caloric intake
Occupational therapist	Evaluation and treatment of sensory processing disorders and fine motor skills
Pediatric gastroenterologist	Evaluation and treatment of gastrointestinal disorders, including the digestive system (esophagus, stomach, small and large intestines)
Pediatrician/family physician	Overall management and referral to specialists; maintenance of developmental history and follow-up; monitoring of growth and development
Physical therapist	Evaluation of motor skills and posture/stability while eating
Psychologist	Evaluation and treatment of behavioral and parent-child interactional aspects that influence feeding disturbance
Pulmonologist	Evaluation and treatment of pulmonary difficulties that affect breathing
Radiologist	Placement of gastrostomy tubes for long-term feeding; evaluation of swallowing difficulties via fluoroscopy
Social worker	Evaluation of family supports, including economic circumstances, family stresses, possible abuse and neglect; location of community and federal resources
Speech-language pathologist	Evaluation and treatment of oral motor deficits that affect swallowing; evaluation and treatment of feeding disorders

What Are Pediatric Feeding and Swallowing Disorders?

Definition

Feeding disorders are a grave and immediate concern in early childhood, because feeding is the route to proper nutrition, healthy growth, and optimal development. The American Psychiatric Association (APA; 1994) defines a *feeding disorder* as a child's "persistent failure to eat adequately" for a period of at least 1 month, which results in a significant loss of weight or a failure to gain weight (p. 98). Feeding disorders are manifested prior to 6 years of age, and in most cases the onset is in the first year of life. Feeding disorders can occur as part of a broader medical or developmental condition, such as cleft palate, or they can occur in apparent isolation and with no clear cause. In addition to the failure to eat adequately, the child with a feeding disorder usually demonstrates one or more of the following:

- Unsafe or inefficient swallowing patterns
- Growth delay affecting height and/or weight
- Lack of tolerance of food textures and tastes
- Poor appetite regulation
- Rigid eating patterns

A *swallowing disorder* is a specific type of feeding disorder in which the child exhibits an unsafe or inefficient swallowing pattern that undermines the feeding process. Swallowing, also called **deglutition**, is the complex neuromuscular act of moving substances from the oral cavity to the esophagus. The substance being moved is generically called the *bolus*. The act of swallowing involves preparation of the bolus in the oral cavity and execution of the swallow to move the bolus from the oral cavity to the esophagus.

Although swallowing is obviously critical to the nutritional purposes of the feeding process, it is also crucial for *safe* feeding. Only a slim margin of error separates the pathway for breathing (i.e., the airway) from the pathway of the bolus. Unsafe swallowing can be a life-or-death matter, as poor management and coordination of swallowing increases a child's risk of penetration or aspiration of food or liquid into the laryngeal area, which serves as the gateway to and the protector of the lungs (see Figure 9-1). With **penetration**, food or liquid enters the larynx, which can cause choking and respiratory distress. With **aspiration**, the food

FIGURE 9-1 An infant's laryngeal area, depicting pathways for nutrition and respiration.

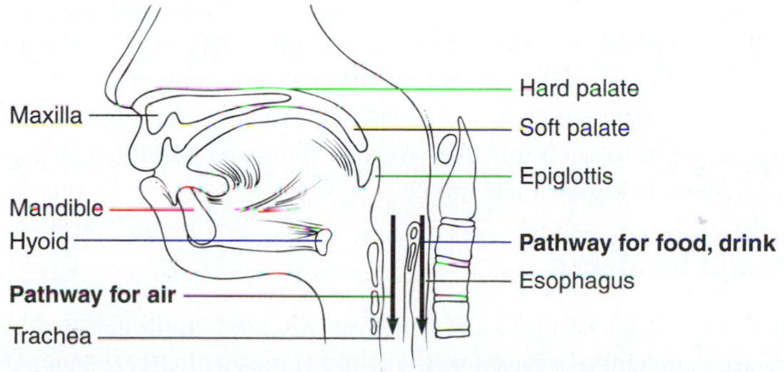

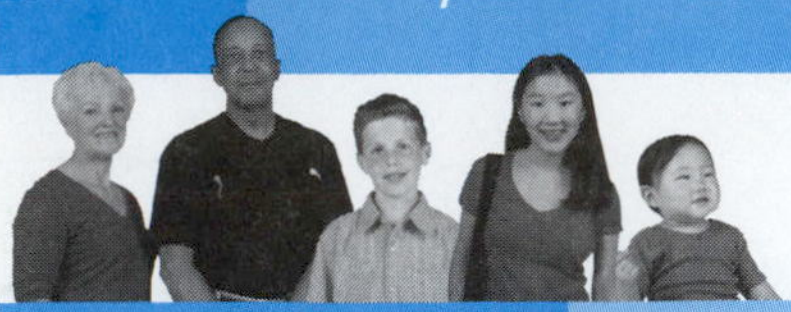

BOX 9-1 Pediatric Feeding and Swallowing Disorders: Case Examples

Lily is a 2-year-old girl living in Omaha, Nebraska. She was born with the umbilical cord tightly wrapped around her neck, resulting in a lack of oxygen during the birthing process and brain damage that led to cerebral palsy and oral motor dysfunction. At birth, Lily could not coordinate a suck-swallow-breathe pattern and demonstrated frequent choking and gagging. A modified barium swallow study at 2 weeks revealed aspiration during bottle feeding and poor coordination of the tongue during sucking. Lily had a gastrostomy tube placed at 3 weeks to provide nutrition. Now, on her second birthday, her parents would like to begin feeding her orally. Lily uses a wheelchair for mobility and positioning and has no functional use of her hands. Cognitively, Lily is delayed but appears to understand some family members' names.

Internet research

1. How common is it for a child to be born with the umbilical cord wrapped around its neck?
2. What kind of community resources are available in Omaha, Nebraska, for Lily's family?
3. How prevalent is cerebral palsy due to perinatal birth trauma?

Brainstorm and discussion

1. How do you think Lily's feeding and swallowing difficulties affect her family?
2. Given that Lily has been on a feeding tube for 2 years, why would her parents want to pursue oral intake at this time?
3. What other aspects of Lily's life might be affected by her dependence on a gastrostomy tube for nutrition?

David is a 3-month-old male who has stayed in the neonatal intensive care unit (NICU) since his premature birth at 30 weeks. He is the youngest of four children born into the Lopez family of Tucson, Arizona. David was originally fed orally but consistently demonstrated coughing and choking while bottle feeding. The NICU feeding therapist thickened David's formula slightly with rice cereal, which decreased his coughing and choking during feeding. However, David then seemed to become very fatigued during feeding and would fall asleep prior to completing his meal. As a result, David had poor weight gain and has since been on a nasogastric tube for supplemental feeding. This tube runs down his nose and into his stomach and allows the nurses to feed him the rest of the formula that he is unable to take in efficiently by mouth.

Internet research

1. Find the Website for a neonatal intensive care unit in a hospital near or in your hometown. How many infants does it see annually? What professionals work in the NICU?

or liquid passes through the larynx and into the lungs, which can interfere with the exchange of air in the lungs and cause asphyxiation or a pulmonary infection, such as pneumonia.

Not all children with feeding disorders have problems with swallowing, but all children with swallowing problems exhibit a feeding disorder. Thus, children with swallowing disorders represent a subset of the larger population of children with feeding disorders. In addition to managing the failure to eat adequately, treatment for a swallowing disorder requires training the child to safely and effectively swallow *and* providing alternative feeding for the period in which swallowing is unsafe.

Prevalence and Incidence

Mild and transient feeding problems are common in young children; 25–35% of parents report that their young children have feeding issues (Linscheid, 1992; Satter, 1986). These

2. How likely is it that David will be discharged from the NICU? Find the statistics on the general rate of discharge for premature infants from the NICU.

Brainstorm and discussion

1. How might David's NICU admittance affect his family?
2. What are some ways that David's parents might be involved with his feeding while he is in the NICU?

Cory is a 2-year-old boy in Parkersburg, West Virginia, with an unremarkable birth history. Starting at 6 weeks of age, Cory began projectile vomiting during breast feeding. He was placed on medication to help decrease the vomiting and went back to eating and growing well. At 6 months of age he was removed from all medications, and his parents introduced baby foods. Cory overtly refused baby foods but continued to breast-feed well. At 9 months his growth was slowing down, and his vomiting increased. He continued to fight the introduction of baby foods, and meals became unpleasant for the whole family. Cory was hospitalized at 11 months for failure to thrive and diagnosed with behavioral feeding aversion. By 14 months of age he had a gastrostomy tube placed and was eating very little orally. Now, at 2 years, Cory's parents are seeking his enrollment in an intensive behavioral feeding program to wean Cory from tube feeding and improve his oral feeding.

Internet research

1. What types of feeding programs are available to children like Cory? How much does a program like this cost?
2. What are some suspected causes of projectile vomiting in infants?
3. How many children in the United States are currently fed using a gastrostomy tube?

Brainstorm and discussion

1. How could Cory's feeding problems affect his family and his own psychological well-being?
2. What are some possible causes of Cory's food aversions?
3. What are some factors that might predict whether Cory will successfully be weaned from the feeding tube?

temporary feeding problems may emerge at certain developmental points, such as the transition to solid foods, but they usually resolve easily with no negative effect on the developing child (Black, Cureton, & Berenson-Howard, 1999). More serious and persistent feeding problems are less common; their prevalence is difficult to estimate. As many as 10% of young children experience malnutrition, although the proportion of these cases accounted for by feeding and swallowing disorders is not clear (Kessler, 1999). Of children admitted to the hospital for failure to gain adequate weight, about half are due to feeding disturbances (APA, 1994).

Discussion Point: *Consider the children described in Box 9-1. Characterize the developmental point at which each child's difficulties emerged. What seemed to trigger each child's feeding problem?*

Feeding disorders become more prevalent in the context of specific risk factors. For instance, about 8% of all babies born in the United States have a very low birth weight—308,470 babies in the year 2000 (Maternal and Child Health Bureau, 2002). These and other conditions described later greatly elevate the likelihood of feeding and/or swallowing disorders in young children (Black et al., 1999; Satter, 1999).

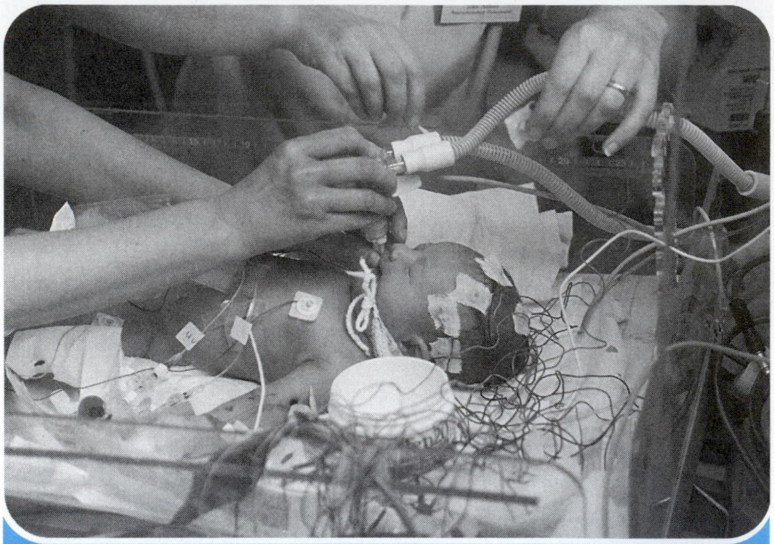

Infants who are born at very low birth weights are at relatively greater risk of developing feeding problems.

Conditions that cause frailty in infants are increasing in their prevalence. In the last decade the likelihood that very low birth weight infants would survive to leave the hospital increased 10%, from 74% to 84% (Lemons et al., 2001). From the very start of their lives, many of these children exhibit significant impairments of feeding and require the earliest of interventions while in the neonatal intensive care unit **(NICU)**. Not only do these children's fragile medical states complicate the feeding process, but the NICU treatments themselves can directly interfere with the development of pleasurable oral experiences—for example, the use of nasogastric feeding tubes for high-calorie nutritional support and ventilators to provide oxygen, as described in Table 9-2.

In addition, children served in the NICU may have limited exposure to foods and thus may have missed out on the

TABLE 9-2 Common neonatal intensive care procedures that can impact feeding and swallowing development

Procedure	Purpose	Description
Enteral (tube) feeding	• Provides a temporary means to improve the child's nutrition and growth when at least 80% of nutritional needs cannot be met orally and weight loss or no gain occurs for 3 months • Used for prematurity, lack of weight gain, gastrointestinal dysfunctions, severe diarrhea, coma, feeding refusal, failure to thrive	• Nasogastric tube passed through nose and esophagus for short-term feeding (<3 months) • Gastrostomy tube surgically placed directly into the stomach for long-term feeding (>3 months) • Jejunostomy tube surgically placed into the jejunum, or small intestine, also for long-term feeding
Tracheostomy	• Provides an alternative airway when the airway is blocked by congenital or acquired airway obstruction • Also used to provide oxygen supplements for cardiopulmonary disease or an infant unable to breathe adequately because of prematurity or trauma and requiring a ventilator	• An incision made into the trachea, or airway • A tracheostomy tube placed into the incision to provide an airway that bypasses the oral/nasal cavity
Ventilation	• Provides an alternative or supplementary source of oxygen when a child cannot breathe because of an immature respiratory system or injury or impairment of the respiratory system (e.g., chronic lung disease) • Supplemental oxygen needed by nearly one fourth of very low birth weight children up to 9 months after birth	• Mechanical ventilation attached to child via a tracheostomy tube

Sources: Based on Kedesdy and Budd (1998); Lemons, Bauer, Oh, et al. (2001), Schauster and Dwyer (1996).

opportunity to progress normally and/or safely in the early stages of feeding development, learn feeding routines, and to experience different tastes and textures. These children may have an inability to manipulate food safely in their mouths and may have increased aversion to foods because of their lack of experience. This may increase the likelihood that these children will demonstrate food refusal, inappropriate meal time behaviors, and/or inefficient ingestion.

Discussion Point: *Consider the case of David in Box 9-1. In addition to having early feeding challenges, explore how being in the NICU might complicate his feeding development.*

Terminology

Nutrition

Nutrition describes an individual's intake of calories and nutrients to meet requirements for energy, growth, development, and learning. Nutrition involves an adequate intake of fats, amino acids, proteins, vitamins, and minerals to support the body's protein utilization, cell growth, blood quality, and overall healthy development (Cunningham & McLaughlin, 1999). The National Academy of Sciences (1989) provides recommended dietary allowances (RDAs), which are standards of nutrition for normal, healthy development. A food guide pyramid depicting these recommendations for young children is shown in Figure 9-2. RDA standards are also available to guide parents and other caregivers of infants and toddlers during their first 2 years of life. This time frame coincides with rapid growth and development; infants triple their birth weight and double their body length in just the first 12 months of life (Cunningham & McLaughlin, 1999).

Undernutrition and **malnutrition** describe conditions in which children's basic nutritional requirements are not being met, most often because of environmental circumstances (e.g., poverty) or developmental disabilities (e.g., cerebral palsy). You might think that in a country as wealthy and prosperous as the United States, pediatric undernutrition and malnutrition would be rare, if not nonexistent. Unfortunately, about one fifth of children and their families in the United States experience regular food shortages (Wehler, Scott, Anderson, & Parker, 1991), necessitating numerous federal and state programs focused specifically on providing nutritional support to families and children—for example, food stamps, soup kitchens, and free/reduced school lunches.

Discussion Point: *What resources are you aware of in your local community to help children and families experiencing food shortages?*

Growth

Nutrition is important because it is the fuel for children's growth. Growth describes children's height/length and weight achievements, as well as the weight-to-length relationship. The greatest detriment to growth is poor nutrition, which undermines children's growth potential, or the amount of growth they could experience given proper nutrition.

As children develop, their height and weight are regularly monitored by health providers using **growth charts**, as shown in Figure 9-3. In this figure the bottom part of the chart depicts seven growth curves for weight over the first 27 months; the top part of the chart depicts seven growth curves for length. These curves correspond to percentile rankings—5th, 10th, 25th, 50th, 75th, 90th, and 95th—to indicate a child's relative standing among all infants. Such rankings are most useful for plotting children's growth trajectory, or growth pattern, over time. By plotting growth, professionals can differentiate between children who are small and those who are *becoming* small—that is, children who are faltering in height and/or weight (Berhane & Dietz, 1999).

The bold dots superimposed on the chart in Figure 9-3 illustrate one child's progress in height and length from birth to 24 months. This child is growing in length at roughly the 50th percentile but falters in weight from the 75th percentile at 4 months to the 5th percentile at 15 months. Thus, 95 out of 100 infants would have weighed more than this child at this stage of development.

FIGURE 9-2 Food guide pyramid for young children.

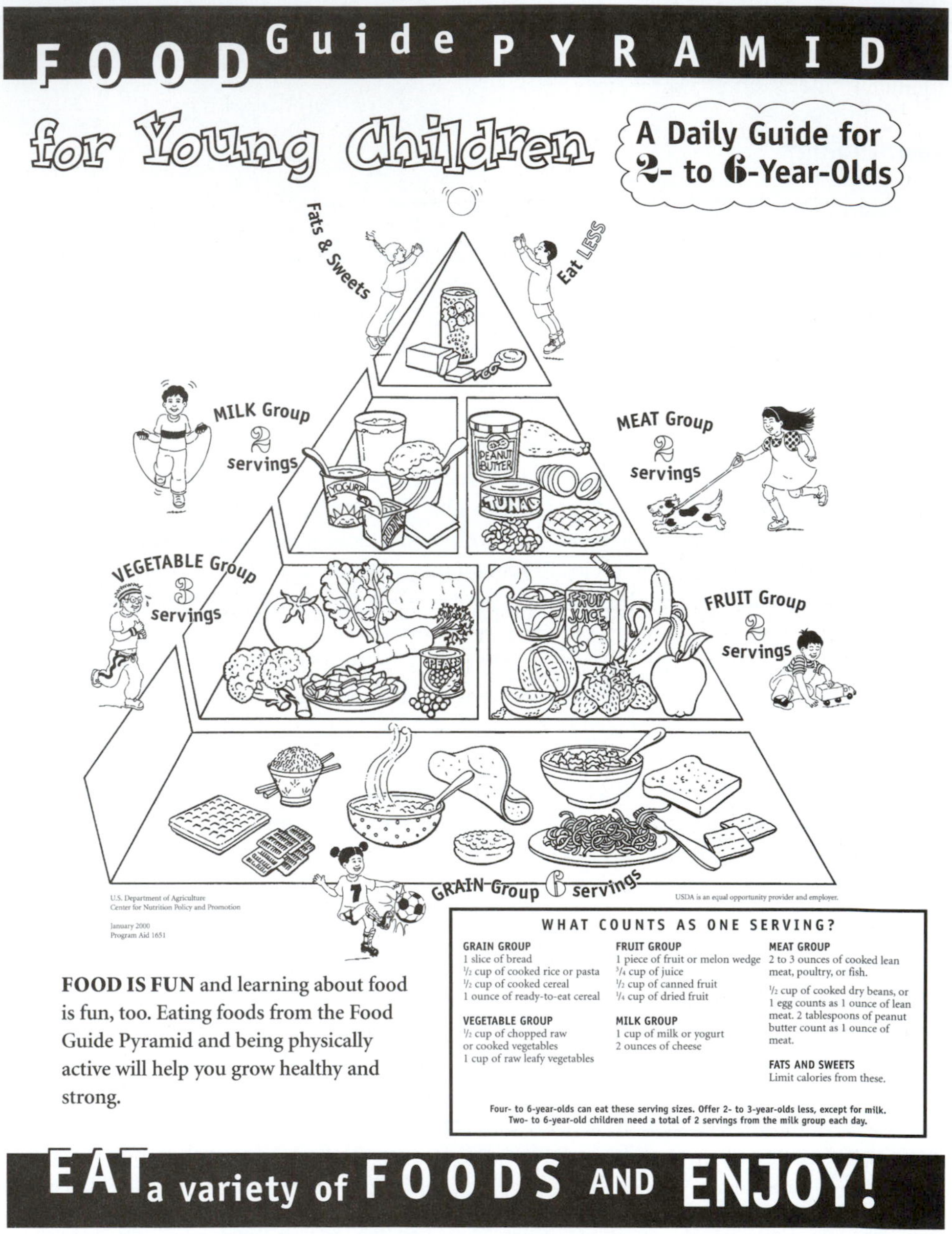

Source: From the U.S. Department of Agriculture.

Experts use three different categories to describe growth deficiencies: underweight, wasting, and stunting. The child who is **underweight** weighs less than expected, based on age. The child who is **wasting** weighs less than expected, based on height; in other words, weight is too low relative to height. This usually indicates an acute situation in which a child has experienced sudden and extreme weight loss, perhaps due to illness (Berhane & Dietz, 1999). The child who is **stunting** is shorter than expected, based on age; this typically signifies long-standing malnutrition or undernutrition.

For children who experience growth deficiencies, interventions can remedy the situation. **Catch-up growth** describes an increase in growth velocity as children recover from a period of growth deficiency, as shown in Figure 9-3 for the child whose length and weight are being monitored (Berhane & Dietz, 1999). Carefully designed interventions in which children take in specific amounts of calories, vitamins, and minerals for an extended period of time can prompt a period of catch-up growth following malnutrition or undernutrition (Cunningham & McLaughlin, 1999).

FIGURE 9-3 Infant/toddler growth curves for length and weight.

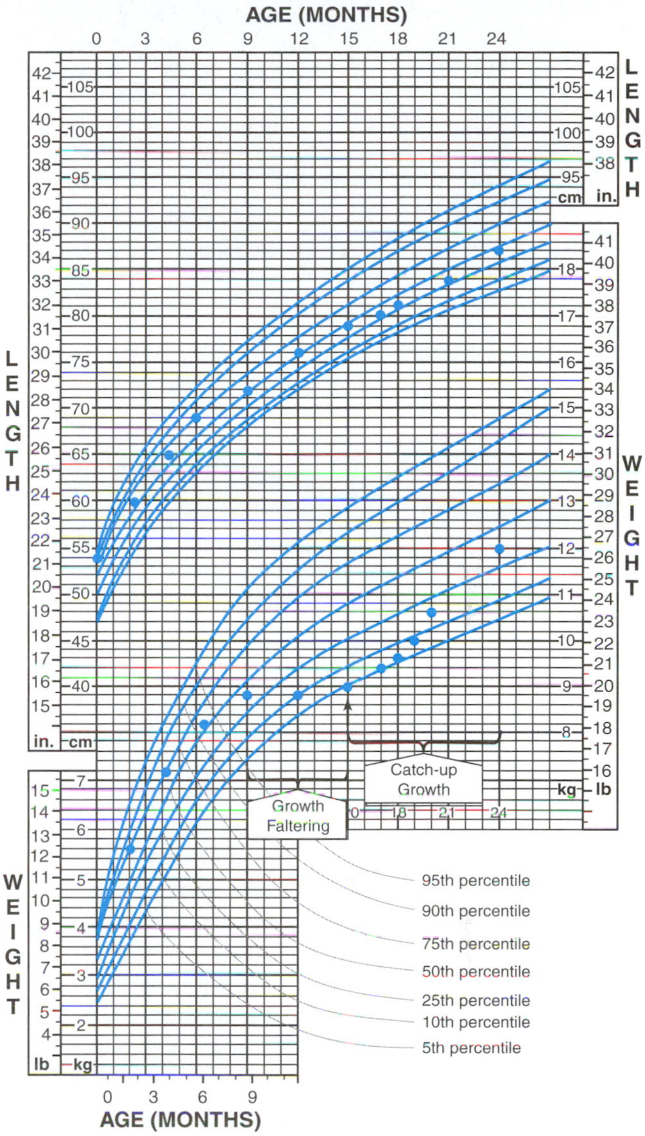

Source: From "Clinical Assessment of Growth" by R. Berhane and W. G. Dietz, 1999, in D. B. Kessler and P. Dawson (Eds.), *Failure to Thrive and Pediatric Undernutrition: A Transdisciplinary Approach* (p. 200), Baltimore: Paul H. Brookes. Copyright 1999 by Brookes. Reprinted with permission.

Feeding and Swallowing Development

The development of feeding skills is a long, complex process that begins at birth. Because infants are born with several reflexes that greatly facilitate feeding, the process *should be* effortless, efficient, effective, and pleasurable. The subsequent 2 years feature many important transitions as the child moves from a reflexive feeder to a self-feeder with specific food preferences. We provide a brief overview of these major transitions here, and Figure 9-4 depicts their timeline.

Birth to Six Months. At birth, babies possess an estimated 27 primitive reflexes, of which four greatly facilitate their ability to feed outside the womb: suckling, rooting, grasping, and gagging (Payne & Isaacs, 1995). The **suckling reflex**, which emerges prenatally, is elicited by stimulating an infant's lips; the infant presses its tongue upward and forward and creates a negative pressure chamber in the oral cavity, which draws fluid in from a nipple. This suck is followed by a swallow, called suck-swallow coordination. Infants are born with sucking pads in their cheeks, which provide for closer contact of the cheeks with the tongue and palate to reduce the amount of pressure needed to pull milk from a nipple. The **rooting**, or search, **reflex** is elicited by stimulating the area around the infant's mouth, causing the infant's head to turn in the direction of the stimulus. This reflex helps the infant locate a source of nourishment. The **grasping reflex**, or *palmar grasp,* enables the infant's fingers to close snugly around a stimulus to the palm. This provides a physical bond between the caregiver and the infant during feeding. The **gagging reflex** is a protective reflex, also present at birth but persisting through the lifespan. In contrast, the suckling, rooting, and grasping reflexes will shift to voluntary rather than involuntary acts by the 3rd month. The gagging reflex is a strong physical reaction to substances entering the laryngeal area, protecting the larynx from foreign entry.

Protection against gagging is important for the infant, as the infant's pharyngeal structures are relatively short in length and the larynx sits relatively high in the neck. The baby's tongue almost completely fills the oral cavity and sits further forward than an adult's. The tightness and close proximity of the infant's tongue, soft palate, pharynx, and larynx obligate the infant to breathe through its nose. The closeness of these features makes it even

FIGURE 9-4 Feeding development from birth to 26 months.

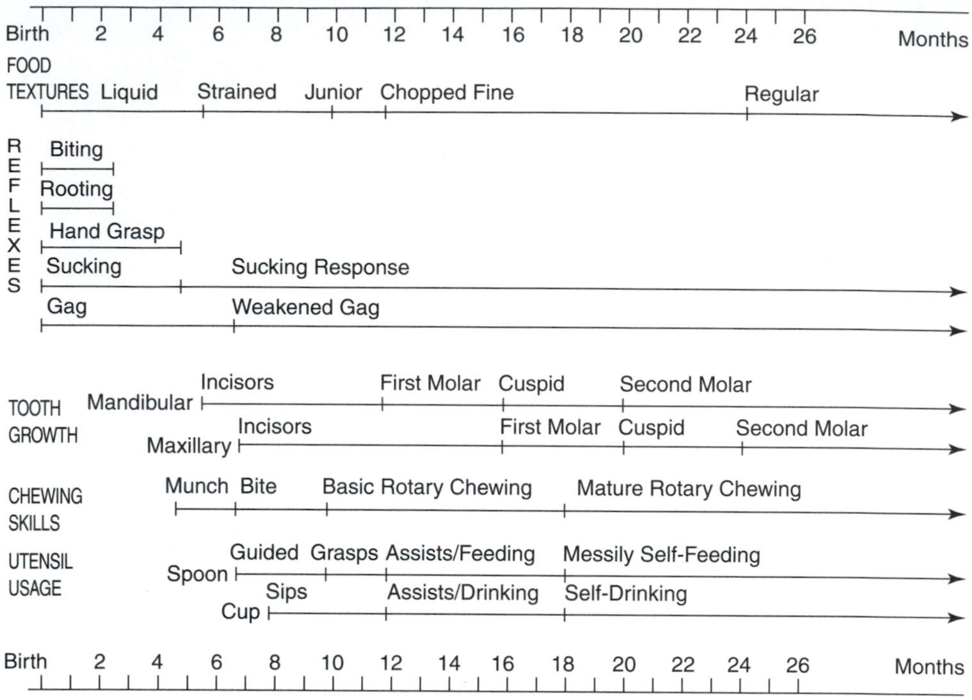

Source: From "Pediatric Feeding Disorders" by S. O' Brien, A. D. Repp, G. E. Williams, and E. R. Christopherson, 1991, *Behavioral Modification, 15,* pp. 394–418. Reprinted with permission.

more important to be able to coordinate safe suckling and swallowing. As a child matures, there is enlargement and forward movement of the mandible, and the tongue's relative proportion becomes smaller as the lips and cheeks enlarge and become firmer.

An important element of early feeding development is the infant's development of **homeostasis**—a quiet, alert, and wakeful state (Satter, 1999). The infant slowly becomes more organized and able to regulate itself, and the caregiver learns how to promote the infant's homeostatic state, not over- or understimulating the child when feeding. Learning to effectively communicate hunger and to safely, efficiently, and effectively ingest enough calories to grow is enough to keep infants busy for several months. For their part, caregivers must learn to accurately read the infant's hunger cues—referred to as *cue sensitivity*—and then further decipher cues about positioning, pacing, and quantity.

Discussion Point: *Why would emotional difficulties between a parent and a child be played out in the feeding context? Explore some possible reasons for this.*

Feeding is one of the first social contacts between parent and infant and is a critical context in which attachment develops. The infant's self-regulation and the caregiver's cue sensitivity both contribute to the caregiver-child attachment, which occurs between 2 and 6 months. Satter (1999) notes that "emotional difficulties between parents and children play themselves out in feeding and may be reflected in the infant's growth" (p. 132). If infant-parent attachment is underdeveloped, the infant may act out during feeding, fail to signal hunger, or resist feeding altogether (Satter, 1999).

Six Months to Twelve Months. When the infant reaches the age of 6 months or so and has increased trunk support and head control for sitting, parents often begin offering solid foods, such as mashed potatoes, soft diced fruits, or rice. At this point the infant's oral-motor patterns begin to transition from mainly anterior-to-posterior (front-to-back) movement to a more up-and-down munching pattern, with more active biting as the infant begins to grow some teeth. This can be an exciting time for caregivers as the change in the infant's positioning from reclining to upright allows for more face-to-face contact, social interaction, and increased reciprocity between caregiver and infant.

By 8 to 9 months, infants are independently sitting and have some trunk rotation. Babies are very curious and very oral at this age and increasingly prefer self-feeding. During this period *everything* goes into the mouth, which is an important way infants explore the world. Now babies are learning to produce a pincer grasp to pick up small foods, such as Cheerios, pieces of banana, and soft cooked vegetables. They have not yet mastered chewing; they usually have only a few teeth and do not have the rotary movements needed to effectively masticate, or chew, tough foods. They are, however, able to chew on more lumpy foods and to break semisoft foods into small enough pieces for safe swallowing. This period of time, the second half of the first year, is a critical determinant of the child's future acceptance of foods (Stevenson & Allaire, 1991).

Twelve Months and Beyond. At 12 months of age, babies are continually delighted by new tastes and textures. They are now manipulating more highly textured foods with their gums and teeth for increased chewing and mashing. They may begin to desire more independence and may no longer wish to be fed with a spoon by a caregiver. Unlikely a coincidence, children at this time also increasingly have the words to express these feelings, as in "No want!" By 18 months most toddlers are effective, efficient eaters and get many of their calories through regular table foods, eating what the rest of the family eats. They are able to handle a variety of food textures and consistencies, although total mastery of all foods is not expected until closer to 24 months.

How Are Pediatric Feeding and Swallowing Disorders Classified?

The effective and efficient treatment of pediatric feeding and swallowing disorders requires careful determination of both descriptive features and etiology. Classification of disorders based on descriptive features focuses on the clinical presentation, or observable symptoms, of the disorder. Classification based on etiology focuses on known or suspected causes of the disorder. Table 9-3 provides an overview of the major classification systems.

Descriptive Features

Transient, Episodic, and Chronic Disorders

One way of describing feeding and swallowing disorders is to describe the time frame or duration of the disorder. A *transient* feeding and swallowing problem is one that is short lived or readily correctable. Take, for example, a baby with a cleft lip that has difficulty maintaining a strong suck because it cannot close both lips tightly around a nipple. This feeding problem may be short lived because it is easily correctable by using an alternative method of oral intake or an adapted nipple. Additionally, once the child's cleft lip is repaired at 3 months, the structural problem is fixed, and the feeding difficulties are likely to resolve.

An *episodic* feeding or swallowing problem is one that occurs periodically. For instance, a child with cancer is likely to have a significant lack of appetite as well as increased vomiting during the course of cancer treatment. This child may have eaten normally while healthy but developed a feeding problem during treatment because of disrupted appetite. Once the treatment is finished, the child is likely to resume normal eating patterns. As another example, some children have significant adverse reactions to food, as in food allergies and food

TABLE 9-3 Classification of pediatric feeding and swallowing disorders

Classification System	Subtypes	Examples
Descriptive features		
Duration	Transient	Cleft palate
	Episodic	Cancer treatment Adverse food reactions
	Chronic	Cerebral palsy
Behavior	Eating too little	Food selectivity
	Eating too much	Hyperphagia
	Eating the wrong things	Pica
Etiology/cause		
Organic	Neuromotor dysfunction	Cerebral palsy
	Mechanical obstruction	Esophageal atresia
	Medical/genetic abnormality	Reflux
Nonorganic	Physical/emotional	Maternal depression
	Educational	Little caregiver knowledge about nutrition and safe feeding
	Environmental	Poverty
	Behavioral	Tantrums

intolerance (James & Burks, 1999). Celiac disease is one type of food reaction, experienced by 1 in 133 Americans (Fasano et al., 2003). These individuals are intolerant of gluten and may experience a host of symptoms, such as diarrhea and reflux, when ingesting gluten. As parents learn to manage their children's gluten intolerance, episodic feeding problems may occur.

A *chronic* feeding or swallowing problem is one that is ongoing over months or years and cannot be resolved easily. A child with oral-motor dysfunction due to cerebral palsy may always be a poor or unsafe oral eater and may require a supplemental feeding tube—a **gastrostomy tube**—placed directly in the stomach. For some children, chronic feeding problems result from a complex of factors that undermine their success with feeding. Consider a very premature infant on a ventilator who receives nutrition solely through a gastrostomy tube (a g *tube*) for the first year of life. During this year the infant develops secondary sensory, experiential, and psychosocial responses to the inability to participate in normal oral-motor and feeding experiences and develops a serious resistance to any oral-motor attention (e.g., stroking of the face). This child's medical issues interfered with normal oral-motor milestones and interrupted the bonding and attachment period with the parents. Even though the acute medical issues have been resolved, this infant now has a chronic feeding disorder and may need many years to transition from tube dependence to oral intake.

Discussion Point: *Consider Lily, David, and Cory, presented in Box 9-1. Characterize each disorder as either transient, episodic, or chronic.*

Behavioral Characteristics of Disorders

Some experts characterize feeding disorders according to the observable behaviors, or symptoms, exhibited. Common characteristics include a refusal to eat, eating nonnutritive substances, and rigidity in eating. A summary of prevalent behaviors that characterize various types of feeding and swallowing disorders is presented in Table 9-4.

TABLE 9-4 Observable behaviors of feeding and swallowing disorders

Behavior	Description
Food refusal	• Resistance to eating and/or drinking that cannot be attributed to a lack of food or a medical condition
Food selectivity	• Severely self-restricted diet based on resistance to certain types, textures, or volumes of food available • May range from mild ("picky eating") to extreme (e.g., refusal to eat all but one color of food)
Rumination	• Persistent regurgitation and reingestion of food for a period of 1 month or longer • Voluntary (self-induced), pleasurable, usually involving small portions, and not associated with nausea
Vomiting	• Persistent voluntary or involuntary expulsion of a typically large volume food and/or drink • Associated with nausea, distress, and acute weight loss
Pica	• Ingestion of nonnutritive substances for 1 month or longer (e.g., clay, soil, insects, animal droppings, paint, pebbles, leaves, hair)
Limited food intake	• Inadequate eating and nutritional intake, perhaps due to passivity, lack of interest or appetite, or excessive selectivity
Excessive food intake	• Persistent overintake of food • May result from an insatiable appetite (hyperphagia)
Oral-motor hypersensitivity	• Excessive sensitivity of the oral-motor structures (e.g., teeth, lips, cheeks, tongue) or functions (e.g., swallowing too soon, gagging)
Oral-motor hyposensitivity	• Inadequate sensitivity of the oral-motor structures (e.g., teeth, lips, cheeks, tongue) or functions (e.g., inability to trigger swallow or detect drooling)
Chewing problems	• Inability to adequately chew or a prolonged chewing of food due to poor coordination, limited muscle control, and/or structural problems
Sucking or swallowing problems	• Weak or ineffective suck and/or swallow, including delayed trigger of swallow and inadequate timing of suck-swallow coordination
Delays in self-feeding and self-drinking	• Slow acquisition of skills in independently transporting food or liquid for eating and drinking • May stem from motor control difficulties, behavioral difficulties, and/or cognitive delays
Disruptive behaviors	• Inappropriate and/or excessive show of tantrums, screaming, kicking, hitting, biting, throwing food, playing with food, talking, and other aggressive behaviors during mealtime • Most often associated with food refusal
Pace of intake	• Inappropriately slow or fast rate of oral intake during mealtime

Sources: Based on American Psychiatric Association (1994); Babbitt, Hoch, and Coe (1994); Ginsberg (1988); Kedesdy and Budd (1998).

Kessler (1966) provided an early scheme that organized the many symptoms into three sets:

1. Eating too little
2. Eating too much
3. Eating the wrong things

Children who have excessive food selectivity and thus have severely restricted diets fall in the first category. Children with excessive overconsumption of food, perhaps due to an insatiable appetite, or **hyperphagia**, fall in the second category. Children with *pica,* a feeding disorder in which children consume inappropriate nonnutritive substances (e.g., pebbles, glass fragments, soap, sponges) for a period longer than 1 month, fall in the third category. Typically, these three categories of behaviors lead parents to professionals for assistance; all three can have detrimental and even fatal consequences for children (Kedesdy & Budd, 1998).

Causal Classifications

As an alternative and a complement to descriptive classification schemes, causal classification focuses on the etiology, or cause, of the feeding or swallowing disorder. Causal classification identifies the elements that originally caused the breakdown in the oral feeding process.

Organic Disorders

Many feeding and swallowing disorders result from known physical, or **organic**, causes. For instance, consider the case of Dwayne, who has cerebral palsy and is unable to successfully and safely execute a swallow. At 6 months Dwayne undergoes surgery to provide an alternative feeding system—a g tube—that bypasses the oral route. Dwayne's feeding and swallowing disorder is attributable to a clear physical challenge, specifically neuromuscular weakness due to cerebral palsy. Because his neuromuscular weakness is severe, he may receive nutrition through a g tube for his whole life.

Other organic causes that can result in feeding and swallowing problems include these:

- *Gastroesophageal reflux:* Regurgitation of stomach contents into the pharynx can cause burning in the throat and gastrointestinal distress.
- *Esophageal atresia:* This congenital condition, in which the infant's esophagus ends in a pouch rather than extending to the intestines, is usually accompanied by a *tracheoesophageal fistula,* a canal that runs between the trachea and esophagus and may lead to choking. Until the problem is corrected surgically, the infant is fed via a g tube or an IV.
- *Lead toxicity:* Elevated levels of blood-lead concentrations can result in poor appetite, vomiting, and refusal to eat (anorexia).
- *Cleft lip and palate:* A cleft, or opening, in the infant's lip and/or palate can result in significant problems with feeding and swallowing, including inadequate nutrition. Prior to surgical repair of the cleft, compensatory approaches to feeding, such as use of special nipples specifically designed for children with cleft palate, are important to ensure adequate nutritional intake (Krebs, 1999).

Experts classify the major organic causes of pediatric feeding and swallowing disorders into three categories (Linscheid, 1992). *Neuromotor dysfunction* describes disorders that result from an impairment of the neurological or motoric systems required for safe and efficient feeding and swallowing, as occurs in some cases of cerebral palsy. *Mechanical obstruction* describes disorders resulting from an obstruction in the feeding and swallowing apparatuses, as occurs with esophageal atresia. *Medical/genetic abnormality* describes disorders resulting from illness, trauma, or disability, such as reflux. Estimates suggest that about 66% of feeding and swallowing disorders stem primarily from these categories of organic causes (Budd et al., 1992).

Nonorganic Disorders

A number of children exhibit disordered abilities for less obvious reasons. About 34% of children with feeding and swallowing disorders exhibit **nonorganic disorders**, in which the cause is not clearly evident or does not stem from a physical impairment (Budd et al., 1992).

Four likely causes that experts have proposed for nonorganic disorders include physical/emotional, educational, environmental, and behavioral factors (Luiselli, 1989). With physical/emotional causes, feeding and swallowing disorders stem from a physical or emotional reaction to the environment, as in cases of abuse or maternal depression. Educational causes include inadequate caregiver knowledge of feeding, eating, and nutrition. Environmental causes are primarily financial constraints, making food under-available. With behavioral causes feeding and/or swallowing deficits result from learned behaviors. For instance, children may exhibit tantrums during eating because they have learned that tantrums effectively control their environments.

A Biopsychosocial Perspective

In the last decade, experts have increasingly come to view pediatric feeding and swallowing disorders as *biopsychosocial disorders*. This term emphasizes the complexities of human nature and pediatric developmental disturbances by referring to the integrative relationships among biology, psychology, and socialization. Rather than providing a single, identifiable cause in feeding and swallowing difficulties, this term emphasizes that, for many children, an early physiological or medical problem may trigger psychological and interactional issues that subsequently spawn maladaptive feeding behaviors (Ramsay, 1995).

Discussion Point: *Consider Lily, David, and Cory in Box 9-1. Consider each disorder from a biopsychosocial perspective, exploring the biological, psychological, and socialization factors that contribute to their disorders.*

To illustrate, let's consider 3-month-old Isabel, who weighed only 1300 grams (about 2.9 pounds) at birth and was born with a cleft palate. Isabel clearly had physical difficulties that directly contributed to poor food intake. Her physical challenges led to a failure to thrive as her growth and development faltered from limited nutrition. Isabel's parents naturally experienced incredible stress and anxiety, which in turn undermined the quality of their feeding interactions with Isabel. Rather than feeding her every 3 hours, they increased the feedings to every hour. And rather than stopping the feedings when Isabel signaled that she was finished, they pushed on in their desperation and used a variety of pressure tactics to get her to continue eating.

With time, feedings turned into ongoing battles in which Isabel was resistant, withdrawn, and agitated and her parents were aggressive, controlling, and persistent. Isabel's refusal to eat contributed to the eventual decision to provide nutritional supplements via a nasogastric tube (an *NG tube*) passed through her nose. Although Isabel's cleft palate was repaired and her oral-motor capabilities were fully functioning by 12 months of age, her feeding disorder would not soon be resolved (see Figure 9-5).

FIGURE 9-5 A biopsychosocial perspective of Isabel's feeding problems.

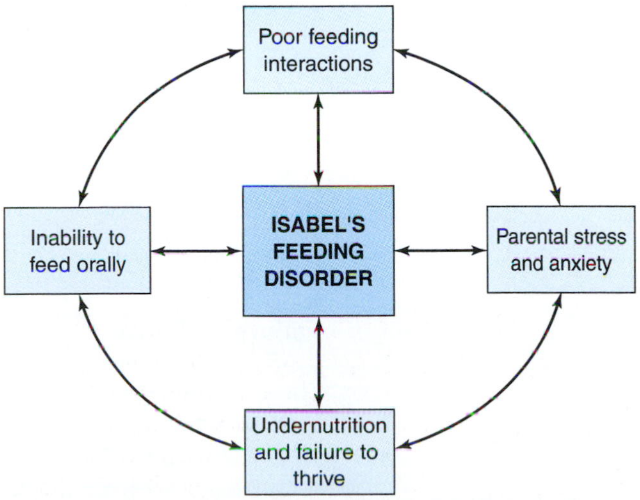

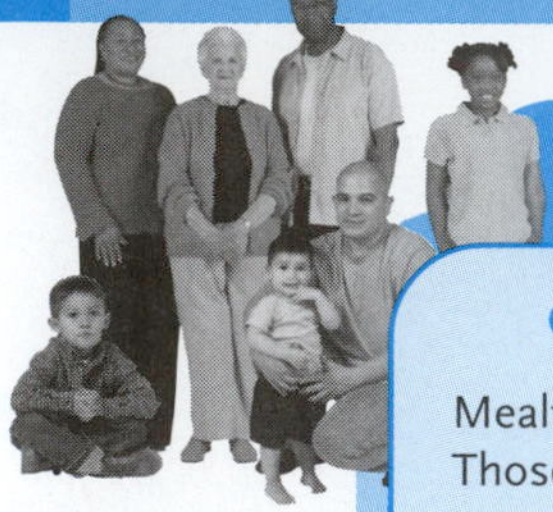

BOX 9-2 Multicultural Focus

Culture and Eating Preferences

Mealtime behaviors and food preferences are highly influenced by cultural background. Those who have traveled outside their native country are well aware of how mealtime customs vary across the world. Chef Anthony Bourdain's book titled *A Cook's Tour: Global Adventures in Extreme Cuisines* provides a humorous look at mealtime preferences across the globe and describes his experiences eating lemongrass tripe in Cambodia, borscht in Russia, and foie gras in France. The particular foods eaten in a cultural community and the way in which these foods are shared provide a unique and enlightening glimpse into a culture's values, beliefs, and history.

Feeding specialists must be knowledgeable about and sensitive to eating and mealtime customs and cultures that differ from their own so that normal behaviors are not mistakenly characterized as disordered interactions. Consider, for instance, the mealtime interactions in one household of children, parents, and grandparents, who are recent immigrants from mainland China. According to Chinese customs, the meal begins with the most senior person, usually the father or grandfather, eating first. The other members of the family wait patiently while the elders eat. In addition, Chinese foods are all served on one plate, and reaching across the table for that plate is acceptable. Because children are expected to eat the same amount of each food, preferences for certain foods are discouraged. Chinese meals consist mostly of the same foods, so there are very few associations between particular foods and the time of day. Beverages and desserts are not served during a meal; the only fluids served are soups, which are eaten at the end of the meal and may be drunk rather than eaten with a spoon. Children are to be quiet and respectful of their elders during meals. Thus, you can recognize how important it is for feeding specialists to both understand and honor the customs and cultures of the families with whom they work.

For Discussion

Consider the different ways that family food preferences and mealtime behaviors might vary as a function of culture. In what ways would knowledge of a family's customs influence the outcomes of a feeding evaluation?

Consider your own family's feeding and mealtime behaviors. What characterizes these behaviors, and how are they influenced by your own culture?

Companion Website

To answer these questions online, go to the Multicultural Focus module in chapter 9 of the Companion Website.

For Isabel and many other children like her, it is nearly impossible to categorize the feeding disorder as organic or nonorganic. Rather, the disorder stems from a complex set of biological, psychological, and socialization influences. Because so many factors can be involved in a pediatric feeding disorder, it is important to look at each child holistically and individually, a principle described later in this chapter.

Failure to Thrive

There is considerable overlap between pediatric feeding and swallowing disorders and the concept of **failure to thrive** (FTT). FTT is a widely used term to describe children whose weight or height deviates significantly from the norm for their age and gender because of nutritional inadequacy (Ramsay, 1995). Other terms used to describe FTT include *growth* *failure* and *undernutrition* (Kessler & Dawson, 1999). Nutritional inadequacy occurs for three major reasons (Kessler, 1999):

1. Inadequate access to food
2. Inadequate intake of food
3. Inadequate retention or absorption of food

Even though the terms *feeding disorder* and *failure to thrive* are often used interchangeably, not all children with feeding disorders have FTT and not all children with FTT have feeding disorders. For example, a child born with a cardiac defect who had a g tube placed early in life because of inadequate oral intake may actually be growing quite well. With the g tube in place, parents can feed the child as many calories as necessary to sustain healthy growth and development. Another child may not have a feeding disorder but may have a medical condition that precludes proper digestion or absorption of ingested foods, and thus the child does not grow properly.

Increasingly, experts view the term *failure to thrive* to be a pejorative term because of its negative connotation for the nonthriving child's parents and because it "obscures the condition's complexity" (Kessler & Dawson, 1999, p. 5). Many experts prefer the terms *pediatric undernutrition* and *growth deficiency,* emphasizing that few cases of pediatric undernutrition result from a single cause.

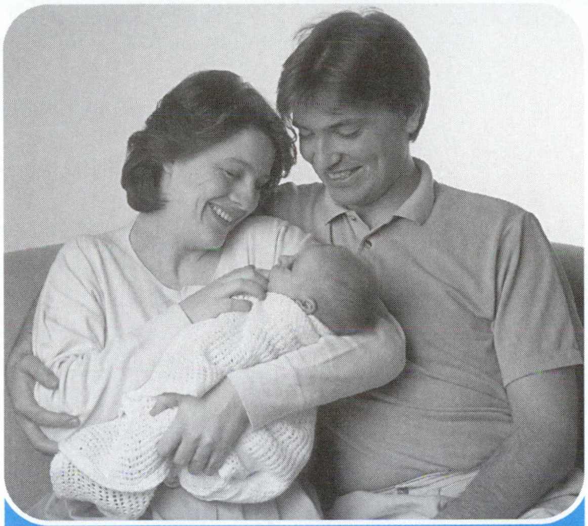

Some experts consider the term *failure to thrive* to be pejorative and to connote that parents are to blame when their children's growth falters.

What Are the Defining Characteristics of Pediatric Feeding and Swallowing Disorders?

Normal feeding and swallowing are safe, efficient, and organized. Whether a feeding or swallowing disorder results from an organic or nonorganic cause, it typically features one or more of these characteristics:

1. Feeding and/or swallowing is unsafe.
2. Feeding and/or swallowing is inadequate.
3. Feeding and/or swallowing is inappropriate.

Unsafe Feeding and Swallowing

Defining Characteristics

At birth an infant must skillfully implement a coordinated pattern of suckling, swallowing, and breathing. This coordination is not always perfect in young infants, but minor deviations do not usually pose a risk (Arvedson & Rogers, 1997). Some children, however, cannot negotiate the suck-swallow-breathe pattern, and feeding and swallowing become unsafe. Feeding and swallowing are unsafe when they pose a risk of penetration or aspiration of the bolus into the airway.

Unsafe swallowing is referred to as *dysphagia,* which typically results from the dysfunction of or damage to a child's **oral-motor system** or an inappropriate eating rate, either too fast or too slow. Swallowing dysfunction can affect planning, timing, coordination, organization, and sensation. Consider, for instance, children who have cardiac or pulmonary issues who may breathe too rapidly to coordinate a suck-swallow-breathe pattern. When liquid is pulled into the oral cavity but allowed to linger, it can create a pool in the *valleculae,* the space created when the epiglottis folds down to cover the trachea during swallowing. If milk pools there, it can easily spill over into the airway before or after a swallow has been triggered, putting the child at risk for aspiration.

Or consider a child born with neurological damage who has oral-motor hyposensitivity. The child may be unaware of substances in the mouth, particularly liquids, which provide little sensory stimulation. Despite a pool of liquid in the oral cavity, there is no trigger of a swallow to move the substance into the esophagus. Children who are very unsafe in their swallowing may receive a physician's order of NPO, which loosely means "nothing per oral." Children who are NPO cannot ingest anything through their mouths and will receive a supplemental feeding tube.

Causes and Risk Factors

Dysphagia frequently accompanies a number of syndromes, particularly those that feature low muscle tone (*hypotonia*), delayed motor development, and physical deformities affecting the oral-motor area (Arvedson & Rogers, 1997). For instance, children with Down syndrome may exhibit hypotonia, contributing to a weak suck, which can result in a swallowing impairment. **Cerebral palsy** (CP), a neuromuscular disorder that affects about 1 in 1,000 children, also presents a significant risk factor for dysphagia (Kuban & Leviton, 1994). CP can result from a variety of causes, including a lack of oxygen to the infant's brain (i.e., anoxia) during birth. During the first year of life, 57% of children with CP have problems with sucking, 38% have problems with swallowing, and 33% exhibit FTT or malnutrition (Reilly, Skuse, & Poblete, 1996). Over time, these problems can become more severe as the child's nutritional needs increase. Children with CP may require supplemental nutrition if they are unable to develop the oral-motor skills needed for oral feeding.

Other conditions in which dysphagia is seen at elevated rates include significant anomalies of the physical structures required for swallowing, including the hard and soft palate, tongue, lips, tonsils, and pharynx; chronic or recurrent respiratory problems, including pneumonia; and cardiopulmonary diseases that cause fatigue during feeding and rapid breathing. Cleft lip or palate is an example of a physical impairment that can affect safe feeding. Children with this condition have an opening, or cleft, in their lip and/or palate. Children with *cleft lip* may be unable to create a strong enough seal around the nipple to efficiently excise the formula or breast milk. Children with **cleft palate** require help achieving a good oral seal, as the hole in the palate creates a loss of pressure during sucking and can result in formula, breast milk, or solid foods entering the nasal cavity. Surgical repair of clefts typically does not occur until after 12 months of age. Thus, during the first year of life, children may require either an adapted nipple or an alternative feeding method for safe and efficient feeding.

Inadequate Feeding and Swallowing

Inadequate feeding and swallowing refers to cases in which the child is unable to achieve the nutrition needed for healthy growth and development. Inadequate nutrition occurs for four primary reasons: (1) inefficiency, (2) overselectivity, (3) refusal, or (4) feeding delay.

Defining Characteristics

Inefficiency. Children who are inefficient at feeding and swallowing are unable to meet their own caloric and nutritional needs because the process of feeding and swallowing is not productive. During feeding, inefficient feeders may fatigue too easily, become breathless, or show disinterest or a lack of persistence. They may be inattentive and frequently off task. These characteristics can contribute to undernutrition and growth delays (Kedesdy & Budd, 1998) as the child's inefficiency does not keep pace with nutritional needs.

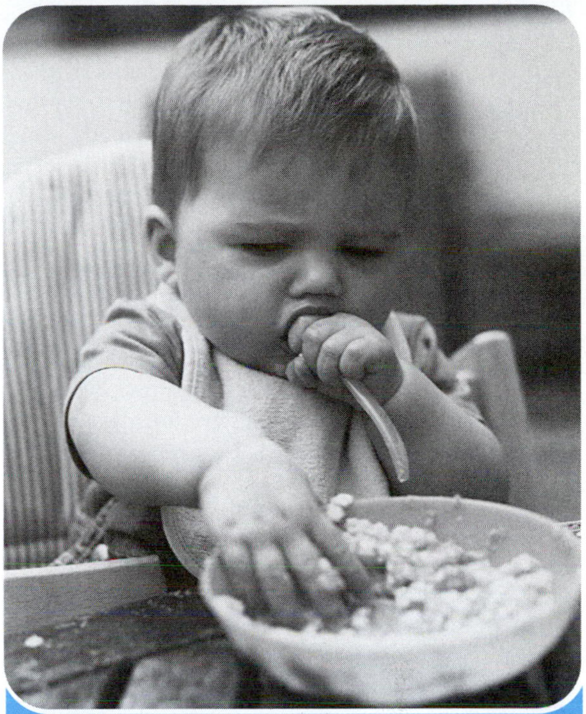

With extreme overselection, children may refuse to eat any food that is not a particular texture or color.

Overselectivity. Some children eat too little because of moderate to extreme **overselectivity**. Children with overselective eating patterns are restrictive in the taste, type, texture, and/or volume of food they will eat (Kedesdy & Budd, 1998). Taste/type restrictions involve rejection of all members of a particular food group because of taste or type—all vegetables or all green foods, for example. Texture restrictions involve resistance to particular textures; the child may eat only one texture, such as liquids. Volume restrictions tend to involve a refusal to eat large portions and can, in the extreme, involve total resistance to eating.

Rigidity in eating is not uncommon in children; parents report about one third of their children to be picky or finicky eaters (Reau, Senturia, Lebailly, & Christoffel, 1996). Pickiness is a problem when it creates significant stress for the family and when it provides a diet that is inadequate in nutrients and calories. For instance, Kedesdy and Budd (1998) describe a 2-year-old child who ate only formula from a bottle, cookies, and sweet dry cereal. One author of this chapter worked with a child who ate only chicken nuggets from a fast-food restaurant. You can imagine the stress on family dynamics as well as the implications for children's growth.

Refusal. Some cases of pediatric undernutrition result from a complete refusal to feed (Kedesdy & Budd, 1998). Although most young children will periodically resist foods (Young & Drewett, 2000), an ongoing refusal to eat is a serious matter that can occur for several reasons. First, the child may have a physical or medical issue that has not been resolved. For example, a child may have poor appetite regulation because of constipation—refusing food on days when stooling has not occurred. Constipation has a significant impact on oral intake because food is not moving through the intestines, resulting in disrupted appetite and hunger.

Discussion Point: *Ask members of your family what you were like as a young eater. Were you finicky or selective? What foods did you like and dislike?*

Second, a child may have gastrointestinal distress, such as reflux. With **reflux**, gastric acid is regurgitated into the esophagus and even the pharynx, resulting in a burning of the esophagus and throat. As many as 40% of infants regurgitate once daily (Orenstein, 1994). When regurgitation is more frequent, significant problems with feeding may occur, including food aversion, loss of appetite, and malnutrition. Because reflux is so painful, children may attempt to avoid eating or may eat only small amounts at one time. Some infants have silent reflux, which produces no visible regurgitation, and hence, no treatment is pursued. Without treatment a child may resist eating or seriously limit intake (Krebs, 1999). The extent to which a child experiences symptoms of gastrointestinal distress—vomiting, diarrhea, and constipation—is strongly associated with refusal to eat and mealtime struggles (Johnson & Harris, 2004).

Third, a child may experience a traumatic experience that results in resistance to eating, described as **conditioned dysphagia**. Some children resist eating after experiences with severe choking, ingestion of poison, or severe allergic reactions (Kedesdy & Budd, 1998).

Feeding Delay. Because of developmental delays, illnesses, or trauma, some children experience delayed development of feeding skills. These children are slow to meet major milestones, such as the transition from a bottle to a cup or the emergence of finger feeding. However, major milestones correspond to increasing nutritional needs, such as the transition to table foods, which provides greater nutritional variety to support growth and development. Thus, when children do not transition, their delays may contribute to insufficient feeding.

Causes and Risk Factors

Insufficient feeding occurs for many reasons, including trauma, abuse, accidents, illnesses, developmental disabilities, oral-motor dysfunction, and the like. Here, we present a few of the more prevalent causes of pediatric feeding disorders that are related to inadequate feeding: low birth weight, developmental disabilities, prematurity, prenatal drug exposure, and diet restrictions.

Low Birth Weight. Children who are born exceptionally small, that is, infants born with low or very **low birth weight**, are at great risk of feeding and swallowing disorders and of failing to achieve adequate nutrition on their own (MacDorman, Minino, Strobino, & Guyer, 2002). More than 80% of children who are LBW or VLBW survive the first 3 months of life, although the survival rate is lowest for the smallest babies (Lemons et al., 2001). Poor postnatal growth in these babies is very common, affecting 99% of infants who weigh less than 1000 grams (about 2.2 pounds) at birth (Lemons et al., 2001).

Developmental Disabilities. Children who exhibit developmental disabilities—such as mental retardation, autism, and cerebral palsy—are more prone to disorders of intake than are other children. Insufficient feeding may occur because of motor or muscular weaknesses, such as hypotonia, which prevent children from ingesting food at the rate needed to grow. Other children, particularly those with autism (discussed in chapter 7), are prone to poor flexibility and excessive rigidity in feeding. These children tend to be easily overwhelmed by sounds, smells, tastes, crowds, movements, or changes in schedules. Children with autism may be very sensitive to sensory input—termed **sensory defensiveness**—which is characterized as overt aversion or defensive reaction to stimuli entering the sensory systems (Wilbarger & Wilbarger, 1991). Children who are sensory defensive are prone to excessively rigid eating and avoid most textures or colors of food, resulting in severe problems with intake.

Prematurity. **Prematurity** occurs when a child is born at or before 37 weeks of gestation. In the year 2000, nearly 12 in 100 births were preterm, and very preterm births (<32 weeks of gestation) comprised almost 2 in 100 births (MacDorman et al., 2002). Children who are born preterm face a complex of challenges, including feeding and swallowing with a neurologically immature system. Children born preterm have many systems that are immature, especially the digestive and respiratory systems. Thus, preterm infants have a diminished ability to coordinate the suck-swallow-breathe pattern, which compromises safe and efficient swallowing (Kedesdy & Budd, 1998).

Prenatal Drug Exposure. Prenatal exposure to alcohol, tobacco, cocaine, heroin, and other toxic substances has been linked to prematurity and low birth weight, as well as to longer-term growth failure and depressed neurological functioning, any one of which can impede a young child's feeding development and swallowing skills (Frank & Wong, 1999). Alcohol consumption by pregnant mothers can result in fetal alcohol syndrome (FAS), alcohol-related birth defects (ARBD), and/or alcohol-related neurodevelopmental disorder (ARND). Current best estimates of prevalence of these three alcohol-related disorders suggest that about 10 in 1,000 infants are affected (May & Gossage, 2001), and symptoms include an increased likelihood of problems with feeding. Prenatal exposure to opiates, such as heroin, increases suckling problems in infants, which in turn impede feeding and nutrition. In addition, maternal drug use can impede the feeding connection between caregiver and child (Frank & Wong, 1999). The development of feeding skills and achievement of coordinated behavioral routines within a stable and structured caregiving context is a critical variable in preventing feeding disturbances (Yoos, Kitzman, & Cole, 1999).

Diet Restrictions. Some children are placed on strict or modified diets in response to diabetes, phenylketonuria, and other metabolic disorders (Kedesdy & Budd, 1998). Diabetes is a disorder in which the body does not produce enough insulin. Nearly 2 in 1,000 children are affected by insulin-dependent diabetes (American Diabetes Association, 1996) and face carefully controlled diets, in addition to insulin injections and blood testing. The challenges of such strict diets—for example, not being allowed to snack and eating meals different from those of other children—can result in feeding issues and a resistance to eating (Kedesdy & Budd, 1998).

Similar challenges are associated with phenylketonuria **(PKU)**, a metabolic disorder characterized by a deficient liver enzyme and elevated levels of the amino acid phenylaline (National Institutes of Health, 2000). PKU affects about 1 in 15,000 infants born in the United States, although the prevalence is much higher in other countries in which PKU screening is not common. PKU management is essential to preventing the growth deficiencies and mental retardation that frequently result from the buildup of unmetabolized amino acids. However, because of strict dietary management, children with PKU may have poor appetite, food aversions, and serious anxieties about eating (Kedesdy & Budd, 1998).

Discussion Point: *Expectant mothers are screened for PKU prior to giving birth to prepare for early interventions if needed. What other kinds of developmental disabilities or metabolic problems are screened for during pregnancy?*

Inappropriate Feeding and Swallowing

Defining Characteristics

Children who exhibit inappropriate feeding behaviors demonstrate undesirable and disruptive behaviors during mealtimes. If the inappropriate behaviors are significant, the children's growth and development may be compromised as successful feeding is disrupted, turning mealtime interactions into serious and stressful struggles between caregivers and children. Inappropriate feeding behaviors include screaming, spitting, throwing, hitting, and other similar actions (Kedesdy & Budd, 1998). Some children may drop food on the floor, let food fall out of their mouths, or eat very, very slowly, resulting in never-ending mealtimes. In contrast, some children may eat excessively fast—as many as 20 bites of food per minute (Kedesdy & Budd, 1998). Eating too slowly can cause nutritional deficiencies, whereas eating too fast can cause choking or aspiration. Some children may wholly resist letting any food touch their faces or mouths, as discussed previously.

Causes and Risk Factors

Anyone who has had the opportunity to engage in feeding interactions with an infant or young child can readily recognize the complexities and challenges of child feeding and can also understand how readily events can spiral out of control. When eating recently in a restaurant with her 2-year-old daughter, one of the authors was approached by a woman who asked, "How do you get your daughter to eat so well in a restaurant? We can't go out to eat with our 2-year-old, because he throws tantrums and refuses to eat, and we have to leave."

For many parents, one of the greatest challenges of bringing home a newborn from the hospital is navigating the intricacies of feeding a baby every several hours. Few parents instinctively know what to do when the infant falls asleep during eating, will not wake to eat, refuses to eat, cannot latch on to a nipple, dislikes the food that is offered, or feeds too much

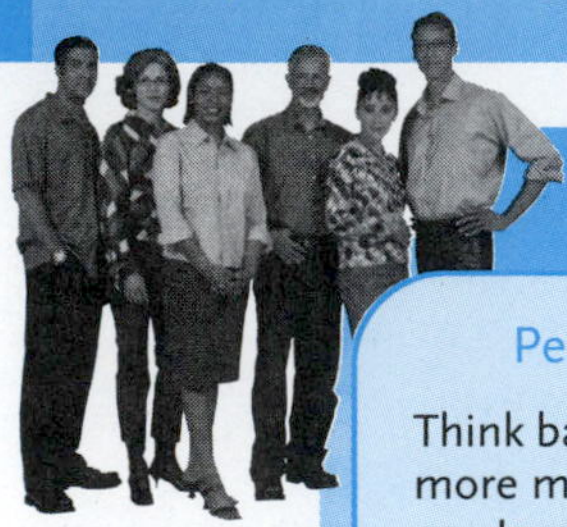

BOX 9-3 Ecological Contexts

Pediatric Feeding and Swallowing Disorders at Home

Think back to life in your home as a child. If you allow yourself to think through several of the more memorable events and occasions, food or eating may be a salient aspect of the memory. In many homes both happy and sad events are commemorated with food and drink.

Now consider how a child's feeding or swallowing disorder might affect a family's life. In working with families of tube-dependent children, one of the most striking outcomes of feeding therapy is its positive impact on the family's quality of life. One parent reported recently with excitement, "Our whole family eats together; we don't play, pick, lick, throw, scratch, bite, arch, gag, or scream, we just EAT; and we are no longer carrying around enough tube-feeding supplies to feed an army."

Parents are excited that their children are no longer tethered to a feeding pump and can explore their environments more readily. Parents also report the freedom and ease of going to a restaurant and actually ordering food for their children. And many families point out that their children no longer stand out at birthday parties, restaurants, church, school, picnics, and the community pool, because there is no longer the need to explain the presence of the tube and why the child doesn't eat. One mother stated how excited her daughter was to be able to finally have a sleepover at a friend's house, now that she didn't require overnight tube feedings. It is important not to disregard the impact that pediatric feeding disorders and tube dependence have on the entire family system, including their ability to participate fully in their communities.

For Discussion

In what other ways might a family be restricted in its community participation because of a pediatric feeding disorder?

For persons who require supplemental feeding across the entire lifespan, what are some physical, social, and educational activities that might be restricted?

Companion Website

To answer these questions online, go to the Ecological Contents module in chapter 9 of the Companion Website.

and too often. For those caregivers who successfully meet the challenges of feeding an infant, the toddler years pose just as great a test as children develop a sense of autonomy that includes controlling what they will and will not eat. Intermittent food refusals and feeding rigidity are not uncommon, and few caregivers always know the best approach to entice their children to finish a meal: punishing? begging? coaxing? offering gifts?

About one third of feeding disorders in young children result from nonorganic causes (Budd et al., 1992). Feeding difficulties can stem from behaviors and attributes of the caregiver and/or the child that become complexly intertwined in the feeding process. During the first year of a child's life, parents and children develop a feeding relationship that has immediate and long-term consequences. Many parent behaviors can undermine or impair the feeding relationship:

- Being overactive and overstimulating
- Being underactive, passive, and unengaged
- Being rigid, directive, and demanding
- Being chaotic, disorganized, and frenzied
- Being overly concerned, anxious, and fearful (Satter, 1999)

Such behaviors may be more prevalent in caregivers who are poor, depressed, drug-dependent, socially isolated, stressed, or undereducated about nutrition (Yoos et al., 1999).

Behaviors exhibited by children can also impair the feeding relationship. For positive feeding relationships to develop, infants must be positive, alert, and calm during feeding; show readable cues to indicate needs and feelings, including fullness; and be willing to experience new tastes and textures (Satter, 1999). As infants develop into toddlers, they must be interested in eating, indicate hunger and satiation, eat at predictable times, and exhibit generally positive behaviors when eating. When any of these behaviors are not present, difficulties can emerge and persist. Table 9-5 presents a summary of important achievements in eating competencies.

Discussion Point: *What kind of cues might an infant give to identify satiation? hunger? specific food preferences?*

At any time in early feeding development, a breakdown can occur that results in power struggles and inappropriate mealtime interactions. In many cases, an organic disorder may first undermine the feeding relationship, but disordered patterns then set in and continue even after the organic difficulties are resolved. For instance, a child with minor reflux during infancy may show resistance to feeding in the first few months of life, which may negatively affect the feeding relationship even when the reflux is resolved.

TABLE 9-5 Achievements in the development of eating competence

Age Range	Stage	Key Achievements
0–3 months	Homeostasis	• Can root, suck, and swallow • Shows readable, moderate feeding cues • Is generally positive, calm, and alert during feeding • Can tolerate the available food
3–6 months	Attachment	• Opens mouth for nipple when hungry • Vocalizes, talks, gestures, smiles with feeder • Looks at feeder • Sustains predictable growth • Shows clear positive signs of fullness
6–12 months	Separation and individuation	• Shows readable, moderate, varied hunger cues • Experiments with cup • Shows positive interest in food and feeder • Experiments with new tastes
12–18 months	Separation and individuation	• Is positive about eating • Tolerates hunger briefly, can wait to eat • Participates in family meals • Eats soft solid foods • Feeds self with hands or utensils • Drinks from a cup
18–36 months	Separation and individuation	• Tastes new foods repeatedly, masters many • Refuses food without becoming upset • Eats and tolerates available food • Takes pleasure in eating • Can accept limits in feeding • Eats to satiety, stops when full
3–6 years	Initiative	• Can refuse food politely • Can make do with less favorite foods • Takes initiative and shows mastery with foods • Eats variety of foods for nutritional adequacy • Experiences and expresses pleasure in eating

Source: From *Feeding with Love and Good Sense: Training Manual for the VISIONS Workshop* by E. M. Satter, 1996, Madison, WI: Ellyn Satter Associates.

How Are Pediatric Feeding and Swallowing Disorders Identified?

Early Identification and Referral

The timely identification of pediatric feeding and swallowing disorders is critical so that immediate intervention can sustain the child's health and nutrition. Typically, newborns stay in the hospital for 48 to 72 hours when there are no complications, and longer when complications are evident or when the child is underweight or premature. Nurses, parents, and physicians are usually well aware when feeding is not progressing well, because the newborn's weight and feeding behaviors are monitored frequently. Interventions are then readily available, ranging from consultation with a breast-feeding specialist to surgical intervention.

However, many children do not demonstrate overt feeding disorders immediately. In those cases it is usually the parent or the pediatrician who identifies a feeding or swallowing difficulty. During the first year of life children's height and weight are carefully monitored to reveal any deviation or faltering. (Remember the growth chart in Figure 9-3?) During routine well-child visits, pediatricians and nurses ask parents to report on feeding and nutrition. Should the parent report any anomaly—excessive feeding time, poor weight gain, rigid eating behaviors, discomfort during feeding—the pediatrician will problem-solve with the parent to prevent early problems from persisting and becoming more serious. Common caregiver concerns about infants under 6 months of age who are bottle or breast fed include arching the back, crying, and turning away from the nipple. Then, around 6 months, some children do not transition well from liquids to solids.

Discussion Point: *What are some possible explanations for the gap between the onset of feeding disorders and referral for treatment of feeding disorders?*

Pediatricians and parents must be extremely vigilant during this period of time. A survey at the Montreal Children's Hospital Failure to Thrive and Feeding Disorders Clinic found that the mean age of onset of pediatric feeding problems was 3 months and the mean onset age of failure to thrive or poor growth was about 9 months. Unfortunately, the mean referral age by the pediatrician to the feeding clinic was 19 months. These results indicate that feeding problems emerge much earlier than referral typically occurs. And when feeding problems persist, problematic secondary behaviors can emerge (Ramsay, Gisel, & Boutry, 1993).

A pediatrician who suspects a feeding or swallowing problem will likely make at least two referrals. First, depending on the symptoms reported, a referral to an ear-nose-throat (ENT) specialist or a gastroenterologist is likely. These two specialists study a child's biological systems to determine the cause of a feeding and/or swallowing problem. For a child who vomits frequently, a **gastroenterologist** will want to rule out a structural problem of the esophagus, stomach, or intestines; an ENT specialist will determine whether reflux is irritating the throat membranes.

The second referral is to a feeding specialist. While other specialists focus on identifying the cause of a disorder, a feeding specialist works closely with parents to promote a child's safe and healthy feeding and nutrition. Prior to implementing any treatment program, of course, a feeding specialist completes a comprehensive assessment, which identifies the characteristics of the feeding and/or swallowing problem and guides treatment.

Comprehensive Assessment

The feeding specialist evaluates the whole child, including the caregiver-child feeding relationship, to study all the systems and factors that influence normal feeding. This is particularly imperative if the feeding difficulty is not easily explained by dysfunction of the oral-motor structures or functions. The comprehensive assessment includes a case history, a physical feeding/swallowing evaluation, and observation of mealtime interactions.

Case History

A careful and detailed history is central in the assessment of children with feeding and swallowing difficulties. The case history gathers information on the child's and family's eating and feeding experiences to explore possible problems, study changes in behaviors over time, and document specific manifestations of the disorder. This history is collected via an interview with the child's primary caregiver and includes prenatal history, perinatal history, a systems review (e.g., cardiac, respiratory), growth history, nutrition history, feeding behavior, developmental and behavioral history, family history, and psychosocial history. A summary of the topics included and sample questions are presented in Table 9-6.

Of particular importance to the feeding specialist is the child's feeding history. A parental report on the length of meals, the quality of intake, and the child's progression from breast/bottle to purees and solids helps the feeding specialist identify where any breakdowns might have occurred. A history of formulas used and volumes tolerated gives the specialist helpful information regarding potential referral to other professionals, such as an allergist or endocrinologist.

Another important aspect of the case history is an in-depth discussion of the child's developmental progression, including current cognitive and language abilities, gross and fine motor skills, sensory processing, and temperament, including the child's flexibility and frustration tolerance. A full understanding of a child's strengths and weaknesses is needed to determine whether feeding skills are delayed or disordered.

Consider, for instance, a 2-year-old child with Down syndrome and mental retardation who demonstrates the feeding skills of a 12-month-old child. Although the child has a feeding delay, that delay is appropriate given the child's mental impairment. Intervention is important to help the child progress, but the level of skills exhibited is not inappropriate. In contrast, consider a 2-year-old child with autism who refuses to eat any food that is not white in color. This is not a typical feeding behavior for a child of any age and is characteristic of a disorder. Identifying a child's strengths, needs, and idiosyncrasies is a vital part of the case history.

Physical Feeding and Swallowing Evaluation

Following the case history, the feeding specialist completes a careful evaluation of the structures and functions of the child's oral-motor mechanism. A complete oral-motor evaluation includes observation of the lips, tongue, jaw, teeth, and hard and soft palates. The structural examination studies the physical nature of these structures, whereas the functional examination assesses how they work together during eating and swallowing. The specialist examines the structures and functions at rest (when not being used for feeding and/or swallowing) and during feeding. The specialist is likely to first watch the child's oral-motor mechanisms during play and other everyday activities. Then the specialist studies these mechanisms as the child eats and drinks various substances—thin liquids (water), thickened liquids (milkshake), purees (applesauce), and solids (crackers).

The structural examination looks for asymmetry, drooling, and abnormal patterns or reflexes (Creskoff & Haas, 1999). Asymmetry refers to an unevenness between one side of the face and the other, which can be a sign of neurological impairment. Drooling can indicate

TABLE 9-6 Information included in the case histories of children with suspected feeding and/or swallowing problems

General Topic	Examples of Questions
Prenatal history	Did the mother use nicotine, alcohol, or medications during pregnancy? Did the mother experience any infections or diseases during pregnancy?
Perinatal history	What was the child's birth weight? What was the child's Apgar score? Were there any delivery complications?
Medical history	Has the child been hospitalized for any reason? Does the child take any medications currently? Has the child had any illnesses or infections? Does the child have any allergies?
Growth history	What is the child's current height and weight? Has the child had any growth difficulties?
Nutrition history	What is the child's current diet? How often does the child eat and drink each day? Are there any food restrictions? When did the child begin to take solid foods? What are the child's favorite and least favorite foods?
Feeding behaviors	Where do mealtimes take place for the child? Does the child show any pain or discomfort during feeding? How easily is the child distracted during feeding? Does the child show any refusals of food?
Developmental milestones	When did the child take its first step? When did the child say its first word? What is the child's activity level? What is a typical day like for the child?
Family history	What is the composition of the family? Do any family members have feeding or nutritional problems? Are there any psychiatric problems in the family? Do any family members have significant health or medical conditions?
Psychosocial history	What are the living conditions like in the home? What are the family's strengths? Is there any history of abuse or neglect? Does the family receive any supplemental resources through community programs?

Source: Based on E. A. Rider and W. G. Bithoney (1999).

oral-motor dysfunction or poor sensory awareness in the oral cavity. Abnormal patterns and reflexes, such as thrusting the tongue forward or having an open mouth in a resting position, can also signal a neurological or motor impairment.

During the functional examination, the specialist ascertains both the safety and the efficiency of feeding and swallowing, as well as the quality of intake. The specialist studies how the child handles substances of various textures and looks for any inability to move food, difficulty breaking down foods, extensive chewing, excessive drooling, swallowing

FIGURE 9-6 Signs to watch for during an oral-motor examination of feeding and swallowing problems.

Oral-motor structures

- Excessive drooling
- Forward thrust of tongue
- Asymmetry of one or more oral or facial features
- Tongue protrusion or low mobility
- Deviation of tongue to left or right
- Enlarged tonsils
- Abnormal height or width of palatal arch
- Weakness of tongue, lips, or jaw
- Abnormal color of pharynx (back of oral cavity)
- Clefting of palate

Oral-motor functions

- Excessive drooling or saliva
- Food falling out of mouth
- Unable to form food into bolus
- Residual food after swallowing
- Difficulty pursing lips for suck
- Easy fatigue
- Extended chewing
- Slow chewing
- Inadequate chewing
- Inability to move food around
- Pocketing food or drink in cheeks
- Spitting out food
- Vomiting or regurgitating from oral or nasal cavity before, during, or after feeding
- Coughing or choking
- Resisting food
- Resisting touch or pressure on oral structures
- Crying during eating or drinking
- Gurgly or wet voice quality after feeding
- Gagging

Sources: Based on Creskoff and Haas (1999); Shipley and McAfee (1998).

whole foods without chewing, and easy fatigue (Creskoff & Haas, 1999). When observing the feeding of an infant or toddler, the specialist must be aware of any signs of aspiration, such as coughing, choking, changes in facial color, vocal stridor, a wet or gurgly voice quality, vomiting, or increased or decreased heart rate. Figure 9-6 lists major signs of oral-motor dysfunction, any one of which may suggest unsafe or insufficient feeding and/or swallowing.

If any of these signs are seen, the feeding specialist will likely refer the child for a **modified barium swallow** (MBS) study. The MBS uses radiography to follow a substance from the child's lips through the pharyngeal and esophageal aspects of the swallow to see whether aspiration or penetration is occurring. Pictures of the child are taken during the oral, pharyngeal, and esophageal stages of the swallow to determine whether swallowing and feeding are safe and efficient. This type of study is conducted by the feeding specialist working closely with a radiologist.

Observation of Mealtime Interactions

An important complement to the case history and oral-motor evaluation is the feeding specialist's live observation of the child during mealtime interactions. Several observations of different meals are recommended, since children's eating behaviors can vary greatly from meal to meal (Young & Drewett, 2000). Observation allows a neutral, outside professional to spot any breakdowns in child-caregiver communication as well any potentially unsafe oral feeding practices. Sometimes simple solutions present themselves that can have far-reaching positive consequences for a child's nutrition.

Consider the case of a young male with profound cerebral palsy who was seen by a feeding specialist for severe oral-motor dysfunction and undernutrition. When asked to feed his child, the father laid the child across his lap and placed crackers in his mouth. Because the child had low muscle tone and was unable to be fed upright in a chair, the father fed him in this reclined manner. Knowing that such a position was highly unsafe, the feeding specialist quickly referred the child to a physical therapist to consult on better positioning for mealtimes. The child began to grow readily once he could be fed in an upright position.

When conducting mealtime observations, the feeding specialist studies the scheduling of meals, the environment, the foods presented, and family traditions. The therapist carefully studies how caregivers interact with their children and how, in turn, the children reciprocate. Figure 9-7 provides a sample form used to study mealtime interactions between infants and their mothers. Information from the observations is then used to set treatment goals and design treatment contexts.

BOX 9-4 Spotlight on Research

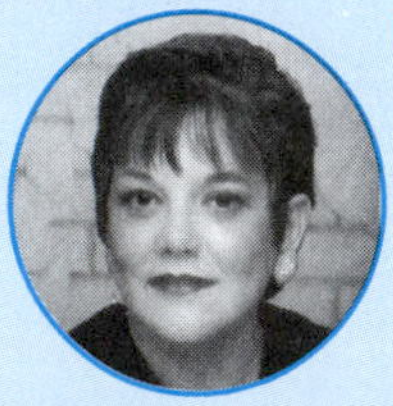

Maria Diana Gonzales, Ph.D., CCC/SLP
Associate Professor
Department of Communication Disorders, Texas State University–San Marcos

I realized as early as eighth grade that I wanted to pursue a health-related profession. This fueled my motivation to earn undergraduate and graduate degrees in speech-language pathology. After earning my SLP credential, I worked as a bilingual speech-language pathologist with an early childhood intervention program and for 18 years provided assessments and intervention for pediatric clients exhibiting communication disorders. During that time, I became frustrated by the limited research available on bilingual speech and language development, which I desperately needed to guide my clinical practice. Because of this frustration and the limited number of bilingual speech pathologists in our profession, I decided to work at a local university as a lecturer and clinical supervisor. I wanted to determine whether I wished to pursue a doctorate in speech-language pathology, and I wanted to help prepare future bilingual speech pathologists.

While employed at the university, I collaborated with an educational psychologist to study the developmental outcomes of Hispanic infants discharged from a local neonatal intensive care unit. We collected longitudinal developmental data on Hispanic premature infants at 1, 4, 9, 12, and 22 months of age. As a result of my participation in this study, I decided to pursue a doctorate because I found research to be just as interesting, challenging, and fascinating as clinical practice. While earning a doctoral degree at Ohio University, I studied how infant birth weights, socioeconomic status, parental generation/acculturation, 12-month mental development, and visual recognition memory related to the language skills of 22-month-old Hispanic NICU graduates. My dissertation suggested a strong relationship between parental acculturation and visual recognition memory and the receptive language outcomes of young Hispanic/Latino infants.

My involvement in the NICU follow-up study resulted in several publications, but more importantly it solidified my belief that clinical practice should always be informed and guided by research. Thus, what began as an eighth-grade interest in a health-related profession resulted in my pursuing a doctorate as well as engaging in research with Hispanic NICU infants and (my other passion) the emergent literacy development of bilingual children.

FIGURE 9-7 An example of an instrument used to study mealtime interactions.

DYADIC RECIPROCITY

MOTHER	None	A little	Pretty much	Very much	Item score
1. Positions infant for reciprocal exchange	0	1	2	3	
2. Talks to infant	0	1	2	3	
3. Makes positive remarks to infant	0	1	2	3	
4. Makes positive statements about infant's food intake	0	1	2	3	
5. Waits for infant to initiate interactions	0	1	2	3	
6. Shows pleasure toward infant in gaze, voice or smile	0	1	2	3	
7. Appears cheerful	0	1	2	3	
8. Appears sad	3	2	1	0	
9. Appears detached	3	2	1	0	
10. Positions infant without needed support	3	2	1	0	
11. Holds infant stiffly	3	2	1	0	

INFANT	None	A little	Pretty much	Very much	
12. Looks at mother	0	1	2	3	
13. Smiles at mother	0	1	2	3	
14. Appears cheerful	0	1	2	3	
15. Avoids gaze	3	2	1	0	
16. Falls asleep and stops feeding	3	2	1	0	

Dyadic Reciprocity Subscale Score

Source: From "A Feeding Scale for Research and Clinical Practice to assess Mother-Infant Interactions in the first three years of life" by I. Chatoor, P. Getson, E. Menvielle, R. O'Donnell, Y. Rivera, C. Brasseaux, and O. Merazek, 1997, *Infant Mental Health Journal, 18,* pp. 76–91. Reprinted by permission.

BOX 9-5 Spotlight on Practice

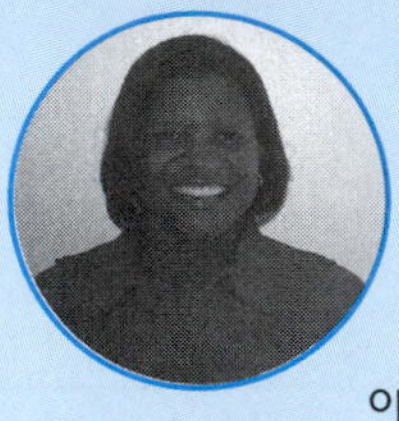

Lisa Moreasun, M.A., CCC-SLP
Speech-Language Pathologist
Detroit Public School District

While attending graduate school at Oklahoma State University on a multicultural grant, my eyes were further opened about how easily children from various ethnic groups are mislabeled, largely because of a lack of knowledge about multicultural differences on the part of the evaluator. Speakers from nontraditional settings have too often been misunderstood and misinterpreted by standardized tests normed on a population unlike their own. I felt that I could best contribute to the field of speech-language pathology and remain grounded in my professional commitment by exerting myself in an area where I could utilize my knowledge of multiculturalism. This ambition inspired me to secure a position with a diversified population in an inner-city school district.

I have practiced as a speech-language pathologist for the past 10 years. My personal experience working in an area of critical shortage has had its rewards, but it has also come with its challenges. The school district in which I work is faced with political, social, and environmental issues that affect the total school system. Implementation of the No Child Left Behind legislation, charter-versus-public-school funding, and the school-board-versus-CEO dispute—all have led to instability in leadership and operational dysfunction. Because of economic conditions, the schools have endured large cutbacks that produced layoffs and contributed further to the teacher shortage.

Speech-language pathologists in this environment are confronted with limited parental support; negative attitudes of students, parents, and staff; lack of available materials; higher than usual caseloads; language barriers and dialectal differences including Spanish, Arabic, Chaldean, Hmong, Romanian, and Bengali; time constraints in the multiple schools served; and a lack of adequate space and room availability. As you can imagine, all of these circumstances have a tremendous impact on the way speech-language pathologists are able to fulfill their job requirements.

These challenges have motivated me to seek alternative methods of service delivery. It is important that the most effective strategies be put into practice to create maximum growth. Consequently, I have focused on integrating many goals simultaneously into one therapy session. I have incorporated literacy goals into speech-language sessions and have found intervention with stories beneficial to improving communication skills. Stories of African folklore in particular hold the interest of the students I serve. Not only do these stories stimulate their motivation to learn, but they also offer great symbolism, a rich vocabulary, and affirmation of high morals. Enhancing students' academic achievement by providing culturally relevant and culturally sensitive practices promotes overall success.

Of course, the treatment provided is not the only factor that promotes student success. Developing and maintaining collaborative relationships with teachers, caregivers, and other specialists effectively bridges the gap between home and school, maximizing learning conditions. Parental and student involvement, completion of homework assignments, counseling, and adaptability all help to foster speech-language development. It is truly a team effort.

How Are Pediatric Feeding and Swallowing Disorders Treated?

Discussion Point: *Identify some barriers to the achievement of a strong working alliance among professionals and parents in treating pediatric feeding and swallowing disorders.*

A Multidisciplinary Alliance

The current standard of care for treatment of pediatric feeding and swallowing disorders is multidisciplinary collaboration (Kedesdy & Budd, 1998). Professionals and parents must also form a working alliance to ensure the effectiveness of treatment; ineffective treatments can result in severe undernutrition and growth deficiency (Kalmanson & Seligman, 1992).

The professionals most intimately involved include the pediatrician, who monitors the child's growth and development during treatment; the nutritionist, who consults on caloric needs and nutrition; and the feeding specialist, who builds the child's capacity for safe and efficient oral feeding. Other professionals may also be involved, some in consultative roles, depending on the specific needs of the children and families. For instance, a radiologist and/or gastroenterologist may place and monitor an alternative feeding system. Or for children with severe behavioral problems, a child psychologist is likely to consult.

Treatment Contexts

The NICU

One context in which feeding specialists are important collaborative partners is the NICU. There, the feeding specialist conducts evaluations of feeding and swallowing for medically fragile infants and provides interventions to enhance their developmental achievements in feeding and communication (American Speech-Language-Hearing Association, 2005b). Specific activities include encouraging communication, stimulating the oral-motor mechanisms, and designing and monitoring feeding interventions.

Special Clinics

A feeding or swallowing problem that seems dangerous or that seriously affects growth may require inpatient treatment in an intensive, hospital-based program. Some hospitals provide inpatient care in specialized growth clinics or feeding programs. For instance, the Kluge Children's Rehabilitation Center of the University of Virginia has a special treatment program called the Encouragement Feeding Program, directed by one of the authors of this chapter. This intensive 3-week program focuses specifically on weaning children from supplemental feeding tubes. Another example is the Kennedy Krieger Institute's Pediatric Feeding Disorders Unit in Baltimore, Maryland, which provides specialized treatment for children with severe feeding disorders, including severe undernutrition and total food refusal.

Many times, hospital- or clinic-based treatment is accompanied by treatment in other contexts, including the child's home, school, or early intervention center. Such treatments tend to occur on a weekly or biweekly basis. *Home visiting* in particular is an important part of treatment (Sturm & Dawson, 1999); it allows the feeding specialist to study food preparation, food options, meal timing, discipline, child behavior, and caregiver-child feeding relationships in authentic and functional contexts. Thus, it is often more effective for "helping parents with difficult feeding interactions, improving dietary habits, and addressing family communication problems" (Sturm & Dawson, 1999, p. 72). Home visiting also provides information on family resources and neighborhood and community characteristics, such as the family's local support network (Sturm & Dawson, 1999).

Treatment Goals and Approaches

The immediate and foremost goals of pediatric feeding and swallowing treatment are to ensure that nutritional needs are met for healthy growth and development and that feeding and swallowing do not endanger a child's life. In some cases this means providing alternative or supplemental nutrition via tube feeding. Once those immediate goals are achieved, specialists focus on improving a child's own ability to meet his or her nutritional needs and to see eating as a psychologically pleasant experience. The feeding specialist may need to increase specific desirable behaviors and skills, such as accepting solid foods, while decreasing undesirable behaviors and skills, such as gagging when chewing. Both physiological and psychological aspects of feeding and swallowing are targeted.

Physiology of Feeding and Swallowing

Physiological targets emphasize the organic and neurodevelopmental aspects of eating and drinking, such as muscle tone, articulator movement and coordination, oral-motor sensitivity, and body posture. For swallowing disorders, treatment focuses on improving the coordination of the swallow to achieve efficiency and safety. Interventions typically feature a hierarchical continuum of training targets, each of which is a small, discreet, and easily attainable behavior or skill. These short-term goals begin at the child's present skill level and

Discussion Point: *What would the long-term goals be for Lily and David, also described in Box 9-1?*

progress toward independent eating, which is typically the long-term goal (Kedesdy & Budd, 1998). For instance, a long-term goal for Cory, the 2-year-old boy described in Box 9-1, is to increase his ability to eat orally. A series of small, measurable steps will be designed by the feeding specialist to help Cory progress from no to total oral intake.

Psychology of Feeding and Swallowing

Psychological targets emphasize the behavioral aspects of eating and drinking, such as accepting certain food types or textures, decreasing resistance and fussiness when eating, following a consistent meal schedule, and the like. For children who receive nutrition supplementally or alternatively, goals correspond to a gradual reduction in tube feedings. Therapists usually utilize behavioral principles to deliver treatment, such as shaping, conditioning and reinforcement, and systematic desensitization (Kedesdy & Budd, 1998).

With *shaping*, the therapist moves a child incrementally toward a desired goal. For instance, if a long-term goal is to increase a child's consumption of foods with texture, the therapist will gradually shape the child's experiences with textured foods—from touching a new texture to the lips without gagging to eating a variety of textured foods during a single mealtime. With *conditioning and reinforcement*, a child learns to associate a stimulus with a particular outcome, such as receiving a preferred food for eating a nonpreferred food. Social approval from a parent ("That was great! I am very proud of you!") is one form of positive reinforcement that then might be paired with the new behavior to increase its frequency. With *systematic desensitization*, the therapist trains a child to accept an aversive sensory experience (e.g., eating a new texture) by breaking down the aversive experience into small steps and showing the child that each step is safe and possible.

Alternative and Supplemental Feeding

Children who are unable to meet their own nutritional needs orally and whose growth is faltering require an alternative solution. Children who are candidates for supplemental or alternative nutrition are those (1) who cannot meet 80% of their caloric needs orally, (2) who have not gained weight or who have continuously lost weight for 3 months, (3) whose weight and height ratio is below the 5th percentile, and/or (4) whose feeding time is greater than 5 to 6 hours daily (Smith & Pederson, 1990).

The most common solution is *enteral*, or tube, feeding, in which liquid nutrition is delivered through a tube. In some cases the tube feeding is supplemental, providing supportive therapy in combination with oral intake (Smith & Pederson, 1990). For instance, a child with cerebral palsy might be able to meet some but not all nutritional needs orally, in which case tube feeding is supplemental. In other cases tube feeding might be the sole avenue for a child's nutrition, as in the case of a child with very low birth weight or one who is very premature.

For short-term treatment a **nasogastric tube** is used, which is passed through the nasal cavity and into the esophagus. No surgery is required, and the tube should not impact communication, although it may interfere with breathing and cause throat irritation. For longer term treatment a *gastrostomy tube* or a *jejunostomy tube* is placed surgically into the stomach or small intestine. Nutritional support is then delivered either intermittently or continuously. With intermittent feeding nutrition is provided four to eight times daily to mimic the timing of normal feeding, whereas with continuous feeding nutrition is provided nonstop. For children requiring enteral feeding, a team of professionals works closely with the families to determine the best approach.

When children receive alternative nutritional support, therapists work to ensure that the caregiver-child feeding relationship also receives special support; it is a special context in which the overall relationship develops, as well as important communicative abilities. In addition, therapists and parents must promote children's oral abilities even when these are not being used for feeding. Children who receive no nutrition orally may become orally hypersensitive or aversive to touch around their mouths, creating significant problems for parents and therapists once these children are more medically stable and ready to eat.

Consider 3-year-old Eva, who received tube feedings her entire life and was so orally hypersensitive that she gagged at the sight or smell of food. Even when oral feeding is possible and safe, children like Eva may resist because of their lack of oral experiences. To prevent oral aversion and hypersensitivity, therapists and parents work closely together to promote pleasurable oral experiences and to encourage oral exploration of fingers and toys. Early positive experiences with the oral-motor structures and functions make later successful weaning from tube feeding more likely.

A return to oral nutrition is an important goal for most children who receive enteral feeding; even when medical complications require lifelong use of enteral feeding, oral intake may still be possible for pleasure or supplemental sustenance. The majority of children who are tube fed are able to return to or begin oral feeding when their nutritional needs and medical conditions are stable. For some who have been tube fed for a long period of time or who have psychological resistance to oral feeding, a special intensive program may be needed for tube weaning. Figure 9-8 provides an overview of such a program for children who are ready for weaning but for whom previous weaning efforts have failed.

FIGURE 9-8 A tube-weaning program: University of Virginia's Encouragement Feeding Program.

The Encouragement Feeding Program is an intensive 2-week inpatient tube-weaning program for children. Children and their parents participate in a variety of therapeutic activities in the hospital during their 14-day stay. The program is based on four key principles that allow children to transition from tube feedings to oral feeding in an effective and efficient process.

Key Principles

- **Creation of internal motivation.** The child must develop an internal motivation to eat. To create this internal motivation, a child needs to experience the feelings of hunger and satiety as much as possible. This occurs by cutting back or rearranging the tube feeding schedule to create feelings of hunger and fullness. Also, a child needs to develop a sense of responsibility toward eating and taking in enough food for growth.
- **Immersion into sensory stimulation.** Many children with feeding difficulties have disordered sensory systems. Oral aversion is usually just one aspect of sensory difficulties; our program emphasizes treatment of sensory difficulties more globally. A successful program must include intensive sensory experiences, including not just oral experiences but a range of developmentally appropriate sensory activities. Planting plants, playing in sand, making peanut butter play dough, playing in water—all address the entire child.
- **Immersion into eating.** Equally important as immersion into sensory experiences is the immersion into oral eating. Children in the program are fed 4 times per day depending on their ages. They are immersed in the oral experience, even if it causes gagging or vomiting or other resistant behaviors. Usually within a day or two, gagging is significantly reduced and intake improves.
- **Determination of primary barrier to normal eating.** We focus intensively on identifying the primary barrier that keeps children from feeding orally. This allows us to individualize therapy. Examples of common barriers include poor hunger/satiety

(continued)

FIGURE 9-8 *(Continued)*

or internal motivation, inexperience with eating, severe sensory/anxiety issues, behavioral issues, and cognitive delays/disorders.

Program Organization

Intake

Objective: To determine the level of current eating readiness, which will regulate how the program is carried out. The feeding therapist evaluates the child's current level of feeding readiness:

- Observation of typical meal with parent and child
- Determination of diet level
- Determination of behavior modification techniques to increase compliance with eating

Objective: To promote normal feeding scheduling and begin to promote development of hunger/satiety cycle. The feeding therapist determines the feeding schedule and feeding environment for the child's days in the program:

- Child is typically fed four to five times per day, 6 days a week, on a strict three-meal, two- to three-snack schedule. Meals last only 30 minutes; snacks last 15 minutes.
- Child is typically fed in a quiet but natural environment, seated in a chair or in a highchair. Parents are included in each meal.
- Child's tube feedings are gradually cut back, as determined by the nutritionist and based on the child's current level of nutrition. Tube feedings are decreased on a daily basis if possible, with the goal of achieving a reduction of 25% of tube feedings at the end of the first week of the program.

Objective: To determine which behavior management methods increase compliance in eating. The feeding therapist determines the most effective approaches to modifying the child's current feeding behaviors, including reinforcers for active eating.

Days 1–3

Objective: To achieve the child's toleration of foods with increased compliance and decreased avoidance behaviors with the feeding therapist. The feeding therapist increases the child's acceptance of pureed foods per meal and may introduce small amounts of highly textured foods. The therapist also works directly with the parent to provide education on techniques that are effective in increasing the child's intake.

Days 4–7

Objective: To achieve the child's active participation in the feeding process with increased amounts of food taken per meal and a reduction in avoidance behaviors with parent. The feeding therapist focuses on increasing the child's intake of pureed foods to 50–75% of those offered during each meal and intake of highly textured foods. The parent receives training in consistent language and behaviors across meals.

Days 8+

Objective: To achieve the child's active participation in the feeding process in less structured meal environments with no change in feeding behaviors. The feeding therapist focuses on increasing the child's intake of foods to 75–100% of those

FIGURE 9-8 *(Continued)*

offered during each meal, including pureed and textured foods. The therapist also focuses on maintaining the child's positive mealtime behaviors in less structured settings and helping the parent to maintain consistent language and behaviors in these settings.

Discharge

Discharge takes place after 2 weeks in the intensive program, with most of our children taking at least 70% of caloric needs by mouth in an efficient and safe manner. A written feeding protocol is provided to families to help with the transition to the home environment. Prior to discharge, community supports are set up as necessary to ease the transition. Weekly weighings are encouraged until adequate weight gain occurs for several months. Parents follow up with their local doctors to determine when the tube can be removed, if appropriate. Follow-up phone calls occur on a weekly basis at first and gradually decrease as parents feel them unnecessary.

Case Study and Clinical Problem Solving

Pediatric Feeding Clinic
Mason Children's Hospital
811 Old Turner Rd.
San Diego, CA

OUTPATIENT TREATMENT ENROLLMENT

Joshua Harvis, 32 months, will be enrolled in the June pediatric feeding clinic for tube weaning. A case history with treatment objectives was developed following an assessment completed 5/2/05, summarized as follows.

Abbreviated History: Joshua was born on 9/12/2002 with a left diaphragmatic hernia. He received a gastrostomy tube and Nissen fundoplication at 4 months. He received feeding therapy through early intervention for 3 months in 2004 during which he progressed from refusing to sit in the high chair and gagging at the presence of foods to happily sitting at the table and exploring most dry foods orally by licking and spitting. Actual consumption of foods, however, was minimal, and the program was halted when the family moved to San Diego in June 2004. Currently, Joshua is medically stable with severe oral aversion and inexperience with all aspects of eating.

Fine and Gross Motor: Low tone with poor trunk stability and general gross motor skills more like those of a 10- to 12-month-old. Delayed fine motor skills. Displayed many characteristics of sensory defensiveness: reluctance to engage in play with any dry or wet foods, frequent gagging.

Oral-Motor Functions: Low tone in face and mouth, hyposensitivity and frequent mouthing of nonfood items. He demonstrated open-mouth posture with drooling. Safety of swallow was judged to be good based on an absence of any clinical signs of aspiration. There was minimal exploration of most foods, and cooperation was minimal at first. When a taste of food was placed on his tongue, his tongue became very rigid, and he was unwilling to close his mouth to trigger a swallow. Most food drooled out.

Speech-Language Status: Joshua demonstrated a delay in expressive language with skills around the 12- to 15-month level. His receptive skills were at the 18-month level. He was very social and demonstrated strong communicative intentions, frequently rejecting, commenting, and requesting objects and actions of his mother.

Behavior: Joshua was extremely motivated by praise, songs, and verbal encouragement.

Growth and Nutrition: Joshua's baseline weight was 12.62 kg, and height was 32.5 inches, putting him slightly under the 50th percentile for weight and between the 10th and 25th percentile for height. Weight-for-height was between the 25th and 50th percentiles. He was receiving 1100 cc of Pediasure daily: 4 4-oz feedings during the day and the rest (650 cc) through an overnight drip. No history of constipation. No allergies. No medications.

Treatment Objectives: Four objectives will be addressed:

1. Increased tolerance of a variety of textures
2. Increased oral-motor function
3. Improved relationship with foods
4. Decreased dependence on feeding tube

CLINICAL PROBLEM SOLVING

1. This report indicates that Joshua was born with a diaphragmatic hernia and had a medical procedure described as a Nissen fundoplication. What is this procedure?
2. At 18 months of age, Joshua's intervention helped him to explore and play with foods, but he would not eat. Why would he have been so averse to eating and enjoying food experiences?
3. Joshua is enrolled in an intensive feeding clinic to wean him from the feeding tube. What are some factors that will influence whether this intensive clinic is successful? Consider family influences, child influences, and treatment influences.
4. This program will be expensive and time-consuming for Joshua's family. Given that Joshua's nutritional needs are being met, why wouldn't his family maintain the status quo?

CHAPTER SUMMARY

A pediatric feeding disorder refers to a persistent failure to eat adequately for a period of 1 month or longer. A swallowing disorder, or dysphagia, is a type of feeding disorder in which safe and efficient swallowing is compromised. Children with feeding and/or swallowing disorders may experience failure to thrive and growth delay, lack of tolerance of food textures and tastes, poor appetite regulation, and/or rigid eating patterns. These may result in undernutrition or malnutrition, both of which can undermine a young child's growth and development.

Pediatric feeding and swallowing disorders are classified by their descriptive features or their etiology. Classification by descriptive features focuses on the timing of the disorder—transient, episodic, or chronic—or the behavioral features. Disordered behaviors fall into three major categories: eating too little, eating too much, or eating the wrong things. Etiological classification focuses on the cause of the feeding or swallowing disorder, which at the broadest level is differentiated as organic or nonorganic. Organic causes include neuromotor dysfunction, mechanical obstruction, and medical or genetic anomalies. Nonorganic causes stem from physical/emotional disturbances, educational causes, environmental causes, and behavioral factors. Current perspectives on etiology emphasize a biopsychosocial view, in which problems emerge from the complex interplay of biology, psychology, and social relationships.

Assessment of pediatric feeding and swallowing disorders emphasizes early identification and referral to promote healthy growth and development in young children. Parents and physicians work together to identify when disordered patterns are emerging and to problem-solve solutions. When problems are more severe, a feeding specialist conducts a comprehensive evaluation that includes a case history, oral-motor examination, and feeding observation.

When treatment is required, behavioral approaches commonly include conditioning, reinforcement, shaping, and desensitization. For very young children, including those in the NICU, ongoing oral-motor stimulation and communicative supports are vital. For some children supplemental or alternative feeding is needed, including enteral feeding systems.

KEY TERMS

aspiration, p. 287
catch-up growth, p. 293
cerebral palsy, p. 302
cleft palate, p. 302
conditioned dysphagia, p. 303
deglutition, p. 287
failure to thrive, p. 300
feeding specialist, p. 285
gagging reflex, p. 293
gastroenterologist, p. 308
gastrostomy tube, p. 296
grasping reflex, p. 293
growth charts, p. 291
homeostasis, p. 294
hyperphagia, p. 298
low birth weight, p. 304
malnutrition, p. 291
modified barium swallow, p. 311
nasogastric tube, p. 316
NICU, p. 290
nonorganic disorder, p. 299
nutrition, p. 291
oral-motor functions, p. 286
oral-motor muscular tone, p. 286
oral-motor sensation, p. 286
oral-motor system, pp. 285, 301
organic disorder, p. 298
overselectivity, p. 303
penetration, p. 287
PKU, p. 305
prematurity, p. 304
reflux, p. 303
rooting reflex, p. 293
sensory defensiveness, p. 304
stunting, p. 292
suckling reflex, p. 293
undernutrition, p. 291
underweight, p. 292
wasting, p. 292

ON THE WEB

Check out the Companion Website! On it you will find

- suggested readings
- reflection questions
- a self-study quiz
- links to additional online resources, including current technologies in communication sciences and disorders

Dysphagia

C. R. O'Donoghue

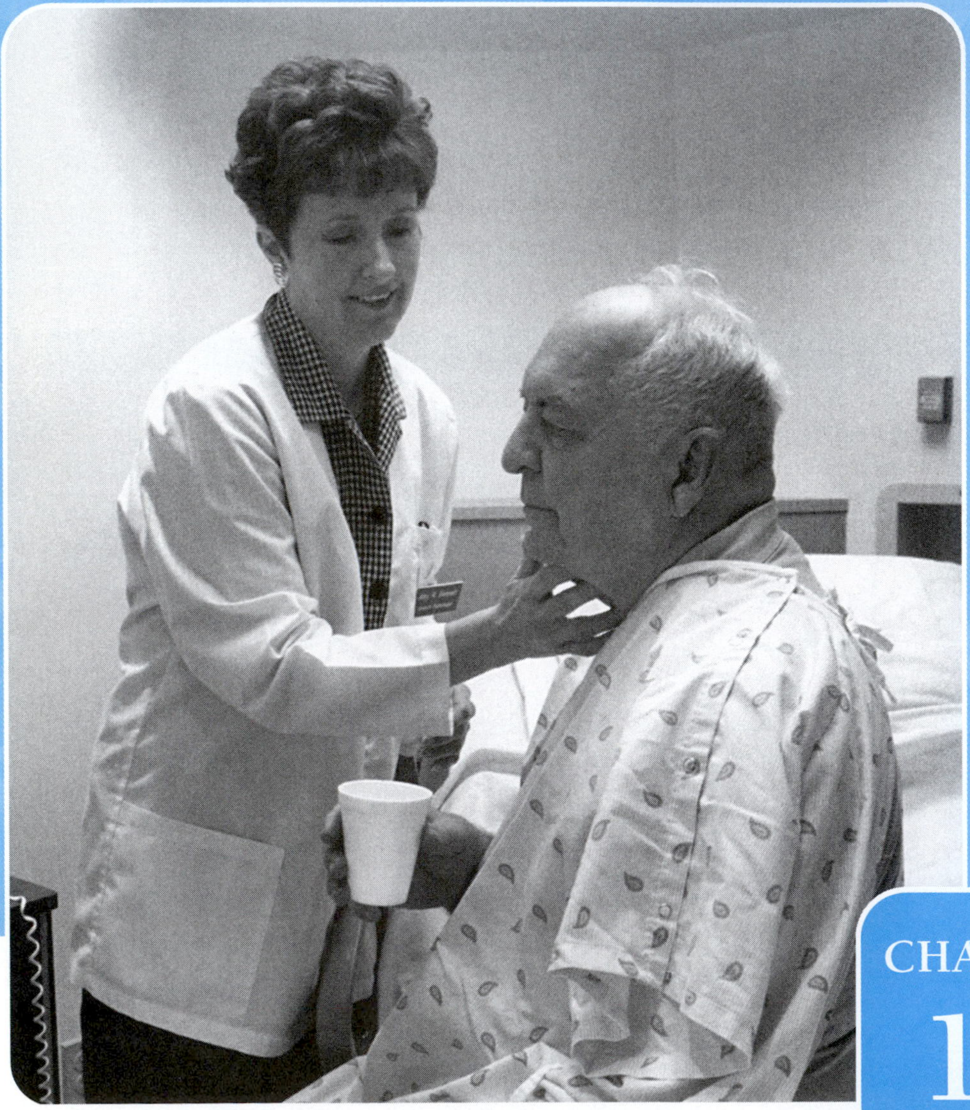

CHAPTER 10

FOCUS QUESTIONS

This chapter will answer the following questions:

1. What is dysphagia?
2. How is dysphagia classified?
3. What are the defining characteristics of dysphagia?
4. How is dysphagia identified?
5. How is dysphagia treated?

INTRODUCTION

Eating cold chocolate ice cream on a hot summer day is a pleasurable experience for most people. However, there are adults whose swallowing mechanism is impaired who are no longer able to enjoy this and many other treats. Individuals with impairments of swallowing may find eating to be a burden, or they may be limited in what foods or liquids they can safely consume. A disorder of swallowing, in which the ability to safely and/or efficiently use the swallowing mechanism is compromised, is called **dysphagia**. Dysphagia occurs in adults because of neurological or structural problems that alter the normal swallowing process. Speech-language pathologists evaluate and treat this disorder, working with individuals to improve their ability to safely and efficiently eat food and drink liquids to promote healthy nutrition and improved quality of life (American Speech-Language-Hearing Association [ASHA], 2002c).

Evaluating and treating persons with dysphagia is a relatively new aspect of the scope of practice for speech-language pathologists (SLPs) (ASHA, 2001); it became a major aspect only in the 1980s. Prior to this time, relatively little was known about swallowing disorders and therapies. However, in the last 2 decades, our knowledge of how swallowing works and how it can be rehabilitated has vastly improved and is now used to improve the quality of life for persons who find their swallowing abilities compromised by stroke, injury, illness, or other causes.

Dysphagia management has grown to be a major component of the SLP's daily professional responsibilities in many settings, including hospitals, rehabilitation centers, nursing homes, and outpatient clinics (ASHA, 2004b). In fact, dysphagia intervention now constitutes close to 50% of the clinical caseload of SLPs who work in medical settings (ASHA, 2002d). SLPs who specialize in dysphagia management are often described as swallowing therapists (Logemann, 1998).

Swallowing therapists require a highly specialized set of clinical skills and knowledge, because clinical mismanagement can have life-threatening consequences. Individuals with swallowing impairments are at risk of choking, aspirating food into their lungs, developing pneumonia, and even dying. Such possibilities may seem overwhelming but must be balanced with the rewards of helping dysphagic clients once

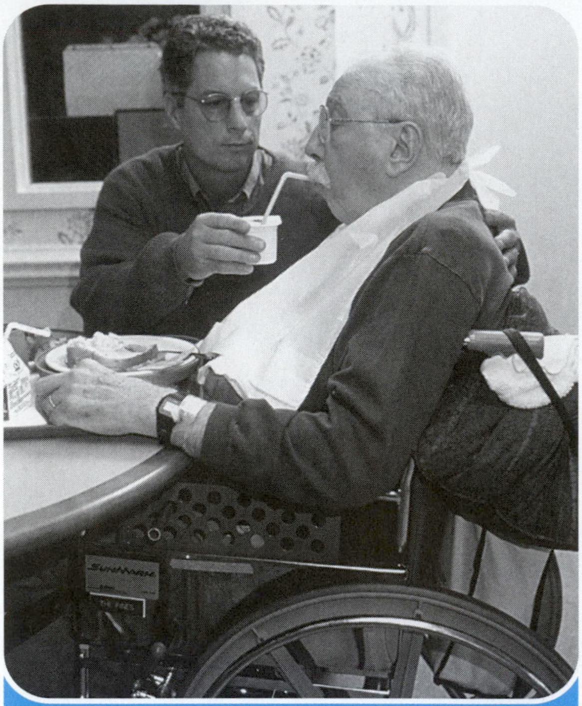

The last decades have seen considerable growth in research on how to rehabilitate swallowing functions.

again assume the skilled and safe swallowing functions that permit eating and drinking to be safe and pleasurable.

What Is Dysphagia?

Dysphagia is a disorder of swallowing. The individual with dysphagia is unable to safely and/or efficiently eat or drink because of impaired structures or functions of the swallowing mechanisms. You may wonder how to pronounce the word *dysphagia:* is it *dys-phah-gia* (with the middle syllable rhyming with "ma") or dys-*phay*-gia (with the middle syllable rhyming with "may")? You are likely to hear both pronunciations, although the current preference is *dys-phay-gia* (and the "ah" vowel is reserved for the adjective *dysphagic*). Why are there two pronunciations? First, American English like all languages allows many regional dialects. Thus, variations are common in the production of any word and, from a linguistic perspective, wholly appropriate and acceptable. Second, the term *dysphasia* (pronounced with a long "a" sound) was long used in the field of communication disorders to describe acquired disorders of language (the term *aphasia* was then used to describe severe variants of dysphasia). In some countries, like Australia, the term *dysphasia* is still used today, although it is seldom used by clinicians in the United States. Nonetheless, because *dysphasia* and *dysphagia* sound quite similar when spoken, as the field of swallowing treatment began to flourish in the 1980s and 1990s, some people began to say *dys-phah-gia* rather than *dys-phay-gia* to differentiate the term from *dys-phay-sia*. Thus, the two pronunciations of *dysphagia* began and persist today. However, given that the term *dysphasia* is rarely used in clinical practice in the United States, the *dys-phay-gia* pronunciation is currently preferred by most U.S. clinicians.

Discussion Point: *Explore the reasons that speech-language pathologists have become involved in the management of swallowing disorders.*

Understanding disordered swallowing requires an understanding of ordered, or normal, swallowing. The next section provides a review of concepts previously introduced in chapter 3.

The Normal Swallow

Swallowing is a basic, life-sustaining function. In fact, it is an innate ability that is present in the developing fetus (Arvedson & Rogers, 1993). Swallowing is so natural that we do it approximately 580 times daily without even thinking about it (Logemann, 1998). Even though we do not consciously think about how to swallow, there are specific physiological components of a normal swallow that occur in a series of unfolding stages. These swallowing stages, also called phases, include the oral preparatory phase, the oral phase, the pharyngeal phase, and the esophageal phase. Each of these phases is essential for safely and efficiently moving food and drink from the oral cavity through the pharynx (i.e., throat) and into the esophagus toward the intestines. As shown in Figure 10-1, the margin of error separating the pathways of food and drink to the esophagus and oxygen to the larynx and pulmonary system is slim. The four phases of swallowing must work seamlessly and efficiently to keep food and drink from possibly dangerous routes.

The Oral Preparatory Phase

The role of the oral preparatory phase is to prepare the substance to be swallowed for swallowing. This phase starts as the food or liquid enters the mouth, and it includes containing the material in the oral cavity by closing the lips and then manipulating and preparing the food or liquid into a cohesive ball, or **bolus**. As food enters the oral cavity, saliva production increases to assist in bolus formation. Also, the soft palate lowers toward the tongue to contain the bolus and prohibit the flow of ingested material into the pharyngeal region until the bolus is adequately prepared. Chewing, or *mastication,* occurs as the lips, tongue, teeth, mandible, and cheeks work cooperatively to grind the food into a manageable texture to swallow. Even with liquids, a bolus is formed that assists in controlling the flow of the liquid.

The time to complete the oral preparatory phase is variable, depending on the substance eaten. Oral preparation for liquids (e.g., tea, milkshake) is more rapid than for foods requiring mastication (e.g., potato chips, popcorn). Throughout the oral preparatory phase, respiration continues with inhalation and exhalation through the nose.

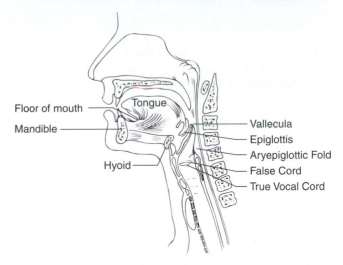

FIGURE 10-1 Cross-section of the head and neck.

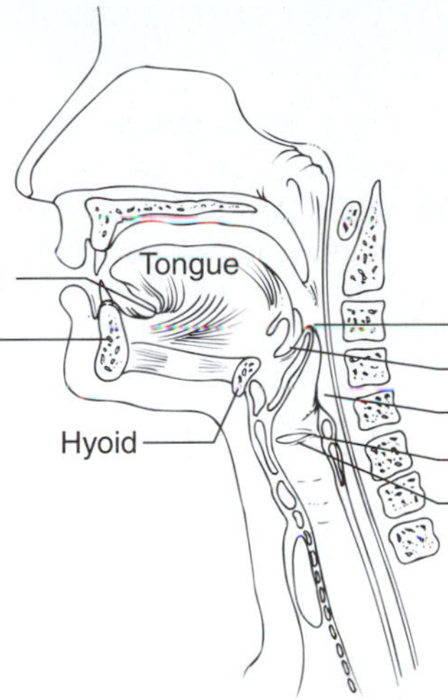

Source: Adapted from Logemann, J. (1998). *Evaluation and treatment of swallowing disorders* (2nd ed., p. 28). Austin, TX: Pro-Ed. Reprinted with permission.

The Oral Phase

The role of the oral phase is to move the bolus to the rear of the oral cavity and prepare it for propulsion down the throat. The oral phase begins as the tongue propels the bolus to the back of the mouth. This "stripping action" is accomplished as the tongue presses upward against the hard palate. This tongue movement, coupled with tension in the cheeks created by the *buccal muscles,* creates a pressure that pushes the bolus backward toward the pharynx. You can experience this yourself by chewing a cracker. Notice that once the cracker is prepared into a ball in the oral preparatory phase, you move it back into the throat by pushing the tongue against the roof of the mouth. The oral phase typically is completed within 1 to 1.5 seconds (Logemann, 1998). In this phase the individual still maintains a normal respiratory pattern, breathing through the nose.

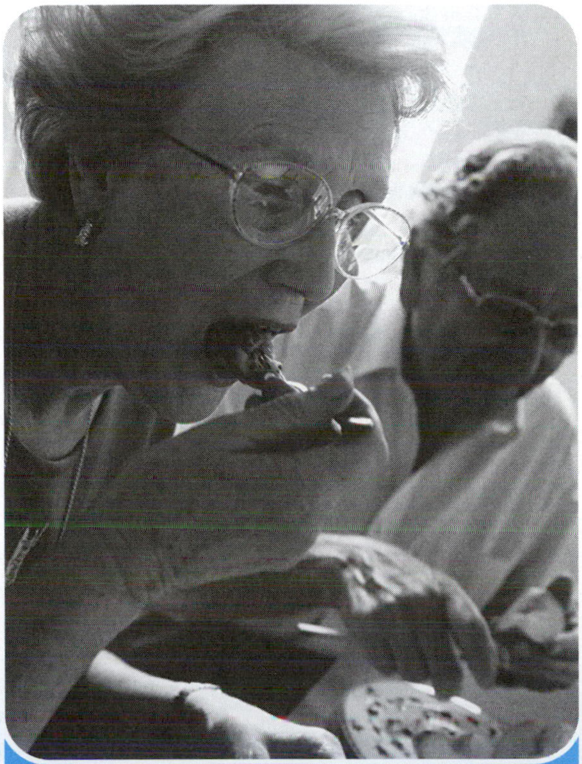

During the oral preparatory phase, the bolus is prepared for transport.

The Pharyngeal Phase

The role of the pharyngeal phase is to propel the bolus downward through the throat to the entrance of the esophagus. The pharyngeal phase begins when the bolus reaches the posterior

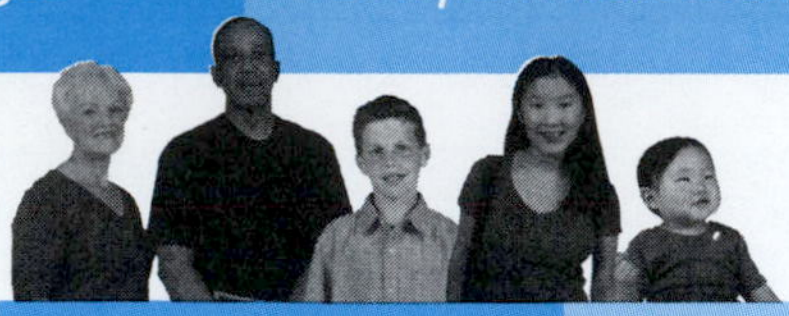

BOX 10-1 Dysphagia: Case Examples

Sylvia Anderson is a 78-year-old female who currently lives at Pleasant Valley Nursing Home. Sylvia has a diagnosis of Alzheimer's dementia, diagnosed approximately 11 years ago. She also has a history of hypertension, diabetes, bilateral hip replacements, osteoarthritis, and intermittent unexplained bronchitis. Sylvia has resided at Pleasant Valley for 2 years, and although she needs supervision for her safety, she is ambulatory with a cane and completes her daily dressing, bathing, and feeding with minimal to moderate assistance.

Recently, the nursing assistants have noted that Sylvia is not finishing her meals and that midway through her meal she has a gurgly voice quality with excessive throat clearing. Three days ago, Sylvia had a severe coughing episode while eating fried chicken. The nursing staff consulted the only speech-language pathologist in the facility to evaluate Sylvia for possible dysphagia. He completed a clinical bedside examination of swallowing and found Sylvia pleasant, cooperative, and able to follow short instructions, although cognitive impairments were evident. Assessment findings suggested that Sylvia has a pharyngeal phase swallowing problem, and an instrumental assessment at the local hospital is scheduled.

Internet research

1. What is the prevalence of Alzheimer's dementia in the United States?
2. What is the percentage of nursing home residents over 65 years of age suspected to have dysphagia?
3. Find a Website that provides information on Alzheimer's disease and support for clients and their families. What kind of supports are prevalent?

Brainstorm and discussion

1. Transporting Sylvia to the local hospital for an instrumental examination of dysphagia is costly. Is this cost justifiable?
2. How will Sylvia's cognitive decline and dementia diagnosis affect treatment of dysphagia?

Lee Chin is a 43-year-old male who is bilingual in English and Chinese and has worked for the past 15 years as a computer analyst in Washington, DC. Lee was diagnosed with cancer of the right buccal space 2 years ago, attributed to his tobacco use for 25 years. Lee underwent radiation treatment for a 3-month period following diagnosis. Several weeks after radiation treatment began, Lee experienced difficulty eating solid foods and consumed mainly liquids and pureed foods. Because of his weight loss and the anticipated duration of his medical treatment, a gastrostomy tube was placed to maintain his normal weight of 140 pounds. Lee had a dysphagia assessment at that time that indicated severe pharyngeal-phase problems with some aspiration of both liquids and purees. Nine months after diagnosis Lee underwent a right type II modified radical neck dissection (MRND). Currently, Lee remains NPO (nothing per oral), taking only water in small sips throughout the day. He reports that his vocal quality is raspy and hoarse. He also has right lower facial weakness and ongoing pharyngeal dysphagia. He has not had any respiratory infections although he does continue to smoke tobacco.

Internet research

1. What structures of swallowing might be affected in an MRND?
2. What are the typical side effects of head and neck radiation, and how long might these symptoms persist?

portion of the oral cavity, specifically the area of the *anterior faucial pillars.* These pillars comprise a band of muscular tissue that extends from both sides of the palate to the tongue. The muscle forms a sphincter that contracts to initiate the pharyngeal phase of the swallow.

The pharyngeal phase is complex, with many important physiological occurrences happening simultaneously and quickly. At the start of this phase, the **pharyngeal swallow reflex** is triggered; the posterior pharyngeal wall and the back of the tongue move toward one another to create a pressure that, in conjunction with the squeezing pharyngeal muscles, moves the bolus downward through the pharynx toward the entrance to the esophagus. The *cricopharyngeus muscle,* also called the *upper esophageal sphincter,* is the

3. What is the incidence of head and neck cancers in individuals who do *not* use tobacco products? and for those who do?

Brainstorming and discussion

1. If Lee is ready to begin dysphagia rehabilitation to move to oral intake, what factors will influence the success of this treatment?
2. Consider why Lee still smokes, given his medical history.

Martin Coleman is a 45-year-old second-generation male of Irish Catholic descent. Martin is married, with two children, aged 12 and 15. Eighteen months ago, Martin began experiencing limb weakness and difficulty in eating. A diagnosis of Amyotrophic Lateral Sclerosis (ALS) was confirmed. Prior to this diagnosis he was a successful corporate lawyer; however, he is now unable to work. Presently, Martin is eating a puree diet with thin liquids with a stringent safety protocol. In the past 2 months, Martin has lost 15 pounds and has recuperated from a serious episode of aspiration pneumonia.

Martin and his family sought out a local swallowing therapist, Ms. Harrow, for guidance on rehabilitation. Her evaluations show severe oral and pharyngeal phase deficits with aspiration on 30% of all swallowing trials, regardless of consistency of the bolus. Compensatory strategies did not alter his performance, and Ms. Harrow notes that swallowing is unsafe and that pneumonia will likely reoccur. Martin and his family are now faced with the decision of whether to place a feeding tube for nutritional purposes. Martin and his wife are concerned that their decision on tube feeding be in keeping with their religious beliefs (whether to sustain life with a tube or to starve by rejecting the tube), and they are seeking counsel from their priest.

Internet research

1. What is the typical life expectancy of an ALS client following initial diagnosis?
2. What is the typical age of onset for ALS, and are there gender differences in incidence?
3. Is there a hereditary predisposition for ALS?

Brainstorming and discussion

1. To what extent should a person's religious beliefs influence decisions about medical interventions?
2. What other factors—beyond religious or spiritual considerations—contribute to the decision-making process for tube feeding?

juncture between the pharynx and the esophagus. It opens to allow passage of the bolus into the esophagus.

The pharyngeal phase of the swallow is an important one; at this point the bolus can potentially enter the laryngeal pathway to the lungs or the nasal cavity to prohibit breathing. However, there are multiple protective mechanisms in place within the pharyngeal phase to prevent either from happening. First, the soft palate elevates to form a barrier between the pharynx and the nasal cavity; this keeps the bolus from flowing upward into the nasal area. Second, the larynx moves forward and higher in the neck, making the risk of material entering the airway less probable. Third, the epiglottis, a leaflike cartilage in the pharynx, folds downward to form a cover over the larynx. Fourth, both the false and true vocal folds approximate (i.e., come together) to close and prevent ingested materials from entering the larynx, or airway.

If for some reason material does go the wrong way, a reflexive cough occurs to propel the material back out. The **reflexive cough** is a protective reflex in which exhaled air is forced upward through the vocal folds to expel any foreign matter. In addition, during the pharyngeal phase of a normal swallow, respiration experiences a brief halt, called an **apneic moment**. This short period of halted breathing further minimizes the risk of material entering the airway. In all, this stage is about 1 second in duration from the time the pharyngeal swallow reflex is triggered until the bolus passes into the esophagus.

The Esophageal Phase

The esophageal phase of the swallow moves the bolus through the esophagus into the stomach. This process starts as the bolus passes through the upper esophageal sphincter (UES). The bolus is propelled through the esophagus by an involuntary wave, or contraction. It then passes through the lower esophageal sphincter (LES) into the stomach. The esophageal phase ranges from about 8 to 20 seconds for adults. Age influences the variation in duration, with esophageal movement slowing as we age—referred to as a decrease in *esophageal motility* (DeVault, 2002). In summary, the normal swallowing process is a complex yet innate ability, as presented in Figure 10-2.

The Disordered Swallow: Dysphagia

Dysphagia is a condition in which an individual exhibits difficulty in at least one of the phases of the swallow, causing swallowing to be inefficient and/or unsafe. When swallowing is inefficient, it does not provide adequate nutrition. For instance, individuals may spend so much time in the oral preparatory phase that they are fatigued and unable to consume enough food to meet their nutritional needs.

When swallowing is unsafe, individuals are at risk of penetration and/or aspiration because of poor coordination or management of the bolus as it moves through the swallowing phases. With **penetration** food or liquid enters the laryngeal area to the level of the true vocal folds (Logemann, 1998). With **aspiration** food or liquid materials, including saliva, move below the level of the true vocal folds into the airway, or trachea. Silent aspiration occurs when there is no sign—such as choking, coughing, or speaking with a wet or gurgly voice—to suggest that aspiration is occurring. Both penetration and aspiration present hazards: penetration can result in choking, causing a loss of oxygen to the brain and leading to brain damage or death, and aspiration can result in pneumonia and pulmonary damage.

When dysphagia is present, affected individuals may be unable to intake certain food consistencies safely and must, as a result, have their diets altered. With such diet changes individuals frequently have difficulty maintaining their hydration and nutrition. If the situation persists, these individuals need to be fed through an alternative means, such as an **enteral feeding tube**, which directs a liquid formula to the stomach and is typically placed through the nose (i.e., nasogastric tube) or directly into the stomach (i.e., gastrostomy tube). The liquid formula provides for nutritional maintenance, and water can also be given to keep persons hydrated.

A Symptom, Not a Disease

Dysphagia is not a disease, but rather a symptom that results from an underlying etiology, or cause. Swallowing problems can result from neurological injuries, progressive disease processes, head and neck cancers, or even the medical treatments prescribed to combat a disease, such as radiation to treat a laryngeal cancer.

Dysphagia is also not a feeding disorder per se. **Feeding** is a more comprehensive term that combines the concept of swallowing with the hand-to-mouth process of eating. Although

FIGURE 10-2 Bolus movement during a normal swallow.

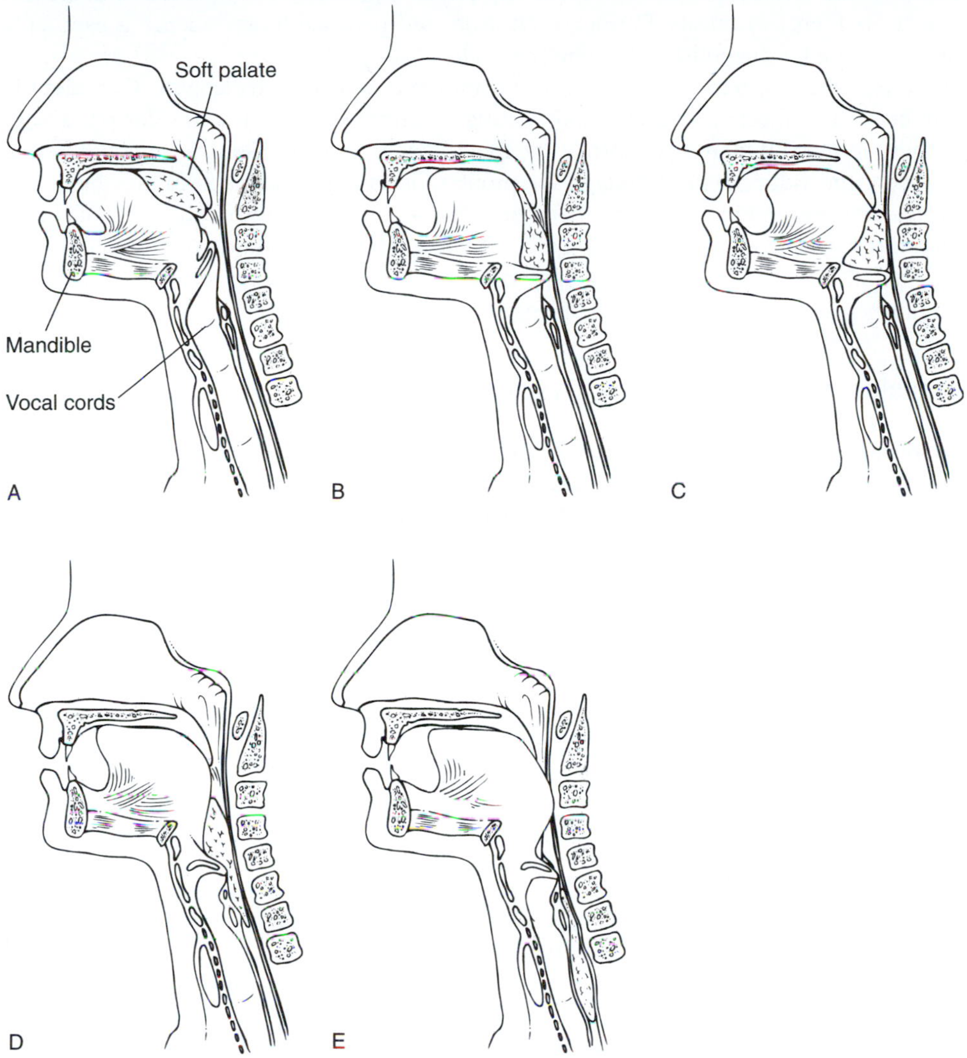

Lateral view of swallow, beginning with initiation of swallow by tongue (A); the triggering of the pharyngeal swallow (B); the bolus in the valleculae area (C); the tongue base retraction against the pharyngeal wall (D); the bolus in the cervical esophagus (E).

Source: Adapted from Logemann, J. (1998). *Evaluation and treatment of swallowing disorders* (2nd ed., p. 28). Austin, TX: Pro-Ed. Reprinted with permission.

the entire feeding process is certainly considered in managing a client with dysphagia, the speech-language pathologist focuses predominantly on assessing and managing the oral and pharyngeal aspects of swallowing.

Social and Psychological Impact

The social and psychological impact of dysphagia is significant. Dysphagic individuals and their families often experience changes in their typical eating routines; changes in diet require alterations in food choices and food preparation. For example, when individuals are unable to safely or efficiently chew meats, these foods need to be chopped finely or even processed to a smooth or pureed consistency. This type of food preparation is burdensome and frequently requires an intensive commitment by a family member or caregiver, because many people with dysphagia have coexisting physical or cognitive limitations and are unable to fix their own meals. Further, such decreased personal independence is especially disheartening for previously self-sufficient adults.

Dysphagia also makes participating in community activities challenging. Consider the number of social activities that involve eating or drinking, such as going for pizza with friends, enjoying buttered popcorn at the movies, or meeting classmates for coffee before an exam. Individuals with dysphagia are prone to isolate themselves from previously enjoyable routines and interactions with others. One recent study showed that 36% of clients with dysphagia avoided eating with others (Ekberg, Hamdy, Woisard, Wuttge-Hannig, & Ortega, 2002). Such changes place dysphagic individuals at risk for feelings of isolation, diminished self-worth, and even depression.

Discussion Point: *Dysphagic individuals have barriers to daily routines and activities. Consider the case of Martin in Box 10-1; what barriers might he face?*

Prevalence and Incidence of Dysphagia

Dysphagia occurs throughout the continuum of health care. About 14% of acutely hospitalized patients experience dysphagia, and 30–35% of patients in rehabilitation facilities have swallowing difficulties (Logemann, 1995). The incidence of dysphagia in nursing home environments can include as many as 50% of the residents at a given time (Logemann, 1995). A recent survey of speech-language pathologists working in adult health care facilities found that 31% of their professional time was dedicated to the delivery of dysphagia services (ASHA, 2004d). Further, 85% of responding SLPs reported that they are not only the preferred providers of dysphagia management, but they are also the only primary providers in the health care setting (ASHA, 2004d).

How Is Dysphagia Classified?

Swallowing impairment is frequently classified in the clinical setting according to three factors: (1) the extent of oral, pharyngeal, or esophageal phase deficits; (2) the underlying pathology or cause; and (3) the severity of the disorder.

Phase Affected

Dysphagia can be characterized by the phase affected to identify the site at which the swallowing system breaks down. This is particularly important for designing interventions, which focus on the site where the breakdown occurs. The swallowing therapist is primarily concerned with disorders in the oral preparatory, oral, and pharyngeal phases, also called *oral-pharyngeal dysphagia.* Gastroenterologists, internists, radiologists, and other professionals study and treat *esophageal dysphagia,* resulting from impairments of the esophageal phase of swallowing. Characteristics of difficulties in the oral and pharyngeal phases are summarized here and are discussed more thoroughly later.

Oral Preparatory Phase

Breakdowns in the oral preparatory phase occur when the structures and functions of the lips, tongue, checks, and mandible do not function as they should. Examples of problems seen in this phase include impaired or reduced labial closure, tongue movement, tension in the cheeks (buccal cavity), mandibular movement, and sensitivity (Logemann, 1998).

Oral Phase

Breakdowns in the oral phase occur when these same structures do not function as they should to get the bolus positioned for the pharyngeal phase. Of greatest impact is the inability to trigger a swallow, which can delay the entire swallow cycle and increase the risk of inadequate intake and penetration.

Pharyngeal Phase

Breakdowns in the pharyngeal phase occur when the pharyngeal structures do not function as they should to move the bolus through the pharynx to the entrance of the esophagus. Common problems seen at this phase include inadequate pharyngeal contractions, malfunction of the upper esophageal sphincter, and inadequate closure of the laryngeal area (Logemann, 1998).

Underlying Pathology

Dysphagia is a secondary disorder, meaning that it results from another primary cause. The most common causes of dysphagia are neurological damage due to a stroke or brain injury, neurological damage due to a disease (e.g., Parkinson's disease), and laryngeal damage due to radiation, surgical removal of the larynx (laryngectomy), or trauma. Figure 10-3 lists

FIGURE 10-3 **Acquired conditions frequently resulting in oropharyngeal dysphagia.**

- Traumatic brain injury
  - Closed-head injury
  - Open-head injury
- Single stroke
  - Lower brain-stem stroke
  - High brain-stem stroke
  - Cerebral cortex stroke (left and/or right hemispheres)
- Multiple strokes
- Head and neck cancer
- Spinal cord injury
- Surgical trauma (e.g., removal of brain-stem tumor)
- Poliomyelitis
- Guillain-Barre disease
- Cerebral palsy
- Riley-Day syndrome
- Multiple sclerosis
- Huntington's disease
- Dementia
- Parkinson's disease
- Wilson's disease
- Infectious disease (e.g., meningitis, Lyme disease)

Sources: Based on Buchholz and Robbins (1997); Logemann (1998).

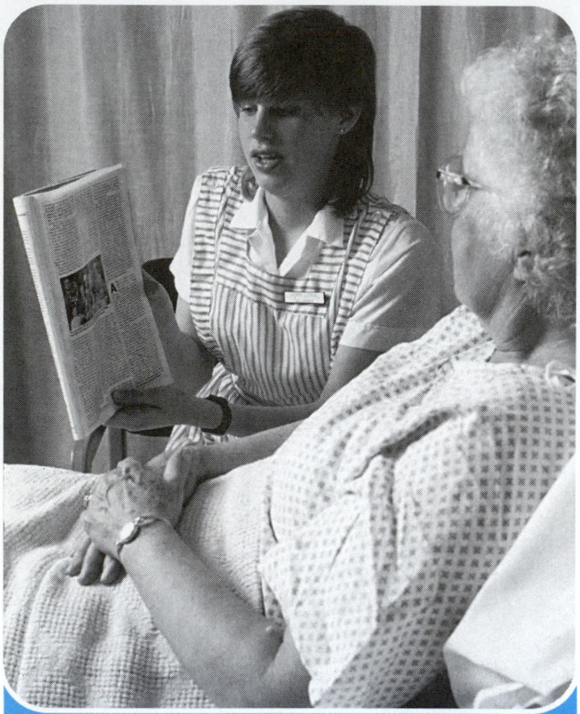

About half of stroke survivors aspirate, placing them at great risk of developing pneumonia and other pulmonary problems.

acquired conditions that commonly result in oropharyngeal dysphagia. Most commonly, speech-language pathologists manage dysphagia cases stemming from brain injury, progressive neurological diseases, and head and neck cancer treatments.

Brain Injury

Stroke. Stroke is a leading cause of disability and even death among adults. The frequency of dysphagia following stroke is relatively high, with incidence figures reaching as high as 50% or even higher (Mann, Hankey, & Cameron, 1999; Martino, Pron, & Diamant, 2000). A stroke results from an interruption in the blood supply to the brain, robbing the brain tissue of required oxygen and nutrients. As a result, brain tissue is damaged. After a stroke individuals are prone to oropharyngeal dysphagia, which increases the risk of malnutrition, aspiration, and pneumonia. As many as 55% of stroke patients aspirate, increasing their risk of developing pneumonia (Ding & Logemann, 2000). Estimates suggest that approximately one third of stroke patients die from pneumonia caused by aspiration (Odderson, Keaton, & McKenna, 1995).

Traumatic Brain Injury. Traumatic brain injuries (TBIs) are caused by car accidents, falls, and physical acts of violence and often result in diffuse brain damage. Dysphagia is a common complication of TBI (Morgan & Mackey, 1999), with incidence figures ranging between one fourth and three fourths of individuals with TBI exhibiting dysphagia (Cherney & Halper, 1996; Mackey, Morgan, & Bernstein, 1999; Schurr, Ebner, Maser, Sperling, Helgerson, & Harms, 1999). Even at the lower estimate, dysphagia is a common concern. The dysphagia commonly seen with TBI includes a significant delay in the pharyngeal swallow reflex, diminished pharyngeal constriction, and oral-motor compromises (Lazarus & Logemann, 1987). In addition, the frequent disturbance in cognitive functioning, such as low level of arousal and attention, can make swallowing further unsafe or inefficient.

Progressive Neurological Disease

Recall from chapter 8 that progressive neurological diseases are disorders of the nervous system producing discoordination and weakness of motor skills as well as decreased sensory abilities. These disorders are called progressive because the neurological problems and resulting symptoms become more disabling over time as the disease follows its course.

Parkinson's Disease. Parkinson's disease (PD) is a progressive neurological disease characterized by gradual depletion of the neurotransmitter dopamine, which hinders functioning of the basal ganglia. This alteration produces a movement disorder characterized by tremors, difficulty initiating movements, and a slow and rigid motion. As the disease progresses, it can also result in cognitive deterioration similar to that of dementia, with confusion and agitation.

Swallowing disorders in PD are common, impacting somewhere between 50% and 92% of individuals (Nilsson, Ekberg, Olsson, & Hindfelt, 1996; Stroudley & Walsh,

1991). This variability in estimates likely results from the fact that many PD clients are unaware of or fail to report dysphagia (Bird, Woodward, Gibson, Phyland, & Fonda, 1994; Bushmann, Dobmeyer, Leeker, & Perlmutter, 1989). Dysphagia in PD affects the oral, pharyngeal, and esophageal phases of the swallow, with common difficulties including drooling, abnormalities in bolus preparation and transport, delayed triggering of the swallow reflex, residual materials in the pharynx, aspiration, and diminished esophageal motility.

Amyotrophic Lateral Sclerosis. Amyotrophic lateral sclerosis (ALS) is more commonly recognized as Lou Gehrig's disease. ALS is a rapidly progressing motor-neuron disease resulting in severe deterioration of the muscles and motoric systems of the body, including the muscles for respiration. Although individuals with ALS experience significant physical deterioration, their cognitive abilities remain intact. At present, the cause of ALS is uncertain, and there is no known treatment.

Dysphagia is prevalent in ALS because of the disruptions in respiratory, phonatory, and articulatory functions. All persons with ALS experience oropharyngeal dysphagia at some point in the disease process. Swallowing dysfunction typically starts in the oral phase and progresses to the pharyngeal stage. Dysphagia may be one of the first symptoms of ALS, leading individuals to seek medical treatment based on changes in their swallowing ability and weight loss (Logemann, 1998).

Dementia. *Dementia* is a global term referring to alterations in cognitive skills. It has numerous etiologies, including Alzheimer's, dementia from multiple strokes, or progressive diseases such as Parkinson's disease or Huntington's chorea. One of the most common causes of dementia is Alzheimer's disease (AD), which is a progressive deterioration in mental capacity and later affects both sensory and motor functions. The incidence of dysphagia in AD is relatively low in the early disease stages. However, as it progresses to moderate and severe impairment levels, dysphagia is a common feature seen in more than one fourth of individuals with AD (Chouinard, 2000; Horner, Alberts, Dawson, & Cook, 1994; Kalia, 2003). Oropharyngeal deficits include the inability to recognize foods as something to eat, resulting from a more general condition of *agnosia,* in which individuals do not recognize things for what they are; difficulty in bolus preparation and transit, often due to apraxia; delayed initiation of the pharyngeal swallow reflex; and poor pharyngeal constriction. The mental decline in these individuals places them at greater risk of aspiration and pneumonia (Wada et al., 2001).

Head and Neck Cancer Treatments

Cancerous growths of the mouth, pharynx, and larynx are currently treated with surgery, radiation, and possibly chemotherapy. Dysphagia is often present prior to medical treatment for these cancers, but it frequently becomes more severe immediately following these interventions, which are necessary for survival. The impact of head and neck cancers on swallowing function relates directly to the type, size, and location of the growth (Colangelo, Logemann, & Rademaker, 2000; Pauloski et al., 2000) and the extent of surgical intervention and radiation therapy. Head and neck cancers often result in oral or pharyngeal stage dysphagia, which can be readily managed for many individuals.

Surgical Management. Since a malignant cancer is potentially life threatening, removal of the diseased tissue or structures is necessary. When components of swallowing are either partially or totally removed, as occurs in *glossectomy* (tongue removal) or *laryngectomy* (larynx removal), changes in swallowing function are probable.

FIGURE 10-4 **Tracheostomy tube placement.**

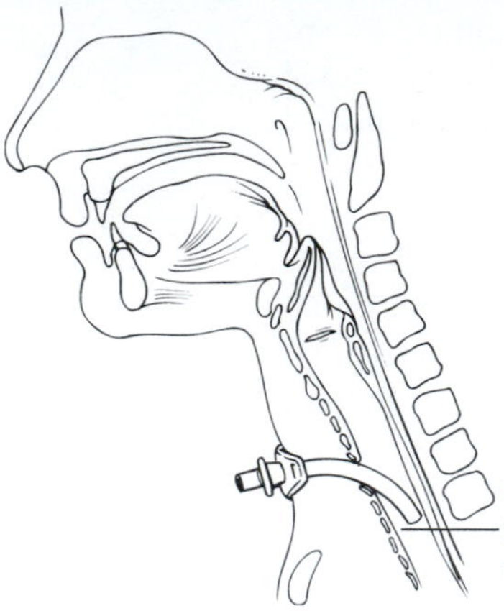

In some cases a tracheotomy is required, either temporarily or permanently. This surgical procedure places a tube through the neck directly into the trachea (see Figure 10-4) to maintain the airway and to allow for pulmonary hygiene. The presence of a tracheostomy tube influences swallowing performance by altering the normal air flow through the nose or oral cavities and vocal folds; air is now inhaled and exhaled through the tube. Physiological changes in the laryngeal muscles also hinder the swallowing process.

Radiation Therapy. Radiation is often used in addition to surgical management. Radiation treatment itself reduces saliva production (known as *xerostomia*) and also results in edema (water retention in tissues), tooth decay, and pain. All of these factors negatively influence swallowing capability.

Discussion Point: *How might the medical interventions to treat cancer make swallowing worse? Consider the case of Lee Chin in Box 10-1.*

Chemotherapy. In certain situations chemotherapy is part of the treatment regimen for head and neck cancers. The side effects of chemotherapy—such as nausea, vomiting, and fatigue—can lead to swallowing concerns, particularly adequate intake to achieve good nutritional status. Fortunately, advances in chemotherapy medications are producing fewer unpleasant side effects.

Severity

As yet, there is no universally accepted classification system of the severity of dysphagia. Several newer instruments, such as the Penetration-Aspiration Scale (Rosenbek, Robbins, Roecker, Coyle, & Wood, 1996) and the New Zealand Index for Multidisciplinary Evaluation of Swallowing (Huckabee, 2004), provide rating systems for certain aspects of the dysphagia profile. The Penetration-Aspiration Scale (Rosenbek et al., 1996) uses an 8-point scale to describe the degree of airway protection during the swallow. A score of 1 indicates that no material enters the airway, whereas a score of 8 indicates that material is aspirated and the individual shows no effort to cough and no gag reflex. A patient with a score of 8 would be at very high risk for aspiration.

The New Zealand Index for Multidisciplinary Evaluation of Swallowing (NZIMES; Huckabee, 2004) provides a comprehensive rating of an individual's swallowing status from the oral phase to the esophageal phase, assessing performance on a variety of indicators (e.g., positioning of bolus in oral phase) and using a scale of 0 (no impairment) to 4 (profound impairment). The NZIMES identifies mild to profound impairments in each function and structure involved in safe swallowing (Huckabee, 2004).

A mild impairment of swallowing includes some difficulties with oral preparation and pharyngeal functioning but overall good mastication and safe, independent feeding and swallowing. A moderate impairment indicates some dangers of aspiration and penetration into the airway. Those may result from such difficulties as problems clearing a spoon of a bolus because of lingual and labial uncoordination or weakness, problems clearing the mouth when creating the bolus, problems masticating solid foods, and a slow trigger of swallow. A severe impairment indicates a serious risk of aspiration and penetration, and a profound impairment indicates that a person is unable to safely swallow, thus requiring an alternative means of nutrition.

What Are the Defining Characteristics of Dysphagia?

The defining characteristics of dysphagia are structural abnormalities or physiological deficits affecting the oral preparatory, oral, pharyngeal, and esophageal phases of deglutition.

Characteristics of Oral Preparatory Phase Dysphagia

In the oral preparatory stage, food or liquid items are intaken, held within the mouth, and prepared for transition to the pharyngeal phase. Some disorders that may result in an oral preparatory dysphagia include strokes, Parkinson's disease, and head and neck cancers. Characteristics of oral preparatory phase dysphagia include the following:

1. Decreased lip closure, resulting in problems intaking foods or liquids from an eating utensil, straw, or cup and allowing food materials to leak from the mouth
2. Problems controlling the ingested materials, such that food or liquid falls in the space between the teeth and gums (i.e., the **sulci**)
3. Difficulty biting or chewing, thus hindering the formation of a bolus
4. Inefficient oral preparation due to reduced range of motion of the tongue and/or weakness of the tongue, requiring increased time to prepare the bolus for swallowing
5. Impaired sensitivity of the tongue, lips, and other oral structures that hinders food positioning and management

Characteristics of Oral Phase Dysphagia

In the oral stage, the formed bolus moves posteriorly in the mouth toward the pharynx to trigger the swallow. Oral phase dysphagia occurs with strokes, progressive neurological diseases such as ALS, and even tooth loss. Characteristics of oral phase dysphagia include these:

1. Difficulty moving the bolus to the pharynx, resulting in food or liquid residuals in the mouth (e.g., in the sulci or adhering to the hard palate)
2. Inability to adequately control the bolus flow, such that some materials spill into the pharyngeal region prematurely
3. Delayed initiation of the bolus movement, increasing the transit time from the oral to the pharyngeal phase

Characteristics of Pharyngeal Phase Dysphagia

The pharyngeal phase of the swallow directs the prepared bolus through the pharynx into the esophagus, while simultaneously making physiological adjustments to protect the airway. This phase is critical because the greatest threat is that of materials entering the airway. Unlike the oral preparatory and oral phases, which are more readily observable at the bedside, pharyngeal phase difficulties are not readily transparent. Pharyngeal phase dysphagia occurs with neurological disorders, as well as with head and neck cancers. Characteristics of pharyngeal stage dysphagia include the following:

1. Incomplete palatal elevation to seal off the nose from the pharynx, allowing foods or liquids into the nasal cavity (i.e., **nasal reflux**)

2. Delayed initiation of the pharyngeal swallow reflex, allowing materials to move deeper into the pharynx or larynx, thus increasing the risk of aspiration
3. Diminished tongue and pharyngeal muscle force to move the bolus through the pharynx, resulting in materials "hanging" in the throat
4. Reduced laryngeal elevation and closure, making the airway more prone to entering materials (i.e., aspiration)
5. Inadequate opening of the cricopharyngeus muscle (i.e., the upper esophageal sphincter), hindering the movement of the bolus into the esophagus and enabling the retention of food residuals within the pharynx

Characteristics of Esophageal Phase Dysphagia

The esophageal phase transports the bolus through the esophagus into the stomach. Typically, the speech-language pathologist's role is focused on oropharyngeal dysphagia, and esophageal dysphagia is managed by a physician specializing in gastrological and intestinal disturbances, the **gastroenterologist**. However, it is important for speech-language pathologists to understand the esophageal phase and its disorders since clients with esophageal dysphagia frequently experience oropharyngeal level problems also (Murry & Carrau, 2001). Diseases such as **reflux** (i.e., the movement of acids from the stomach into the esophagus) and certain cancers produce esophageal dysphagia. Characteristics of esophageal phase dysphagia pertinent to the speech-language pathologist include these:

1. Structural alterations in the esophagus (e.g., strictures or narrowed areas) that inhibit the flow of material to the stomach
2. Diminished esophageal motility or contraction, making it difficult to move the bolus to the stomach
3. Inadequate opening of the lower esophageal sphincter, affecting the movement of the bolus into the stomach
4. Excessive opening of the lower esophageal sphincter, allowing the backward flow of contents from the stomach into the esophagus (i.e., reflux)

How Is Dysphagia Identified?

The speech-language pathologist is the key professional responsible for evaluating clients with suspected dysphagia. This assessment process includes a clinical swallowing examination and, when indicated, an instrumental dysphagia evaluation. These are the goals of assessment:

1. Determine the presence or absence of dysphagia and the underlying causes if swallowing problems are present
2. Assess the severity of the swallowing impairment
3. Make recommendations regarding ability to eat by mouth; if oral intake is acceptable, recommend the appropriate diet and any strategies to optimize safe feeding and adequate nutrition
4. Design and implement an individualized dysphagia rehabilitation regimen
5. Share information gained with the interdisciplinary swallowing team (e.g., dieticians, physicians, nurses, occupational and physical therapists) and the family of the client

All therapy decisions should include the client and the client's family. The speech-language pathologist works closely with the client and the family to design a swallowing program in which the client has minimum risk of aspiration but achieves adequate nutrition in the least restrictive manner. The speech-language pathologist must balance decisions concerning safety with quality of life concerns.

FIGURE 10-5 Warning signs in dysphagia screening.

- Coughing or choking
- Frequent throat clearing
- Wet or gurgly voice quality
- Thick or copious secretions
- Drooling or leakage of foods from the mouth
- Recurrent pneumonia or upper respiratory infections
- Fatigue during eating
- Altered cognitive status
- Presence of a tracheostomy tube
- Excessive time required to complete a meal
- Unexplained weight loss

Referral

The speech-language pathologist first receives a consult request from a referral source, such as a physician or a nurse who suspects a swallowing impairment in a patient. Staff members in health care facilities are routinely trained by speech-language pathologists to recognize possible signs of dysphagia. This interdisciplinary approach is necessary since speech-language pathologists are not able to independently screen all clients admitted to hospitals, rehabilitation centers, and other health care facilities. Professionals are trained to spot dysphagia warning signs, as identified in Figure 10-5. When any of these signs are present, a referral to a speech-language pathologist typically occurs.

Discussion Point: *Consider the case of Martin in Box 10-1. How would you characterize his quality of life?*

The Clinical Swallowing Examination

The clinical swallowing examination is also referred to as a **bedside swallow examination**, because it typically occurs at a client's bedside. In this procedure speech-language pathologists do the following:

1. Review current and past medical records
2. Complete a comprehensive interview of the client to learn medical, social, and family history, with particular attention to the history of the swallowing problem (e.g., When did the problem start? What foods are most troublesome?)
3. Conduct a thorough oral mechanism examination of the mouth and throat to determine structural and functional adequacy for swallowing

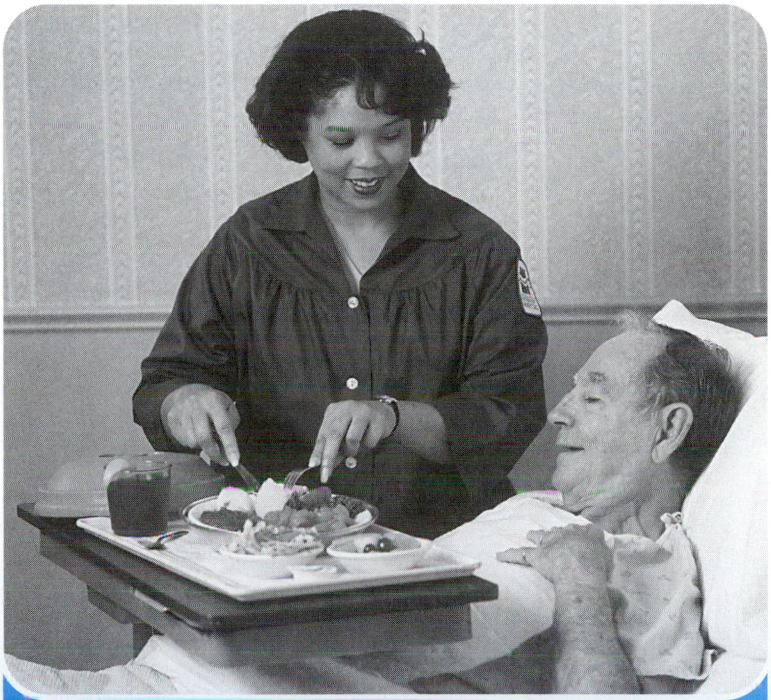

During the bedside examination, a therapist studies how an individual takes in food and drink and considers the safety and efficiency of swallowing.

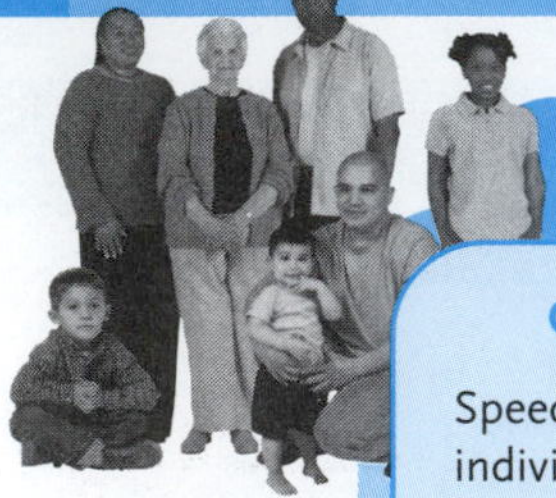

BOX 10-2 Multicultural Focus

Consideration in Dysphagia

Speech-language pathologists are responsible for dysphagia management for a wide range of individuals, varying in age, native language, and social and ethnic backgrounds. The ways in which these individuals and their families respond to the disease process vary immensely as a function of their individual differences. Given the newness of the field of dysphagia treatment, a great deal remains unknown about differentiating assessments and interventions to be culturally responsive. This is, indeed, a ripe area for research in the coming decade.

Nonetheless, there are some best practice suggestions to follow in working with clients and families whose cultural backgrounds differ from that of the therapist. These three suggestions come from Westby (2000).

1. *Use an interpreter:* When working with families who speak a different language, an interpreter is an important resource. The interpreter should not be just anyone, however; a good interpreter is familiar with the topic of dysphagia and is acceptable to the family.
2. *Include the extended family:* Include as many extended family members as a client desires to be involved. Facilitate this by specifically inviting clients and their families to bring as many friends or family members as they wish to meetings and sessions.
3. *Get to know the culture:* When working with someone of a different culture, get to know that culture. Talk to people of the culture and research it in books and other resources. Culture has a great influence on the way information is shared, and it is easy to offend out of ignorance. Because dysphagia management can be a life and death matter, sensitive information sharing is essential.

As a profession, we need to know more about the treatment of dysphagia and the ways its effectiveness can vary for persons of different cultural, linguistic, ethnic, religious, and racial groups. Future research should address these questions:

1. Are there variations in normal swallowing performance across culturally and linguistically diverse populations?
2. Are there evaluation and treatment approaches better suited to certain culturally and linguistically diverse populations?
3. How do we attract more culturally and linguistically diverse individuals to become swallowing therapists?

For Discussion

What language or cultural challenges might an English-speaking speech-language pathologist encounter when treating dysphagia in someone who speaks little English?

What are some approaches that might improve the diversity of swallowing therapists?

Companion Website

To answer these questions online, go to the Multicultural Focus module in chapter 10 of the Companion Website.

4. Attempt trial feedings or observe the client during a meal
5. Make feeding recommendations if appropriate
6. Refer the client for instrumental assessment of swallowing if indicated
7. Refer the client to other professionals for any specialized testing that is needed

Figure 10-6 provides an outline of a clinical swallowing examination and subsequent report.

FIGURE 10-6 An outline of a clinical swallowing examination and report.

CLINICAL SWALLOW EXAMINATION

Client:
Date of Birth:
Date of Exam:
Diagnosis:
Referral Source:
Client Identification Number:

History. This section includes all relevant past medical, social, and family history, as well as current medical diagnoses, procedures and results, medications and allergies. Specific interview questions include these:

- What is your chief complaint and the nature of the problem?
- How long has this been a problem?
- Do you experience this problem more at certain times of day? (e.g., better at breakfast and worse at dinner?)
- Are there certain food textures (e.g., liquids, soft foods) that make the problem better or worse?
- When you experience swallowing problems, what happens?
- Have you found things that make you swallow better?
- Have you had a change in weight? If so, how much and over what time span?

Oral Mechanism Exam. This section includes observation of oral structures at rest and in use. Rate, strength, and direction of the movements of structures used in articulation, phonation, and resonance are noted. If a tracheostomy tube is present, the type, size, and duration of tube placement are determined.

Feeding Trials. This section reports observations of swallowing performance for various consistencies. Optimally, this includes liquids, purees, soft foods, foods requiring much chewing, and pills. Problems across the phases of the swallow are identified. In addition, techniques to compensate for or improve swallowing performance are attempted, and benefits, if present, are noted. If the client is not taking foods or liquids by mouth, this is noted, and the type of feeding tube, current formula, and feeding schedule are listed.

Clinical Impressions. This section summarizes findings on the presence of dysphagia, its severity, specific swallowing deficits, and prognosis for improvement.

Recommendations. This portion outlines the recommendations for oral intake, optimal diet, and safety strategies. Referrals for instrumental assessment or professional services are indicated. If therapy is indicated, an intervention plan is suggested that includes the frequency and duration of treatment, measurable goals, and specific treatment techniques.

Signature of speech-language pathologist
Credentials
State license number

CC: Others receiving a copy of this report

If the clinical swallowing examination cannot clearly determine the nature of the swallowing problem, an instrumental assessment of dysphagia is required to study the swallowing phases more throughly. This assessment uses radiography and other instrumentation and should be used only when it is necessary for further diagnosis. These five indicators suggest the need for instrumentation to quantify swallowing problems (ASHA, 2000b):

1. Clinical bedside findings are inconsistent with reported signs and symptoms of dysphagia.
2. Instrumentation is needed to assist in determining the medical diagnosis.
3. Dysphagia diagnosis or the safety and efficiency of the swallow require confirmation.
4. Nutritional or pulmonary compromises are present, and oropharyngeal dysphagia is suspected as a contributing factor.
5. Specific swallowing information is required to design and implement a treatment plan.

Discussion Point: *Consider whether Sylvia in Box 10-1 meets the five indicators presented here for instrumental evaluation.*

When instrumental evaluation is required, the speech-language pathologist initiates the referral process through the appropriate physician. Most instrumental procedures require a physician's prescription if they are to be paid for by the insurance company. Speech-language pathologists are typically responsible for actually conducting the instrumental dysphagia examination, but they work closely with other professionals, especially radiologists, in carrying out and interpreting the assessment.

Instrumental Dysphagia Examination

Evaluation of swallowing problems using technology, or instrumentation, typically provides a more objective and quantifiable measure of swallowing functions, including the safety of those functions. Commonly used instrumentation includes fiberoptic endoscopic evaluation, ultrasonography, and videofluoroscopy.

Fiberoptic Endoscopic Examination

The **fiberoptic endoscopic examination of swallowing**, commonly referred to as FEES, provides direct visualization of the swallowing mechanism. A fiberoptic endoscope, or flexible tube containing a small camera, is passed through the nose and into the pharynx, yielding a real-time picture of swallowing, both before and after the swallow. However, pharyngeal movement during the swallow makes imaging impossible during the actual swallow itself. FEES is videotaped so that replay of the test is possible, and it has no radiation exposure. Complications can include nasal laceration, hemorrhaging, or allergic reaction to topical anesthetics.

Ultrasonography

Ultrasonography, or ultrasound, is the same technology long used to visualize a fetus in the mother's womb. In dysphagia evaluation, ultrasound uses high-frequency sound waves to create a black-and-white picture of the structures targeted. A transducer, placed either at the chin or at the thyroid area at the front of the neck, generates sound waves to create the image. Ultrasound is most beneficial in oral phase evaluation; pharyngeal phase assessment with ultrasound is poor. Ultrasound is without known risk and is noninvasive. Further, it is portable, so it can be used at bedside.

Videofluoroscopy

Videofluoroscopy is the most commonly used instrumentation for swallowing evaluation and is the gold standard in most cases. Videofluoroscopy couples fluoroscopy, a radiographic imaging technique, with videotaping, to produce a real-time image of the swallow as it occurs from the oral preparatory through the pharyngeal and esophageal phases. This procedure is typically referred to as a modified barium swallow (MBS) study or, occasionally, as a video swallow study. Speech-language pathologists conduct the MBS by having clients ingest a variety of food consistencies and using fluoroscopy to watch the functioning of the swallow. MBS is sometimes called a cookie study because clients chew and swallow a variety of different foods, often including a cookie.

Since MBS uses fluoroscopy, a radiopaque contrast material, such as barium, must be mixed with the foods for visualization. Clients are administered liquids and foods in graduated and controlled trials to optimize safety and to ascertain swallowing competency. Generally, the procedure flows in the following steps:

1. A baseline picture of structures, including the posterior portion of the mouth, the soft palate, the pharynx, the larynx, and the upper esophageal sphincter

2. Administration and observation of liquids and foods in the following order:
   a. Thin liquids (e.g., apple juice)
   b. Thick liquids if indicated (e.g., tomato juice or apricot nectar)
   c. Purees (e.g., applesauce)
   d. Mechanical soft items (e.g., Rice Krispies)
   e. Regular foods (e.g., graham cracker)
   f. Pills
3. Study of different compensatory strategies to assess their impact on swallowing efficiency and safety while different textures are ingested (e.g., a chin tuck, leaning, or a head turn)

Although this procedure yields information on all phases of the swallow, there are certain drawbacks. The MBS uses radiation, so client exposure must be considered and minimized. Further, the MBS is not readily portable in most environments, so client transport and positioning needs should be considered. Finally, MBS is an expensive procedure that requires highly specialized instruments and skilled professionals. Not all facilities are equipped with both.

Discussion Point: *Consider the case of Lee in Box 10-1. What MBS findings indicate that swallowing is unsafe?*

How Is Dyspahgia Treated?

Dysphagia rehabilitation is best accomplished through an interdisciplinary team, generally including speech-language pathologists, occupational therapists, physical therapists, dieticians, nurses, physicians, and family members of the individual being treated. The team members work cooperatively, bringing their expertise to the process of feeding recovery and balancing safety and nutrition with quality of life.

Consider an individual with paralysis affecting one side of the body who may have difficulty sitting in a chair and eating independently. The speech-language pathologist determines the safety and efficiency of the client's eating and determines approaches to promote both, but other professionals are also involved in related aspects of the rehabilitation process. The physical therapist evaluates the positioning issues and recommends a seating system that provides support so that the individual is upright for feeding. The occupational therapist evaluates the hand-to-mouth aspect of the individual's eating and designs adaptive utensils to optimize independence and efficiency. The dietician evaluates nutritional support and develops a dietary plan to ensure adequate nutrition. Thus, many professionals have essential skills and knowledge to offer in dysphagia rehabilitation.

The Speech-Language Pathologist's Role

The speech-language pathologist works to remediate oropharyngeal dysphagia, using two types of rehabilitation strategies: compensatory and restorative approaches.

Compensatory Approaches

Compensatory techniques are, as the name implies, strategies that compensate for a specific problem in order to make swallowing safe and efficient. For example, for clients who experience oral leakage of foods or the packing of foods in the cheeks, the speech-language pathologist might place a mirror in front of them during meals so that they can monitor and correct this problem. Or the SLP might help clients with left facial weakness place food on the stronger right side of their mouths during the oral preparatory phase.

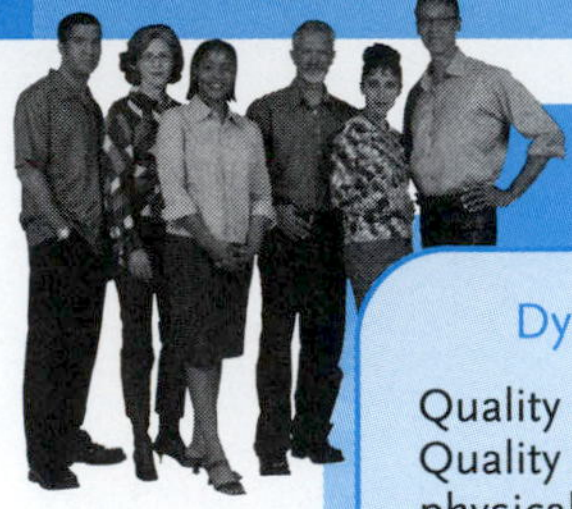

BOX 10-3 Ecological Contexts

Dysphagia in the Home, at Work, and in the Community

Quality of life (QOL) is a phrase that receives great attention in the dysphagia literature. Quality of life relates to one's satisfaction with life, goal achievement, social well-being, physical ability, and independence (Dedhiya & Kong, 1995; McKevitt, Redfern, LaPlaca, & Wolfe, 2003). QOL is a critical issue in the management of dysphagia; persons with dysphagia tend to eat less, lose weight, and view eating as unenjoyable. About one third of those with dysphagia avoid dining with others (Ekberg, Hamdy, Woisard, Wuttge-Hannig, & Ortega, 2002). The case of Joe, described here, is not uncommon among individuals with dysphagia.

Joe is a 49-year-old stroke survivor who is wheelchair bound with right-sided hemiparesis involving both his arm and leg. He lives at home with his wife and teenage children. Joe is on a mechanical soft diet with thickened liquids, which he hates, and he is reliant on his family members to select and prepare his foods. Prior to his stroke, Joe worked as a plumber and was active at his children's sporting events, attended church regularly, and played cards with his friends every third Tuesday of the month. Now Joe feels isolated and unmotivated to interact outside the home.

Like many whose lives are turned upside down by a serious disease and its aftermath, Joe is depressed and often angry. Although he has never received psychological intervention to help him and his family cope with his dysphagia and other impairments, it is likely warranted to help him accept his disability and to become reengaged in his community. Psychological support would be best provided by a trained psychologist working as part of a health care team that includes the speech-language pathologist.

For Discussion

What are some barriers that Joe's dysphagia places on him in his daily living activities at home and community settings? Which can be overcome and which cannot?

How might therapists intervene to optimize Joe's success at home and in the community?

Companion Website

To answer these questions online, go to the Ecological Contexts module in chapter 10 of the Companion Website.

In addition to modifications in the way individuals take in food, SLPs use diet modifications as a compensatory approach. For example, if chewing is difficult for a client, meals can be customized to use chopped rather than whole meats. Or if an individual is at risk for aspirating on thin liquids, like water, a thickening agent can be added. Additional compensatory techniques are listed in Figure 10-7.

Restorative Techniques

Restorative techniques are intended to improve or restore swallow function. Examples include oral and pharyngeal exercises and biofeedback. For an individual with a delayed swallow reflex, the therapist might use thermal stimulation to improve the sensitivity of the oral area and the timeliness of the swallow reflex. In the case of a weak swallow, the therapist might train the client to use an effortful swallow in the pharyngeal phase to help propel the bolus downward without leaving residue behind. However, this requires considerable muscular effort and an ability to follow directions, so it might not be suitable for some clients with language impairment, cognitive decline, or muscular fatigue (Logemann, 1998). Figure 10-8 lists these and other commonly used restorative treatments.

FIGURE 10-7 Compensatory strategies.

- *Diet modifications*
  - Change the consistency of foods and drinks
  - Change the temperature of foods and drinks
- *Altered positioning during swallowing*
  - Have client tuck chin in (chin tuck)
  - Place client on side
  - Have client turn head to the left or right side
- *Intake modifications*
  - Alternate solids and liquids
  - Encourage extra swallows per bite
  - Change food placement in the mouth
  - Alter bite size
- *Meal set-up/environment*
  - Minimize distractions
  - Monitor tray placement
  - Use adaptive feeding equipment, such as high-rimmed bowls, feeding utensils, nonslide placemats to secure plates, cups that control the rate of liquid flow
  - Have staff monitor and assist
- *Prosthetic devices or appliances*

Evidence-Based Treatment

Interventions must be individualized, appropriate to each client's needs, and reflective of current scientific evidence on what are and are not effective treatments. In **evidence-based treatment**, the professional carefully examines the client's needs and preferences and matches these with approaches supported by empirical or quantitative research on effectiveness.

Discussion Point: *Consider the cases in Box 10-1. Which interventions are likely compensatory? Restorative? Are any both? Explain.*

FIGURE 10-8 Restorative strategies.

- *Thermal stimulation:* The therapist rubs a cold laryngeal mirror on the faucial pillars to improve the timeliness of the swallow reflex.
- *Effortful swallow:* The client tries to swallow hard using the swallowing muscles.
- *Mendelsohn maneuver:* The client learns to catch the swallow during elevation of the larynx, increasing the duration of the upper esophageal opening.
- *Supraglottic swallow:* In this multistep maneuver clients hold their breath before swallowing, then swallow, and finally cough to improve the closure of the airway.
- *Oral motor exercise:* The client completes exercises of the swallowing structures to improve strength and efficiency.
- *Electromyography (EMG):* This biofeedback approach enhances awareness and self-monitoring of performance.

BOX 10-4 Spotlight on Research

Bonnie Martin-Harris, Ph.D.

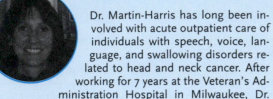

Dr. Martin-Harris has long been involved with acute outpatient care of individuals with speech, voice, language, and swallowing disorders related to head and neck cancer. After working for 7 years at the Veteran's Administration Hospital in Milwaukee, Dr. Martin-Harris sought out the professor at Northwestern University whose name was becoming familiar to speech-language pathologists—Dr. Jeri Logemann. Dr. Logemann was calling for evidence-based practices long before the term became popular in the clinical literature during the late 1990s. At Northwestern Dr. Martin-Harris developed her passion for teaching as she observed and assisted Dr. Logemann in laboratory and classroom instruction.

After completing her doctorate, Dr. Martin-Harris was recruited to an academically oriented, tertiary care hospital in Atlanta, Georgia—St. Joseph's Hospital. There she collaborated with a pulmonary physician, Dr. Ralph Haynes, because of their mutual interest in the relationships between breathing and swallowing functions. Together, they had the opportunity to treat a successful businesswoman with chronic obstructive pulmonary disease and voice and swallowing problems. This Atlanta Businesswoman of the Year and WWII pilot, Evelyn Trammell, lost her battle with her disease in the late 1980s, but a trust was established in her name and her husband's—the Mark and Evelyn Trammell Trust Fund. Through a proposal to that fund, clinical service and research endeavors found a home in the Evelyn Trammell Voice and Swallowing Center at St. Joseph's Hospital. Dedicated in 1993 and directed by Dr. Martin-Harris, the center was the first to combine voice and swallowing services in a seamless continuum of care for patients with overlapping disorders of voice and deglutition.

Nutrition and Dietary Considerations

The importance of nutritional health to an individual with dysphagia cannot be overestimated. Because dysphagia results from an underlying disease, individuals must achieve adequate nutrition to promote healing of and recovery from the underlying disease. For example, persons recovering from neurological injuries such as stroke or traumatic brain injury have greater nutritional needs than they did prior to their illness. Unfortunately, however, swallowing dysfunction places them at a higher risk of malnutrition and dehydration. A

BOX 10-5 Spotlight on Practice

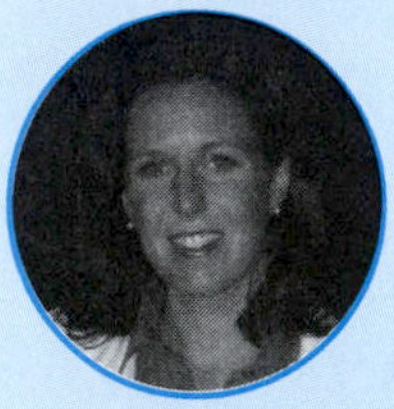

Katherine Walsh Sullivan, M.S., CCC-SLP
Speech-Language Pathologist
Walter Reed Army Medical Center

Walter Reed is the flagship hospital of the United States military system, caring for all branches of active-duty military personnel, retirees, and their families. Walter Reed is also the most active, comprehensive center for evaluation, treatment, and research of communication disorders in the Department of Defense. My clinic's primary population is the young men and women injured in military activities, including war. In a recent 11-month period of the War on Terrorism, we saw 74 casualties, 48 of which (65%) had some type of swallowing difficulty. These were patients with trauma to the head and neck due to gunshot wounds, blast injuries from land mines and rocket-propelled grenades, and motor vehicle and helicopter accidents. Frequently, we follow casualties from admission to the intensive care unit, where they are often tracheotomy- and ventilator-dependent, to their discharge to a rehabilitation center or home. Because of our unique setting, we are able to carefully examine our caseload and outcomes to advance the field's knowledge of dysphagia. Our researchers collect and analyze data in the hope that patients everywhere will someday benefit from a higher standard of care. Few careers offer the gratification of helping people in need, serving a profession with clinical research, and working in a field you love. Right now, at the bedside of our nation's wounded soldiers, I can testify that speech-language pathology provides all that and more.

Note: The opinions expressed herein are not to be construed as official or as reflecting the policies of the Departments of the Army or Defense.

FIGURE 10-9 Typical diet levels.

- *NPO (non per os):* This level indicates that no liquids or foods are to be consumed orally. These clients require intravenous or tube feedings to maintain their nutritional needs.
- *Thin liquids:* This level allows thin liquids such as juices and water. It also includes foods that melt to a liquid consistency, such as gelatins.
- *Thickened liquids:* This level allows liquids that are more viscous, such as tomato juice or nectars. If clients are unable to tolerate thin liquids, commercial thickening agents are added to achieve the required thickness.
- *Puree:* These items have well-blended, smooth consistencies that require relatively little oral preparation (e.g., applesauce or pudding).
- *Mechanical soft:* These foods require oral preparation but are soft, so that chewing demands are limited. Examples include soft cooked vegetables, canned fruits, and moist, tender meats that are sometimes ground or finely chopped.
- *Soft:* This level includes most foods except those that are difficult to manage orally, such as peanuts, raw apples, and hard candy.
- *Regular:* This is an unrestricted level that allows all foods.
- *Medications:* Many dysphagia clients experience difficulties swallowing needed medications. In these cases medications can be given in liquid form or crushed, if not contraindicated.

speech-language pathologist works closely with a registered dietician to assess diet and adjust recommendations to meet nutritional demands. Figure 10-9 describes the typical diet levels.

Despite dietary modifications and compensatory strategies, some clients are unable to meet their nutritional requirements orally. In these cases alternative nutritional means, such as a feeding tube, are necessary to supplement intake by mouth; it is not unusual for dysphagia clients to receive both oral intake and tube feedings. Feeding tubes may be *nasogastric* (inserted through the nose and down to the stomach) or *gastrostomy* (surgically inserted directly into the stomach). For individuals with digestive problems, a *jejunostomy tube* can be surgically inserted into the small intestine, bypassing the dysfunctional gut. The type of tube is determined by a client's physician, who consults with the swallowing team about the nature of the dysphagia, the comprehensive clinical profile, and the anticipated duration of tube placement. The goal is to ensure proper nutrition but to decrease a client's reliance on nonoral feeding over time and to return to solely oral intake if possible.

Discussion Point: *Why might some clients be unable to meet their own nutritional needs, despite dietary modifications and compensatory strategies?*

Measuring the Effects of Therapy

It is imperative that a client's response to dysphagia intervention, either positive or negative, be measured. Measurement begins with the initial evaluation, during which both subjective and objective information is gathered to formulate a *baseline status*. That baseline describes an individual's swallowing capabilities before treatment begins. Then, treatment effects are monitored with each session, and treatment goals and approaches shift in response to the data collected. For some individuals, swallowing performance may increase rapidly, or they may be able to be independent, safe eaters with only slight modifications to their diet or the use of other compensatory approaches. For other individuals, swallowing performance may improve gradually, requiring considerable rehabilitation. Individuals with cognitive decline or serious cognitive or linguistic impairment may progress slowly or even decline over time. By constantly evaluating swallowing functions, a clinician can readily adjust therapeutic approaches to maintain safety and meet the client's changing needs and capabilities.

Case Study and Clinical Problem Solving

SPEECH-LANGUAGE PATHOLOGY MODIFIED BARIUM SWALLOW REPORT

Client: Joseph Runger
Date of Birth: 4 March 1947
Date: 20 March 2005
Diagnosis: Left CVA
Referral Source: Dr. Ruth Anderson
Account: P248956

History

Joseph Runger is a 58-year-old Caucasian male referred for a videofluoroscopic modified barium swallow (MBS) examination to assess dysphagia status and determine the appropriateness of oral intake. Mr. Runger suffered a large left cerebrovascular accident March 18, 2005, and remains on the acute medical floor. He has a moderate right hemiparesis. Past medical history includes hypertension, cardiovascular disease with a myocardial infarction in 2000, glaucoma, tobacco use, and limited alcohol use (3 drinks per week). Prior to this episode, Mr. Runger was independent and resided at home with his wife. He is employed as a chemical engineer. At present he is hydrated via intravenous fluids and remains NPO.

Examination

Mr. Runger was transported to the fluoroscopy suite and positioned in the Vess fluoroscopy chair. He was able to independently maintain a feeding position and alignment appropriate for the swallowing investigation. Mr. Runger was administered graduated trials of various consistencies mixed with a barium medium for contrast. Performance was as follows:

1. *Liquid*—With 1/4 teaspoon of liquid barium administered via medicinal spoon, during the oral phase Mr. Runger exhibited mild premature spillage to fill the valleculae, with aspiration prior to the initiation of the swallow. Latency in the pharyngeal swallow reflex was 6 seconds. Mr. Runger exhibited a weak throat clearing and did not self-initiate a reflexive cough. With verbal cues from the examiner, he produced a strong reflexive cough. A chin tuck was tried, which stopped aspiration for all subsequent trials, including sips from a straw.

2. *Puree*—Mr. Runger was given 1/3 teaspoon of applesauce mixed with barium paste. Oral motor performance was adequate to move the bolus to the pharyngeal stage. A delay in the pharyngeal swallow was noted. He had moderate amounts of residue in the pharyngeal area after the swallow. The upper esophageal sphincter adequately opened to allow passage of the bolus into the esophagus. He self-initiated extra swallows that effectively cleared the pharynx.

3. *Mechanical Soft*—Mr. Runger was given 1/2 teaspoon of cereal coated in barium liquid. Moderate to severe deficits in the oral preparation of the bolus were noted, including uncoordinated bolus formation and packing of the material in the right cheek. The pharyngeal phase followed a delayed swallow reflex (5 seconds) with filling of the valleculae. Once the reflex was triggered, approximately 60% of the material moved into the esophagus. He independently attempted repeated swallows to clear the material, with little success. He was given water and instructed to use a chin tuck and take a sip. With this technique the majority of the residue moved into the esophagus. Larger bite sizes were not attempted.

4. *Soft/Regular*—Given the deficits noted with the mechanical soft food, these consistencies were not administered.

Clinical Impressions

Mr. Runger suffered a left CVA 2 days ago and currently exhibits moderate to severe oropharyngeal dysphagia. Oral and pharyngeal stage deficits include difficulty in bolus formation and transport, slow triggering of the pharyngeal swallow reflex, and inadequate airway protection. He is aspirating both before and during the swallow reflex on liquids but can compensate with a chin tuck.

Susan E. Hinton, M.S., CCC-Sp
Virginia license number #R000342
CC: Dr. Ruth Anderson

CLINICAL PROBLEM SOLVING

1. Mr. Runger experienced dysphagia after a stroke. How commonly does stroke result in dysphagia?
2. Given the case history and findings, are any other referrals needed for this client?
3. What were some of the techniques used to improve the safety and efficiency of Mr. Runger's swallowing?
4. In your opinion, what is the prognosis for Mr. Runger's eating safely on his own at home with his wife?

CHAPTER SUMMARY

Swallowing is an innate behavior that is present in early fetal development and continues through the lifespan. Normal swallowing has distinct, yet coordinated, physiological stages: the oral preparation phase, the oral phase, the pharyngeal phase, and the esophageal phase.

When diseases such as stroke, traumatic brain injury, Parkinson's disease, ALS, dementia, or head and neck cancer occur, swallowing impairment or dysphagia is possible. Management of oropharyngeal dysphagia in these cases requires an interdisciplinary rehabilitation team approach. The team includes physicians, nurses, dieticians, occupational therapists, physical therapists, and speech-language pathologists. A speech-language pathologist is recognized as the primary interventionist for both the evaluation and the treatment of oropharyngeal dysphagia.

The evaluation of dysphagia includes a clinical swallowing or bedside examination and, when indicated, instrumental assessment using fiberoptic endoscopy, ultrasonography, or videofluoroscopy. Results of a comprehensive dysphagia evaluation should identify the presence or absence of dysphagia, the nature of the swallowing disturbance, the appropriate treatment strategies, and recommendations for current diet, other indicated procedures, and professional consultations.

Treatment plans incorporate both compensatory and restorative interventions to optimize current performance and future recovery. Strategies implemented should be evidence based and measurable in terms of client progress. The rehabilitation plan must be sensitive to the client's quality of life and ethnocultural background.

KEY TERMS

apneic moment, p. 328
aspiration, p. 328
bedside swallow examination, p. 337
bolus, p. 325
dysphagia, p. 323
enteral feeding tube, p. 328
evidenced-based treatment, p. 343
feeding, p. 329
fiberoptic endoscopic examination of swallowing, p. 340
gastroenterologist, p. 336
nasal reflux, p. 335
penetration, p. 328
pharyngeal swallow reflex, p. 326
reflexive cough, p. 328
reflux, p. 336
sulci, p. 335
ultrasonography, p. 340
videofluoroscopy, p. 340

ON THE WEB

Check out the Companion Website! On it you will find

- suggested readings
- reflection questions
- a self-study quiz
- links to additional online resources, including current technologies in communication sciences and disorders

Voice Disorders

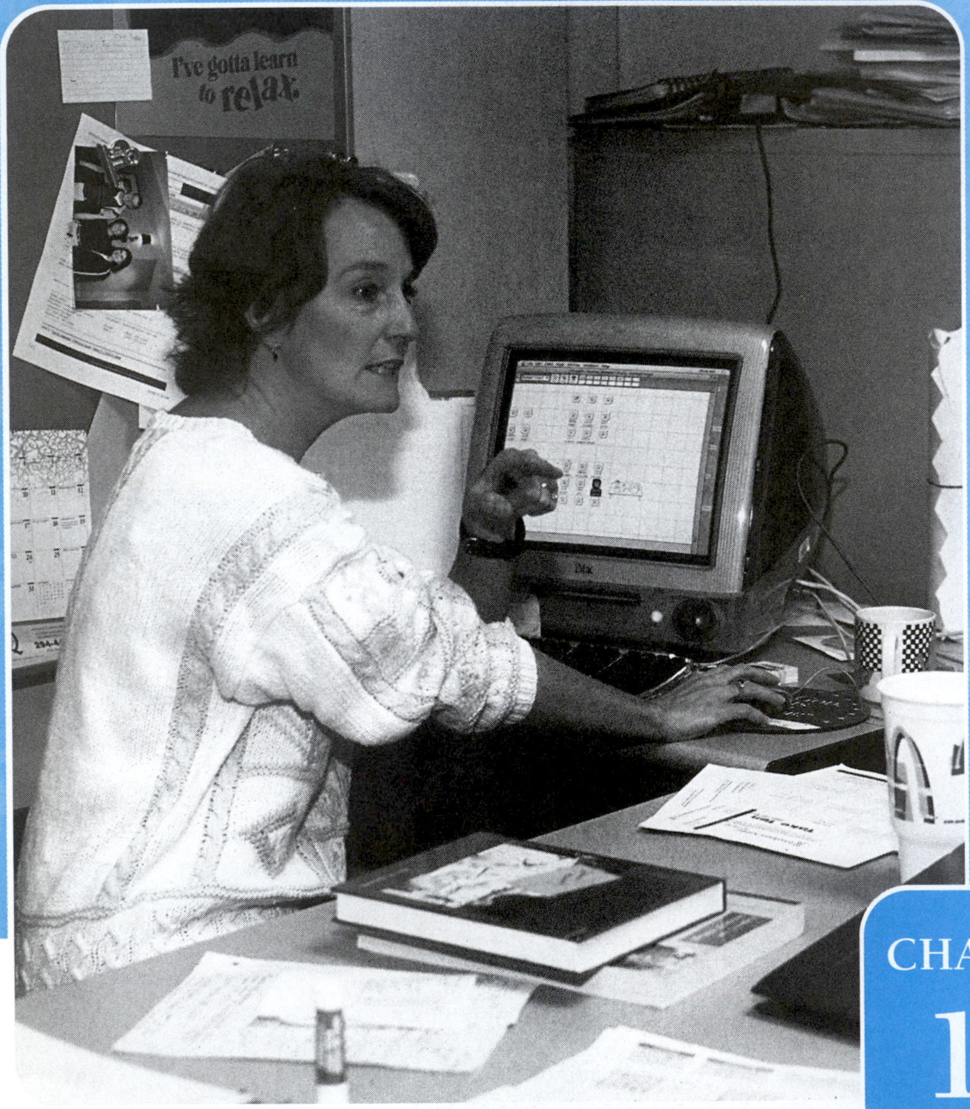

CHAPTER 11

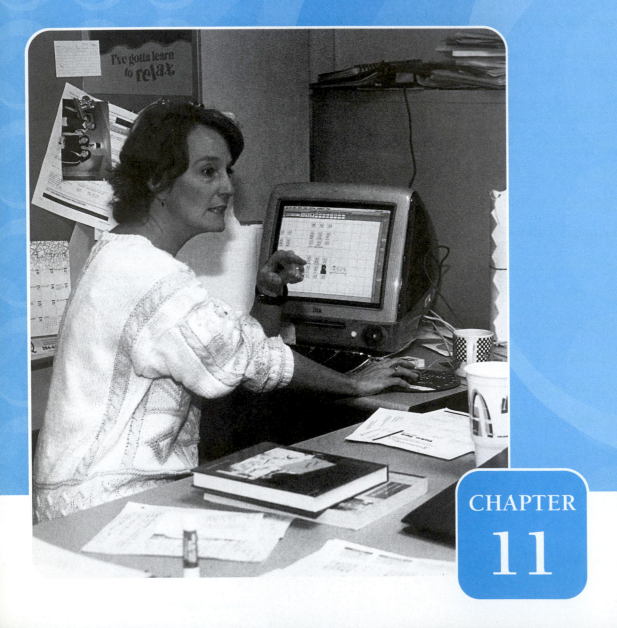

FOCUS QUESTIONS

This chapter answers the following questions:

1. What is a voice disorder?
2. How are voice disorders classified?
3. What are the defining characteristics of voice disorders?
4. How are voice disorders identified?
5. How are voice disorders treated?

INTRODUCTION

You may recall from chapter 3 that the larynx sits deep in the neck at the base of the pharynx; it cannot be seen without some type of technological assistance. Prior to the advent of these technologies, knowledge of the larynx required dissections of human cadavers, which obviously did not permit scientists or physicians to see the larynx at work or to study its function. The well-hidden larynx avoided careful scrutiny until the 16th century.

The first book on laryngeal structures appeared in 1600, and by the 18th century scholars had achieved a relatively well-developed understanding of the way in which the vocal folds vibrate to produce the human voice (Karmody, 1996). Technological innovations furthered this understanding in the early 19th century. The **glottiscope**, invented in 1829, coupled a tongue retractor with a mirror to provide a crude glimpse of the laryngeal cavity. An 1853 improvement attached a gaslight to a more sophisticated glottiscope to project a beam of light down onto the vocal folds (see Figure 11-1). The most elegant, novel, and simple innovation, which contributed to a vast improvement in understanding the laryngeal function, occurred in 1854 when voice teacher Manual Garcia devised the concept of the laryngeal mirror, also called a *laryngoscope*. A **laryngeal mirror** is essentially a small, round dental mirror that is placed at the back of the oral cavity to look down on an individual's vocal folds.

These early technologies gave way to increasingly sophisticated approaches to looking at the larynx and its structures in action, including the 21st century's embrace of *endoscopy* and *videostroboscopy*. These tools, discussed later in the chapter, allow clinicians and scientists to watch the vocal folds in action by lowering a flexible tube through the oral and nasal cavity into the laryngeal area.

Long ago, clinicians and scientists had few resources to study a person's larynx compared to those available today. In 1888 Friedrich III, who reigned only briefly as Germany's emperor, died of laryngeal cancer. The professionals then relied on subjective acoustic evaluation (listening to the Emperor's hoarse voice quality) and indirect examination of the laryngeal cavity with a laryngeal mirror (Karmody, 1996). Now, clinicians and scientists have numerous resources to study the larynx.

FIGURE 11-1 The 19th century glottiscope.

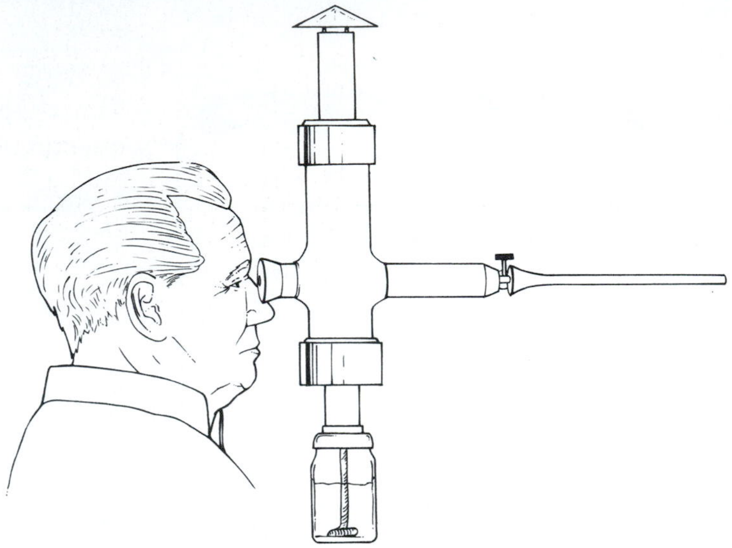

Discussion Point: *Consider your own voice. How would you characterize it? Is its pitch high or low? Is its intensity loud or soft? What gives it your own vocal signature?*

This chapter describes disorders of voice, in which an individual's vocal quality is in some way compromised. Some voice disorders are mild and transient and require no treatment, as you may have experienced after a night of cheering for your favorite sports team. In other cases, voice disorders are severe and persistent, and require ongoing treatment. In the most serious cases, an individual's larynx may need to be removed, as is sometimes required with laryngeal cancer.

What Is a Voice Disorder?

Definition

Defining Voice

Voice is the complex, dynamic product of vocal fold vibration that allows us to vocalize (i.e., make sounds) and verbalize (i.e., produce language through speech). An essential tool for both speech and communication, voice is also a major tool for personal expression, creativity, and art. Consider the opera singer, the actress, the professor, the minister, the talk show host, the stock trader, the politician. Could these professions exist without voice?

The human voice resides in the vibratory patterns of the larynx's tiny vocal folds. Humans can volitionally set their vocal folds into a vibratory pattern, referred to as *phonation,* using airflow from the lungs as fuel. Pause for a moment to phonate—try "ooo" and "ahh." Contrast these two sounds with some that are *not* phonated in their production, such as "sss" and "fff." Now take a moment to compare whispering with talking. Whisper a short phrase, such as "My dog is brown," followed by the same phrase at a conversational level. Think about your voice and where and how it is produced.

As you may recall from earlier chapters, phonation is one of several systems critical to the process of speech production. To phonate, the vocal folds must be closed, or *adducted,* at midline. Such a state is called **adduction**. (When not producing voice, the vocal folds rest in an open, or *abducted,* position so that one can breathe—a state called **abduction**.) For phonation to occur, air is exhaled from the respiratory system upward against the adducted vocal folds, which are then blown apart and set into a rapid vibratory pattern. Once voice is produced, it is modified as it travels up through the pharynx, or throat, and into the oral and nasal cavity, a process called *resonation.* **Resonance** refers to the actual vibration of the air within the pharyngeal column, which impacts the quality of the voice. The voice is also manipulated within the oral cavity in a process of *articulation.*

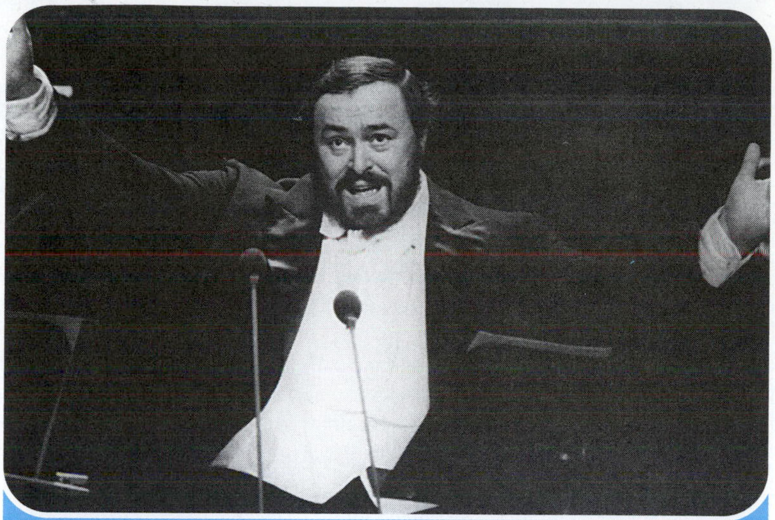

Voice is a tool not only for communication but also for art and creativity.

Individual voices seem very distinct. When familiar people call us on the telephone, they often do not have to introduce themselves because we know their voices so well. The voice that each of us calls our own arises from the complex interaction of three vocal characteristics: frequency, intensity, and phonatory quality (Stemple, Glaze, & Gerdeman, 1995).

Frequency is the rate of vocal fold vibration, expressed as cycles per second, or hertz (Hz). Frequency is an objective, physical measurement of vibratory rate, whereas **pitch** is the psychological or perceptual equivalent (Case, 1996), even though these terms are often used interchangeably. When the vocal folds vibrate, they actually vibrate at several different frequencies simultaneously. *Fundamental frequency,* notated as F_0, is the arithmetic mean of the rates of vibration for the vocal folds (Robb & Smith, 2002). If an individual's vocal folds vibrate 250 times in a second, the F_0 is 250 Hz, which is the average F_0 for kindergarten girls and boys (Awan & Mueller, 1996). For adult women the F_0 ranges from about 180 to 220 Hz, and for adult men the F_0 ranges from about 120 to 140 Hz (Morris, Brown, Hicks, & Howell, 1995; Russell, Penny, & Pemberton, 1995).

A person's fundamental frequency relates to three characteristics of the vocal folds:

1. *Length:* Longer vocal folds contribute to a lower F_0.
2. *Mass:* Thicker vocal fold mass contributes to a lower F_0.
3. *Tension:* Greater tension contributes to a higher F_0 (Case, 1996).

The fundamental frequency of our voices changes as we age because of the impact of physical growth and change on the length, mass, and tension of the vocal folds. The greatest amount of change occurs between birth and puberty, when the vocal folds lengthen from 2 mm to an average of 9 mm for females and 16 mm for males (Titze, 1994). As these physical changes occur, fundamental frequency decreases, most significantly for males. Fundamental frequency then plateaus for several years, but at midlife it begins to decrease again, particularly for women. Toward the end of the lifespan, a woman's fundamental frequency has decreased from an average of 220 Hz to 180 Hz (Russell et al., 1995).

Intensity is the physical measurement of sound pressure reported in decibels (dB), which corresponds to the perception of loudness. Intensity is determined by how far the

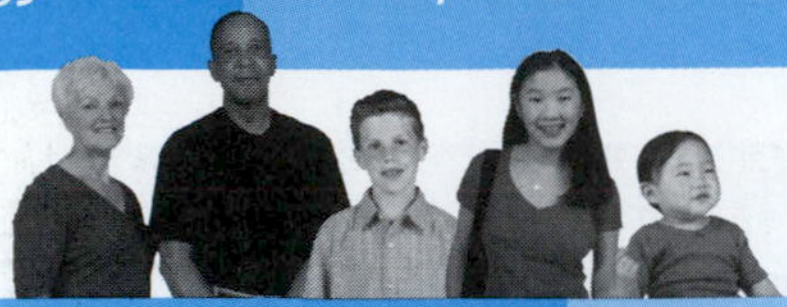

BOX 11-1 Voice Disorders Across the Lifespan: Case Examples

Ms. Chin is a 42-year-old television personality in Houston, Texas. She is the coanchor for the 5:00 PM news show on the local CBS affiliate, a position that she reached after about 18 years at the station. Ms. Chin has begun to experience intermittent problems with her voice; it seems to start and stop and feel strangled. Three times while on the air she had to stop what she was saying and allow her coanchor to take over. On the not-so-gentle advice of her producer, Ms. Chin consulted her primary care physician, who referred her to an otolaryngologist at the Houston Medical Center. During the appointment, her voice never broke down, but the otolaryngologist made a preliminary diagnosis of spasmodic dysphonia (SD). The otolaryngologist did not know any local speech-language pathologists who specialized in SD but referred her to a therapist who had treated his child's vocal nodules. Ms. Chin has an appointment next week to discuss treatment options. Meanwhile, Ms. Chin's producer has suggested that she take a disability leave or at least be reassigned until her voice problems are resolved.

Internet research

1. How many people are affected annually by spasmodic dysphonia? Does it affect women and men at similar rates?
2. What other media personalities have been affected by voice problems? How did this impact their careers?

Brainstorm and discussion

1. Do you agree with Ms. Chin's producer that she should be off the air until her voice problem resolves?
2. Ms. Chin has an appointment soon with a speech-language pathologist who may not be skilled in treating spasmodic dysphonia. How important is it to see a clinician who has worked with this condition before?
3. What other professionals should be involved with Ms. Chin's voice treatment?

Kate Mitchell, M.D., is a 46-year-old former trauma surgeon and mother of four in Salt Lake City, Utah. Dr. Mitchell was in a car accident 2 years ago after a night of emergency surgery. She swerved to avoid a deer, suffered a severe spinal cord injury, and became a paraplegic. Dr. Mitchell is unable to breathe on her own and is ventilator dependent. She was extremely depressed and did not speak for over a year, even when a speaking valve was placed on the ventilator. However, after 1 year, Dr. Mitchell began to work with a speech-language pathologist and a psychologist to use her voice. She began to speak at home to her four daughters and her husband and then increasingly used her voice in public. She recently gave a brief speech to members of the trauma surgery department, who held a ceremony on her behalf. Dr. Mitchell's speech-language pathologist has set up a voice-activated computer so that eventually Dr. Mitchell can use the speaking valve to interact with the computer for typing and even accessing the Internet.

Internet research

1. Annually, how many vehicular accidents result in severe spinal cord injuries?
2. Dr. Mitchell received a speaking valve, specifically a Passy-Muir ventilator speaking valve. How many different kinds of speaking valves are on the market?

vocal folds separate laterally and how quickly they come back together in a vibratory cycle. **Loudness** relates to two features of vocal production: (1) the amount of airflow from the lungs and (2) the amount of resistance to the airflow by the vocal folds (Case, 1996). An increase in airflow from the lungs results in increased loudness; shouting is a good example. When you shout, you first take a large gulp of air, which is then exhaled forcefully through the vocal folds. The greater volume of air results in a wider excursion, or separation, of the vocal folds, contributing to a loud shout. Increased resistance by the vocal folds—achieved through compression of the vocal folds at the midline—also results in increased loudness. You can experience this by clenching together the vocal folds, as if you

Brainstorm and discussion

1. What community activities might be possible for Dr. Mitchell, now that she uses her voice?
2. How might Dr. Mitchell be involved with her profession as a quadriplegic?

Anton is a 68-year-old military veteran in Atlanta, Georgia. Although Anton never smoked, he was diagnosed with laryngeal cancer at the age of 62. Following two unsuccessful surgical resections, Anton had his larynx surgically removed 2 years ago. Anton worked closely with a speech-language pathologist to learn to produce esophageal speech but was never successful. Now, he uses an artificial larynx, which he places against his neck to provide an artificial sound source; he learned to use it just a few days after his laryngectomy.

Anton has become very interested in helping other laryngectomees like himself and has begun to visit them in the hospital immediately after surgery, to support them as they relearn to communicate. On a recent visit to the hospital, the wife of a laryngectomee Anton visited told him that they were pursuing a laryngeal transplant, which they had heard about on television. Apparently, a man had recently received the larynx of another individual and was able to produce voice again using this larynx. Anton is very interested in this option, too, and has contacted his speech-language pathologist for information on laryngeal transplants.

Internet research

1. See what you can find out about laryngeal transplants. Is this really possible?
2. How many laryngectomies occur annually in the United States? What is the major cause of laryngeal removal?

Brainstorm and discussion

1. Given that Anton already has a way to produce speech via the artificial larynx, why would he dream about a laryngeal transplant?
2. Anton's hobby after his laryngectomy was to counsel other laryngectomees. In what ways would Anton's counseling be superior to that of a clinical professional, like a psychologist?

were about to lift something heavy. This tightening creates resistance to the air pressure under the vocal folds; when the pressure is released, it is louder than it would have been without the resistance. Even though vocal loudness is under volitional control, every individual has a baseline loudness, or intensity level, that characterizes that person's conversational speech.

Phonatory quality is a more difficult concept to define but is no less important in constructing a definition of voice. As Case (1996) notes, the numerous terms used to describe phonatory quality suggest its importance: mellow, rich, harmonious, velvety, reedy, whiney, whispery, whining, harsh, shrill, flat, breathy, pleasing.

Phonatory quality relates to how well the two vocal folds work during the vibratory cycle (Stemple et al., 1995). When the vocal folds work together symmetrically and harmoniously, the voice is pleasant, clear, and unremarkable. When the relationship between the two folds is compromised in some way, phonatory quality is compromised. For instance, a growth on one of the two vocal folds impedes the union of the two folds as they come together, resulting in a breathy or hoarse quality.

Discussion Point: *Consider other terms used to describe variations in voice. For each term you come up with, decide whether it references frequency, intensity, or phonatory quality.*

Phonatory quality can also be influenced by the resonation of the voice as it travels up from the vocal folds through the pharynx and into the oral and nasal cavities. Fran Drescher's character in the long-running television sit-com *The Nanny* had an unmistakably nasal voice quality, which Drescher made an essential part of her character's personality. She produced that quality by manipulating the column of air in her nasal cavity.

Defining a Voice Disorder

Individuals exhibit a voice disorder when their pitch, loudness, or phonatory quality differs significantly from that of persons of a similar age, gender, cultural background, and racial and/or ethnic group (Stemple et al., 1995). The difference must be serious enough to draw attention and to detract in some way from performance in ecological contexts, such as school, home, community, and/or work.

Many people exhibit vocal characteristics that differ significantly from those of peers. We all vary in our pitch, loudness, and other vocal qualities, and this variation gives us our unique voices. For some public personalities, unique vocal characteristics are an intrinsic part of their personae. For instance, former president Bill Clinton often had a hoarse vocal quality, resulting from both innate laryngeal characteristics and constant overuse of his voice. Actresses Kathleen Turner and Marilyn Monroe and singers Jamie O'Neal and Billie Holiday are also well known by their breathy and/or hoarse vocal qualities. Thus, when an individual's voice qualities differ from those of others, it does not always signal a disorder. For a disorder to be present, the voice should call attention to the speaker in a negative way and should detract from the person's ability to function in society.

Discussion Point: *Why is a voice disturbance considered attractive in some cases, as with Marilyn Monroe, but detrimental in other cases, as with Ms. Chin in Box 11-1?*

For some public personalities severe breathiness and hoarseness resulted in a loss of livelihood. Julie Andrews, whose voice become world famous from her role in *The Sound of Music,* lost her singing voice after surgery on her vocal folds in 1997 to remove vocal nodules that were restricting her range and voice quality. The surgery further compromised the elasticity of her vocal folds, and Andrews did not perform publicly for several years after the surgery. Diane Rehm, host of the *Diane Rehm Show* on National Public Radio, developed **spasmodic dysphonia**, a voice problem characterized by a strained, broken, and breathy

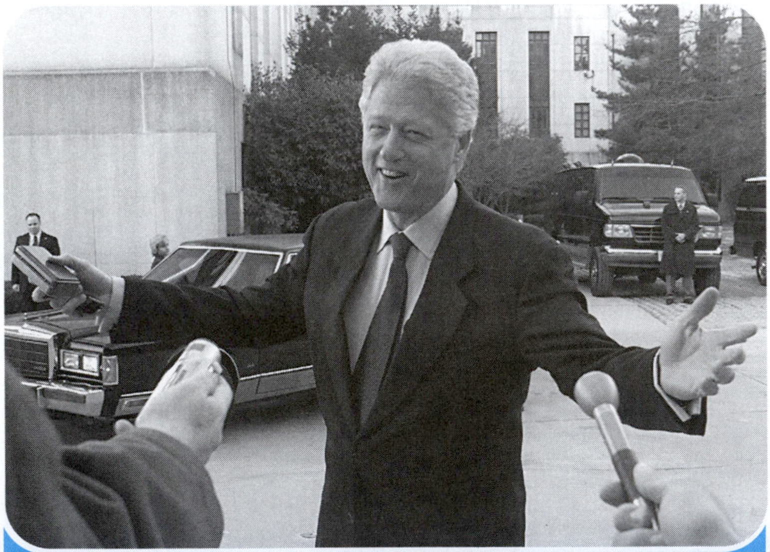

Former President Bill Clinton is an example of a public personality with a well-known and unique vocal signature.

quality. Rehm is currently treated with Botox injections into her vocal folds, which allow her to maintain her daily radio program. (Rehm shares her experience in the 1999 memoir *Finding My Voice*.)

Terminology

Voice Quality

Numerous terms are available to describe aberrations in vocal quality. **Dysphonia** is the umbrella term used to refer to a voice that is disordered in some way (*dys* is a common prefix meaning abnormal or impaired, and *phonia* refers to voice). **Aphonia** refers to the total loss or lack of voice. In addition, many other terms are used to describe the ways in which a voice differs from the norm. Most of these terms are subjective—terms like *breathy*, *hoarse*, *rough*. These and other less familiar terms are described in Table 11-1. Some of these terms describe variations in pitch and frequency, such as *jitter* and *diplophonic*. Other terms

TABLE 11-1 Terms used to describe voice and its many variations

Descriptive Term	Perception
aphonic	No sound or little sound; may cut out or whisper
biphonic or diplophonic	Two pitches produced simultaneously
breathy	Excessive air escaping voice folds
covered	Muffled sound
creaky	Sounding like two hard surfaces rubbing against one another
glottal attack	Harsh, rapid initiation of voicing at beginning of words
glottal fry	Voice pulsing in and out at low frequency; rough, low-pitched, tense voice quality
hoarse (raspy)	Harsh, grating, bumpy sound
honky/hypernasal	Excessive nasality; nasal emissions possible
hyponasal	Reduced nasal resonance; sounds flat
jitter	Rough-sounding pitch
monotonic	No variation in pitch or loudness
pressed/strident	Harsh, loud quality
rough	Noisy, uneven, bumpy vocal fold vibration
shimmer	Crackly, buzzy
soft	Difficult to hear; sounds fatigued
strained	Effortful, hyperfunctioning; neck and jaw perhaps appearing tense
tremorous	Voice shaking during phonation
twangy or ringing	Sharp, bright sound
wheezy	Turbulent airflow when inhaling or exhaling; may sound like asthma or troubled breathing
wobble	Wavering or irregular variation

Sources: Based on Lee, Stemple, and Glaze (2003); National Center for Voice and Speech (2004).

focus on loudness and intensity, such as *pressed* or *strident,* whereas some focus specifically on resonance, such as *nasal* and *ringing.* Some terms focus more broadly on general phonatory quality, describing voices that *flutter* or that *creak.* All of these terms provide more precise ways of describing dysphonia and aphonia.

Vocal Fold Functioning

Many problems with vocal quality result from a malfunctioning of the vocal folds in which the relationship of the folds during vocal production is undermined in some way (Case, 1996). Two terms that describe the most common malfunction are hypofunction and hyperfunction. **Hypofunction** describes vocal folds that are underfunctioning and have inadequate tension. With hypofunction the vocal folds do not come together adequately or evenly, allowing air to escape through the vocal folds and resulting in a breathiness or hoarseness. With complete hypofunction no voice is produced at all, and the person either does not speak or must whisper. In some voice disorders hypofunction affects only one vocal fold and the other works normally.

The opposite of hypofunction is **hyperfunction**. Hyperfunctioning vocal folds are overly tense and compress together too tightly. Thus, the hyperfunctioning voice may sound too loud, too high, and/or too strained. Excessive tension in the neck or jaw may accompany the hyperfunctioning voice. In some cases the hyperfunctioning vocal cords completely impede the production of voice, resulting in *spasticity,* in which the voice stops and starts intermittently.

Diplophonia is a particularly interesting type of vocal fold malfunction. *Diplophonia* means "double pitch" and describes a vocal quality in which the vocal folds produce two different pitches simultaneously. The primary cause of diplophonia is that the two vocal folds have different mass characteristics and therefore vibrate at different rates (Case, 1996). It can also occur if one vocal fold is paralyzed or hypofunctioning.

Voice Without a Larynx

A **laryngectomy** is a procedure in which a person's larynx is surgically removed. It occurs for two primary reasons: laryngeal cancer and laryngeal trauma (Case, 1996). Laryngeal cancer, one of the most serious causes of voice disorders, affects an estimated 11,000 persons each year (Meyerhoff & Rice, 1992). The larynx may be removed to stop the spread of the cancer. For a person who sustains severe trauma to the larynx, as might occur in a car accident, the larynx might be removed if it is too damaged to protect the respiratory system or if the damage impedes breathing. People who have no larynx must develop an alternative way to produce speech, which is called **alaryngeal communication**. In alaryngeal communication, different types of which are described later in this chapter, speech is produced outside the larynx.

Discussion Point: *Anton, described in Box 11-1, uses alaryngeal communication. How does he produce speech?*

Prevalence and Incidence

Voice Disorders in Adults

The prevalence and incidence of voice disorders in both children and adults is relatively high compared to other disorders of communication. Epidemiological research on the rate of voice disorders among adults indicates prevalence and incidence rates of about 29% and 6%, respectively (Roy, Merrill, Thibeault, Parsa, Gray, & Smith, 2004). These numbers show that the number of persons who have ever exhibited voice disorders is relatively high, although at a given point in time only about 6 in 100 persons exhibit a voice disorder. Incidence rates are higher for women (7%) compared to men (5%), they tend to peak between the ages of 40 and 60 years, and they are significantly higher among persons with frequent respiratory allergies, asthma, colds, and sinus infections (Roy et al., 2004).

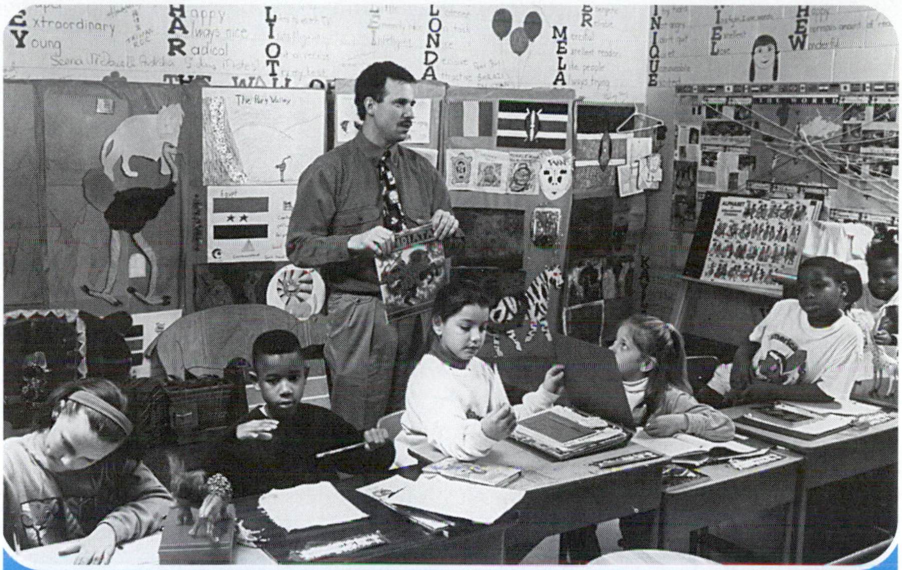

People such as teachers who must use their voices to perform their jobs often experience short-term but recurrent voice problems.

The most common causes of adult voice disorders include vocal nodules (22% of cases), edema/swelling (14%), polyps (11%), carcinoma (10%), and vocal fold paralysis (8%); in about 10% of cases the cause is unknown (Herrington-Hall, Lee, Stemple, Niemi, & McHone, 1988). Many more adults experience recurrent but short-term problems with vocal quality or production. Consider Mr. Grey, a fourth-grade teacher in Albuquerque, New Mexico. Mr. Grey has experienced a 3-week bout of laryngitis each of the last three winters, during which time he has had no voice at all. His laryngitis typically accompanies colds and respiratory infections. Of the nearly one third of adults who have experienced voice disorders, most cases resemble that of Mr. Grey—a short-term problem that appears on several occasions.

Mr. Grey's case also brings up an interesting point about voice disorders: people in some professions exhibit much higher rates of voice disorders (Roy et al., 2004). Whereas about 29% of the general adult population reports a voice disorder at some time, the rate doubles to 58% for teachers. Studies consistently show that some work conditions are causally linked to an increased rate of vocal problems (e.g., Sala, Laine, Simberg, Pentti, & Suonpaa, 2001). The combination of constant voice use (or overuse) and a noisy environment seems to pose the greatest risk of vocal problems. The Center for the Voice at the New York Eye and Ear Infirmary reports that the most frequently seen professionals in that clinic, other than teachers, are vocal performers, sales representatives, customer service personnel, restaurant workers, police officers, and machine shop or factory workers (Center for the Voice, 2004).

Voice Disorders in Children

Researchers estimate that nearly one fourth of children exhibit significant vocal problems, with about 40% of these cases reflecting ongoing rather than transient problems (Powell, Filter, & Williams, 1989). For some of these cases, the voice problem reflects a congenital problem with the vocal apparatus, such as vocal fold paralysis. For a larger number of children, the problem is acquired, resulting from overuse or misuse of the voice. The most common cause of voice dysfunction in children stems from **vocal nodules**, which affect more than 1 million children annually (von Leden, 1985). The nodules, or protuberances, that appear bilaterally on children's vocal folds impede the smooth meeting of the folds at midline, typically resulting in a breathy or hoarse vocal quality and, in some cases, complete loss of voice. Vocal nodules can result from physiological factors—such as gastroesophageal reflux, low blood circulation, dehydration, and laryngeal tension—but are most often associated with psychological and social factors, such as anger, anxiety, distractibility, frustration, interpersonal problems, hyperactivity, and loud talking (see Sapienza, Ruddy, & Baker, 2004).

Prevalence and Treatment

Although the rate of voice disorders is relatively high, many of these cases go undiagnosed and untreated. For instance, although some estimates suggest that about one fourth of all children exhibit voice disorders, only about 6–9% of school children receive voice therapy (Andrews & Summers, 2002). Given that voice disturbances sometimes serve as the outward manifestation of a significant life-threatening disease, such as carcinoma, voice professionals work hard to raise the public's awareness of the importance of diagnosis and treatment for voice problems.

Experts point to several reasons that children and adults with voice disorders may not receive treatment. The first relates to treatment access. Even though children with communication disorders can receive voice therapy through their school's speech-language pathologist, they might not be eligible for treatment if the disorder does not adversely impact educational performance. Also, the American Speech-Language-Hearing Association (ASHA, 1997) requires that children and adults receive a medical evaluation from a physician prior to beginning voice therapy with an SLP. Some parents or adults may not follow up on a referral to a physician for a medical evaluation, and thus an SLP cannot deliver treatment. In addition, the cost of a medical evaluation may be prohibitive, particularly if medical insurance does not cover the evaluation or an individual does not have insurance.

The second reason for nontreatment relates to knowledge. Some individuals may believe that voice difficulties will disappear spontaneously (Andrews & Summers, 2002). Further, the general public may not be well informed about voice disorders and may not understand how the voice works or that treatment can correct vocal problems. This is particularly true for children. Experts argue that a child's early abuse and misuse of the voice, such as being habitually loud, can trap the child in inappropriate habits that result in negative listener reactions and can greatly impact later life ambitions (Andrews & Summers, 2002).

For adults, voice problems can undermine many aspects of

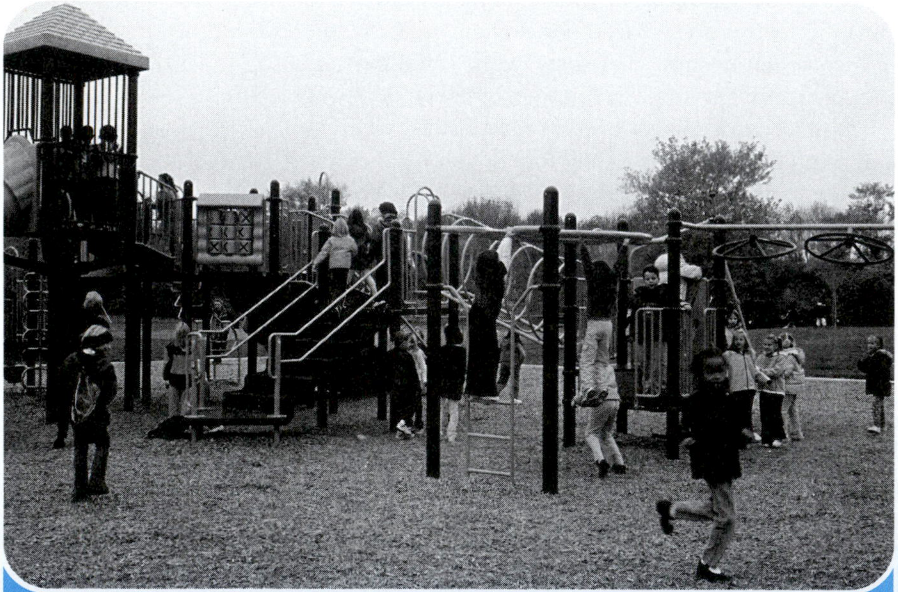

Early misuse of the voice can trap a child in inappropriate vocal habits that result in negative reactions from others.

life, including work performance, employment opportunities, and communication with friends and family. Vocal problems can also impact how others perceive us: "a voice that draws attention to itself and results in negative listener reactions is a significant lifetime handicap, although at times an insidious one" (Andrews & Summers, 2002, p. 63). Ensuring that the general public has information about how the voice works and how treatment can improve vocal quality is important for ensuring that people who need treatment are able to access treatment.

Discussion Point: *Consider the three cases in Box 11-1. What could these individuals do to raise public awareness about their particular voice disorders?*

The third reason for nontreatment relates to social perceptions about vocal quality. In American society a breathy or hoarse vocal quality is sometimes considered an attractive attribute, particularly for women. Marilyn Monroe's breathy voice quality was one of her most frequently acknowledged assets. A breathy voice quality is also viewed as a social marker of the female gender (Hillenbrand, Cleveland, & Erickson, 1994). Thus, a breathy voice quality may bring an individual positive social attention, which is quite different from the possibly negative impact of other communication disorders. However, a breathy vocal quality is also one of the most prominent features of serious voice pathologies, including vocal fold paralysis and carcinoma (Hillenbrand et al., 1994).

Discussion Point: *We all misuse our voices sometimes. What are some ways you have misused your voice? Do any of these ways occur chronically? If so, brainstorm some strategies for eliminating your own chronic voice misuse.*

How Are Voice Disorders Classified?

Experts typically classify voice disorders according to their cause. This etiological classification organizes disorders into four different causal categories (Case, 1996): vocal abuse, neurogenic disorders, psychogenic disorders, and alaryngeal communication.

Vocal Abuse

The vocal folds are a well-used part of the human body; in a given minute of speaking, the vocal folds strike together over 9,000 times. And even when we are not speaking, the vocal folds are often hard at work, as Case (1996) points out in describing the "aerodynamic turmoil" of coughing:

> The tissues of the larynx are tossed about as though caught in a hurricane. The arytenoid cartilages are in chaotic and frenzied motion, matched by the turbulent actions of the vocal folds . . . . It is impossible to watch this coughing episode without realizing how vulnerable laryngeal tissues are to this and other forms of abuse. (p. 127)

The vulnerability of the laryngeal tissues is readily apparent in the regular appearance of scratchy voices during flu season, congested voices during allergy season, and even the loss of voice (laryngitis) during basketball season.

The most common cause of voice disorders in both children and adults is **vocal abuse**, which describes the chronic or intermittent overuse or misuse of the vocal apparatus. Consider your own experience with these vocally abusive behaviors (Case, 1996; Shipley & McAfee, 1998):

- Talking in noisy environments
- Coughing or clearing the throat frequently
- Using caffeine products
- Yelling, screaming, and cheering
- Giving speeches or lectures
- Spending time in smoky environments

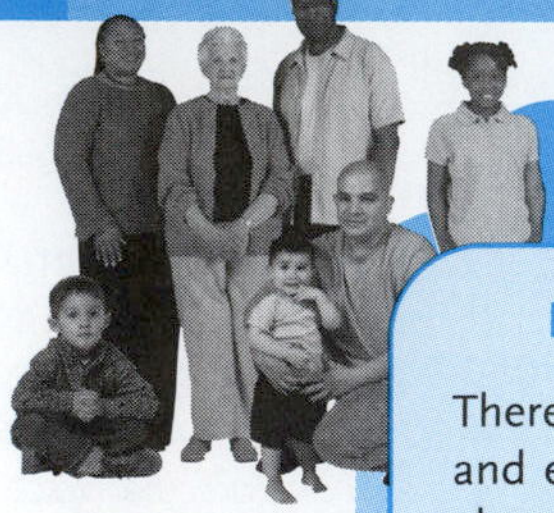

BOX 11-2 Multicultural Focus

Increasing the Number of Diverse Professionals in Speech-Language Pathology

There is a great need to increase the number of persons from traditionally underrepresented racial and ethnic backgrounds in the field of communication sciences and disorders (CSD). In 2003 about 7% of the members of the American Speech-Language-Hearing Association were members of racial/ethnic minority groups (ASHA, 2003b); at that same time about 30% of the U.S. population belonged to racial/ethnic minority groups. Although the reasons for this disparity are complex and numerous, the fact remains that students of racial/ethnic minority backgrounds have historically had unequal access to higher education opportunities and, accordingly, advanced training in CSD (ASHA, 2003b).

ASHA has, in recent years, taken direct actions to respond to the need to diversify the CSD disciplines. ASHA has sponsored many initiatives to promote the diversity of its own membership. One strategy has been to work closely with institutions of higher education to encourage the diversity of students in undergraduate and graduate programs in CSD. Universities receiving recognition for their efforts in this area include Hampton University, Howard University, San Diego State University, Southern Connecticut State University, and the University of Akron. (See http://asha.org/about/leadership-projects/ for additional details on these and other programs.) Here are some examples of current innovations:

- Long Island University (Brooklyn campus) developed a bilingual specialization as part of its CSD curriculum. Students take courses on bilingualism and complete clinical practicum experiences in settings that utilize their bilingual skills.
- The University of Texas at Austin features a specialized training sequence in bilingual speech-language pathology and audiology. Four bilingual faculty members serve as mentors for students in the bilingual program.
- The Department of Communication Disorders at Southern Connecticut State University developed a mentorship program with the local chapter of the National Black Association for Speech, Language, and Hearing (NBASLH). Incoming minority students are partnered with local NBASLH members to provide mentoring and professional networking opportunities.
- Temple University in Philadelphia, Pennsylvania, developed a Hispanic Emphasis Program that prepares students to address the speech, language, and hearing needs of Hispanic and Latino populations.
- The University of Illinois at Champaign-Urbana developed specific multicultural courses to increase the focus on diversity issues within the curriculum. All master's students take the

Figure 11-2 provides a list of the more common misuses and abuses of the voice. Two common conditions associated with vocal abuse include vocal nodules and contact ulcers and granuloma.

Vocal Nodules

Sometimes called teacher's nodules and singer's nodules because of their increased prevalence among these professionals, vocal nodules are small, bilateral protuberances or calloused growths on the inner edges of the vocal folds (see Figure 11-3). Described for the first time in the 1880s, vocal nodules are one of the most frequent causes of hoarseness in adults and children (Benjamin & Croxson, 1987; Goldman, Hargrave, Hillman, Holmberg, & Gress, 1996). Among the estimated 23% of children who have experienced chronic hoarseness at some time in their lives, vocal nodules are to blame in the majority of cases (Benjamin & Croxson, 1987).

departmental multicultural course Clinical Sociolinguistics, and independent study is available through both Advanced Clinical Sociolinguistics and Multicultural Issues in Communications Sciences.

- The University of Northern Iowa (UNI) and Xavier University in New Orleans (a historically black college) developed a collaborative partnership to support the recruitment of African American students from Xavier into graduate-level training in speech-language pathology at UNI.
- The University of Wisconsin–Milwaukee developed a program called Project DUIT (Diverse Urban Interdisciplinary Teams). Project DUIT features a partnership between the university and Milwaukee Public Schools to encourage academic students from traditionally underrepresented backgrounds to consider a career in CSD.

These innovative strategies represent an important inroad into recruiting and retaining students from diverse ethnic and racial backgrounds into the CSD disciplines.

For Discussion

What are additional recruitment and retention strategies that might be used to build a more diverse membership in the CSD professions?

What are some barriers that might prohibit persons from diverse ethnic and racial backgrounds from pursuing a career in CSD?

Why is it important to promote diversity among the professionals who do research and practice in CSD?

The following resources provide additional information on multicultural practices:

American Speech-Language-Hearing Association. (2003a). *Compendium of exemplary practices by colleges and universities in the recruitment, retention and career transition of communication sciences and disorders (CSD) professionals.* Retrieved December 10, 2003, from http://asha.org/about/leadership-projects/multicultural/diversity-fi/compendium.htm

American Speech-Language-Hearing Association. (2003b). *Minority student recruitment, retention, and career transition practices: A review of the literature.* Retrieved December 10, 2003, from http://asha.org/about/leadership-projects/multicultural/diversity-fi/litreview.htm

Companion Website

To answer these questions online, go to the Multicultural Focus module in chapter 11 of the Companion Website.

Vocal nodules come in two varieties, acute and chronic. Acute nodules are essentially bruises on the vocal folds, which over time will thicken and harden as they become a chronic condition and advance to becoming fibrous protuberances. Vocal nodules represent the body's response to an irritant, which in this case is the vocal folds' repeated hard contact at midline. The protuberances impede the vocal folds from seamless contact and allow air to escape during phonation, resulting in a breathy or hoarse vocal quality.

Nodules are most prevalent in young children and in adults who engage in vocal overuse and misuse (Goldman et al., 1996). Research on high school and college cheerleaders described by Case (1996) found that nearly 50% of high school cheerleaders showed emerging vocal nodules after a 1-week cheerleading camp (none had any evidence of vocal pathology before the camp started), and 75% of the college cheerleaders had emerging nodules after only several weeks of practice. The characteristics of cheerleaders who

FIGURE 11-2 Common misuses and abuses of the voice.

Yelling and screaming	Alcohol use
Hard glottal attack	Speaking during menstrual cycle
Abusive singing	Excessive speaking
Hydration concerns	Inadequate breath support
Speaking over noise	Laughing hard
Coughing/throat clearing	Aspirin (drugs)
Grunting in exercise	Cheerleading, aerobics instruction, pep clubs
Calling at a distance	Making toy/animal noises
Inappropriate pitch	Athletic activity (coaching, etc.)
Excessive talking with allergy or upper respiratory infection	Intense personality
Muscular tension	Arguing
Smoking factor	

Source: From *Clinical Management of Voice Disorders* (4th ed.) by G. L. Case, 2002, Austin, TX: Pro-Ed. Copyright 2002 by Pro-Ed. Adapted with permission.

developed nodules included excessive laryngeal tension when cheering, hard glottal attacks when beginning a cheer, cheering at too low or too high a pitch, and general misuse of voice (e.g., cheering during a cold or infection). An individual's temperament and general health may also come into play in elevating the risk of nodules. Adults with vocal nodules have greater anxiety and bodily complaints, such as trouble sleeping or stomach ailments (Goldman et al., 1996).

FIGURE 11-3 Vocal nodules.

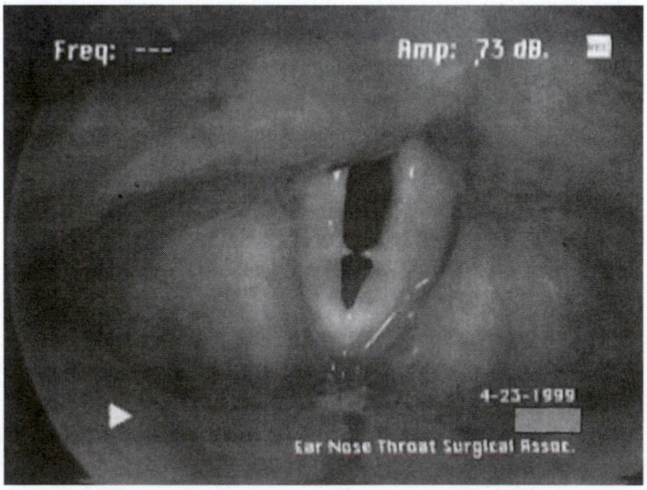

Source: From "Laryngeal Structure and Function in the Pediatric Larynx: Clinical Applications" by C. M. Sapienza, B. H. Ruddy, and S. Baker, 2004, *Language, Speech, and Hearing Services in Schools, 35*, p. 303. Copyright 2004 by ASHA. Reprinted with permission.

FIGURE 11-4 A contact ulcer with granuloma.

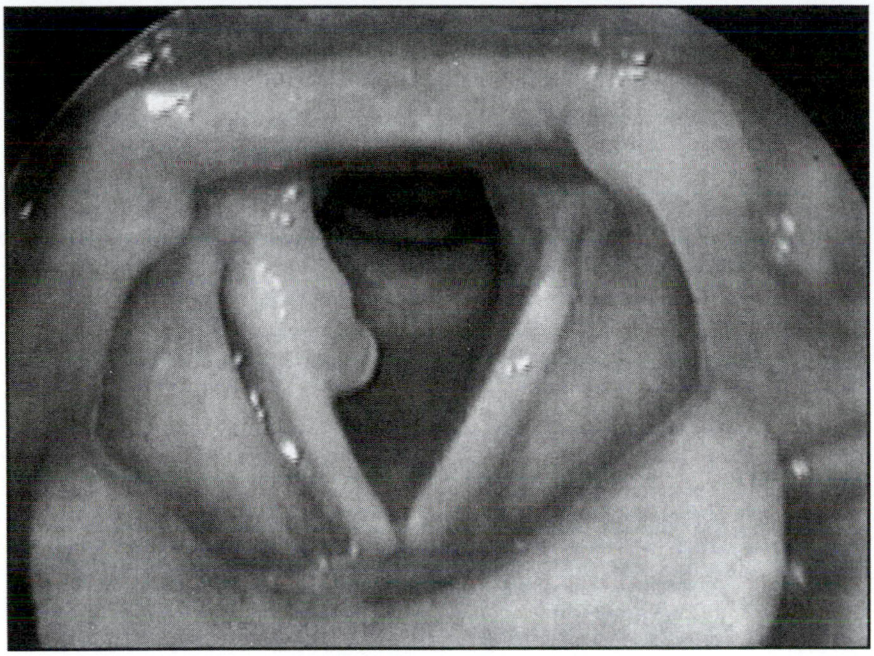

Source: From *Clinical Management of Voice Disorders* (4th ed., p. 171) by J. L. Case, 2002, Austin, TX: Pro-Ed. Copyright 2002 by Pro-Ed. Reprinted with permission.

Contact Ulcers and Granuloma

Contact ulcers are inflamed lesions, or ulcers, that develop on the arytenoid cartilages in the posterior region of the larynx. These lesions develop from repeated forceful contact of the vocal folds and progress from tissue irritation to necrosis, or death of the tissue. The body's healing process then generates a mass of tissue, or *granuloma,* at the site of the ulcer (see Figure 11-4) (Case, 1996). Although a major cause of granuloma is vocal abuse and chronic irritation of the laryngeal cartilages, it can also result from acidic irritation to the laryngeal area because of chronic reflux or from tubal intubation (e.g., during surgery; Hirano, 1990).

Contact ulcers and granuloma, which typically result in a breathy, low voice quality, affect both men and women in a ratio of roughly 4:1 (Watterson, Hansen-Magorian, & McFarlane, 1990). The ulcers result from persistent vocal abuse and overuse and can affect persons in a variety of professions. Case (1996) reports that he has treated vocal nodules in a Buddhist chanter, a school superintendent, a high school physical education teacher, and a politician—all of whom rely on voice in their everyday life and work.

Neurogenic Disorders

Neurogenic voice disorders result from illness, damage, or disease to the neurological systems associated with voice production. Both the central nervous system (CNS) and the peripheral nervous system (PNS) are involved in managing the motor and sensory functions of the larynx, and damage to either can cause dysfunction of the vocal mechanisms. Figure 11-5 illustrates the complex interplay of the CNS, the PNS, and the larynx. One of the most important nerves involved in the smooth functioning of the larynx is the **vagus nerve** of

FIGURE 11-5 The nervous system and voice production.

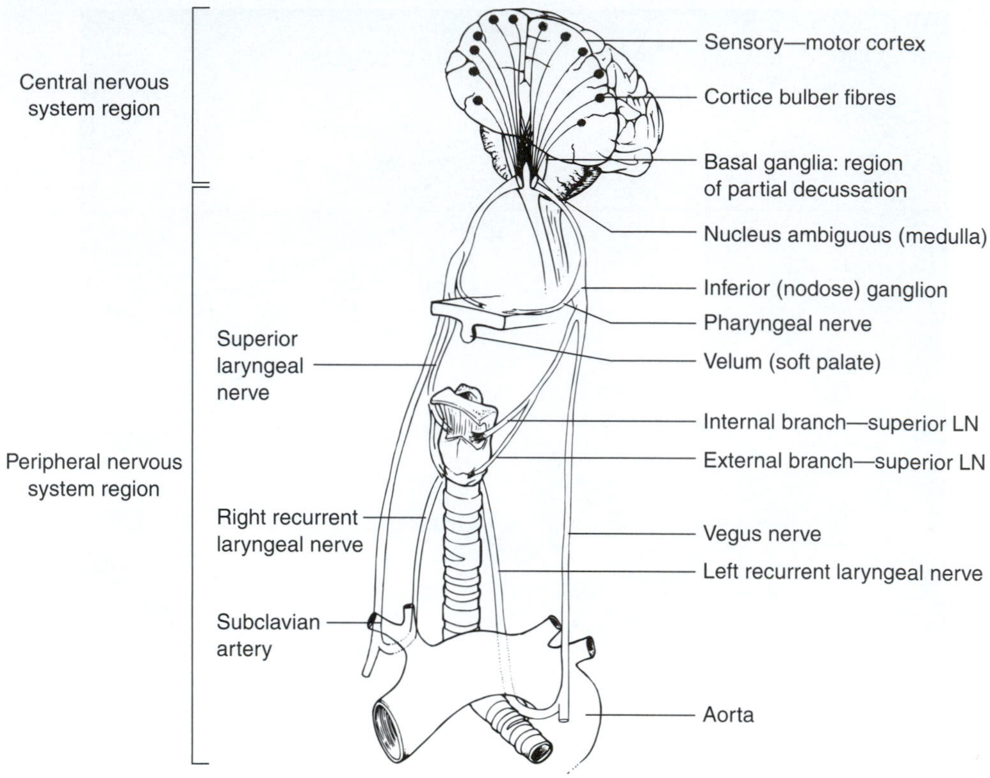

the PNS, also described as cranial nerve X. The vagus (which means "wandering") nerve runs from the cranium down and around the heart and has several branches departing from the main nerve to innervate the pharynx and the larynx. The first branch is the pharyngeal nerve, which communicates sensory and motor information to the pharynx and the soft palate. The next branch is the superior laryngeal nerve (LN), which departs from the vagus above the larynx to innervate parts of the tongue, pharynx, and larynx. Yet another branch, the recurrent laryngeal nerve, departs from the vagus below the larynx to innervate the larynx, esophagus, and trachea (Zemlin, 1988).

If the nerves of the CNS or PNS that innervate the voice-production system are disrupted in some way, a voice disorder can result. Disorders of this type are called neurogenic because their etiology stems from neurological malfunctioning. Several of the more well-known types of neurogenic voice disorders are described here.

Vagus Nerve Lesions

Lesions to the vagus nerve can occur for a variety of reasons, including surgical damage (particularly thyroid surgery), trauma, and viral infections (Case, 1996). The most serious outcome of vagus nerve damage is vocal fold paralysis, which typically is unilateral, affecting only one vocal fold. When the vocal fold is paralyzed in an adducted position—called *abduction paralysis* because the vocal fold cannot open—the voice is usually not affected because the other fold can press against it to phonate. However, in these cases a person will struggle with breathing because of the closed position of one fold. When the vocal fold is paralyzed in an abducted position—called *adduction paralysis* because the vocal fold does not close—vocal production is compromised because the two vocal folds do not meet at midline. This causes a hoarse or breathy vocal quality. In some cases of vagus nerve damage, complete paralysis of the vocal folds occurs, leaving them completely opened or completely blocking the airway. In the latter case a **tracheostomy** is performed, in which an artificial airway is placed below the larynx so the individual can breathe.

Spasmodic Dysphonia

Spasmodic dysphonia (SD), also called *spastic dysphonia,* is a disorder affecting motor control of the larynx. Vocal spasms that result in intermittent voice stoppages are the hallmark of this disorder. A diagnosis of SD has these characteristics:

- An occasionally normal voice
- Intermittent breaks in voicing
- A normal-sounding whisper
- Improved voice at high pitches
- Worsening voice with stress
- Periods of significant dysphonia (Cannito et al., 1997)

Terms used to describe the voices of people with SD include *jerky, grunting, squeezed, groaning,* and *stuttering-like* (Aronson, 1990). Although SD was historically viewed as a voice disorder of psychological origin—early described as nervous hoarseness (Cannito et al., 1997)—current theories recognize SD as a neurologically based **laryngeal dystonia**, which affects the movement patterns of the laryngeal muscles (Brin, Fahn, Blitzer, Ramig, & Stewart, 1992). *Dystonia* describes abnormal movements of the body (Case, 1996), and *laryngeal dystonia* identifies this condition as it affects the larynx. For people with laryngeal dystonia, vocal tremors are common.

SD appears in several different forms and can range from mild to severe. The adductor type is the most common, representing about half of SD cases (Blitzer & Brin, 1992; Cannito et al., 1997). In this type a person exhibits a hyperfunctioning voice that seems strangled, strained, and squeezing (Cannito et al., 1997). The abductor type of SD is less common and features a hypofunctioning voice that is breathy and open. Some people show a mixed SD, in which they intermittently experience both adductor and abductor characteristics.

ALS

Amyotrophic lateral sclerosis (ALS), also called Lou Gehrig's disease, is a progressive, degenerative, neuromuscular disease resulting in muscular weakness, fatigue, and atrophy as well as muscular spasms, tremors, and cramping (Renout, Leeper, Bandur, & Hudson, 1995). The cause is unknown, and the impact of the disease is significant, with most individuals surviving fewer than 10 years (Case, 1996). Because of its widespread impact on muscular functioning, voice disorders are a common symptom of ALS, and voice functioning deteriorates over time (Strand, Buder, Yorkston, & Ramig, 1994). The voice of an individual with ALS is usually soft, breathy, low in pitch and loudness with limited variability, and hypernasal. In addition to voice disturbances, people with ALS have difficulty clearly articulating speech sounds because they cannot precisely and strongly coordinate the motor processes needed to articulate (Case, 1996).

As Case (1996) notes, the cognitive abilities of people with ALS remain intact even while muscular processes are rapidly deteriorating. In the later stages of the disease, a person is unable to produce voice or speech yet is aware of this loss of function. Augmentative communication devices, such as those described in chapter 15, can provide a person with ALS an alternative way to communicate with others.

Parkinson's Disease

Parkinson's disease is, like ALS, a progressive, degenerative neurological disease, one that is caused by dopamine depletion (Ramig, Countryman, Thompson, & Horii, 1995). The majority of people with Parkinson's disease exhibit impaired communication abilities, including a significant disorder of voice, which occurs because of the impact of the disease on the respiratory and laryngeal systems. A person with Parkinson's disease is unable to produce a strong voice because of a weakened respiratory system, resulting in reduced loudness and a breathy, weak voice. The disease also results in a more rigid muscular tone, which restricts the movement of the laryngeal muscles so that the vocal folds can no longer forcefully adduct (Ramig & Dromey, 1996), resulting in hoarseness and a monotonic pitch. The Lee Silverman voice treatment program (Ramig, Pawlas, & Countryman, 1995) is effective in improving respiratory strength and vocal fold adduction for people with Parkinson's disease, helping them have a stronger voice even as the disease progresses.

Psychogenic Disorders

Our voices often carry information about our emotional and psychological states, as when we speak angrily and produce voice forcefully with tightly contracted muscles or when we speak tenderly and produce voice with smooth and light contact of the vocal folds (Andrews & Summers, 2002). Most of us can remember a time when our voices gave our feelings away, perhaps conveying our excitement, fear, anxiety, or shock. The human voice also serves as a more permanent marker of our personalities. For instance, consider the macho, tough personality of Tony Soprano in the HBO hit show *The Sopranos* and the way his vocal characteristics convey this part of his personality. The voices of individuals who experience significant disorders of personality or psychological health can be impacted. **Psychogenic disorders** of voice, also called *nonorganic disorders,* result from or are linked to emotional and psychological characteristics. *Psychogenic dysphonia* is the diagnostic term used to describe disordered voice quality that results from an emotional or psychological event.

Discussion Point: *Consider the cases of Dr. Mitchell and Alton in Box 11-1. What are some explanations for their very different psychological responses to the loss of voice?*

Psychological or Emotional Triggers

Some individuals develop a chronic voice disorder as a result of a vocal injury. People who rely on their voice professionally—such as actors, singers, and teachers—are particularly vulnerable to a vocal injury. However, once the injury is resolved, these individuals may experience a sense of vulnerability and anxiety about their voice, which can translate into hypochondria and chronic worry that a brief lapse is the signal of a serious disorder. The anxiety that can follow a vocal injury can result in disturbances in memory, concentration, and emotional well-being, all of which can then further exacerbate vocal problems (Rosen & Sataloff, 1997).

Voice disorders can also result from traumatic experiences, such as being treated for cancer, being robbed or raped, or having throat surgery (Case, 1996; Rosen & Sataloff, 1997; Stemple et al., 1995). Case (1996) describes his work with a 45-year-old woman who exhibited dysphonia for several months, stemming from an intense fear of having laryngeal cancer. Delving into the patient's history, Case found that she had already been treated for uterine cancer and breast cancer and had a friend who was diagnosed with laryngeal cancer. Although her fears were understandable given these circumstances, examination of her larynx showed them to be unfounded, and her dysphonia resolved soon after.

Psychopathology

A variety of psychopathological conditions can also affect the quality of the voice. Several of the more common psychological disturbances—such as stress, anxiety, and depression—can detract from voice quality, as can more serious disturbances, such as conversion disorder.

Stress, Anxiety, and Depression. Stress, anxiety, and depression are relatively well-known psychological disturbances, which, in their more severe forms, can have a significant impact on an individual's well-being. Sometimes an individual's vocal patterns provide the first clue of severe stress, anxiety, or depression. *Acute stress disorder* develops within 1 month of a traumatic experience, such as a sexual or violent assault or diagnosis of a life-threatening illness (American Psychiatric Association [APA], 1994). The chronic distress that results includes a cluster of symptoms, including exaggerated startle responses, motor restlessness, and irritability, all of which can be reflected in a person's voice.

Anxiety conditions, such as generalized anxiety disorder and performance anxiety, are generally less serious psychological disturbances but can also be reflected in vocal characteristics. A person with *generalized anxiety disorder* is excessively anxious and worried, is easily fatigued and irritable, and experiences long periods of general restlessness (APA, 1994). Common symptoms also include muscle tension, which results in trembling, twitching, shakiness, and muscular aches, all of which can extend to the muscles of the larynx. Someone with *performance anxiety,* also called stage fright, experiences anxiety in the context of specific triggers, such as speaking to a large group of people or performing a task (e.g., surgery) in front of an audience. The context triggers a fight-or-flight response that features heart palpitations, sweatiness, vocal tremors, and voice breakages. Successful treatment for stress, anxiety, and depression can alleviate voice-related symptoms as a byproduct of resolving the primary disorder, although in some cases specific targeting of communication and voice production is beneficial.

Conversion Disorder. **Conversion disorder** is a psychological disturbance in which an individual exhibits symptoms of a physical disease or disorder. The physical symptoms reflect emotional stress or conflict. One possible symptom of conversion disorder is dysphonia or aphonia, characterized by a weak, breathy voice with little or no voicing. A person with conversion disorder is not malingering, or feigning illness; rather it appears the physical symptoms result from severe anxiety or stress (APA, 1994). Some experts suggest that the loss of voice for people with conversion disorder provides them a way to reduce communication with persons of importance—such as parents, spouse, or others—particularly if communication is psychologically painful (Case, 1996). Despite the serious impact of conversion disorder, the person affected may be indifferent to vocal problems (called *la belle indifference)* or may exhibit a dramatic or histrionic response (APA, 1994).

Vocal Tics and Tourette's Disorder. Two additional psychopathological conditions that impact voice production are vocal tic disorder and Tourette's disorder. The individual with **vocal tic disorder** produces sudden, rapid, recurrent vocalizations, including clicks, yelps, snorts, and coughs. These occur many times a day for a period of longer than 1 year, causing significant stress and impairment in key areas of functioning, including interpersonal relationships and occupational or academic performance (APA, 1994). With *Tourette's disorder,* vocal tics occur simultaneously with other motor tics affecting the head, torso, and extremities. These might include eye blinking, twirling, or deep knee bends, for instance (APA, 1994). The vocal tics seen in both vocal tic disorder and Tourette's syndrome are not linked to any known physical cause.

Mutational Falsetto and Juvenile Voice

Two additional categories of psychogenic voice disturbances require mention; both describe vocal characteristics that are inconsistent with an individual's age and gender. **Mutational falsetto**, also called **puberphonia**, describes a male child or adolescent who exhibits an inappropriately high voice. During puberty hormonal changes greatly impact the male voice, and fairly sudden and dramatic changes in voice quality and pitch occur. Case describes that in a period of only a "few short months, the boy's voice becomes a man's" (1996, p. 243). However, for some boys, the changes do not occur easily, and their voices maintain an unusually high pitch, which may resemble or even exceed that of pre-puberty. Voice therapy is usually quite effective in helping the adolescent male shift his voice to a more appropriate pitch. When specific organic factors, such as undergrowth of the larynx or endocrine imbalance, are to blame for an overly high pitch in adolescent or adult males, the condition is considered an *organic mutational falsetto,* and medical treatment is likely needed.

Juvenile voice disorder, in which women maintain a juvenile voice into adulthood, is the female companion to mutational falsetto. The female voice also changes dramatically during puberty, reducing its pitch to a more adultlike level. Juvenile voice disorder describes cases in which females do not drop their pitch but maintain the pitch of a child. Often accompanying the childlike pitch is a low intensity, nasality, and breathiness (Stemple et al., 1995).

Alaryngeal Communication

Some individuals must produce voice without the benefit of a larynx; theirs is called *alaryngeal communication,* which most often results from a tracheostomy or a laryngectomy.

Tracheostomy

When a person's respiratory system is compromised, mechanical ventilation and respiration are needed to preserve life. The most common reasons for mechanical ventilation are progressive neuromuscular conditions, spinal cord injury, genetic syndromes, and premature birth. A tracheostomy is a surgical procedure in which a tracheostomy tube, or trach, is inserted through the neck below the vocal folds to direct air into the lungs (see Figure 11-6). Some people receive a trach because their vocal folds are not functioning well, as in the case of laryngeal cancer and bilateral vocal fold paralysis. These individuals are at risk of aspiration or penetration of substances into the lungs, increasing the risk of pneuomonia and other respiratory ailments.

FIGURE 11-6 A standard tracheostomy tube placed in the upper airway.

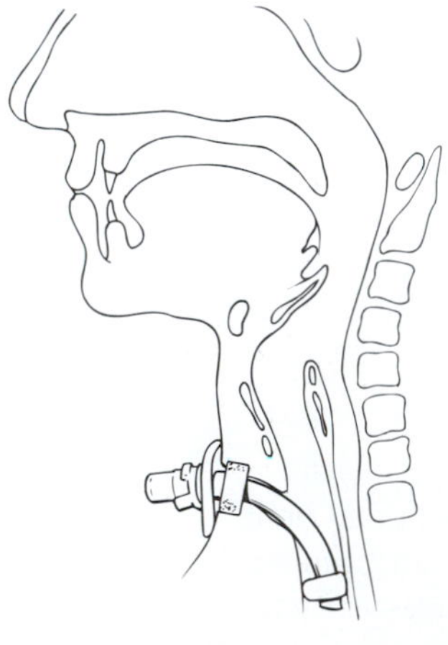

A person with a trach is unable to talk because the air that is typically expelled over the vocal folds to produce phonation is directed outward through the trach tube. As you can imagine, this creates a "multitude of adverse physical and psychological experiences for the critically ill patient" (Bergbom-Engberg & Haljamae, 1989), not the least being the inability to communicate. One study of adults who had received respiratory treatment showed that their inability to talk was second only to general anxiety and fear in their list of discomforts (Bergbom-Engberg & Haljamae, 1989). For children, being on a trach for an extended period of time can undermine their ability to develop speech, language, and communication abilities. This is particularly true for children who receive a trach at birth and have never been able to use their voices.

Fortunately for these children and adults, David Muir, a young man with muscular dystrophy, invented a speaking valve that enabled him to produce speech while on a trach tube. Now commercially available as the Passy-Muir tracheostomy speaking valve, it uses a valving system that sends air downward into the pulmonary system during inhalation but directs exhaled air over the vocal folds to produce speech. Thus, the valve allows adults to speak while ventilated and infants (see Figure 11-7) to vocalize and communicate (Torres & Sirbegovic, 2004).

FIGURE 11-7 An infant fitted with a Passy-Muir speaking valve and tracheostomy tube.

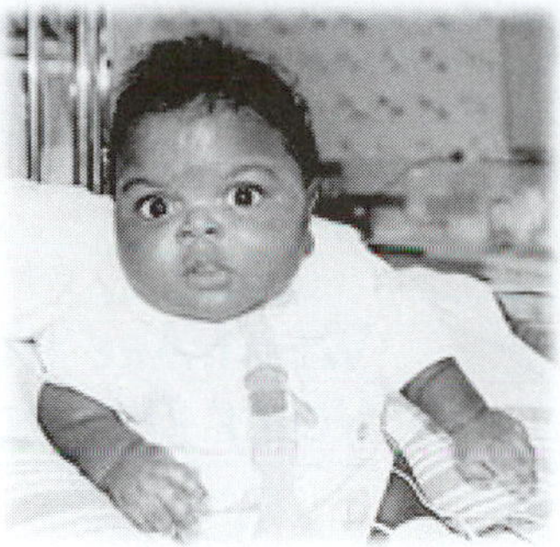
Kylon / Premature 31 weeks,
Bronchomalacia, Aspiration
Pneumonia, Necrotizing Enterocolitis

Source: Courtesy of Passy-Muir, Inc.

Laryngectomy

For adults the most common reason for alaryngeal communication is the removal of the larynx. This can occur because of trauma, such as a car accident in which the larynx is seriously damaged, but commonly the larynx is removed because of laryngeal cancer. To prevent the spread of cancer or to treat an advanced cancer, the larynx is removed in a procedure called laryngectomy; a person whose larynx has been removed is called a **laryngectomee**. Speaking and voicing is possible through a variety of procedures described later in this chapter. Here is an overview of the etiology, symptoms, and treatment of laryngeal cancer.

Etiology. Laryngeal cancer accounts for about 1–2% of all cancers, or about 12,000 cases annually in the United States. It affects men at much higher rates than women (Surveillance, Epidemiology, and End Results [SEER], 2004) and older African American males at the highest rates. In general, the rate of laryngeal cancer has declined since the 1970s, most dramatically for African American and European American men. However, current rates of diagnosis remain high for men, affecting about 11 in 100,000 African American men and 6 in 100,000 European American men, as compared to about 1.5 to 2 per 100,000 African American and European American women (SEER, 2004).

Laryngeal cancer is linked to tobacco use; as tobacco use goes up, so does the risk of developing laryngeal cancer (Cann, Rothman, & Fried, 1996). About 15 of 100,000 smokers develop this form of cancer, as compared to fewer than 1 of 100,000 nonsmokers (Cann et al., 1996). Alcohol use also increases the risk of laryngeal cancer; that risk is elevated exponentially when alcohol and tobacco use are combined (Cann et al., 1996). Additional risks include nutritional inadequacies and occupational exposures, particularly exposure to asbestos and certain man-made fibers, like glass wool production.

Symptoms. Successful treatment of laryngeal cancer requires early identification. The most consistent early symptom is hoarseness. As a general rule, no one should ever allow hoarseness to continue for longer than 2 weeks without a medical evaluation (Brodnitz, 1988). Additional symptoms that may emerge as cancer progresses include *stridor* (i.e., hearing the voice when inhaling), laryngeal pain, discharge, and swelling in the neck (Case, 1996).

Treatment. The first goal in cancer treatment is always to rid the body of the malignancy. The second goal is to maintain the body's functions and structures. With laryngeal cancer it is likely that some of the body's functions and structures will be adversely impacted because the malignancy sits squarely in the path of breathing and speaking (Fried & Lauretano, 1996). When the malignancy is removed surgically, most often the surgery affects one or both of these abilities.

Many oncologists use *conservation approaches* when treating laryngeal cancer to preserve the larynx as much as possible. With a conservation approach the larynx remains, with portions of it removed. With *cordectomy* one of the vocal folds is surgically removed, and with *hemilaryngectomy* portions of the laryngeal cartilages are removed. When the larynx cannot be conserved, it is removed in a near-total or total laryngectomy. Alternative ways of communicating are then possible, although they will never replicate the quality of the natural voice.

Discussion Point: *Consider all three cases in Box 11-1. Identify the etiology, or cause, of each type of voice disorder.*

What Are the Defining Characteristics of Voice Disorders?

A voice disorder impacts one or more of the following perceptual characteristics of voice: resonance, loudness and pitch, or phonatory quality. Table 11-2 identifies the perceptual aspects of voice affected by the specific voice disorders described in this chapter.

Resonance

As the voice travels up from the vocal folds, it vibrates as a column of air within the nasal and oral cavities. The extent to which the column of air is allowed to enter the nasal and oral cavities is controlled at the **velopharyngeal port**, or the back of the oral cavity where the oral and nasal cavities meet. The velopharyngeal mechanism is the coupling of the velum, or soft palate, and the back of the pharynx to channel the vibrating air into the oral and nasal cavities. The velopharyngeal port typically rests in an open position with the velum lowered, as it is when we are breathing through the nose. When we speak, the velum rises to close the port, channeling the airflow and voice into the oral cavity, with no airflow

TABLE 11-2 The impact of specific voice etiologies and disorders on perceptual characteristics

Etiology	Specific Disorder	Resonance	Pitch/ Loudness	Phonatory Quality
Vocal abuse	Vocal nodules		X	X
	Contact ulcers/ granuloma		X	X
Neurogenic	Vagus nerve lesion		X	X
	Spasmodic dysphonia		X	X
	ALS	X	X	X
	Parkinson's disease		X	X
Psychogenic	Psychological/ emotional experience		X	X
	Psychopathology	X	X	X
	Vocal tics			X
	Mutational falsetto/ juvenile voice	X	X	

released into the nasal cavity. Only during the production of the three nasal consonants—/n/, /m/, and /ŋ/—and adjacent vowels is the velopharyngeal port open to allow air into the nasal cavity (Case, 1996).

Disorders of resonance result from problems with control of the velopharyngeal port due to velopharyngeal inadequacy. **Velopharyngeal inadequacy** occurs when there is imperfect closure of the port because of structural or muscular problems (Case, 1996). There are several common causes of velopharyngeal inadequacy:

1. *Cleft palate and cranio-facial anomalies:* This congenital malformation often affects the functioning of the velopharyngeal port. Even after surgical repair, the velum may be weakened or stiff because of scar tissue.
2. *Iatrogenic problems:* These result from surgery, particularly removal of the tonsils and adenoid tissues, which are located in the velopharyngeal region.
3. *Allergies:* Allergic rhinitis can cause hyponasal speech and impact the smooth functioning of the velopharyngeal port through swelling and congestion.
4. *Neuromuscular impairment:* Disorders that undermine neuromuscular functioning often affect control of the velopharyngeal port. Common causes of neuromuscular disturbance include cerebral palsy, head injuries, meningitis, tumors, neck trauma, nerve trauma, and muscular dystrophy (Dworkin, Marunick, & Krouse, 2004).

Velopharyngeal inadequacy causes either hypernasality or hyponasality. With hypernasality, the velopharyngeal port remains open, allowing too much resonance in the nasal cavity. Often, nasal emissions are present—that is, air emits from the nose during speech. The lowered pressure in the oral cavity also degrades the production of some oral speech sounds, particularly the pressure consonants—such as /b/, /p/, and /t/—which require a large build-up of air for their production.

Hyponasality describes a condition in which there is too little nasal resonance. When the nasal cavity is blocked in some way and thus is not available to serve as a resonating chamber, sounds that require nasal resonation, such as /m/, become denasalized. These are some conditions that can cause hyponasality:

- *Acute rhinitis:* Nasal inflammation and congestion, both of which are symptoms of the common cold
- *Allergic rhinitis:* Nasal inflammation due to environmental allergies
- *Papilloma:* Wartlike growths, potentially caused by a virus, which grow in the nasal cavity
- *Tonsilitis:* Inflamed tonsilar tissue due to infection (Case, 1996)

These and other conditions can make it difficult to breathe through the nose and to use the nasal cavity for the production of speech. In such cases the voice may sound denasalized, stuffy, and congested.

Pitch and Loudness

Appropriate vocal pitch and loudness—alternatively, frequency and intensity—relate directly to how well the vocal and speech production mechanisms work together as a system. Too much or too little tension or force in voice production can result in aberrational pitch or loudness, such as a voice that is too loud, too soft, too high, or too low. Pitch changes are one of the most common symptoms of vocal pathologies (Stemple et al., 1995).

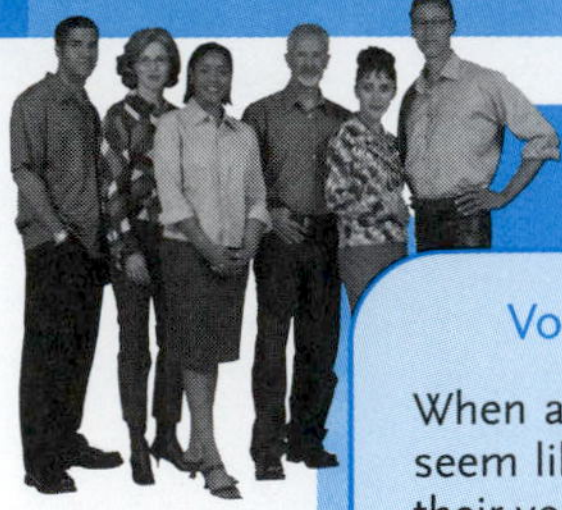

BOX 11-3 Ecological Contexts

Voice Disorders at Home, at Work, and in the Community

When a person's voice is lost, how much of that individual's personality is lost? This may seem like an esoteric question, but it is an important one to consider for people who lose their voice forever through laryngectomy. Helping these individuals regain their sense of self and personality through rehabilitation and counseling is just as critical as teaching specific techniques to produce voice.

Three aspects of life that help to define us are our friends, our work, and our hobbies. Consider your own social circle, work, and hobbies. How much is your voice involved in these? How would they be impacted if you lost your voice? The individual with a laryngectomy suddenly cannot call his friends on the telephone, cannot lead meetings at work, and can no longer conduct storytime at the local library. Everything changes. Some relationships will be lost, responsibilities at work will shift, and new hobbies will need to be found.

For Discussion

Some people with laryngectomy feel marginalized by their difference. How accepting is our society of physical and vocal differences among people?

For people with no voice, what are some physical, social, and educational activities that may be restricted for them?

Companion Website

To answer these questions online, go to the Ecological Contexts module in chapter 11 of the Companion Website.

Pitch

When vocal pitch is aberrational, it brings undesirable attention to the voice of the speaker. For instance, when a young adult male speaks with a functional falsetto voice or a young adult female speaks with a juvenile voice, both pitches are inappropriately high, with hyperfunctioning laryngeal muscles. More common is the pitch disturbance described as **glottal fry**, in which the pitch is unusually and chronically low, produced on tightly approximated vocal folds and sounding like a "poorly tuned motorboat engine" (Stemple et al., 1995, p. 50).

Several concepts are important in understanding pitch disturbances:

1. ***Habitual pitch**:* Also called *vocal idle,* the pitch used in normal speaking situations without applying any extra physiological effort
2. ***Optimal pitch**:* The pitch at which one's voice is the least abusive, least effortful, and most efficient
3. ***Basal pitch**:* The lowest steady pitch a person can produce without pitch breakages or glottal fry.
4. ***Ceiling pitch**:* The highest pitch at which a voice can be sustained without pitch breakages
5. ***Vocal range**:* The difference between a basal and a ceiling pitch, normally covering two to three octaves (Case, 1996)

A pitch disturbance is present when a person's habitual pitch differs significantly from the optimal pitch and/or when vocal range is overly limited.

Loudness

Voice disorders can also affect loudness, resulting in a voice that is insufficiently or overly loud or one in which loudness does not vary, referred to as **monotonic**. Excessive shouting, loud talking, and screaming are several types of vocal abuses that are overloud. To produce an overly loud voice, the air pressure under the vocal folds must build up. Excessive loudness is sometimes seen in persons who are deaf or hard of hearing because they are unable to monitor the loudness of their own voices.

Other people are not loud enough, and listeners must strain to hear them. Underloudness can result from a lack of respiratory force due to neurological injury or disease, such as traumatic brain injury, Parkinson's disease, or multiple sclerosis, all of which can undermine the muscular processes required to produce a strong voice. Researchers Solomon, McKee, and Garcia-Barry (2001) recently described a 23-year-old man, JN, who sustained a severe traumatic brain injury in a motor vehicle accident. In addition to other cognitive, language, and speech problems, JN's neurological damage compromised his ability to produce a loud, strong voice: "In connected speech, [JN's] vocal quality was breathy and rough, accompanied by decreased vocal pitch and monopitch/monoloudness" (p. 54).

Underloudness can also occur for social or psychogenic reasons. Some homes value quietness, and children may develop early patterns of speaking softly. Other reports suggest that underloudness can occur for psychological reasons. Case (1996) reports a case in which a woman was virtually aphonic (i.e., unable to produce an audible voice) because of a traumatic incident in which she was robbed at knifepoint. In less obvious cases, an adult or a child might experience serious vocal or throat pain and then be hesitant to exert the pressure needed to produce a strong voice. Like overloudness, speaking too softly is a type of vocal abuse; persistent underloudness can cause vocal strain and fatigue because the vocal muscles must work harder, given the inadequate force of the air stream.

Phonatory Quality

Phonation is the production of voice via the vocal folds. The vocal folds must work together easily and harmoniously to produce a normal voice quality that does not draw attention to itself. Several of the more common disturbances to phonatory quality are described here:

1. *Hard glottal attack:* Voice is produced with a hard vocal burst, created by building up air pressure below the vocal folds and tensing them together, after which they burst apart and then bang back together.
2. *Glottal fry:* Referenced previously as a pitch disorder, glottal fry also represents a disordered phonatory quality in which pitch is held at an unusually low level and is produced on tightly approximated vocal folds.
3. *Breathy phonation:* Voice is produced without complete closure or approximation of the vocal folds, resulting in a weak and breathy voice.
4. *Spasticity:* Voice is produced with too much vocal tension and effort, resulting in intermittent stoppage of the voice.
5. *Hoarseness:* Voice is produced with noise introduced into the sound spectrum and a loss of the higher frequencies (Stemple et al., 1995).

How Are Voice Disorders Identified?

The Voice Care Team

The identification and management of voice disorders require the close collaboration of a variety of professionals, called the *voice care team* (Harvey, 1996). Voice management is a holistic process that requires close attention to an individual's physical health and psychological well-being. The professional team includes medical professionals, including the primary care physician (PCP) and an otolaryngologist, as well as allied health professionals, including a speech-language pathologist and perhaps a psychologist or psychiatrist. For children, educators are essential members of the voice care team, including classroom teachers and special educators. For patients who use their voices professionally for performance art, including singers and actors, the voice care team may involve a voice teacher and a voice coach (Harvey, 1996).

Involving a range of professionals in the management of voice disorders results in a more accurate and thorough diagnosis of the voice disorder and a more comprehensive description of how the voice disorder affects the individual both physiologically and psychologically. It also enhances the design of comprehensive and coordinated treatment approaches (Nuss, Hillman, & Eavey, 1996).

The Assessment Process

The assessment process for a voice disorder begins with the identification of warning signs that suggest a possible disturbance of resonance, pitch, loudness, or phonatory quality. It is important for professionals who work with children (e.g., general and special educators) and those who work with adults (e.g., primary care physicians and nurses) to be aware of warning signs of voice disorders.

Warning Signs of Voice Disorders

Figure 11-8 presents a comprehensive list of warning signs of possible voice disorders in children and adolescents. Some of these warning signs are indicative of vocally abusive behaviors, such as "yells, screams, or cries frequently." Other warning signs suggest that an underlying medical condition may warrant attention; for example, "loses his/her voice every time s/he has a cold" or "uses a lot of effort to talk." Several warning signs focus on the child's psychological well-being (e.g., "seems tired or unhappy a lot of the time"), acknowledging the intricate relationship between an individual's psychological and physical health.

For adults the warning signs include many of those identified for children and adolescents. However, adults are better able than children to notice changes in resonance, pitch, loudness, and phonatory quality on their own—even though they will not necessarily seek treatment for those problems! Many adults may assume that a disturbance in voice quality will go away on its own, or they may fail to recognize that the disturbance could signal a more serious underlying problem. Whenever a change in the resonance, pitch, loudness, or general phonatory quality of an individual's voice lasts for longer than 2 weeks, consultation with a primary care physician (PCP) is needed.

Discussion Point: *Sometimes a person may exhibit warning signs of a voice disorder but resist seeking a medical evaluation. What are some ways to raise public awareness of how important it is to get a medical evaluation?*

The PCP will examine the quality of the voice and likely make two referrals. The first is to an otolaryngologist, who will take a careful look at the structures of the laryngeal system and determine whether a potentially serious underlying medical condition exists. The second referral is to a speech-language pathologist who specializes in voice treatment. The speech-language pathologist will work closely with the individual to assess and treat cases of vocal abuse or misuse, neurogenic voice disorders, psychogenic voice disorders, and alaryngeal communication.

Assessment Protocol

This section focuses on the assessment completed by the speech-language pathologist, even though other professionals, such as the otolaryngologist, are also completing an assessment using a variety of complementary but different techniques. The speech-language pathologist's role in assessment is to (1) characterize the general features of the voice (i.e., resonance,

FIGURE 11-8 Warning signs of possible voice disorders in children and adolescents.

Coughs, clears throat, or chokes frequently
Has difficulty breathing or swallowing
Complains of a sore throat often
Voice sounds rough, hoarse, breathy, weak or strained
Loses his/her voice every time s/he has a cold
Always sounds "stuffed up," like during a cold; or sounds like s/he is talking "through the nose"
Voice sounds worse at different times of the day (morning, after school, evening)
Sounds different from his/her friends of the same age and gender
Voice sounds worse after shouting, singing, playing outside, or talking for a long time
Uses a lot of effort to talk; or complains of vocal fatigue
Yells, screams, or cries frequently
Likes to sing and perform often; participates in acting and/or singing groups
Participates in sports activities or cheerleading activities that require yelling and calling
Has difficulty being understood by unfamiliar listeners
Can't be heard easily in the classroom or when there is background noise
Talks more loudly than others in the family or classroom
Voice problem is interfering with his/her performance at school
Doesn't like the sound of his/her voice; or is teased for the sound of his/her voice
Attends many loud social events (parties, concerts, sports games)
Seems tired or unhappy a lot of the time
Is facing difficult changes, such as death, divorce, household financial problems
Does not express his/her feelings to anyone
Lives with a family that uses loud voices frequently
Smokes, or is exposed to smoke at home or at a job
Uses alcohol
Eats "junk food" frequently; or complains of heartburn or sour taste in the mouth
Drinks beverages that contain caffeine; or drinks little water
Has allergies, respiratory disease, or frequent upper respiratory infections
Has hearing loss or frequent ear infections
Takes prescription medications
Has a history of injuries to the head, neck, or throat
Has had surgeries
Was intubated at birth or later
Has a chronic illness or disease

Source: From *Functional Indicators of Voice Disorders in Children and Adolescents*, by L. Lee, J. C. Stemple, and L. Glaze, 2003, Gainesville, FL: Communicare. Copyright 2003 by Communicare. Adapted with permission.

pitch, loudness, and phonatory quality), (2) establish whether any of these features differ significantly from normal, (3) identify the cause of any disorder, and (4) identify the most beneficial approach to improving the client's voice. Clinicians use a variety of different tools, including case history and interview, oral-motor examination, clinical voice observation, and instrumental voice observation.

Case History and Interview. The case history and interview with the client are indispensable in learning more about the client, including how the voice is used for daily living activities and how the client perceives the voice in terms of resonance, pitch, loudness, and phonatory quality. The clinician carefully questions the client about the entire history of voice use including:

- The client's medical history
- The chronological history of the problem
- The symptoms and possible etiology of the problem
- The way in which the client uses the voice at home, school, or work and in the community
- The client's motivation for seeking help (Stemple et al., 1995)

For young children who cannot reliably serve as informants, their primary caregivers are carefully questioned.

Oral-Motor Examination. The oral-motor examination is used to rule out or identify a structural problem—to identify the condition of the structures involved in speech production, study the amount of tension and sensation involved in speech and voicing, and examine possible swallowing problems (Stemple et al., 1995). The clinician carefully studies the motion of all of the articulators and questions the client as he or she engages in oral-motor activities about any sensations associated with these motions, such as tickling, burning, or aching (Stemple et al., 1995).

Given the importance of the velum and the velopharyngeal port for modulating resonance, the clinician carefully studies the appearance and functioning of the velum, examining it for symmetry and signs of atrophy, edema, or swelling. The clinician may ask the client to engage in a few oral-motor activities (e.g., saying "ahh") to see that the velum does not deviate to the right or left or show signs of weakness (Dworkin et al., 2004). The clinician also determines whether the velopharyngeal port is closed to nasal airflow by holding a laryngeal mirror under the nostrils while the client produces speech that should not produce nasal emissions (Dworkin et al., 2004). The clinician attends carefully to any abnormal nasal emissions or snorting-like sounds that suggest velopharyngeal insufficiency.

Clinical Observation. The voice specialist carefully studies the client's voice during a variety of speaking and vocal activities, to document the characteristics of the voice. Also called perceptual observation, the clinical observation documents how the client's voice sounds. Figure 11-9 provides one tool that clinicians use to document the voice across a variety of measures, including pitch and loudness. Because many of the descriptive terms on this rating scale are highly subjective, relying heavily on the ear of the listener, it is important that the clinician be knowledgeable and experienced in working with voice clients so that the subjective observations are valid. (Recall from chapter 4 that validity describes the certainty of findings.) The validity of subjective observations of voice quality is improved when clinicians bring a wealth of experience to their observation, allowing them to differentiate between normal and abnormal voice characteristics.

FIGURE 11-9 A rating scale for clinical observation of voice characteristics.

High pitch	1	2	3	4	5	6	7	8	9	Low pitch
Loud	1	2	3	4	5	6	7	8	9	Soft
Strong	1	2	3	4	5	6	7	8	9	Weak
Smooth	1	2	3	4	5	6	7	8	9	Rough
Pleasant	1	2	3	4	5	6	7	8	9	Unpleasant
Resonant	1	2	3	4	5	6	7	8	9	Shrill
Clear	1	2	3	4	5	6	7	8	9	Hoarse
Unforced	1	2	3	4	5	6	7	8	9	Strained
Soothing	1	2	3	4	5	6	7	8	9	Harsh
Melodious	1	2	3	4	5	6	7	8	9	Raspy
Breathy voice	1	2	3	4	5	6	7	8	9	Full voice
Excessive nasal	1	2	3	4	5	6	7	8	9	Insufficient nasal
Animated	1	2	3	4	5	6	7	8	9	Monotonous
Steady	1	2	3	4	5	6	7	8	9	Shaky
Young	1	2	3	4	5	6	7	8	9	Old
Slow rate	1	2	3	4	5	6	7	8	9	Rapid rate
I like/voice	1	2	3	4	5	6	7	8	9	Don't like/voice

Source: From *Clinical Management of Voice Disorders* (4th ed., p. 180) by J. L. Case, 2002, Austin, TX: Pro-Ed. Copyright 2002 by Pro-Ed. Reprinted with permission.

The clinical observation examines the client's voice in a variety of activities designed to elicit different vocal behaviors, such as:

1. Counting from 1 to 40 softly and then loudly
2. Sustaining the vowel /a/ for as long as possible
3. Sustaining the consonants /s/ and /z/ for as long as possible
4. Humming at different pitches
5. Repeating multisyllabic words (e.g., *Mississippi*)
6. Repeating sentences that do and do not contain nasal sounds (e.g., "She keeps cheese chips" versus "My mommy makes me mad") [Andrews & Summers, 2002]

The clinician also engages the client in conversations on various topics to study vocal quality during normal speaking situations. Children might be asked to describe an ideal pet or a perfect birthday party, whereas adults might be questioned about what they would do if they won the lottery. On the basis of these observations, the clinician can document ways in which voice is disordered in resonance, pitch, loudness, and phonatory quality.

The clinician also studies the systems that support vocal production, particularly respiration. The clinician studies how long the client can sustain inhalation and exhalation during different tasks. The client might be asked to inhale as long as possible to keep a piece of tissue on the end of a straw or to exhale through a straw into a glass of water for as long as possible. The clinician also studies how the client modulates breath support when speaking to determine whether inhalation and exhalation are appropriately coordinated and whether airflow is adequate to support phonation.

Instrumental Observation. Objective measures of vocal functioning are an essential part of the clinical voice assessment to complement more subjective procedures. Objective evaluation uses four types of clinical instrumentation to examine how the larynx is functioning during phonation and other speech activities: acoustic assessment, aerodynamic assessment, electroglottography, and videostroboscopy (Nuss et al., 1996).

Acoustic assessment documents the frequency (pitch) and intensity (loudness) of the voice, including the maximal range and habitual levels of each. It also documents **jitter** and **shimmer**, which refer respectively to perturbations, or changes, in frequency and intensity in a phonatory cycle. In addition, acoustic assessment can document nasal and oral sound pressure during speaking to quantitatively characterize a client's resonance. Clinicians must be comfortable with the technologies used for acoustic assessment (see Figure 11-10). The information obtained can help determine whether frequency, intensity, and resonance characteristics differ from normative references.

Aerodynamic assessment provides an objective measure of airflow, air pressure, and vocal fold resistance against airflow from the lungs, called *subglottal airflow*. Several devices are commercially available for this assessment, in which clients wear a face mask and have their airflow carefully studied by computer hardware and software (Case, 1996). The data provided tell about the flow of air through the laryngeal mechanism and how well the vocal folds resist the airflow.

Electroglottography, or EGG, provides an objective examination of vocal fold contact during voicing (Nuss et al., 1996). The clinician places electrodes on the surface of the client's neck to monitor voltage changes in the vocal folds as they vibrate (Case, 1996). The EGG provides a graphic representation of the vocal folds as they close and open to show whether contact is normal, overadducted (too tightly pressed together), or underadducted (inadequately pressed together; Nuss et al., 1996).

FIGURE 11-10 Clinical instrumentation for objective voice assessment.

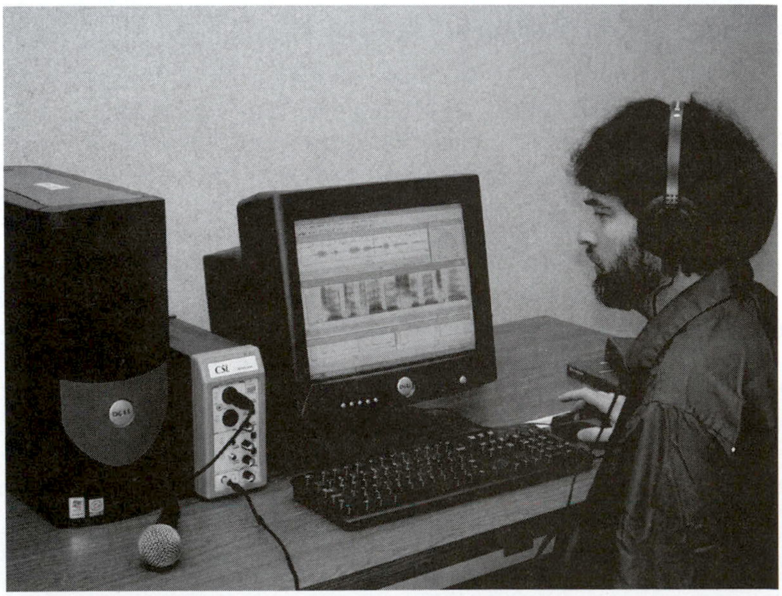

Source: Photo courtesy of Kay Elemetrics.

BOX 11-4 Spotlight on Practice

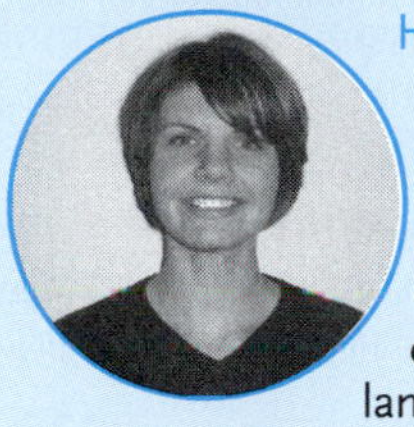

Heather L. Draheim, M.S., CCC-SLP
Speech-Language Pathologist
Early Childhood Intervention

After graduating from Pennsylvania State University, many of my colleagues chose to work as speech-language pathologists for school systems in suburban areas. In contrast, I worked for a special education cooperative serving five rural school districts in east Texas. Instead of working with a specific age group or area, I worked with children from 3 to 23 with a wide variety of challenges, including voice disorders and disorders of phonology, fluency, and even dysphagia.

I was responsible for evaluations, therapy, developing IEPs, writing progress notes, and attending team meetings. I found that I needed my knowledge base in every disorder category to work as a public-school clinician. I also quickly learned how to best distribute my services while utilizing new resources. I consulted with both regular and special education teachers, many of whom had never worked directly with a speech-language pathologist, to develop ways to implement IEPs in the classroom. The teachers informed me about the strengths, weaknesses, and learning styles of each student. I also contacted parents and asked about their concerns and goals at home. And I read the literature about what *should* be done, assessed what the reality was and made modifications to implement any necessary changes.

Although I often felt as though I was not doing enough, the teachers and parents reminded me otherwise, thanks in part to these collaborative relationships. This position may have seemed overwhelming at times to a new graduate, but it allowed me to use and sharpen the majority of my skills, rather than focus on a few skills associated with a specialized area. A speech-language pathologist can provide services in a multitude of environments, each with different challenges, interactions, and personal rewards. And this variety of settings and services promises to pique my interest for years to come.

Laryngoscopy is the examination of the vocal folds and laryngeal system using a flexible endoscope passed through the nasal cavity. The endoscope is connected to a camera to present the images of the larynx on a color monitor. Laryngoscopy is an important tool because it provides a close-up view of the vocal folds, allows several people to study the larynx simultaneously, and provides permanent video documentation to monitor change

BOX 11-5 Spotlight on Research

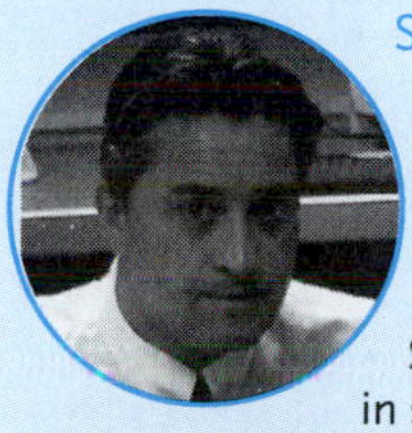

Shaheen N. Awan, Ph.D., CCC-SLP
Professor of Speech-Language Pathology
Bloomsburg University

Shaheen Awan received his doctorate in speech-language pathology from Kent State University in 1989 and taught at the University of North Texas and Northern Michigan University. For the last 10 years, he has been a faculty member at Bloomsburg University of Pennsylvania, where he is currently professor and graduate coordinator of speech-language pathology.

Dr. Awan is a recognized expert in the treatment of voice, resonance, and swallowing disorders. He is the author of *The Voice Diagnostic Protocol: A Practical Guide to the Diagnosis of Voice Disorders*. His research interests focus primarily on the development of computer applications for voice analysis. In particular, his interest is in developing clinically applicable tools that will be available to the practicing clinician, not just to the researcher. It is his opinion that clinicians should have access to objective methods of voice analysis to guide them in their diagnostic decision making and to provide essential data for documenting patient characteristics and change. This interest has led him to develop tools such as the EZVoicePlus voice analysis program and the NasalView program for analysis of resonance disturbances.

Dr. Awan's skills and interest in computer applications have provided him with a unique niche within the field of speech-language pathology. One of the key reasons he became interested in this field was that the diversity of clinical and research possibilities within the field allowed for a wide variety of contributions. Dr. Awan hopes to continue work that will address some of the research and clinical issues of speech-language pathology for many years to come.

of the vocal mechanism over time (Nuss et al., 1996). Even with this technology, however, the human eye cannot see how the vocal folds move because they vibrate so quickly—as many as 200 cycles in a second. But by coupling endoscopy with a pulsing light directed onto the vocal folds—a procedure called **videostroboscopy**—vocal fold movement is slowed down, and the vibratory cycle can be closely observed. Videostroboscopy is used by both speech-language pathologists and otolaryngologists. The otolaryngologist uses it to study the structures of the larynx, whereas the speech-language pathologist studies how the larynx functions and how that function might be improved through therapy (Nuss et al., 1996).

How Are Voice Disorders Treated?

A voice assessment provides a speech-language pathologist with essential information concerning both the etiology of an individual's voice disorder and the perceptual features of the disorder. Whenever possible, treatment goals target the etiology to eliminate the cause of the disorder, which, in turn, should eliminate the disordered features of voice. Such a goal may be attainable in the case of vocal abuse, but in other cases the cause of the disorder may not be so easily resolved. For people who have had their larynx removed or for those who have spasmodic dysphonia, for instance, the SLP must help the individual compensate for a cause that is not easily eliminated. In those cases the SLP works with the individual to develop improved or alternative ways to produce voice. Often, the speech-language pathologist works closely with other professionals as medical solutions are pursued, such as placement of a voice prosthesis for laryngectomized patients or the use of Botox injections for individuals with spasmodic dysphonia.

In general, treatment for voice disorders has three possible goals:

1. To teach a vocal behavior that is absent
2. To substitute an appropriate vocal behavior for an inappropriate one
3. To strengthen vocal behaviors that are weak or inconsistent (Andrews & Summers, 2002)

To achieve these general goals, the SLP first develops a treatment plan to identify a set of short-term goals and one or more long-term goals, or terminal objectives (Andrews & Summers, 2002). The long-term goal is the functional, meaningful, and concrete outcome of treatment—for example, "Melissa will use a pitch level that is appropriate for her age and gender when speaking spontaneously with others." The set of short-term goals is the carefully arranged hierarchy of steps needed to achieve the long-term goal.

Treatment for Vocal Abuse

The symptoms of vocal abuse—such as vocal nodules and contact ulcers—can be treated through surgery on the vocal folds. If a person has no voice or a severely disordered voice, surgery may provide the most efficient route to improved voice (Mori, 1999). However, individuals can often avoid surgery by completing treatment programs that promote better vocal behaviors and improved knowledge about the voice (McFarlane & Watterson, 1990). For adults voice treatment that focuses on changing vocal behaviors is typically at least as successful as surgical intervention for vocal nodules and ulcers (Ramig & Verdolini, 1998). These *vocal hygiene programs* guide the individual to identify each specific vocal abuse, understand its effect on the voice, identify specific occurrences of the abuse, and then modify, replace, or eliminate the behavior (Stemple et al., 1995).

Specific voice therapies that incorporate laryngeal massage, biofeedback, voice-production exercises, and counseling are often coupled with general vocal hygiene treatment, all of which are effective ways to promote better voice use (Ramig & Verdolini, 1998). Some clinicians use computer programs designed specifically to provide feedback on voice behaviors, such as the rate of airflow (Blood, 1994). Computer software provides an objective way to monitor progress toward certain goals, such as "demonstrating correct breathing patterns during speech" (Blood, 1994, p. 65).

Voice therapies that systematically train improved vocal behaviors seem especially important for children, for whom teaching general vocal hygiene does not seem to have great effect. In contrast, completing a course of voice therapy, typically 3 to 6 sessions, results in an improved or normal voice quality for about 50% of children (Mori, 1999). Even for people who elect surgical treatment for the symptoms of vocal abuse, treatment focused on better use of voice is essential to keep those symptoms from reappearing.

Treatment for Neurogenic Disorders

Neurogenic voice disorders result from a specific physiological cause that negatively impacts the voice-production system in some way. Those disorders are often treated with a combination of medical interventions and voice therapy. Medical intervention focused on the improvement, alteration, or restoration of the voice is called *phonosurgery* (Ford, 1996). One type of phonosurgery is *thyroplasty,* which involves modification of the thyroid cartilage of the larynx. Modifications to the thyroid cartilage impact the tension and position of the vocal folds and provide a way to improve their functioning in some cases (Ford, 1996). This is the prevailing surgical approach for treatment of breathy dysphonias resulting from vocal fold paralysis or other vocal fold damage (e.g., scarred folds or bowed folds; Ford, 1996). Vocal outcomes are excellent with this surgery, resulting often in improved vocal intensity and frequency. Although surgical complications of thyroplasty occur relatively infrequently (10% of cases), they can be serious and even life-threatening (Ford, 1996).

Injections into the vocal folds, using Teflon or botulinum toxin Type A (Botox), are also used to treat vocal fold disturbances, such as spasmodic dysphonia (Fisher, Scherer, Guo, & Owen, 1996). A disadvantage of Teflon is that it is irreversible and can evoke a foreign-body reaction; a disadvantage of Botox is that its effects are temporary, necessitating regular reinjections (Ford, 1996).

Whether or not surgical intervention is used, voice therapy is an essential part of voice management. Voice therapy helps an individual cope with voice disturbances and develop compensatory or alternative ways to produce a better voice. One of the better known programs for treatment of neurogenic voice disorders is the Lee Silverman voice treatment (LSVT) program. LSVT is an intensive 1-month program using repeated exercises informed by theories of motor learning. It is designed to improve the phonatory strength of people with Parkinson's disease, although positive effects are seen in other populations as well (e.g., stroke, multiple sclerosis; Fox, Morrison, Ramig, & Sapir, 2002). This treatment increases the intensity and frequency of the voice and the general rate and articulation of speech.

Treatment for Psychogenic Disorders

Persons who exhibit psychogenic voice disorders require a multidisciplinary treatment program involving a speech-language pathologist and other mental health professionals. Therapy focuses on determining the emotional and psychosocial cause of the voice

FIGURE 11-11 Anatomy of the larynx following a laryngectomy.

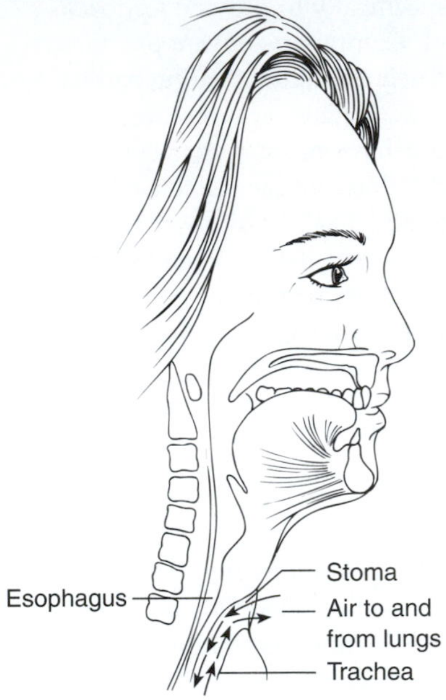

disturbance, as resolution of the cause may reduce the voice disturbance (Stemple et al., 1995). Therapy focuses primarily on counseling, reducing tension, and eliminating any voice abuses or misuses (Ramig & Verdolini, 1998).

Alaryngeal Communication

Individuals whose larynx has been removed must develop alternative ways to produce voice. When the larynx is removed, the airway between the lungs and the mouth is closed, and the airflow is shunted out the front of the neck via a *stoma,* or hole in the neck (see Figure 11-11). An essential aspect of treatment for alaryngeal communication is communication counseling, which explores all the options possible for voice and helps clients make the best choices for their needs and interests (Wagner, 1996). Typically, an artificial larynx is introduced immediately to provide at least a temporary solution. An artificial larynx is a vibrating power source placed against the neck or in the mouth; sound is shaped through articulation. Some users do not like the artificial larynx because of its mechanical sound and its poor differentiation of similar-sounding consonants, such as *f* and *v*, *b* and *p* (Wagner, 1996).

The most commonly used alternative for alaryngeal communication is **esophageal speech**, with which the individual traps air in the esophagus and then uses that air to produce voice. However, it is not easy to get enough air into the esophagus to produce voicing, and learning to use esophageal speech can be very difficult for some people. Consequently, a surgical procedure called a *tracheoesophageal puncture* can be used to create a channel between the trachea and the esophagus, into which a prosthetic device is inserted. The individual then takes a deep breath, covers the stoma, and forces the air into the esophagus, providing an air source for speaking. This type of speech is called **tracheoesophageal speech** and allows an individual to speak longer and more loudly as compared to esophageal speech (Wagner, 1996).

Case Study and Clinical Problem Solving

SCREENING SUMMARY

Speech and Hearing Associates
222 River Road
Phoenix, AZ

Client:	Arthur Pena	**Parent:**	Claudia Pena
Age:	4 years, 6 months	**Referral Source:**	Reevaluation
		File No:	06-09-09-8877
		Date of Birth:	05-22-01
		Screening Date:	11-11-05

Background and History

Arthur Pena received treatment for vocal nodules for 6 months from 01/04 to 07/04 by Jason Clovis, CCC-SLP. At the start of treatment, Arthur's voice quality was hoarse, breathy, and at times completely inaudible. However, Arthur showed rapid progress in treatment, and a series of modifications were made in his home and day care environments to reduce identified vocal abuse. Arthur was discharged when his vocal quality returned to normal and laryngeal examination by an ENT physician showed no signs of vocal nodules. Arthur was seen on 11-11-05 for a follow-up reevaluation. He was supposed to have been seen at 6 months following discharge, but his mother did not keep the appointment. Ms. Pena called in 9/05 to request the follow-up screening as Arthur was having some hoarseness and breathiness again. Ms. Pena has scheduled an appointment with an otolaryngologist (Dr. Dell of Phoenix Children's Hospital) for 12/1/05 because of congestion, allergies, and complaints of sore throat, and Dr. Dell requested that we conduct a screening prior.

Oral Examination

An oral examination was conducted. All structures were normal except tonsilar region was swollen and red. Velar activity was normal. Velopharyngeal mechanism appeared normal; normal gag reflex. Arthur complained of pain and burning in the neck region during laryngeal palpations.

Vocal Abuse Questionnaire

Ms. Pena completed a vocal abuse questionnaire for Arthur. Remarkable behaviors reported included frequent screaming and yelling; frequent crying and tantrums; frequent respiratory complaints; complaints of throat pain and vocal fatigue; loud talking at home and school.

Clinical Observation

Arthur completed a series of activities designed to clinically assess respiration, resonation, pitch, loudness, and phonatory quality. Observations showed the following abnormal vocal behaviors:

1. Jerky and nonrhythmical coordination of inhalation and exhalation when speaking, particularly when agitated or excited
2. Moderate to severe dysphonia characterized by hoarseness and breathiness worsening with ongoing communication
3. Frequent vocal straining
4. Consistently excessive loudness and an inability to modulate loudness even with cues and models
5. Habitual pitch lower than optimal
6. Pervasive coughing, throat clearing, and hard glottal attacks

Arthur refused the use of clinical instrumentation, including the Visi-Pitch and EGG, to document intensity and frequency and provide jitter and shimmer estimates. We provided counseling to Ms. Pena regarding the need for improved vocal habits and supplied the pamphlet *How to Care for Your Child's Voice*. Our opinion is that more direct ongoing counseling will be necessary. We have scheduled a follow-up appointment to discuss therapy approaches in 1/06 following Dr. Dell's evaluation.

If Arthur's voice changes in any way or if you have questions about this report, please feel free to contact me immediately.

Andrew Chance, MEd, CCC-SLP
Speech-Language Pathologist

CLINICAL PROBLEM SOLVING

1. Arthur was discharged following a course of treatment, but his mother did not follow up as requested. What reasons might account for this lack of adherence to the plan?
2. Arthur's original diagnosis was vocal nodules. What are vocal nodules? What causes them?
3. This case represents collaboration between a speech-language pathologist and an otolaryngologist. What are some barriers to successful collaboration? What are the benefits of this type of collaboration?

CHAPTER SUMMARY

The human voice is a complex, dynamic product of the vocal folds. It is also an essential tool for personal expression, creativity, and art. The human voice is characterized by four different parameters: resonance, loudness, pitch, and phonatory quality. When one or more of these vary significantly from normal, based on age and gender, a disorder may be present.

Voice disorders are relatively common, affecting about 29% of the population at one time or another. In many cases disorders are transient, resulting from respiratory problems, colds, sinus infections, and the like. Some professionals, such as teachers and singers, experience voice disorders at relatively higher rates than others do.

Experts classify voice disorders in four causal categories. Vocal abuse describes the chronic or intermittent overuse or misuse of the vocal apparatus. Common abuses include talking in noisy environments, coughing or clearing the throat frequently, and yelling, screaming, and cheering. Neurogenic disorders result from illness, damage, or disease to the neurological systems associated with voice production. Spasmodic dysphonia and vocal fold paralysis are two examples of neurogenic voice disorders. Psychogenic voice disorders describe disorders that stem from a psychological or emotional cause. Examples are conversion disorder and generalized anxiety disorder. Alaryngeal communication is the fourth category and describes voice without a larynx. The most common reason for removal of the larynx is laryngeal cancer. Regardless of etiology, the defining characteristics of voice disorders include aberrational resonance, pitch, loudness, or phonatory quality.

Treatment for voice disorders is a multidisciplinary process. Those involved typically include a speech-language pathologist, a primary care physician, medical specialists such as an otolaryngologist, mental health specialists such as a psychologist, and educators. The speech-language pathologist's assessment focuses on vocal function and ways it might be improved through treatment. The comprehensive assessment process includes case history and interview, oral-motor examination, clinical voice observation, and instrumental voice observation.

Treatment for voice disorders differs based on etiology. In general, three goals are addressed: (1) to teach a vocal behavior that is absent, (2) to substitute an appropriate vocal behavior for an inappropriate behavior, and (3) to strengthen weak or inconsistent vocal behaviors. Treatment for vocal abuse emphasizes vocal hygiene and modifying or eliminating vocally abusive behaviors. Treatment for neurogenic disorders may include medical management, such as thyroplasty, coupled with intensive therapy designed to improve phonatory behaviors. Treatment for psychogenic disorders uses counseling to address the underlying emotional issues. Individuals who require alaryngeal communication receive therapy to teach them alternative means of producing speech, including the use of an artificial larynx, esophageal speech, or tracheoesophageal speech.

KEY TERMS

shimmer, p. 378
spasmodic dysphonia, p. 354
tracheoesophageal speech, p. 382
tracheostomy, p. 365
vagus nerve, p. 363
velopharyngeal inadequacy, p. 371
velopharyngeal port, p. 370
videostroboscopy, p. 380
vocal abuse, p. 359
vocal nodules, p. 357
vocal range, p. 372
vocal tic disorder, p. 367
voice, p. 350

ON THE WEB

Check out the Companion Website! On it you will find

- suggested readings
- reflection questions
- a self-study quiz
- links to additional online resources, including current technologies in communication sciences and disorders

Fluency Disorders

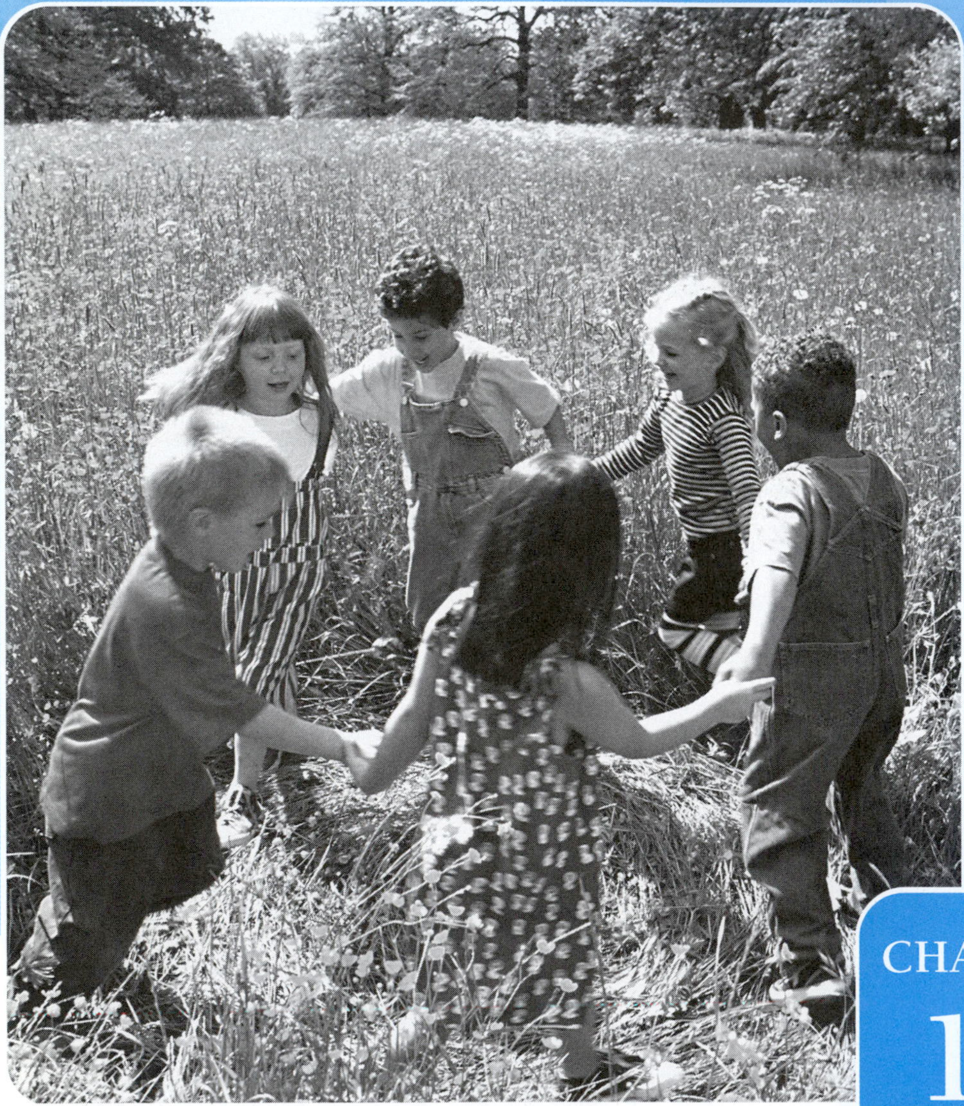

CHAPTER 12

FOCUS QUESTIONS

This chapter answers the following questions:

1. What is a fluency disorder?
2. How are fluency disorders classified?
3. What are the defining characteristics of fluency disorders?
4. How are fluency disorders identified?
5. How are fluency disorders treated?

INTRODUCTION

This chapter describes disorders of fluency, in which an individual's ability to produce speech effortlessly and automatically is seriously compromised. Fluency disorders are better known as **stuttering**, an onomatopoeic word that well captures the stops, starts, and hesitations in the speech of persons with fluency disorders.

Fluency disorders affect a relatively small number of people, compared to other disorders of communication; about 1–2% of the population are affected at any given time (Craig, Hancock, Tran, Craig, & Peters, 2002). Despite their generally low incidence, fluency disorders seem to be the communication disorder with which the general population is most familiar—for a variety of reasons.

- Fluency disorders have perhaps the longest documented history of any communication disorder. Bobrick (1995) reports that "stuttering is probably as old as speech itself" (p. 49), with documented reports going back to ancient times. For instance, two famous Greek contemporaries who lived from 384 to 322 B.C., Demosthenes and Aristotle, were both purported to have significant fluency disorders. Obviously, neither Demosthenes, a great orator, nor Aristotle, a revered philosopher and scientist, allowed his speech difficulties to hold him back.
- Fluency disorders have affected some very famous people, including such contemporary celebrities as John Stossel (ABC reporter), Annie Glenn (wife of astronaut and former senator John Glenn), James Earl Jones (film and theater actor), Nicholas Brendon (television actor, known for his role on *Buffy the Vampire Slayer*), and diver Greg Louganis (Stuttering Foundation of America, 2004). Not only have these individuals learned to manage their communication difficulties, but many have also used their positions to advocate for stuttering treatment and research.
- Fluency disorders are often used as a comedic device in the media or, alternatively, as a dramatic, metaphoric technique. A recent comic example was Adam Sandler's character in the 1998 film *The Waterboy*. (However, one CNN reviewer did not find his stuttering a humorous device: "The biggest impediment to this movie is Sandler's speech. His stammering and stuttering prevents the classic Sandler from shining through" [Rickett, 1998].) A dramatic, metaphoric example is the character

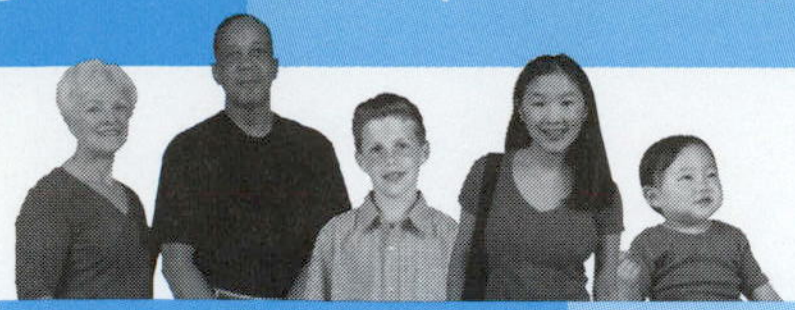

BOX 12-1 Fluency Disorders Across the Lifespan: Case Examples

Kaimon is a 7-year-old boy just starting second grade in Detroit, Michigan. Kaimon is in the same class as his twin sister, Kaida. Kaimon received treatment for a fluency disorder in kindergarten and first grade but was dismissed from therapy at the end of first grade. (In contrast, Kaida has never shown any problems with fluency.) Kaimon's new second-grade teacher, Mr. Damon, reports to Kaimon's parents that Kaimon is still stuttering and that he thinks Kaimon should be referred to the school speech-language pathologist again.

In their fall conference, Mr. Damon reported that earlier in the day, Kaimon changed seats three times to avoid reading during a round-robin reading activity in which each child in the class read aloud a page of a book. Mr. Damon also reported that Kaimon asked to use the restroom seven times during the day, which he suspects is an avoidance tactic. Kaimon's parents noted that they had not seen these behaviors or indicators of disfluency at home and that Kaimon absolutely does not want to go to therapy again because he is afraid the other kids will make fun of him and he doesn't want to miss class. In addition, he doesn't think it's fair since Kaida doesn't have to go to therapy. Mr. Damon agrees to try different strategies in class over the next 3 months, and Kaimon's parents agree to the speech-language referral if the stuttering doesn't decrease by winter.

Internet research

1. Approximately how many second graders in the public school system in the United States receive special services for speech-language disorders? Of these, what proportion of the children receive services specifically for fluency disorders?
2. How likely is it for only one member of a twin set to have a fluency disorder?
3. What is one example of a treatment program available for an elementary-school child who stutters?

Brainstorm and discussion

1. What are some strategies that Mr. Damon might use to promote peer acceptance of children with communication disabilities in his classroom?
2. What are some strategies that Mr. Damon might use to increase Kaimon's fluency and decrease his disfluency within the classroom?
3. Why do you agree or disagree with Kaimon's parents for keeping him out of therapy for the next few months?

Ralston Weber is a 4-year-old child attending a private day care center in Charleston, West Virginia. Ralston has two younger siblings (3-month-old Veronica and 2-year-old Renaro) and two older siblings (6-year-old Houston and 9-year-old Donald) and lives with his mother and father in a 2-bedroom apartment in subsidized housing in downtown Charleston. Ralston is a very social and communicative child who gets along well with the other children in the day care center.

His day care provider, Ms. Henry, has noted lately, however, that Ralston seems to be stuttering and is having problems communicating his needs and interests to her and the other children. This has coincided with a series of temper tantrums over the last 3 weeks when Ralston arrives or leaves the center. Ms. Henry has sent several notes home to Ralston's mother sharing her concerns, but Mrs. Weber reported to Ms. Henry that her two older children also went through stuttering stages and she didn't see it as a problem. Ms. Henry is frustrated because she thinks the stuttering might cause Ralston to stop interacting with the other kids and it might be related to his temper tantrums. Ms. Henry is beginning to log when Ralston stutters, including what seems to cause it and how it affects his communication with others.

Discussion Point: *What are your perceptions about stuttering? In what ways have you had exposure to persons with fluency disorders?*

Billy Bibbit in Ken Kesey's award-winning *One Flew over the Cuckoo's Nest*. Confined to a mental institution, Bibbit is fearful and anxious, particularly toward his overbearing mother. Kesey seems to use Bibbit's stuttering as a window into his internal psychological turmoil.

What the general population may not know, however, are other interesting facts about stuttering: (1) Most young children go through a period of normal disfluency in which as

Internet research

1. What kind of information is available to day care providers on the warning signs of early stuttering?
2. What community resources are available for children like Ralston if his stuttering becomes a problem?

Brainstorm and discussion

1. What warning signs should Ms. Henry look for when documenting Ralston's stuttering behaviors?
2. What are some strategies Ms. Henry might use to promote Ralston's ability to communicate effectively?
3. What are some events or challenges in Ralston's life that might be related to the emergence of disfluencies?

Mr. Cho is a 39-year-old man who recently had a stroke during heart surgery. Although the heart surgery was successful, the stroke has left Mr. Cho both paralyzed on his right side and significantly impaired in his ability to communicate. Mr. Cho's communicative difficulties include a severe motor-speech disorder, in which he has difficulty planning and coordinating the motor movements needed to produce speech, as well as a severe fluency problem marked by frequent pauses, interjections, word and phrase repetitions, and sound prolongations. Fortunately, Mr. Cho has no fear of or embarrassment toward his disfluencies, and he works closely with his daughter to keep track of his disfluencies and to try to decrease their rate. Upon his recent release from the hospital, Mr. Cho's insurance approved him for only 12 sessions of outpatient therapy, including both physical and speech therapy. Mr. Cho decided to use these 12 sessions for physical therapy and to pay out-of-pocket for an experimental treatment offered by a local rehabilitation specialist. His daughter saw the advertised treatment in the newspaper; it reported 100% cure for acquired stuttering using a 3-month vitamin treatment, which is designed to improve neurological functioning following disease. Mr. Cho purchased the 3-month treatment for $1,200 and is pleased with his decision: 2 months into the treatment his communication difficulties began to improve.

Internet research

1. What are the policies of major health insurance carriers for coverage of speech-language therapy for acquired disorders of communication?
2. What evidence (if any) supports vitamin therapy as a therapeutic rehabilitation tool for acquired communication disorders, including fluency impairment?

Brainstorm and discussion

1. Do you agree with Mr. Cho's decision to forfeit the outpatient speech therapy in favor of the physical therapy and to pursue the vitamin treatment? Why?
2. Mr. Cho selected a rehabilitation treatment from the newspaper under the guidance of his daughter. How can a consumer differentiate between those treatments that are effective and those that are questionable?
3. What other explanations might explain Mr. Cho's improved fluency following 2 months of a special vitamin regimen?

much as 5% of their speech may be disfluent (Ambrose & Yairi, 1999) (2) The majority of cases of stuttering in children are resolved either spontaneously or through treatment (Yairi & Ambrose, 1999) (3) Many of the perceptions the public holds about stuttering are not accurate, such as stutterers being timid, fearful, and anxious. This chapter delves into these and other topics concerning fluency disorders in children, adolescents, and adults.

What Is a Fluency Disorder?

Definition

Defining Fluency

Fluency is a descriptive term used to characterize the flow of speech during communication. Speech that is fluent moves along at an appropriate rate with an easy rhythm; it is smooth, effortless, and automatic. By contrast, speech that is disfluent is disrupted in one or more of these elements—rate, rhythm, smoothness, effort, or automaticity. A **disfluency** is the speech behavior that disrupts the fluent forward flow of speech, such as pauses, interjections, and revisions.

The speech of many adults contains a number of typical disfluencies:

> ***You know, I think we should, um, well, I know you don't want to, but I really think we should consider giving it—the money—back.***

The speech of young children also often contains a great number of disfluencies:

> ***I want, I want ice cream, too. Daddy, mommy, daddy, daddy has ice cream.***

Although the disfluencies in these two snippets seem considerable, they are examples of normal disfluencies that typically do not detract from the communication between two people. These disfluencies reflect a combination of personal dialect ("You know"), hesitation in imparting an idea ("I know you don't want to"), and moments of mental processing or thought gathering ("um, well" or "I want, I want"), which are entirely normal in the complex process of communication.

Defining a Fluency Disorder

A fluency disorder describes speech with an unusually high rate of stoppages that disrupt the flow of communication and are inappropriate for the speaker's age, culture, and linguistic background, including dialect. The disorder must be significant enough that it impacts social communication and educational or occupational performance (American Psychiatric Association [APA], 1994; Guitar, 1998). Formal definitions of fluency disorders emphasize the presence of both these features:

- Disturbance in the normal fluency and timing patterns of speech that is inappropriate for the person's age and is characterized by at least one of the following: sound and syllable repetitions, sound prolongations, interjections, words broken by pauses, pauses in speech (i.e., blocks), word substitutions to avoid problematic words, and excess physical tension in producing speech
- Disturbance in social communication, academic performance, or occupational achievement as a result of the fluency disturbance

Identifying Core and Secondary Features

Speech disfluencies are the **core features**, or primary characteristics, of a fluency disorder. Three types of disfluencies predominate: repetitions, prolongations, and blocks. A **repetition** occurs when a sound, syllable, or word is repeated several times to the point of interrupting the flow of speech, as in "I want-want-want more milk." A **prolongation** refers to a sound being held longer than is normal. With a prolongation, the airflow continues but the articulators seem to be stuck, as in "I wwwwwant more cake." A **block** occurs when the airflow and the articulatory movement completely stop during production of a sound; the block can last as long as 5 seconds (Guitar, 1998).

Accompanying these core features are the **secondary features**, which are also important characteristics of a fluency disorder. These result from an individual's excessive mental and physical efforts to promote fluent speech and to disrupt disfluent speech (Guitar, 1998). They are called secondary, or associated, features because they emerge in response to the core behaviors. A person with a fluency disorder develops secondary features to avoid and escape moments of disfluency. Common secondary features include physical/motor behaviors such as eye blinks, lip tremors, and head jerks and speaking behaviors such as fillers, pauses, and word changes.

Another secondary feature is negative feelings and attitudes, which reflect an individual's emotional reactions to disfluency. People who stutter may have negative feelings about speaking; they worry about speaking situations, view speaking as difficult, and believe that others do not like the way they talk (Vanryckeghem & Brutten, 1997). These negative feelings and attitudes reflect the everyday challenges that accompany communication for someone with a fluency disorder. An adult whose fluency disorder resolved after an intensive 3-week treatment program described it this way (Anderson & Felsenfeld, 2003): "You just feel naked, you just feel so vulnerable, especially when you are in the midst of the speaking problem" (p. 248).

Discussion Point: *Consider the case of Kaimon in Box 12-1. What signs suggest that he is already manifesting some negative feelings about communication?*

Terminology

Stuttering and *stutterer* are two terms that are used to describe a fluency disorder and the person exhibiting the disorder. However, in describing anyone affected by disorder or a condition, the use of person-first language helps to give the individual primacy over the disorder. Thus, Kaimon, in Box 12-1, is not described as the *stutterer* or the *stuttering child* but as the *child who stutters*.

Discussion of stuttering and fluency requires careful use of vocabulary. Some key descriptors are explained in Table 12-1.

Prevalence and Incidence

Fluency disorders affect relatively few individuals, with an incidence rate of about 1 in 100 persons and a prevalence rate of about 5 in 100 persons (Bloodstein, 1995). Thus, although about 5% of people have stuttered sometime in their lives, only about 1% have a fluency disorder at the present time. Fluency disorders affect children most between 2 and 10 years of age, with estimates showing an incidence rate of about 1.5% for children under 10 as compared to about .5 to .7% for adolescents and adults (Craig et al., 2002). Males are affected at higher rates than girls, with a ratio of about three or four boys to every one girl affected (Craig et al., 2002).

Discussion Point: *Did you or any family member go through a period of stuttering? How long did it last?*

Discussion Point: *Consider these statistics in light of the case of Ralston in Box 12-1. Is his day care provider right to be so concerned? Why?*

Recovery from Stuttering

The difference between incidence and prevalence rates indicates that the majority of people who stutter do recover, either spontaneously (i.e., without treatment) or therapeutically (i.e., with treatment; Yairi & Ambrose, 1999). Thus, for a given child or adolescent who exhibits a fluency disorder, a parent might reasonably ask whether treatment is needed if the likelihood of recovery is high. Scientists have pursued the answer to this question over many years, using a variety of techniques. The body of research is complicated, however, by a lack of consensus on how to define *recovery,* when to measure it (e.g., 12 months after stuttering begins or 5 years), and whether to withhold treatment from young children to determine who might recover spontaneously.

Recent estimates from epidemiological research at the University of Illinois at Champaign-Urbana indicate that about 74% of preschool or early school-age children who exhibit persistent stuttering behaviors (4 years or longer) will recover (Yairi & Ambrose, 1999). Further, girls

TABLE 12-1 Terminology used with fluency disorders

Term	Explanation
Block	A complete pause in the production of a syllable or a word; the airflow stops and the articulators become stuck in place. A block can last 1 to 5 seconds and may be accompanied by jaw tremors (Peters & Guitar, 1991). A block is represented in writing with a #, as in "He was #wrong," with a block occurring before the word *wrong.*
Broken word	A word interrupted by a pause, prolongation, or block; the location of the break in the word is notated with a #, as in "My name is Lau#ra."
Circumlocution	Talking around a word or substituting another word or phrase for it, as in "We went to the, uh, the, uh, the city where they make cars," in which the word *Detroit* is avoided.
Filler word, interjection	A word(s) inserted into utterances or phrases, such as *um, uh, I mean,* and *like* ("I, like, think we should go").
Prolongation	A consonant or vowel sound held for a longer-than-normal time, ranging from a fleeting moment to several seconds. During a prolongation, the airflow continues, but the articulators seem stuck in place. Prolongations are represented in writing as a repeated letter, as in *"thaaaat"* or *"mmmmommy."*
Rate	An individual's pace of speaking, which is often measured as the total number of words produced in a minute or the total number of syllables produced in a second (Hall, Amir, & Yairi, 1999). Fluency disorders negatively impact rate, with persons who stutter producing fewer words per minute and fewer syllables per second.
Repetition	The replication of a sound (*b-b-b*), a syllable (*an-an-animal*), or a word (*that-that-that*). The repetition of part of a word, as in the first sound, is called a part-word repetition (*th-th-that*). The repetition of a whole word (*that-that-that*) is called a whole-word repetition, and repetition of a phrase (*I want-I want-I want)* is a phrase repetition.
Revision	Changing or abandoning an utterance during its delivery, as in "He cooked/he made me dinner" or "I really can't/I just don't think we should go."

are more likely to recover (85%) than boys are (69%). However, even though fluency treatments have excellent outcomes—some treatment programs show nearly all children achieving normal speech (Lincoln & Onslow, 1997)—it is not clear how many children would have recovered spontaneously.

Some experts provide persuasive commentaries against early intervention for stuttering (e.g., Curlee & Yairi, 1997), but three points warrant comment. First, children who recover from fluency disorders have often experienced stuttering for relatively long periods of time. One study showed the duration of their stuttering to have ranged from 6 to 35 months (Yairi & Ambrose, 1999). During this time these children likely experienced significant challenges and frustrations when communicating with others, feelings probably shared by their caregivers.

Second, when children begin to stutter, there is no way to know whether they will eventually recover or not. Even though many children do recover, the percentage of those who do not (estimated at about 25%) is consequential. The children who do not recover will need ongoing support to develop their communicative skills and to mitigate their negative feelings about communication.

Third, among children who stutter, there is a relatively high rate of co-occurring speech and language problems beyond the fluency disorder. These may include, for instance, a phonological disorder (described in chapter 5) or a language disorder (described in chapter 7). One study of children who stutter showed 44% to have a concomitant language disorder (Arndt & Healey, 2001). Thus, although children might resolve their stuttering problems, other speech and language challenges might be present.

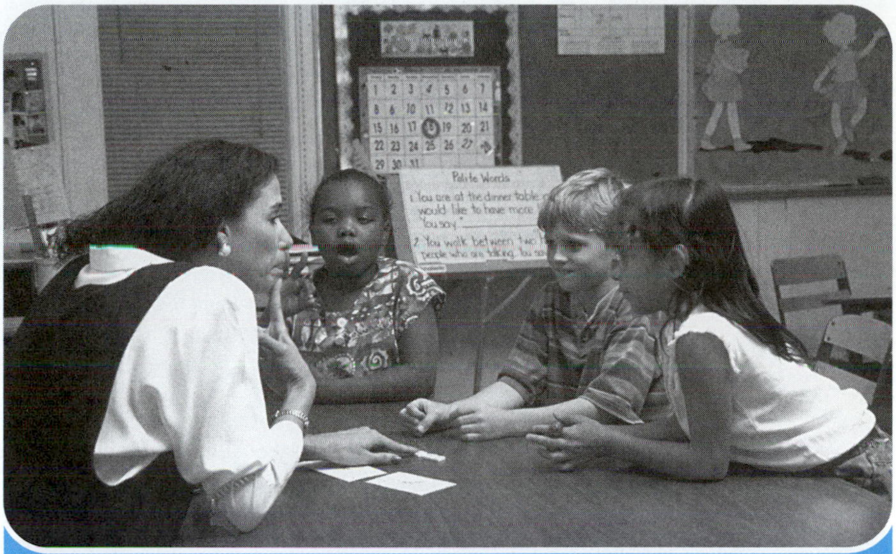

Girls recover from stuttering at higher rates than boys do.

Even though we can be optimistic that many young children with persistent stuttering problems *will* recover from this disorder, this likelihood should not be interpreted to mean that children and adolescents with fluency disorders do not need special supports to enhance their recovery. All of these children should be supported using the best means possible, as "once recovery has been achieved and maintained for several months, chances are very high that it will be permanently sustained" (Yairi & Ambrose, 1999, p. 1109).

How Are Fluency Disorders Classified?

Fluency disorders are typically classified in one of two ways, using either an etiology focus or a symptom focus. Etiology-focused classification focuses on the cause of the fluency disorder, whereas symptom-focused classification focuses on the impact or appearance of the disorder, including its severity.

Etiology Focus

Developmental Disorders of Fluency

For the majority of people who experience a fluency disorder, it emerges in early childhood, and its cause is unknown. When stuttering emerges in early childhood, typically when children are between 2 and 5 years of age, it is called a developmental disorder of fluency, or **developmental stuttering** (Peters & Guitar, 1991). Children who exhibit developmental stuttering may stutter for only several months, or they may stutter for several years. The longer a child's stuttering persists, the less likely it is that the stuttering problem will be resolved on its own (Yairi & Ambrose, 1999). Roughly 25% of children who exhibit developmental stuttering will continue to have a fluency disorder 4 years following its onset (Yairi & Ambrose, 1999); the other 75% of children will resolve their stuttering within 4 years either spontaneously or as a result of treatment.

Developmental stuttering needs to be differentiated from the normal disfluencies seen in most young children. Nearly all children go through a period in which disfluencies are prevalent in their speech, particularly during the toddler and preschool years. The key to

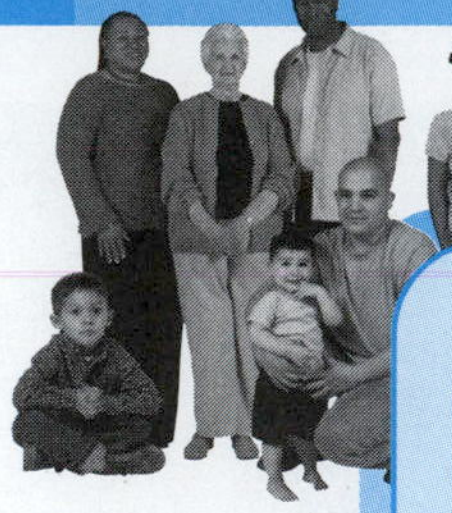

BOX 12-2 Multicultural Focus

Cultural Awareness and Stuttering Treatments

For treatments of communication disorders to be maximally effective, they must be individualized to respect and integrate the cultural values and beliefs that individuals and their families bring to the treatment process. This is particularly true for stuttering; a person's perspective on the cause, treatment, and seriousness of stuttering is likely to be highly influenced by the individual's cultural system and environment (Robinson & Crowe, 1998). And the clinician's orientation to stuttering may not be shared by the individual and the family. For instance, cultural perspectives may prompt a parent to think that treatment is moving too slowly because the child is not trying hard enough. Or perhaps a family is reluctant to pursue conventional treatment because of a preference for home remedies.

Moreover, all individuals have their own identities. We cannot assume that an individual who is a member of a specific racial or ethnic group shares the cultural values of that group (Robinson & Crowe, 1998). Consequently, a clinician must work closely with every individual to fully understand the cultural system that is brought to the treatment process. Robinson and Crowe (1998) describe specific strategies for improving cultural awareness through the assessment and treatment process for fluency disorders:

1. *Explore the cultural identity of clients:* Do this through specific queries concerning their background, their beliefs and values, and their perceptions of communication. Do not assume that the race or ethnicity of a client is synonymous with the individual's identity. Explore how various aspects of communication are viewed, such as interruptions, pauses, turn-taking, and silence.
2. *Learn about the language used to discuss communication:* Listen to clients to learn their terminology to describe aspects of communication and stuttering. It is important that clinicians and clients use the same terminology so that clients can share information in other environments. Explore what terms mean explicitly.
3. *Learn about causes and consequences:* Find out what clients consider to be the causes of their stuttering. Clinicians must remember that stuttering emerges from a complex interplay

differentiating between developmental stuttering and normal disfluencies in young children is to examine the type of disfluencies that are present. Developmental stuttering is characterized by the appearance of **stuttering-like disfluencies** (SLDs), which include (1) part-word repetitions, (2) single-syllable-word repetitions, (3) sound prolongations, (4) blocks, and (5) broken words. For children who exhibit developmental stuttering, SLDs are seen at higher rates than for children who are developing typically. For instance, children with developmental stuttering produce about 5 part-word and 3 single-syllable-word repetitions per 100 spoken syllables, as compared to about 0.5 and 0.7, respectively, for other children (Ambrose & Yairi, 1999).

As a general rule of thumb, part- and single-syllable-word repetitions are viewed as a hallmark of developmental stuttering, particularly when 3 or more are seen within 100 words of conversational speech (Yaruss, 1997). Children without developmental stuttering may occasionally produce part-word and single-syllable-word repetitions, but they do so relatively infrequently. Table 12-2 gives examples of stuttering-like disfluencies and indicates their rate of occurrence in children with and without developmental stuttering.

In contrast, other types of disfluencies in the speech of young children are considered to be quite normal. These include interjections, revisions, and multisyllabic word and of predisposing and precipitating factors, and the sharing of information between client and clinician is useful for understanding these complexities. The clinician must also explore clients' and parents' perceptions about the negative and positive consequences of stuttering. For instance, a parent might feel a child is stuttering to get attention, or perhaps a child is angry about having a new sibling in the home. The extent to which these various causes and consequences relate to treatment outcomes is an important topic for parent-clinician counseling.

4. *Counsel clients on hindrances to treatment progress:* Explore possible myths, beliefs, and attitudes about stuttering. For instance, a father might believe he caused his daughter to stutter because he tickled her too much (Robinson & Crowe, 1998), or a mother might think she corrected her daughter's speech too harshly. Discuss how these myths, beliefs, and attitudes might prevent or hinder treatment progress.
5. *Know the rules for interacting:* As a final suggestion, Robinson and Crowe (1998) emphasize the need for clinicians to know the rules of interacting with persons of different cultural backgrounds. Cultural rules dictate whether it is acceptable to interrupt, to talk loudly, to touch, to stand close, to maintain eye contact, and the like. Treatment is not apt to progress well if the client or the clinician feels uncomfortable. When in doubt, it is best to honestly question what is and is not acceptable behavior when communicating.

For Discussion

What are some cultural myths that explain why children begin to stutter?

What are some cultural myths that suggest treatment approaches to stuttering?

What cultural beliefs or values might influence whether a family seeks treatment for a child who shows signs of stuttering?

Companion Website

To answer these questions online, go to the Multicultural Focus module in chapter 12 of the Companion Website.

TABLE 12-2 The rate of stuttering-like disfluencies in 2- to 5-year-old children

	Rate of Occurrence	
Type of Disfluency	**Typical Children**	**Children Who Stutter**
Single-syllable-word repetitions ("I want-want-want lemonade")	0.7 per 100 syllables	3.3 per 100 syllables
Part-word repetitions ("Give me the pu-pu-puzzle")	0.5 per 100 syllables	5.3 per 100 syllables
Prolongations ("That's my mmmmommy") and blocks ("Here it i#s")	0.09 per 100 syllables	1.8 per 100 syllables
Total stuttering-like disfluencies	1.3 per 100 syllables	10.4 per 100 syllables

Source: From "Normative Disfluency Data for Early Childhood Stuttering" by N. G. Ambrose and E. Yairi, 1999, *Journal of Speech, Language, and Hearing Research, 42*, 895–909. Copyright 1999 by ASHA. Reprinted with permission.

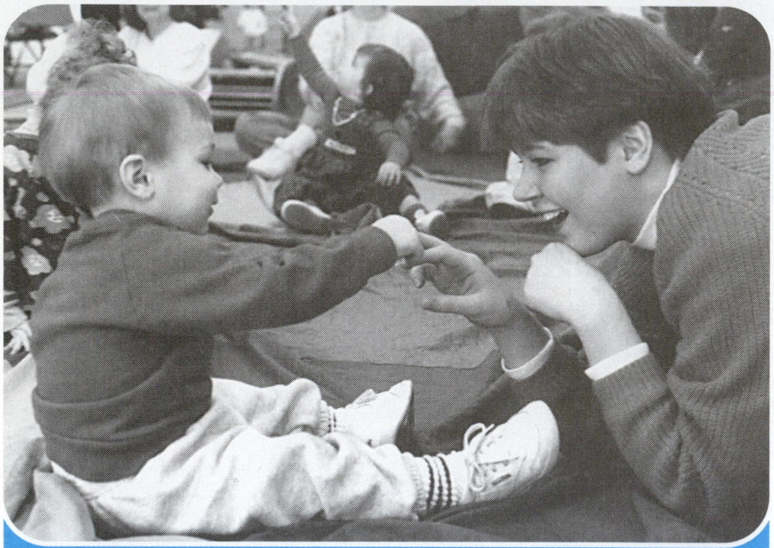

Nearly all young children go through a period in which disfluent speech increases; this is a normal part of communication development.

phrase repetitions, as shown in Table 12-3. These types of disfluencies can occur at high rates for young children, averaging about 4 per 100 spoken syllables. The most common type of normal disfluency is the interjection, which is seen on average in 2 of 100 spoken syllables (Yairi & Ambrose, 1999).

Acquired Disorders of Fluency

Unlike developmental disorders of fluency, acquired fluency disorders do not necessarily emerge in early childhood. Rather, they can emerge at any time across the lifespan, resulting from illness, trauma, or accident affecting the brain or, occasionally, from psychological trauma. Stuttering that results from brain injury or neurological insult is called **neurogenic stuttering**, whereas stuttering resulting from psychological trauma is called **psychogenic stuttering**. Both occur less frequently than developmental stuttering, with psychogenic stuttering being the rarest of the three types. Possible causes of neurogenic stuttering include stroke, traumatic brain injury, brain infections (e.g., meningitis), and brain tumors (Mysak, 1989). Possible causes of psychogenic stuttering include serious abuse and conflict (Roth, Aronson, & Davis, 1989).

Acquired disorders of fluency show many of the same symptoms seen in developmental stuttering, but their onset is more dramatic. Also, neurogenic disorders of fluency are

TABLE 12-3 The rate of normal disfluencies in 2- to 5-year-old children

Type of Disfluency	Rate of Occurrence: Typical Children	Rate of Occurrence: Children Who Stutter
Interjection ("I want, uh, that one")	2.1 per 100 syllables	2.5 per 100 syllables
Revision ("It's on yellow, red paper")	1.8 per 100 syllables	2 per 100 syllables
Multisyllable word repetition ("It's the elephant-elephant") or phrase repetition ("I want the I want the blue one")	0.4 per 100 syllables	0.9 per 100 syllables
Total normal disfluencies	4.3 per 100 syllables	5.4 per 100 syllables

Source: From "Normative Disfluency Data for Early Childhood Stuttering" by N. G. Ambrose and E. Yairi, 1999, *Journal of Speech, Language, and Hearing Research, 42*, 895–909. Copyright 1999 by ASHA. Reprinted with permission.

often accompanied by other disorders of communication, such as aphasia, an acquired impairment of language functioning, or dysarthria, an acquired impairment of speech functioning. When accompanied by significant brain damage, as may be the case following a stroke, people with neurogenic stuttering may be unaware of their disfluencies and thus may not exhibit the associated emotional reactions seen in individuals with developmental disorders of fluency.

Discussion Point: *Consider the cases of Kaimon, Ralston, and Mr. Cho in Box 12-1. Characterize each as having either a developmental or an acquired disorder of fluency.*

Symptom Focus

For most people with developmental stuttering, the symptoms of the disorder change over time as the communicative impairment persists. For about 65% of those with a developmental fluency disorder, their primary or core symptoms gradually become more severe over time. As this change occurs, the individuals develop secondary behaviors, such as tremors and head nods, and are likely to begin to feel fear in anticipation of moments of disfluency (Yairi & Ambrose, 1992). Less frequently, corresponding to about 35% of people with a developmental fluency disorder, symptoms emerge suddenly and do not follow a pathway of increasing severity (Yairi & Ambrose, 1992). Regardless of the course, several classification systems have evolved to describe fluency disorders in terms of how far they have advanced (e.g., Bloodstein, 1995). These classification systems focus on the symptoms exhibited.

Peters and Guitar's Five-Level Classification System

Theodore Peters and Barry Guitar (1991) presented a five-level system to capture the symptoms of a fluency disorder as it progresses. As described in Table 12-4, the five levels include normal disfluency, borderline stuttering, beginning stuttering, intermediate stuttering, and advanced stuttering.

Normal Disfluency. Most children exhibit normal disfluencies between the ages of 18 months and 6 years. The extent to which a particular child is disfluent can ebb and flow over time and across contexts. For example, a child may be disfluent in particularly demanding situations, as when asked to tell a story to a grandparent, but fluent in less demanding circumstances. The most common types of disfluencies are interjections and revisions, although word repetitions, phrase repetitions, and part-word or sound repetitions also are evident. Such repetitions do not typically go beyond two repetitions (e.g., "I-I want my babydoll"). Peters and Guitar (1991) note that children at this level may stutter on as many as 10 out of 100 words. Importantly, the child who is normally disfluent does not exhibit any struggle with or tension toward these moments of disfluency and seems to take them in stride as a normal part of communication.

Borderline Stuttering. The second level of Peters and Guitar's classification system is **borderline stuttering**. It identifies children who are beginning to show disfluent behaviors that may signal the beginning of a fluency disorder. Children at this level are between 18 months and 6 years old, just like those who are normally disfluent, and in many ways look like children who are normally disfluent—with two important exceptions.

First, children who are borderline stutterers produce more disfluencies than do those who are normally disfluent. Borderline stutterers produce more than 10 disfluencies per 100 words, whereas normally disfluent children produce fewer than 10 disfluencies per 100 words. Second, children who are borderline stutterers produce a higher rate of certain types of disfluencies, as compared to normally disfluent children. Particularly prominent are part-word repetitions (e.g., "b-b-b-baby"), word repetitions (e.g., "He-he-he said"), and phrase repetitions (e.g., "I want-I want-I want-I want that one"),

TABLE 12-4 Peters and Guitar's five levels of stuttering

Level	Characteristics
Normal	• No more than 10 disfluencies per 100 words • Typically only one unit repeated in repetitions • Most common disfluencies are interjections, revisions, and word repetitions • Child unaware of disfluencies
Borderline	• More than 10 disfluencies per 100 words • Typically more than two units repeated in repetitions • More repetitions and prolongations than revisions or incomplete phrases • Loose and relaxed disfluencies • Child unaware of disfluencies
Beginning	• Signs of muscle tension and hurry in stuttering • Rapid and irregular repetitions, with abrupt terminations of each repeated unit • Sound prolongations emerging, usually first sound of a syllable • Some blocks observed; may be momentary stoppages • Possible increase in pitch at end of repetition or prolongation • Escape behaviors beginning to emerge: physical behaviors (eye blinks, head nods) and speech behaviors (interjections) • Aware of difficulty, feelings of frustration, but no strong negative feelings of self as a speaker
Intermediate	• Most frequent core behaviors are blocks, although repetitions and prolongations also occurring • Escape behaviors common to terminate blocks • Word avoidance emerging to avoid blocks; situation avoidance when speaking is required • Fear before stuttering, embarrassment during stuttering, and shame after stuttering
Advanced	• Most frequent core behaviors are long, tense blocks coupled with tremors of lips, tongue, or jaw • Complex patterns of avoidance and escape; may suppress stuttering with extensive avoidance behaviors • Very strong emotions of fear, embarrassment, and shame; negative feelings about self as helpless and inept when stutterering; self-identified as a stutterer

Source: From *Stuttering: An Integrated Approach to Its Nature and Treatment* (2nd ed.) by B. Guitar, 1998, Baltimore: Lippincott Williams & Wilkins. Copyright 1998 by Lippincott Williams & Wilkins. Adapted with permission.

which are likely to have more than two units repeated. Borderline stutterers also show some sound prolongations (e.g., "mmmmommy"). These types of disfluencies are more prevalent in the speech of borderline stutterers, occurring in about 10% of spoken syllables, than in the speech of normally disfluent children, where they occur in about 1% of spoken syllables (Yairi & Ambrose, 1999). These disfluencies comprise about 66% of all disfluencies produced by borderline stutterers, as compared to about 20% for children with normal disfluencies (Yairi & Ambrose, 1999).

Like children who are normally disfluent, children who are borderline stutterers show little tension toward their own disfluencies, although children in this age range are capable of differentiating between disfluent and fluent speech (Ezrati-Vinacour, Platsky, & Yairi, 2001).

Beginning Stuttering. Peters and Guitar's third level is **beginning stuttering**, a level that characterizes a true fluency disorder. Some children enter this level from the borderline stuttering level, although others enter it spontaneously, without demonstrating borderline behaviors. The beginning stuttering level describes children between 2 and 8 years of age who look like true stutterers—with core behaviors, secondary behaviors, and the emergence of negative feelings and attitudes toward stuttering. The core behaviors of the beginning stutterer include the repetitions of words and sounds, as seen in borderline stuttering, and an increase in sound prolongations. Importantly, the beginning stutterer demonstrates an additional core behavior not seen in borderline stutterers, namely, the block. You may recall that a block is a speech disfluency characterized by a complete stoppage of the airflow and the articulators. For the beginning stutterer, blocks do not last long and may be hardly noticeable. Nonetheless, they are an important marker of the beginning stuttering level.

In addition to these core behaviors, the beginning stutterer also develops secondary behaviors to escape and avoid moments of disfluency. These include, for instance, head nods, eye blinks, and interjections. The core and secondary behaviors of the beginning stutterer may prompt the beginning of negative emotions and feelings (e.g., frustration) toward stuttering and communication. As Peters and Guitar note, however, these feelings are not overly strong.

Intermediate Stuttering. Peters and Guitar's fourth level is **intermediate stuttering**, which is entered between 6 and 13 years of age and marks a significant impairment of fluency for the individual. Children and adolescents who are intermediate stutterers have likely stuttered for a long time, perhaps since their toddler years, and have developed significant levels of fear and frustration toward stuttering.

Prolongations and blocks are the prevalent core behaviors of the intermediate stutterer, with blocks becoming increasingly prevalent and lasting up to several seconds. Secondary behaviors that help the intermediate stutterer to avoid a block (e.g., substituting words or phrases) and to escape a block (e.g., nodding the head and blinking the eyes) become more evident and habitual. The real hallmark of this level, however, is the intermediate stutterer's fear of and frustration with stuttering. At this level intermediate stutterers may increasingly fear and avoid situations in which they are called on to talk which can bring about feelings of helplessness and embarrassment.

Discussion Point: *What kind of speaking situations might the person who is an intermediate stutterer avoid?*

Advanced Stuttering. **Advanced stuttering** is Peters and Guitar's fifth and most advanced level of stuttering; it characterizes a significant fluency impairment for persons over 14 years of age. The core and secondary behaviors of the advanced stutterer are similar to those of the intermediate stutterer, the greatest difference between them being the age of the individual and the likelihood of self-identification as a stutterer. For some advanced stutterers, core behaviors are not very evident, for they have honed their secondary behaviors to completely avoid or escape the appearance of prolongations and blocks.

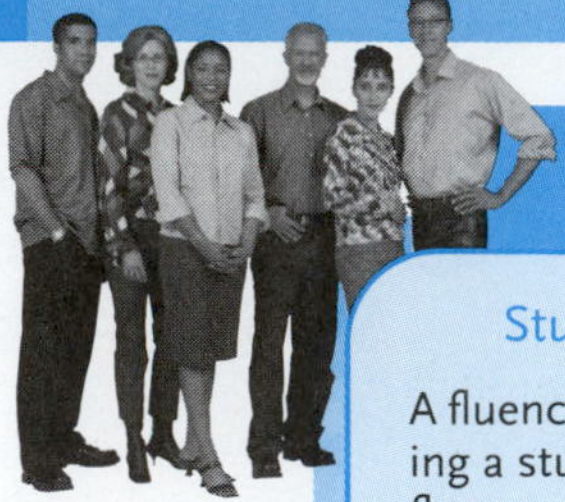

BOX 12-3 Ecological Contexts

Stuttering and Its Impact on Life

A fluency disorder can have a profound influence on an individual's life. For some people, being a stutterer negatively affects their employment aspirations. For example, a person with a fluency disorder who is interested in helping others might resist being a teacher, a social worker, or a psychologist because these professions involve communicating often with others. However, this is not the case for everyone who stutters, and in the communication disorders disciplines there are numerous scholars and practitioners who themselves have a fluency disorder. In fact, much of what we know today about stuttering comes from the research labs of people with fluency disorders who developed an interest because of their own struggles. Pioneers in the field of stuttering research, most notably Charles van Riper, did not develop a self-image that kept them from progressing academically and occupationally.

For Discussion

What makes one person who stutters succeed in career aspirations when another does not? What experiences might make the difference in the lives of people who stutter, pushing them forward academically instead of letting them falter because of a disability?

Companion Website

To answer these questions online, go to the Ecological Contexts module in chapter 12 of the Companion Website.

Stuttering Versus Cluttering

This chapter thus far has emphasized stuttering as the primary type of fluency disorder. One other type that affects children, adolescents, and adults warrants mention. **Cluttering** is a type of fluency problem that can considerably affect intelligibility. It is a pattern of disfluency characterized by breakdowns at the word or phrase level, such as incomplete phrases ("I want to go to, oh, that's not a good idea"), poor cohesion and coherence in expressing thoughts and organizing sentences ("Well, we went to the shop, oh, but first we had to get gas"), and a fast and spurty speaking rate (St. Louis & Myers, 1995). Unlike someone who stutters, the person who clutters does not seem inhibited or anxious about speaking, does not experience any physiological or psychological struggle when speaking, and does not exhibit prolonged sounds or tense pauses. Like stuttering, however, cluttering can reduce speech intelligibility and cause problems with effective communication.

Some individuals exhibit both cluttering and stuttering simultaneously, with cluttering behaviors emerging as the individual attempts to escape and avoid moments of stuttering. However, cluttering can also exist on its own. Some people may also show borderline cluttering behaviors, in which they exhibit the characteristics of cluttering, such as a fast speaking rate and frequent revisions or interjections, but intelligibility and communication are not compromised.

What Are the Defining Characteristics of Fluency Disorders?

The most readily apparent characteristic of a fluency disorder is the disruption of speech with disfluencies, which for the intermediate and advanced stutterer include primarily sound and word repetitions, sound prolongations, and blocks. These speech disfluencies represent the core features of a fluency disorder. As discussed previously, however, secondary features also emerge—escape and avoidance behaviors such as head nods and word substitutions, as well as negative feelings and attitudes about disfluency and communication. This section provides greater detail on core and secondary features and also describes the causes of and risk factors for stuttering.

Core Features

Their Dynamic Nature

The core features of fluency disorders are the speech disfluencies that disrupt an individual's ability to effectively communicate at home, school, work, and in the community. For most persons with a fluency disorder, the disorder emerges in early childhood during the toddler and preschool years, and for those who do not resolve the impairment either spontaneously or through treatment, the symptoms of the disorder will gradually change.

The hallmark characteristic of stuttering is the presence of an abnormally high rate of speech disfluencies and the presence of specific types of disfluencies, namely sound repetitions and sound prolongations. As stuttering progresses and a child moves from borderline to beginning and then intermediate stuttering, the types of disfluencies are dynamic, changing to reflect the individual's physical and cognitive maturation, self-awareness of stuttering, and development of compensatory strategies to avoid and escape moments of stuttering. The early sound repetitions and brief sound prolongations give way to longer sound prolongations and serious blocks. For individuals who reach the level of advanced stuttering, these disfluencies may all but disappear as they learn to avoid and escape the majority of speech disfluencies (Peters & Guitar, 1991).

Description of Core Features

The term *core feature,* or *core behavior,* emphasizes speech disfluencies as the original and primary source of communicative difficulty experienced by individuals with fluency disorders (Guitar, 1998). Core features represent the original manifestation of the speech impairment, which may give way to secondary features if the core features are not resolved. For borderline stutterers or beginning stutterers, core features are often called *stuttering-like disfluencies* (SLDs; Ambrose & Yairi, 1999). Although this term is controversial—the word *like* emphasizes a resemblance to stuttering rather than stuttering per se (Wingate, 2001)—it is used often to differentiate the disfluencies of stuttering from normal disfluencies.

The core features of fluency disorders include four types of speech disruptions (Ambrose & Yairi, 1999; Pellowski & Conture, 2002):

1. *Part-word repetition.* During part-word repetitions, part of a word, typically a sound or a syllable, is repeated, as in "It's my b-b-b-baby," "Judy is my ba-ba-ba-baby," or "Thi-thi-this is my baby." For young children who are borderline or beginning stutterers, part-word repetitions represent about one third of all disfluencies, occurring at a rate of about 5 times in 100 syllables (Ambrose & Yairi, 1999). In contrast, part-word repetitions are only one tenth of all disfluencies seen in typically developing children, occurring at a rate of about 0.5 times in 100 syllables. The number of part-word repetitions in a single moment of stuttering—referred to as *repetition units*—ranges from 2 to 4, with an average of about 2.5 units (Zebrowski, 1994).

2. *Single-syllable-word repetition.* In a single-syllable-word repetition, a single-syllable word is repeated two or more times, as in "My-my-my-my friend is here" or "and-and-and-and-and then we went on". Although single-syllable-word repetitions characterize a normal

speech disfluency seen in children, this type of disfluency occurs at much higher rates for children who are borderline or beginning stutterers. Children who stutter average more than 3 word repetitions in 100 syllables, as compared to typical children, who produce fewer than 1 per 100 syllables (Ambrose & Yairi, 1999). Nonetheless, it is important to note that this type of disfluency is common in young children, comprising about 12% of speech disfluencies for typical children. Thus, the occurrence of single-syllable-word repetitions in the speech of a young child is not necessarily cause for alarm, although it is a core feature of a fluency disorder.

3. *Sound prolongation.* A sound prolongation occurs when the duration of a speech sound is lengthened. During the prolongation the movement of one or more of the articulators stops in its place, but the airflow serving as the source of the speech sound continues (Guitar, 1998). For instance, in the prolongation of the sound /r/ in "He went to rrrrrun," the mandible and the tongue are held in place while the /r/ sound continues for half a second or longer. This type of core behavior includes both inaudible and audible prolongations. For the former, the speech sound is prolonged quietly and inaudibly followed by a hard attack when the sound is forced forward. For the latter, the speech sound is prolonged constantly and audibly. Persons who stutter produce both types of prolongations about equally.

This type of disfluency can occur fairly frequently in the speech of the stutterer. For instance, one study recorded an average of 31 prolongations during 45 minutes of speech for 14 children with fluency disorders (Zebrowski, 1994). The sound prolongations of stutterers range in duration from about .4 second to 1 second, with an average duration of .7 second (Zebrowski, 1994). Sound prolongations are unusual as a normal disfluency and represent an important and early sign that a child is stuttering.

4. *Block.* Blocks represent the core behavior most frequently associated with stuttering. In a block the articulators and airflow completely stop during the production of a sound, syllable, or word. Blocks can last for less than a second or for several seconds, and the duration and severity of blocks can increase as stuttering develops (Guitar, 1998). The block can also be accompanied by physical tension, including tremors of the jaw or the neck. Blocks are not typically seen in borderline or beginning stuttering but are a core feature of intermediate and advanced stuttering. Many adolescent and adult stutterers learn to compensate for blocks by avoiding them with word substitutions and pauses or escaping them through various means.

Within-Word and Between-Word Disfluencies

The types of core features just described are quite different from speech disfluencies that are not stuttering-like (Yaruss, 1997). Researchers classify disfluencies in two categories: those that are stuttering-like, or of a stuttering type, and those that are normal-like or of normal type (Yaruss, 1997). The best way to differentiate between disfluencies is to consider whether the disfluency affects the internal structure of a word. Those that do are called **within-word disfluencies**; these include sound repetitions, sound prolongations, and blocks. These disfluencies characterize problematic speech behaviors, or stuttering. When a disfluency does not affect the internal structure of a word, it is called a **between-word disfluency**—that is, the disfluency occurs between words rather than within a word. Between-word disfluencies include phrase repetitions (e.g., "He is in the—in the—in the house"), interjections (e.g., "Put it in the, uh, um, drawer"), and revisions (e.g., "I gave it to, uh, wait a minute, I gave it to Frances"). These types of disfluencies are perfectly normal unless they occur at inappropriately high rates, characteristic of cluttering.

Note that the core feature of single-syllable-word repetition was not included in either the within-word or the between-word category. Single-syllable-word repetitions technically fall into the between-word category, which is more or less synonymous with normal disfluencies. Single-syllable-word repetitions *are* a normal disfluency, but when seen at higher than expected rates in young children, they are also characteristic of borderline and beginning stuttering. Thus, some researchers place single-syllable-word repetitions in the category of within-word disfluencies because they are characteristic of early stuttering behavior (e.g., Conture, 1990).

Secondary Features

As an individual's stuttering progresses, secondary features emerge. Secondary features include **escape behaviors**, which an individual develops to get out of a moment of stuttering; **avoidance behaviors**, which an individual develops to evade moments of stuttering; and feelings and attitudes about stuttering, which develop over time with the experience of stuttering. Because these behaviors develop secondarily, they tend not to be seen until people have experienced the core features for a period of time. Thus, those who are borderline or beginning stutterers tend not to exhibit secondary features. But for intermediate and advanced stutterers who have stuttered for years and for whom secondary features are well developed, secondary features can be even more prominent and difficult to treat than the core disfluencies.

Escape Behaviors

Escape behaviors develop in a person with a fluency disorder as a response to moments of stuttering. These are, in essence, volitional strategies to cope with disfluencies. Whereas stuttering itself seems to be involuntary—that is, out of an individual's control—escape behaviors are within a person's control, used strategically to break out of a disfluency. Typical escape behaviors include head nods, eye blinks, hand tensing, and leg movements. These and some other physical behaviors used to escape disfluencies are listed in Figure 12-1. Sometimes physical behaviors are combined with verbal behaviors, such as interjections.

Escape behaviors tend to change over time as their effectiveness decreases. Bobrick (1995) provides an apt description of how escape behaviors change over time:

> There was a student at Harvard, for example, who discovered one day that he could break his blocks by stamping on the floor. It worked for a while, we are told, but then he found he had to stamp harder and longer to release a word. Finally, the whole house in which he lived seemed to shake from his pounding. (pp. 33–34)

For persons who are very experienced at stuttering, escape behaviors can be molded to look like natural speaking behaviors.

It is not hard to imagine how escape behaviors might emerge. Consider, for instance, what you might do if you were introducing yourself to someone unfamiliar and

FIGURE 12-1 Examples of physical escape behaviors.

- Blinking eyes
- Closing eyes
- Shifting eyes (up/down)
- Widening eyes
- Flaring nostrils
- Wrinkling nose
- Licking lips
- Pursing lips
- Tensing lips
- Trembling lips
- Clicking tongue
- Clenching jaw
- Trembling jaw
- Nodding head
- Shaking head
- Rubbing fingers
- Tapping fingers
- Clenching hands
- Tapping foot
- Crossing/uncrossing legs
- Bunching shoulders

Sources: Based on Guitar (1998); Shipley and McAfee (1998); Zebrowski (2000).

became stuck on the first sound in your name. In my own simulation, I can see myself extending my hand to introduce myself to the friend of a friend: "Good to meet you, I'm L# . . . ." As I put myself through this, blocking on the /l/ in my name for several seconds, I can feel the air swell in my chest, my neck tense, my eyes bulge, and my jaw jut forward as I try to push the sound out. I am embarrassed and feel as if I might pass out as my friend and her friend look at me. Nothing happens—the block doesn't give. Suddenly, I jerk my head to the side, and finally the block is released. Thus, I have developed a strategy that seems to dislodge the block, and it is adopted for future use.

Avoidance Behaviors

Although escape behaviors might be useful for breaking out of a moment of stuttering, you can imagine that a person with a fluency disorder would prefer to simply avoid those moments of stuttering altogether. People who stutter are often able to anticipate moments of stuttering, based on their experiences in certain speaking situations or with certain words or phrases; they might be more likely to stutter on certain sounds or words. For instance, some people might always stutter on words that start with /m/ or on the name of their hometown, perhaps Chicago. Knowing this and not wanting to subject themselves to a moment of stuttering, these individuals might try to avoid their probable pitfalls. Avoidance behaviors commonly used include both word and sound avoidance and situation avoidance (Guitar, 1998).

Word and Sound Avoidance. With **word** and **sound avoidance** a person with a fluency disorder uses several strategies to avoid a disfluency (Guitar, 1998; Van Riper, 1982). A substitution occurs when a word or phrase is substituted to avoid a word or sound. For example, the person who stutters on the word *Chicago* might say, "I am from Ch-Ch. . . the Windy City." A **circumlocution** occurs when a person tries to delay a potential disfluency by putting it off or avoid it by talking around it, as in "He told me, uh, when we met, uh, we were at the mall, and . . . ." With a postponement, the person pauses or uses filler words prior to producing a potential disfluency, as in "I would like . . . (pause) bacon."

Situation Avoidance. Few people find public speaking easy and enjoyable; some of us may even find it frightening or anxiety producing. This is not uncommon, particularly in demand situations, when we are put on the spot, as on the first day of a class when we all have to introduce ourselves to the group. For people who stutter, one strategy that emerges as a secondary feature is **situation avoidance**, in which the individual steers clear of circumstances in which stuttering is probable. The number of such situations is endless—answering the phone at home, introducing oneself at a party, ordering food in a restaurant, asking a price in a store, asking for directions when lost.

Discussion Point: *What are some opportunities an individual might lose out on because of situation avoidance? Consider the case of Kaimon in Box 12-1.*

Avoiding situations that cause discomfort is a common, if not normal, behavior among children (e.g., going to the dentist), adolescents (e.g., calling someone for a date), and even adults (e.g., sending food back at a restaurant). But for people who stutter, situation avoidance can have an extraordinarily negative impact on their achievements at home, school, and work and in the community. Anxiety, mood disturbances, and stress can all result as a function of chronic avoidances (Blood, Blood, Bennett, Simpson, & Susman, 1994).

Feelings and Attitudes

It is probably not surprising that people with long-term fluency disorders may develop negative feelings toward communication. Whereas the beginning stutterer has moments of fear, frustration, and embarrassment, the intermediate or advanced stutterer may experience these feelings all day long, both within and beyond direct communicative activities.

As the experience of stuttering accumulates, "these experiences pile up like cars in a demolition derby to create the entanglement of fear, embarrassment, and shame that accompanies moments of stuttering" (Peters & Guitar, 1991, p. 99). Peters and Guitar note that negative feelings toward stuttering increase as fluency problems move from being "an annoyance to a serious problem" (p. 99), illustrated by this adult's description of her own experiences with stuttering:

> I just couldn't get anything out, but you could tell that my mouth was trying. It would be like my cheeks were puffed like I was trying to blow a trombone without any air coming out . . . . And you could see my jaw tightening and my lips tightening, but not any word would come out. (Anderson & Felsenfeld, 2003, p. 248)

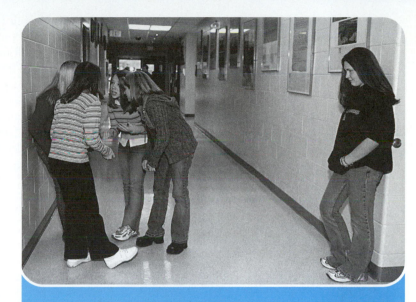

Avoiding situations that require speaking can have a negative impact on the social and educational achievement of an adolescent who stutters.

It is through the accumulation of disfluent experiences that stress, tension, and negative emotions emerge (Ezrati-Vinacour et al., 2001). This is not to say that young children do not recognize stuttering; even children as young as 3 are able to differentiate between fluent and disfluent speech, preferring fluent speech over disfluent speech (Ezrati-Vinacour et al., 2001). However, as an interesting tribute to the sensibilities of 3-year-old children, they are no more likely to choose a friend who is fluent over a friend who is disfluent. But by 4 and 7 years of age, 69% and 94% of children, respectively, would choose a friend who is fluent over one who is disfluent (Ezrati-Vinacour et al., 2001).

Adolescents and adults who have stuttered for years are likely to identify themselves as stutterers, view communication with negativity, and use myriad techniques to avoid speaking situations. They may have experienced people laughing at them, treating them harshly, or avoiding talking to them altogether because of their stuttering. Surveys do suggest that the general public has negative attitudes toward people who stutter, viewing them as tense, anxious, withdrawn, fearful, and emotional (Kalinowski, Stuart, & Armson, 1996). Although these perceptions may stem from the tensions inherent in moments of stuttering, they are not appropriate descriptions of the character of those who stutter (Kalinowski et al., 1996).

Discussion Point: *Strong negative feelings toward speaking can emerge with the repeated experience of stuttering. Why do you think Mr. Cho in Box 12-1 doesn't seem to have these feelings?*

Causes and Risk Factors

What causes the emergence of the core features of fluency disorders, which lead to secondary features? This question has long been a focus of stuttering researchers, particularly those who study developmental stuttering. Nonetheless, the cause of developmental stuttering remains very elusive. In fact, for the majority of children, stuttering begins for no obvious reason. Van Riper (1973), a researcher who spent most of his career studying the development of stuttering in children, noted that for most children, "stuttering seemed to begin under quite normal conditions of living and communicating" (p. 81) with no apparent conflicts, illnesses, shocks, or other types of disturbances to explain the fluency disorder.

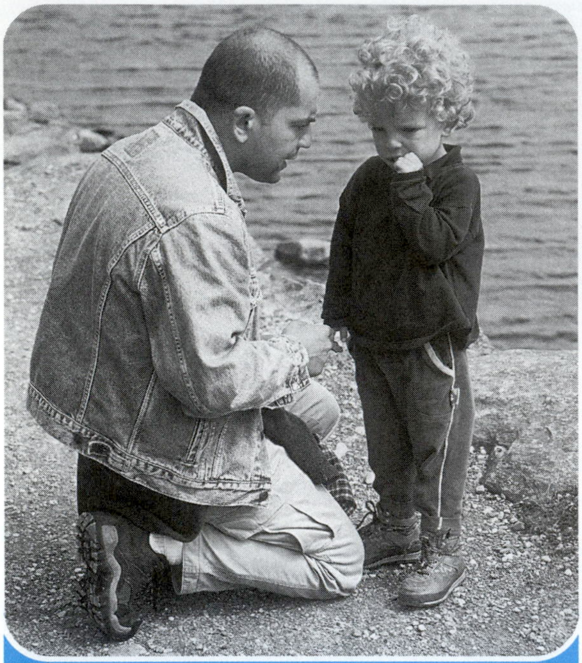

About 50% of young children who stutter have an immediate family member who stutters also, such as a sibling or a parent.

The inability of researchers, practitioners, and parents to pinpoint a cause is likely due to the fact that stuttering does not result from a single identifiable cause. Rather, stuttering results from the complex interaction of a variety of predisposing factors and precipitating factors (Peters & Guitar, 1991), which emphasize an integrated model of stuttering development (Guitar, 1998). **Predisposing factors** are constitutional factors that make an individual susceptible to a fluency disorder, such as carrying a genetic trait (Yairi, Ambrose, & Cox, 1996) or having an overly sensitive temperament (Guitar, 1998). **Precipitating factors** include both developmental and environmental factors that can worsen stuttering, such as age and/or stress. These two sets of factors must interact in such a way as to disturb the developmental trajectory of a child, with predisposing factors contributing about 70% of the likelihood to stutter and precipitating factors accounting for 30% of the liability (Andrews, Morris-Yates, Howie, & Martin, 1991). Thus, an individual may have one or more significant predisposing factors for a fluency disorder, yet not develop a disorder. Or an individual may experience several salient precipitating factors and not develop a disorder. Figure 12-2 identifies key predisposing and precipitating factors in fluency disorders; Figure 12-3 shows how their interaction can result in developmental stuttering.

Predisposing Factors

Predisposing factors, also called *constitutional factors,* make a child more vulnerable than other children to developing a fluency disorder. Considered here are four important predisposing factors: family history, gender, processing ability, and motor speech coordination.

Family History. Fluency disorders tend to run in families, suggesting that genetics are a particularly important predisposing factor. Of young children who stutter, nearly half have

FIGURE 12-2 Key predisposing and precipitating factors in the development of fluency disorders.

Predisposing factors	Family history Genetic predisposition Gender Processing ability Motor-speech coordination
Precipitating factors	Age Stressful adult speech models Stressful speaking situations Stressful life events Self-awareness/temperament

Source: Based on Guitar (1998).

FIGURE 12-3 Predisposing factors interacting with precipitating factors to worsen stuttering.

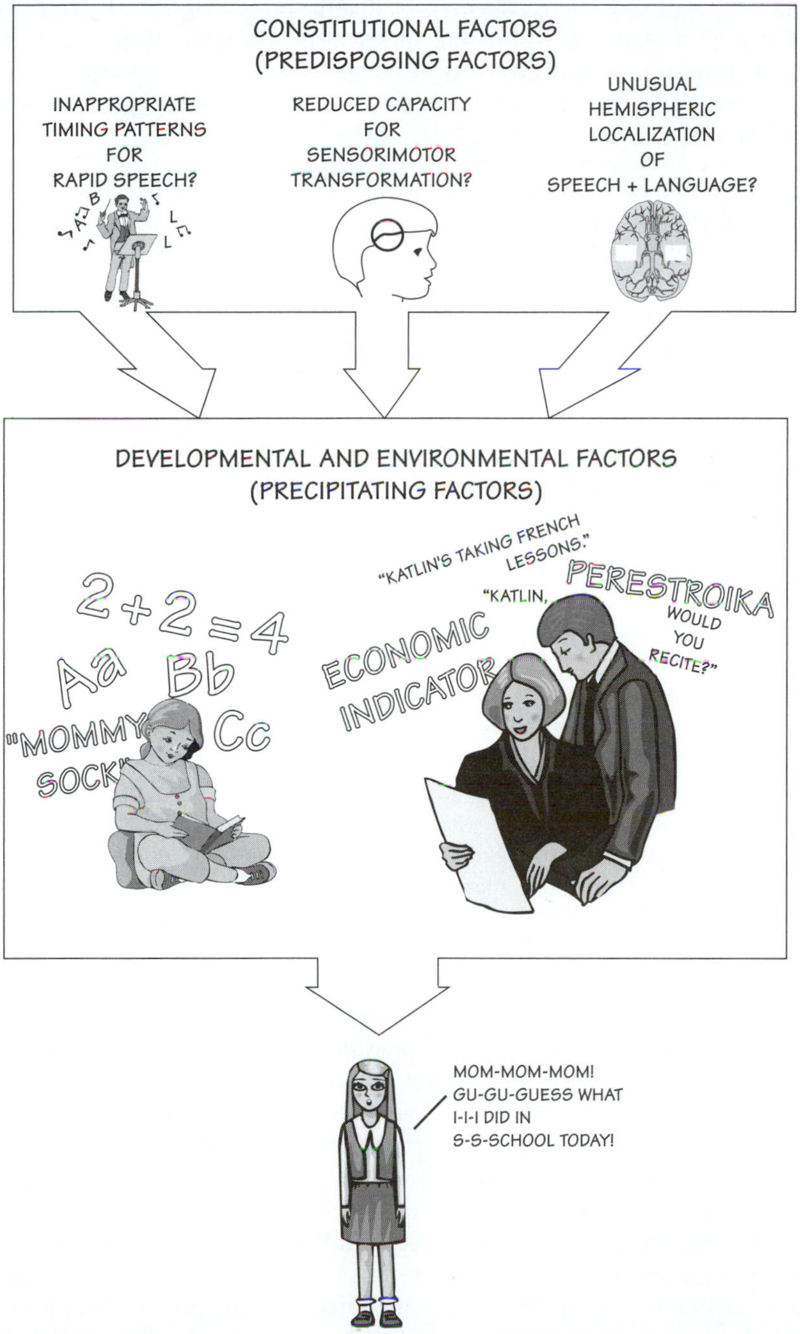

Source: From *Stuttering: An Integrated Approach to Its Nature and Treatment* (2nd ed.) by B. Guitar, 1998, Baltimore: Lippincott Williams & Wilkins. Copyright 1998 by Lippincott Williams & Wilkins. Reprinted with permission.

an immediate family member who stutters, and about 70% have an extended family member who stutters (e.g., grandmother, uncle; Yairi et al., 1996). A genetic transmission is also suggested by twin studies, which show that when one twin stutters, there is an increased likelihood (estimates range from 20% to 90%) that the other twin will also stutter (Yairi et al., 1996). Given this genetic linkage, one might wonder whether stuttering is perhaps a gene-linked dominant or recessive trait. Although this may be too simplistic a picture, studies from the 1990s have suggested that a susceptibility to stuttering may be linked to a single specific gene (Ambrose, Yairi, & Cox, 1993).

Gender. Gender is a second predisposing feature, with boys more likely to develop a fluency disorder than girls. Among children in the early stages of developmental stuttering, the gender ratio is about 3 boys to 1 girl (Ambrose, Cox, & Yairi, 1997). Among adolescents and adults who have not resolved their stuttering, the gender ratio shifts to about 7 boys to 1 girl affected. Therefore, while boys are not only more likely to experience a fluency disorder, they are also more likely to persist in the disorder once it is manifested. And about 77% of boys who stutter will recover, as compared to 87% of girls (Ambrose et al., 1997). Reasons for these gender differences have been explored for decades, focusing on environmental differences in social pressures on boys and girls. More recent data suggest that explanations may be found in genetic research examining how girls and boys may vary in their susceptibility to an expression of genetic traits (Ambrose et al., 1997).

Processing Ability. Among persons with fluency disorders, additional communicative impairments are likely to co-occur, including language disorder, phonological disorder, and language-based reading disability (Arndt & Healey, 2001). A predisposing factor that makes theoretical sense in explaining the co-occurrence of these disorders is an underlying problem with linguistic processing, that is, how language is processed in the brain.

The efficiency and effectiveness of processing abilities relate to both capacity (how much processing can an individual handle?) and demand (is the processing within the individual's capability?). A demand-and-capacity model of linguistic processing explains that language and speech are likely to break down when processing demands exceed capacity (Arndt & Healey, 2001). This discrepancy between capacity and demand can result in a problem with any one of a number of aspects of speech and language production, including fluency. Researchers noting that children who stutter produce speech at slower rates than children who do not stutter suggest that this may result from slower processing of language, which results in slowed production of speech (Hall, Amir, & Yairi, 1999).

What might cause a child to have a problem with linguistic processing? Recent data using brain imaging techniques provide some interesting possibilities (Riley, Maguire, Franklin, & Ortiz, 2001). These data suggest that processing limitations may be caused by poor or inappropriate hemispheric specialization. Recall from chapter 3 that the left hemisphere is specialized in humans for language processing. However, studies of the brain activities of people who stutter show greater activity in the right hemisphere during stuttering and decreased metabolic activity in the left hemisphere, particularly in those areas critical to language processing (i.e., Broca's and Wernicke's areas). Specifically, the primary motor area of the right hemisphere appears to be overactive in persons who stutter (Riley et al., 2001). It is likely that these brain differences compromise the production of fluent speech and present an important predisposing factor to the development of fluency disorders.

Motor Speech Coordination. People who stutter may have an underlying difficulty in coordinating and timing the motor activities required to produce fluent speech (McClean & Runyan, 2000). Observations of differences in various aspects of speech timing (e.g., rate of tongue movement) and coordination (e.g., movement of tongue in relation to lips) suggest that difficulties in motor speech production may make persons who stutter vulnerable for fluency breakdowns (McClean & Runyan, 2000; Kleinow & Smith, 2000).

Unlike the other predisposing conditions described, this one is located directly within the motor speech apparatus itself, placing the cause of the fluency problem somewhere in the muscular and/or articulatory systems involved with fluent speech production. However, the exact site of the breakdown remains speculative, with research continuing to rule out possibilities. For instance, theories that the muscles of the larynx are overactivated (or hyperactive) during stuttering, and thus a cause of disfluencies, have not held up in laboratory studies (Smith, Denny, Shaffer, Kelly, & Hirano, 1996).

It is possible that early in the development of stuttering, the rate and coordination of these children's speech exceed their capacity to produce fluent speech, resulting in disfluencies (van Lieshout, Hulstijn, & Peters, 1996). This predisposing factor is also based on the demand-and-capacity model but emphasizes discrepancies between a child's demands on coordination and timing for speech production (potentially fueled by a desire to communicate) and the capacity of the speech system. This early disruption in the coordination and timing of the speech system may undermine the development of well-coordinated and well-timed speech, setting the stage for ongoing problems with fluency.

Discussion Point: *What are some possible predisposing factors in the cases of Kaimon and Ralston in Box 12-1?*

Precipitating Factors

For an individual to develop stuttering, a predisposing factor must be present, which may account for as much as 70% of the likelihood that a child develops stuttering (Yairi et al., 1996). But what about the other 30%? It represents the precipitating factors, which influence whether an individual's predisposition, or susceptibility, to stuttering will actually manifest itself as a fluency disorder. Many children may have a constitutional predisposition to a fluency disorder but nonetheless follow a path to healthy fluency development. Predisposing and precipitating forces must align in a way that is sufficient to steer a child onto the path to stuttering, as shown in Figure 12-4. Three categories of precipitating factors may contribute to the likelihood of developing a fluency disorder: age, developmental stressors, and self-awareness.

Age. Age is, interestingly enough, a significant risk factor in the development of a fluency disorder. The average age of onset in one study of children with fluency disorders showed the average age of stuttering emergence to be 3 years for boys and 2.5 years for girls (Yaruss, LaSalle, & Conture, 1998). The likelihood of developing a fluency disorder beyond 6 years is negligible; thus, it seems safe to say that everyone reading this book need not worry about this particular precipitating factor.

To understand why age is a significant risk factor, let's consider the normal challenges for a young child in achieving fluent speech and language. About 2 years after birth, children move into a period of remarkable speech and language growth, in which their ever-developing urge to communicate is accompanied by a dramatic increase in speech and language capabilities. As children produce more phonologically complicated words (e.g., "hippopotamus") and more syntactically complex utterances (e.g., "Mommy sit here and Daddy sit there."), the speech and language mechanisms are repeatedly taxed, compromising the fluency of communicative acts. The challenges of picking precise words, conveying appropriate intent, organizing sentence structure, and articulating strings of sounds result in considerable disfluency in the speech of most youngsters—about 6 disfluencies in 100 syllables (Ambrose & Yairi, 1999).

Now let's consider the child whose genetic endowment includes a susceptibility to stuttering. For reasons that remain unknown, this child's communicative system is already vulnerable to a weakness in fluency. With the repeated taxing of the system that occurs between 2 and 5 years, the systems of a number of these children give way to a more serious problem with disfluencies than other children experience. These children produce about

FIGURE 12-4 The developmental pathway to stuttering.

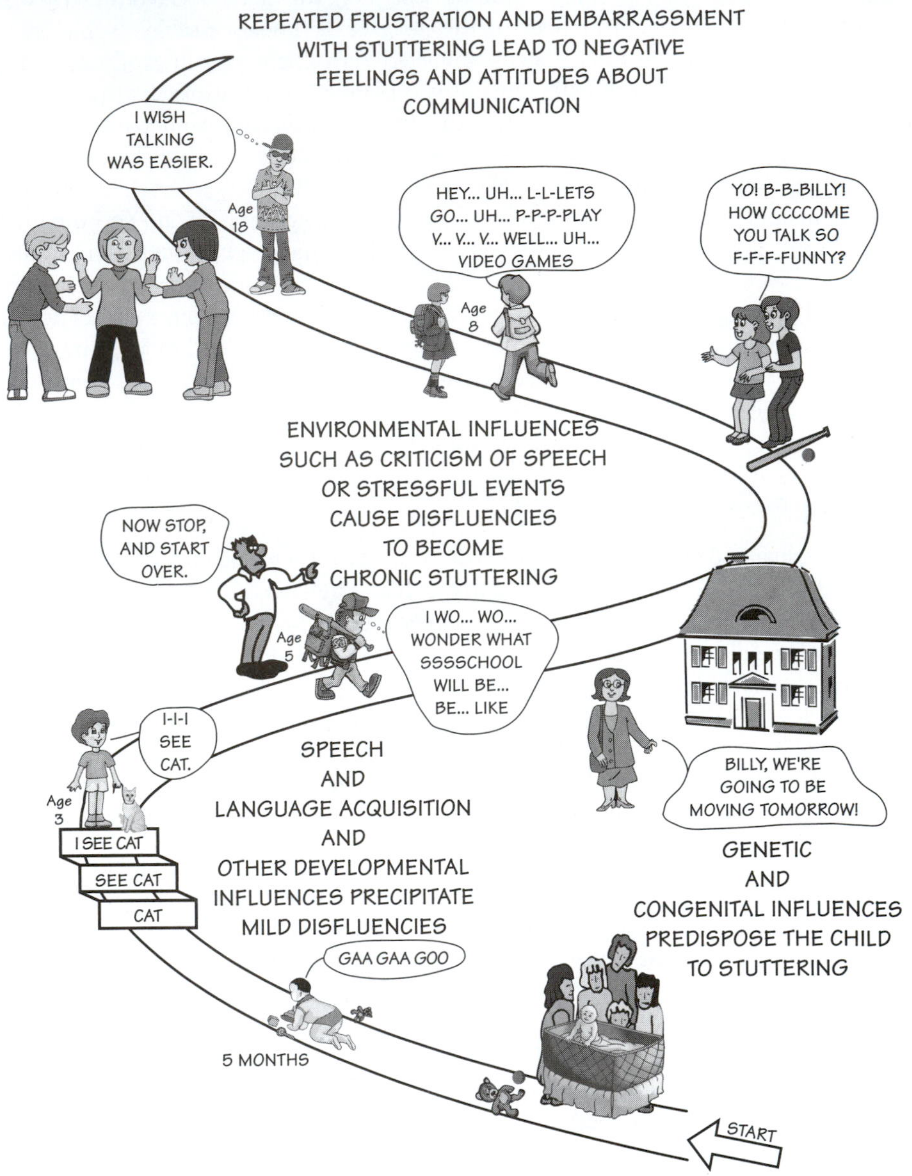

Source: From *Stuttering: An Integrated Approach to Its Nature and Treatment* by T. J. Peters and B. Guitar, 1991, Baltimore: Williams & Wilkins. Copyright 1991 by Williams & Wilkins. Reprinted with permission.

16 disfluencies in 100 syllables (Ambrose & Yairi, 1999). Fortunately, the majority of these children—about 75%—will not stutter into adulthood, although their stuttering may last for months if not years. The longer the child's stuttering continues, the less likely it is to be resolved and the more likely it is to increase in severity (Ambrose & Yairi, 1999; Pellowski & Conture, 2002).

Developmental Stressors. Stress does not promote fluency, as we have all probably found out at least once in our lives. Accordingly, some evidence suggests that a variety of developmental stressors may serve as precipitating factors in the emergence of stuttering in children, specifically for those children who are already susceptible to a fluency disorder. Guitar (1998) describes three categories of stressors that can influence stuttering in children.

Stressful adult speech models describe adult speech that is not well-tuned to children's speech, language, or cognitive capabilities. Features that may be stressful include a rapid speech rate, use of complex syntax and complicated vocabulary, interruptions of child speech, overuse of questions and directives, and short wait times following questions (Rustin & Cook, 1995).

Developmental researchers have long shown the value of parental speech and language input that is sensitive and well-tuned to a child's developmental functioning. Well-tuned parental input is not too simple nor too challenging; rather, it mirrors and is sensitive to a child's own capabilities. Exposure to sensitive and well-adjusted speech models serves as a powerful accelerant to children's early speech and language development (e.g., Hoff, 2003). However, when children with a susceptibility to fluency disorders consistently experience adult speech in the home or other caregiving environment that is too demanding or complicated, that may precipitate disfluencies. Yet there is little evidence showing that parents of children who stutter are overly or inappropriately demanding of their children during communicative activities. Indeed, many parents of children who stutter are sensitive to the communicative skills of their children and adjust their own language accordingly (Miles & Bernstein Ratner, 2001).

Stressful speaking situations are the second type of stress that may precipitate fluency challenges for children. These situations include competing to speak, hurrying when speaking, and having many things to say (Guitar, 1998). Although these stressors can be influenced by external events, such as being interrupted often when speaking or being asked many questions, it seems more likely that these stressors arise from internal sources within the child. For instance, a child may be trying to hurry and share a thought but may not have the capacity to meet that demand. Or a child may be producing a particularly long sentence and again may not have the capacity to produce it fluently. *Cross-talk* describes the challenge to the child's developing but still immature nervous system when the expression of emotion interfaces with speech and language production (Guitar, 1998). In such cases fluent speech production can become compromised and over time may result in chronic fluency breakdowns.

Stressful life events are a third precipitating factor in fluency disorders. Possible stressors include moving, divorce of parents, loss of a parent or close family member, illness, or accident (Guitar, 1998). Transitions such as these may impact development of any young child in a variety of ways, fluency abilities notwithstanding. For some children these and other types of stressors can provide the catalyst for the emergence of stuttering.

Self-Awareness. Researchers and clinicians have longed viewed young children as being unaware of their own disfluencies, even children who are borderline and beginning stutterers. A newer perspective of the last 2 decades is that children who stutter are aware of their disfluencies at an early age (Ezrati-Vinacour et al., 2001). Researchers Rustin and Cook (1995) of London, England, describe an interview with a 4-year-old who stuttered, in which she noted, "Oh, it's so hard sometimes; the words won't come out." In this same interview, the child reported that the one thing she would change about herself if given some magic would be to "make her voice better" (p. 130). By 6 years of age, children who stutter have more negative attitudes toward their speech than do children who do not stutter (Vanryckeghem & Brutten, 1997).

Some experts believe that children who stutter have an atypically high awareness of their own disfluencies (Bernstein Ratner, 1997), which may serve as a precipitating factor in the emergence of fluency disorders. For children with a predisposition to fluency disorders, this atypically heightened awareness of their own fluency may create a tension toward communication that builds with each disfluency.

Discussion Point: *What are some possible precipitating factors in the cases of Kaimon and Ralston in Box 12-1?*

BOX 12-4 Spotlight on Research

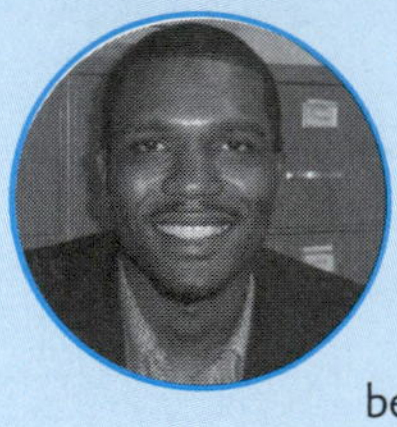

John Spruill, III, M.A.
Doctoral Student, Audiology and Speech Sciences, Purdue University

While in the process of receiving a bachelor's degree in political science, I became attracted to the field of speech-language pathology through an elective that I chose, Voice and Stuttering, during my senior year. I eventually received a master's degree in communicative sciences and disorders from Hampton University, an education that allowed me to acquire required clinical hours and experience. I am currently a Ph.D. student attending Purdue University in the Department of Audiology and Speech Sciences.

At the present, I am working with Dr. Chris Weber-Fox, who, as my advisor, is committed to training me and other students in our lab in an area that addresses the development of neural subsystems for language processing. More specifically, this requires the measuring of event-related brain potentials, which are obtained from speakers possessing a variety of communication experiences and abilities, ranging from typically developing children to individuals who stutter.

As a doctoral student, I assist in the training of new students who enter the lab and coordinate many of the day-to-day activities that constitute the research process. For example, my duties include identifying research participants, conducting research with participants, and data analysis. These training tools are serving as preparation for me to become an effective independent researcher.

Our current research, which focuses on individuals who stutter, has allowed me the opportunity to present our data at national conferences, an important experience to acquire. To be able to come face-to-face with individuals I've read about in the field's literature is a priceless opportunity, especially when they make themselves available for suggestions and/or comments on how our research can become more effective. It is also extremely gratifying when individuals who are the focus of our research view our results as hope.

Working with this population is preparing me for independent research, which will be geared toward the elderly population. I plan to follow in the footsteps of those responsible for training me, in order that I am able to give back what they have given me: invaluable experiences on the road to becoming an effective, independent researcher.

How Are Fluency Disorders Identified?

The identification of fluency disorders is complicated by the fact that nearly all persons are disfluent in their speech at least some of the time. Thus, professionals must carefully study an individual's disfluencies to determine whether their quality and/or quantity is significantly different from what is normal.

As an exercise in studying the quality and quantity of disfluencies, you can record yourself during a conversation with a friend and then count the number of disfluencies in your own speech. Count the number of sound and word repetitions, prolongations, blocks, interjections, revisions, and longer-than-normal pauses or hesitations. You can then calculate two common metrics to arrive at an estimate of your level of disfluency:

1. *Average number of disfluencies per 100 words:* Count the total number of disfluencies produced, divide this by the total number of words, and then multiply the result by 100. For example, a sample of 300 words containing 22 disfluencies results in an average number of 7.3 disfluencies per 100 words.
2. *Average number of disfluencies per 100 syllables:* Count the total number of disfluencies produced, divide this by the total number of syllables, and then multiply the result by 100. For example, a sample of 622 syllables containing 34 disfluencies results in an average number of 5.5 disfluencies per 100 syllables.

You should also examine the quality or type of disfluency. For most students, I would expect that interjections and revisions will predominate and that repetitions, prolongations, and blocks will be infrequent, if not nonexistent.

BOX 12-5 Spotlight on Practice

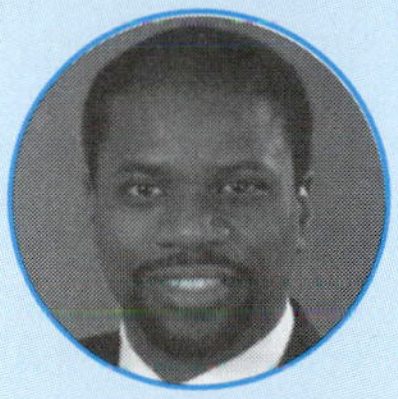

Tommie L. Robinson, Jr., Ph.D.
Speech-Language Pathologist
Scottish Rite Center for Childhood Language Disorders
Children's Hearing and Speech Center, Washington, DC

As the director of the Scottish Rite Center in Washington, DC, I find so much joy in my everyday responsibilities as an administrator, clinician, researcher, and teacher. You can say that I really have the best of all four worlds, but the best for me are my roles as an administrator and a clinician. My favorite part is creating new clinical service programs. As a practicing clinician, I often have first-hand knowledge of the needs of the patients that we serve. The things that I must do as an administrator are to determine whether there is a clinical need for a program, develop the program's content and target audience, utilize a feasibility study, seek funding sources for support, and set up an evaluation component. Through these programs lives are touched and differences are made.

This center has been in existence since 1989. During that time we have expanded the staff and developed parent training programs, summer enrichment programs for language and stuttering, and most recently, Head Start screening programs. In addition, I direct a public schools program in which I employ speech-language pathologists who are housed in the public schools and who deliver high-quality clinical services while increasing community relations and establishing trust and partnerships with principals, teachers, parents, and students. This has been one of the highlights of my career.

There is another part of my job that some might find sterile, but I like to think of it as an ongoing learning experience—monitoring the day-to-day operations of a very diverse program. I oversee an autonomous two-story building that needs daily monitoring, and it is my job to do so. My position is responsible for monitoring the budget, recruiting and retaining staff, supervising the professional and administrative staffs, meeting with a foundation board, developing and implementing marketing and public relations plans, and performing quality checks. My job has been made easier by the knowledge and skills that I have gained in leadership positions in professional societies such as the American Speech-Language-Hearing Association, the District of Columbia Speech-Language-Hearing Association, the National Black Association for Speech, Language and Hearing, and the list goes on.

When I look back on my life, I can think of nothing that brings me greater joy than knowing that I have made a difference in the lives of children, adolescents, and their families, whose outlook on life has been changed by the diminishing of a communication disorder. What other profession can bring such satisfaction?

If you prefer to practice on someone other than yourself, have a friend read the following statement of 43 words and calculate the average number of disfluencies per 100 words:

> ***Um, yesterday I picked her, uh, up from daycare and we, then, uh, we walked to my office to see if Becky was there, she wasn't, but, um, but uh, oh what's her name, Linda was there and had the key, so, uh we got to pick up the candy.***

This type of careful study of speech disfluencies characterizes the assessment process for identifying fluency disorders.

The Assessment Process

Referral

Speech-language pathologists (SLPs) are the professionals who are specially trained for assessing, diagnosing, and treating fluency disorders. Other professionals—such as special and general educators, psychologists, and physicians—often play an important role in referring individuals to SLPs for fluency assessment, informing the diagnostic process, and executing treatment plans. Thus, it is important for these and other professionals to be familiar with the warning signs of possible fluency disorders to make timely and appropriate referrals.

Warning Signs for Developmental Fluency Disorders. Professionals who work with young children should be aware of the following warning signs of a possible developmental fluency problem, particularly for children between 2 and 6 years of age (Guitar, 1998), the period in which most cases of developmental fluency disorders emerge.

1. Repetition of parts of words, such as the first sound ("b-b-ball") or the first several sounds ("ba-ba-ball"), including repetitions in which the vowel sound "uh" is substituted ("cuh-cuh-cuh-cake")
2. Repetitions of words or parts of words involving three or more repetitions of the unit ("I-I-I-I do it")
3. Prolongation of a sound or appearance of being stuck on a sound ("It is mmmine")
4. Feelings of frustration or embarrassment toward speaking and communication

Professionals who work with young children should also be aware of three epidemiological facts in conjunction with these warning signs. First, fluency disorders tend to run in families, with children more likely to be affected if they have an immediate or extended family member with a fluency disorder. Second, fluency disorders occur more often in boys than in girls. Third, fluency disorders often co-occur with other disorders of communication, such as phonological impairment. Thus, professionals should be particularly vigilant for warning signs in children who have one or more of these general vulnerabilities.

Additionally, professionals should recognize that fluency disorders become less likely to resolve the longer they persist. Although some cases of developmental stuttering do resolve spontaneously without treatment, there is no crystal ball that can identify those fortunate youngsters. Thus, when warning signs are present, consultation with an SLP who can provide further input on the possible disorder and the need for treatment is always the best approach.

Warning Signs for Acquired Fluency Disorders. Acquired disorders of fluency can result from various types of trauma, illness, or injury that affect the brain. For instance, stuttering can follow a brain injury caused by a stroke or dementia from a progressive disease of the brain. In these persons stuttering can result from the loss of automaticity in retrieving language (Mysak, 1989). As an example, an elderly person with dementia might not be able to remember the word for *table,* thus compromising fluency: "I put it on the, the, the, the . . . I don't know." A small minority of acquired cases of stuttering result from psychological causes, such as severe abuse or a mental illness (National Institutes of Health, 2002). Warning signs for a possible acquired fluency disorder include these:

Discussion Point: *Early childhood educators and day care providers should be well aware of signs of possible fluency disorders. What are some approaches to increase this awareness for these professionals?*

1. Presence of stuttering-like disfluencies, such as part-word or whole-word repetitions and sound prolongations
2. Presence of cluttering-like disfluencies, such as overuse of interjections, revisions, and abandonment of phrases or sentences (e.g., "He told me he would, uh, uh . . . He said, um . . . Do you want to sit down?")
3. Inability to effectively communicate, which may or may not be coupled with frustration and/or embarrassment toward communication

Assessment Protocol

Assessment by the speech-language pathologist is designed to answer four main questions (Zebrowski, 2000): (1) Is the individual stuttering or at risk of stuttering? (2) Does the individual exhibit any other communicative risk factors or disabilities? (3) Is therapy for stuttering warranted? (4) What therapy approach would be most beneficial? Answers to these questions are obtained using a variety of different tools, including case history and interview, speech observation, questionnaire and survey, and direct testing.

Case History and Interview. The case history is an indispensable part of the fluency assessment process; it is a detailed questionnaire and interview in which the clinician gathers information about the individual. As implied by its name, the case history is designed to clarify the history of the perceived fluency problem and place it within the context of the individual's life. For children the case history informant is typically the primary caregiver; for adolescents and adults the informant is typically the person experiencing the fluency problem.

A child's case history examines family demographics (e.g., number of siblings), developmental milestones in all areas (e.g., motor, self-care, communication, social, cognitive), medical history, educational history, and history of the fluency problem, including parental perceptions of the child's specific difficulties and the ways the problems have changed over time. The clinician asks the informant to provide details on what was happening in the child's life when the disfluencies were first noticed and to discuss changes in the disfluencies since the problem began.

The adolescent's and adult's case history is similarly organized but encourages greater detail on how fluency has changed over time and how it affects their lives, including educational and occupational performance. For instance, the informant is asked about specific situations in which fluency becomes more compromised and the details of strategies used in such situations to promote fluency (Guitar, 1998).

Additional informants are often interviewed to complement the case history. For preschool children the clinician is likely to interview any individual who cares for the child, such as day care providers. These persons can provide important information on the ways a child's disfluencies are manifested in different environments and the extent to which these affect the child's communicative performance in everyday activities. For older children and adolescents, teachers are likely to be interviewed to determine how disfluencies affect the child's performance in the classroom and whether stuttering interferes with academics. For adults, interviews might be conducted with an individual's family members, including spouses and/or children, as well as employers and colleagues. Each of these individuals can provide a unique and important perspective in determining the extent to which fluency problems affect a person's life in diverse contexts.

Speech Observation. Observation of a child's, adolescent's, or adult's speech in a variety of situations is the most important part of the fluency assessment. The clinician observes and records the individual's speech in as many activities as possible, including home, classroom, work, and social situations. The clinician uses a fluency charting grid, which is a tool for counting the total number and different types of disfluencies that occur within a speech sample. By calculating the number of disfluencies within a sample, the clinician can estimate the percentage of disfluent speech in a given speaking situation. For instance, in a sample of 500 words during play with a peer, if a child produces 30 repetitions, 10 sound prolongations, and 4 blocks, the clinician's calculations can show that about 9% of the child's speech is disfluent in peer-play context.

By calculating the exact amount and type of disfluent speech, the clinician can then determine whether it is sufficiently different from normal expectations *and* whether it sufficiently detracts from effective communication. If one or both of these conditions exist, a fluency disorder may be present. The clinician can also use the speech observation to determine the presence of secondary features (e.g., escape and avoidance behaviors). These emerge as stuttering progresses and thus may provide a useful index of the extent of the problem.

Questionnaire and Survey. The clinician uses questionnaires and surveys to study an individual's feelings and attitudes about stuttering and communication. These questionnaires are particularly helpful for estimating the extent to which experiences with stuttering have resulted in the accumulation of negative feelings about speaking. One such questionnaire is the Communication Attitude Test by Brutton (1985; cited in Vanryckeghem & Brutten, 1997). It contains 35 true/false statements that explore an individual's attitudes toward communication; examples include "I like to talk" and "People don't seem to like the way I talk." By 6 years of age, children who stutter have more negative attitudes toward communication than do other children, and these tend to increase in magnitude for older children (Vanryckeghem & Brutten, 1997). The Adolescent Communication Questionnaire (Bray, Kehle, Lawless, & Theodore, 2003) examines adolescents' confidence and sense of self-efficacy related to specific communication activities, such as ordering food at a restaurant or telling a joke. This questionnaire is shown in Figure 12-5. Adolescents who stutter give lower ratings on individual items on this questionnaire than do adolescents who do not stutter (average 3.5 vs. 4.6; Bray et al., 2003).

Direct Testing. The clinician also uses formal norm- and criterion-referenced tests to study an individual's speech and language skills. Such tests examine an individual's skills in syntax, vocabulary, phonology, and pragmatics and compare performance against expectations. Speech and language performance is an important part of the fluency assessment, given the prevalence with which speech-language impairments coexist with fluency disorders in children, adolescents, and adults.

Diagnosis

After the clinician administers a comprehensive fluency assessment, a diagnosis is made, based on all of the accumulated evidence. As a general rule, a fluency disorder is more likely to be diagnosed when the following are observed during assessment (Guitar, 1998):

1. Ten or more total disfluencies in 100 words
2. Three or more stuttering-like disfluencies in 100 words, summed across monosyllabic word repetitions, sound repetitions, prolongations, and blocks
3. Physical escape behaviors, such as head nods and eye blinks
4. Verbal avoidance behaviors, such as word substitutions

In addition to determining whether a disorder is present, assessment findings also characterize the severity of the disorder. A common estimate of stuttering severity is the Stuttering Severity Index (SSI; Riley, 1972). It estimates severity based on three variables, to each of which the clinician assigns points. The first variable is the frequency of disfluencies—the percentage of disfluencies within a 100-word sample. Frequency estimates range from 1% (2 points) to more than 29% (18 points). The second variable is duration of blocks, ranging from none (0 points) to longer than 60 seconds (7 points). The third variable is physical concomitants, which encompass distracting sounds (e.g., sniffing), facial grimaces (e.g., jaw jerking), head movements (e.g., turning away), and extremity movements (e.g., foot tapping). To each the clinician assigns points, ranging from none (0 points) to severe (5 points). The clinician then sums the points allocated to each variable and produces an SSI score and a severity rating: very mild, mild, moderate, severe, or very severe.

Prognosis

The prognosis describes the likelihood that the symptoms of a disorder will be resolved with time and/or treatment. A good prognosis predicts that a disorder will be resolved or will reverse its course, whereas a poor prognosis predicts that resolution is unlikely. The prognosis

FIGURE 12-5 Adolescent communication questionnaire.

We are interested in learning more about your speaking ability. Your responses are confidential.

DIRECTIONS: How much confidence do you have about doing each of the behaviors listed below? Circle the number that best represents your confidence.

No way, I would be too uptight to speak — 1 2 3 4 5 — No problem, I would be very confident speaking

No way … No problem	
1 2 3 4 5	1. Talking with a parent about a movie.
1 2 3 4 5	2. Talking to a brother or sister at the dinner table.
1 2 3 4 5	3. Talking with three friends during lunch at school.
1 2 3 4 5	4. Talking with a large group of friends during lunch at school.
1 2 3 4 5	5. Answering the telephone.
1 2 3 4 5	6. Talking with the teacher during class.
1 2 3 4 5	7. Talking with the principal.
1 2 3 4 5	8. Asking a friend to come to your house after school.
1 2 3 4 5	9. Arguing with a brother or sister.
1 2 3 4 5	10. Asking a parent if you can spend the night at a friend's house.
1 2 3 4 5	11. Telling a new friend about your family.
1 2 3 4 5	12. Telling your teacher your birth date.
1 2 3 4 5	13. Calling your friend on the telephone.
1 2 3 4 5	14. Asking your parent if you can go to bed later than usual.
1 2 3 4 5	15. Talking to a family member on the telephone.
1 2 3 4 5	16. Explaining how to play a game to your friends.
1 2 3 4 5	17. Asking a librarian for help in finding a book.
1 2 3 4 5	18. Talking with a friend alone.
1 2 3 4 5	19. Asking a sales clerk how much an item costs.
1 2 3 4 5	20. Telling a police officer your home address.
1 2 3 4 5	21. Calling a store to find out what time it opens.
1 2 3 4 5	22. Talking to a teacher alone after class.
1 2 3 4 5	23. Reading aloud to a whole class.
1 2 3 4 5	24. Reading aloud to 5 classmates.
1 2 3 4 5	25. Reading aloud to your family.
1 2 3 4 5	26. Speaking to your pet.
1 2 3 4 5	27. Raising your hand to ask the teacher a question.
1 2 3 4 5	28. Answering a question in class.
1 2 3 4 5	29. Asking a question in class.
1 2 3 4 5	30. Ordering food at a restaurant.
1 2 3 4 5	31. Telling a joke.
1 2 3 4 5	32. Giving a book report in front of the class.
1 2 3 4 5	33. Taking a speaking part in a school play.
1 2 3 4 5	34. Reading aloud just to your teacher.
1 2 3 4 5	35. Talking with a large group of your friends.
1 2 3 4 5	36. Talking aloud to yourself with no one else there.
1 2 3 4 5	37. Talking with the school secretary.
1 2 3 4 5	38. Reading a book aloud with no one else in the room.
1 2 3 4 5	39. Talking to your teacher on the telephone.

Source: From "The Relationship of Self-Efficacy and Depression to Stuttering" by M. A. Bray, T. J. Kehle, K. A. Lawless, and L. A. Theodore, 2003, *American Journal of Speech-Language Pathology, 12*, 425–431. Copyright 2003 by ASHA. Reprinted with permission.

is a subjective decision make by the clinician, based on careful scrutiny of the complex body of information aggregated through the assessment process. For fluency disorders prognosis is complicated; the likelihood of resolution relates to many factors, including the age of stuttering onset, length of time since onset, type and number of core features, type and number of secondary features, and presence of such individual risk factors as gender, family history, coexisting speech and language disorders, and available support systems.

Treatment Recommendations

Discussion Point: *To what extent would you consider the treatment pursued by Mr. Cho in Box 12-1 to be an evidence-based treatment?*

When a fluency disorder is diagnosed, the SLP recommends a specific course of action derived from (1) in-depth knowledge of the client, (2) clinical experience with fluency disorders, and (3) knowledge of the current scientific research on fluency disorders. Treatment recommendations derived from these information sources are called **evidence-based practice** (Ingham, 2003; Justice & Fey, 2004), a term that emphasizes the clinician's use of the scientific literature when making treatment decisions.

How Are Fluency Disorders Treated?

The pursuit of effective approaches to eliminating stuttering has a long history. As described so colorfully in Bobrick's (1995) *Knotted Tongues: Stuttering in History and the Quest for a Cure,* historical treatments included Demosthenes' placement of stones in his mouth to reduce his stuttering, which was undoubtedly less painful than the bloodletting of the tongue practiced by physicians in the Middle Ages. Other treatments included electroshock therapy, tongue lozenges, beetroot nose drops, tongue wrapping, and immersion of the head in cold water followed by eating and vomiting horseradish. Many of these historical treatments were based on faulty understanding of both fluency and disfluency. For instance, one treatment approach from more than 1,000 years ago involved drying out, because experts thought that excess moisture and humidity caused stuttering (Bobrick, 1995). In one approach to drying out, the tongue was rubbed with salt, honey, and sage, and the neck and ears were cauterized and blistered.

Fortunately, scientific knowledge of stuttering causes and treatments continues to grow, and the tenets of scientific reasoning and empirical evidence have become the norm when making treatment decisions for fluency disorders. Described here are the current treatments based on the best available scientific evidence for borderline, beginning, intermediate, and advanced stuttering.

Borderline Stuttering

As mentioned earlier, there is some controversy as to whether young children who show characteristics of borderline stuttering should be provided with treatment and early intervention or whether a wait-and-see approach is more appropriate. This argument focuses specifically on children who are between 2 and 5 years of age and who show stuttering-like disfluencies in their speech but are not advanced in stuttering beyond borderline characteristics (Curlee & Yairi, 1997).

Professionals who argue for early intervention for these children emphasize that treatment is needed to prevent them from progressing to more advanced levels of stuttering. These professionals stress that (1) it is impossible to know for sure which children will recover from early stuttering without treatment, (2) the consequences of an established stuttering disorder can be both devastating and consequential to the life of the child and the family, and (3) early treatments do no harm and are more likely to be effective than later treatments are (Zebrowski, 1997).

Other professionals advocate withholding treatment for 6 months or longer after stuttering begins (Curlee & Yairi, 1997). These experts emphasize research showing that (1) the majority of children spontaneously recover from stuttering within a year or two after onset, (2) little evidence supports the effectiveness of earlier rather than later treatment, and (3) treatment should be based on clear indicators that a child is likely to progress as a stutterer (Curlee & Yairi, 1997). This wait-and-see approach is not a new concept: as Bobrick reported (1995), Mercurialis' 1583 *Treatise on the Disease of Children* argued that children should not be treated for stuttering until at least 7 years of age "since before that time it cannot be known whether their speech is defective or not" and many children are spontaneously cured.

Discussion Point: *As you might guess, the debate over early treatment versus wait-and-see is a heated one. If you were a parent, which would be your preference? If you were a clinician, which would you endorse? Why?*

Future research will undoubtedly determine the costs and benefits of early intervention for borderline stuttering. Currently, treatment decisions are based largely on the clinical judgment of the professional consulted, with input from the family of the child and other involved professionals. When treatment is pursued, indirect treatment models are often used rather than direct treatment delivered by a therapist.

Indirect Treatments

Treatments implemented by parents within the home environment are frequently used for borderline stuttering. These parent-implemented treatments are often called *indirect treatment*, because the clinician provides the treatment indirectly through the parents. Two popular models of indirect treatment are environmental modification and operant training.

Environmental modification models emphasize reduction of the mismatch between environmental demands and the child's capacity for fluent speech. These models typically involve training parents to both reduce environmental demands and promote fluency models. Parents are counseled about ways to reduce demands on fluency, such as frequent interruptions, questions, and a lack of listening, especially when children are fatigued, excited, or anxious (Gottwald & Starkweather, 1995; Rustin & Cook, 1995). Clinicians provide parents with specific suggestions:

- Avoid putting the child on the spot during social situations
- Repeat what the child says to show that you are listening
- Make comments when talking with the child rather than asking questions
- Modify activities that seem particularly stressful to the child (Nelson, 1985)

Clinicians are also likely to give parents specific guidance on how to provide improved models of fluency for their children. Many clinicians recommend regular periods of quiet time, in which parents devote a special length of time to their children that is characterized by undivided attention, no time pressures, and the pleasure of talking together. During this time the parent focuses on positive communication qualities of the child, such as selection of words or conversational participation (Gottwald & Starkweather, 1995). And the parent models speech that is comfortable, smooth, and unhurried, as in the last example here:

1. Haveyoufinishedyourdinner?
2. Have you finishedyourdinner?
3. Have you finished yourdinner?
4. Have you finished your dinner (Graham, Conture, & Schwenk, 2004)?

To assist the parent in making these changes, the clinician is likely to provide ongoing and periodic support to the family. The clinician might see the family monthly to monitor the child's fluency, discuss progress in the home treatment, and counsel the parent, particularly if the parent is anxious about the child's fluency (Zebrowski, 1997). Some families might participate in a parent fluency group, in which parents share the strategies they use to promote fluency.

Operant training models take a different approach, viewing stuttering as a learned behavior that can be eliminated through contingent stimulation (Onslow, Andrews, & Lincoln, 1994). *Contingent stimulation* refers to the way in which adults respond to children's disfluencies and uses these responses to stimulate children's production of fluent speech. In operant training models, such as the Lidcombe Program of Sydney, Australia, parents receive training in three techniques they use to shape their child's use of fluent speech (Onslow et al., 1994):

1. *Identify disfluencies and provide positive input:* Parents learn to identify disfluencies and to correct disfluent speech in a nonpunitive and positive manner, as in "Oops, that was a bumpy word" (Onslow et al., 1994, p. 1246). Parents also learn to praise fluent speech, as in "You said that very smoothly."
2. *Prompt fluent speech:* Parents prompt the child to produce fluent speech in normal everyday speaking situations, as in "Let's see if you can have really smooth speech while we are at the grocery store."
3. *Prompt self-correction:* Parents help the child identify when disfluencies occur and self-correct, as in "I heard a bumpy word. Did you hear it? See if you can say it again."

When used with children between 2 and 5 years of age, operant training programs appear to be effective in reducing the likelihood of ongoing fluency problems (Lincoln & Onslow, 1997).

Beginning Stuttering

For those who show characteristics of beginning stuttering, treatment goals focus on eliminating the core disfluencies, which are most likely to be repetitions and prolongations. At this level secondary features, including negative feelings toward communication, have not yet emerged and thus are not typically addressed in treatment. Treatment approaches utilize direct treatment as well as indirect treatment, including parent counseling.

Current Approaches to Stuttering Treatment

Two approaches to stuttering treatment predominate in the field today (Guitar, 1998): stuttering modification therapy and fluency shaping therapy. These two approaches differ not only in the methods used to treat fluency disorders, but in the overall goal of treatment (see Table 12-5). The goal of **stuttering modification** therapy is to help the person who stutters to better manage the moment of stuttering—that moment when an individual repeats, prolongs, or blocks on a sound. As stuttering progresses, these moments become more intense and long-lasting; they are what the person with a fluency disorder fears and strives to avoid or escape. Stuttering modification therapy focuses on helping the individual manage these moments and stutter more effortlessly and less tensely. Thus, the outcome of treatment is *controlled stuttering,* coupled with careful attention to feelings and emotions toward stuttering and communication. The end goal is for moments of stuttering to be hardly noticeable and completely manageable. Disfluency is viewed as a problem that one can learn to manage.

The goal of **fluency shaping** therapy is to help the person who stutters produce fluent speech more often, potentially eradicating disfluencies completely. This therapy focuses on increasing the amount of fluent speech produced as an individual progresses through a highly structured program. Fluency shaping pays little attention to the individual's feelings and emotions toward stuttering; the end goal is for fluent speech to predominate and moments of stuttering to disappear, resulting in *controlled fluency.* Completely fluent speech is the therapeutic goal.

TABLE 12-5 Key principles in stuttering modification and fluency shaping therapy

	Stuttering Modification	Fluency Shaping
Goal	To manage and modify the moment of stuttering (i.e., controlled stuttering) and reduce fear and anxiety associated with stuttering	To increase the amount of fluent speech and eliminate moments of stuttering (i.e., controlled fluency)
Focus	To teach how to modify disfluencies using cancellations and pull-outs, to reduce escape and avoidance behaviors, and to reduce anxiety and fear	To establish fluent speech by using a slower speech rate, more relaxed breathing, easy onsets into speech, and soft contact while speaking
Approach	Involves counseling; loosely structured; practice with different techniques in clinic and then in different settings	Highly structured; practice with different techniques in clinic and then in different settings

Source: Based on B. Guitar (1998).

Stuttering Modification. Charles Van Riper, who died in 1994 at the age of 88, was one of the greatest authorities on stuttering and the original champion of stuttering modification. For this reason this approach is sometimes called the Van Riper method. Stuttering modification used with beginning stutterers emphasizes positive fluency models, fluency-building techniques, and desensitization (Guitar, 1998; Van Riper, 1973). The therapist provides positive fluency models during comfortable, well-paced interactions, in which the therapist uses simple words and phrases intermixed with generous pauses and periods of silence. The therapist introduces the child to fluency-building techniques through games focused on improving the child's rhythm and timing during talking, such as chanting familiar rhymes. The therapist also focuses on desensitizing the child to disruptors of smooth speech and increasing the child's ability to manage disfluencies. The therapist uses specific exercises designed by Van Riper that build the capacity to handle fluency disruptors.

Fluency Shaping. Like stuttering modification, fluency shaping focuses on building the beginning stutterer's capacity for and experience with fluent speech. However, fluency shaping uses different techniques to reach this goal. The Lidcombe Program described earlier is an example of a fluency shaping approach based on operant procedures; it emphasizes positive reinforcement of fluency and negative reinforcement, or correction, of disfluencies. Parents or therapists provide regular reinforcement of periods or instances of good fluency (e.g., "That was terrific—you didn't stutter at all") in conjunction with correction of disfluencies (e.g., "That word was bumpy—say it again for me") (Lincoln & Onslow, 1997). Over time, with appropriate amounts of reinforcement, the child's production of fluent speech increases and disfluent speech decreases (Jones, Onslow, Harrison, & Packman, 2000).

Intermediate and Advanced Stuttering

Intermediate or advanced stutterers have experienced stuttering for a longer time than beginning stutterers have. Secondary features, including a complex host of escape and avoidance behaviors and negative feelings toward communication, characterize these two levels of stuttering (Guitar, 1998). Intermediate and advanced stutterers are likely to be adolescents or adults who go in and out of treatment as disfluencies change in type and severity and respond to life's challenges.

Treatment for Adolescents

Providing stuttering treatment to adolescents who are intermediate or advanced stutterers is not for the fainthearted. A number of experts have commented on the challenge of working with adolescents who stutter, noting that these are among the toughest clinical cases (Daly, Simon, & Burnett-Stolnack, 1995). In addition to the well-known social, academic, psychological, and physical challenges of the adolescent period, stuttering therapies are complicated by the fact that the most well-established therapies were designed for either children or adults, not for adolescents (Blood, 1995). The treatments for adolescents need to contend with the specific challenges of this period of life—peer pressure, time commitments, the drive for autonomy and individuality, academic demands, self-doubt, self-esteem, and the like (Blood, 1995; Daly et al., 1995). Several important considerations are listed in Figure 12-6.

Both stuttering modification and fluency shaping approaches are useful for adolescents (see Ramig & Bennett, 1995). Stuttering modification emphasizes teaching the adolescent about stuttering (i.e., getting to know your stuttering) to demystify the disorder. This approach teaches adolescents how to work through instances of disfluency, using different techniques such as cancellations and pull-outs. In cancellations individuals pause after a word containing a disfluency, wait until they have control, and then repeat the word with a gentle, easy stutter, as in "He said he w-w-w-wanted . . . wanted it." In pull-outs individuals stop during a disfluency, wait until they have control, and then gradually and lightly produce the rest of the word. With both cancellations and pull-outs, the individual practices moving easily, gently, and voluntarily through disfluencies (Guitar, 1998). While learning these skills, an adolescent also learns to reduce anxiety, fear, and tension about stuttering.

Fluency shaping with adolescents, sometimes called *smooth speech treatment,* emphasizes an increase in fluent speech using a combination of operant conditioning techniques (Craig et al., 2002). Fluent speech is promoted by training the adolescent to use several techniques characteristic of smooth, or fluent, speech, including easy onset, soft contact, and continuous airflow. With *easy onset* an individual releases a soft flow of air prior to initiating

FIGURE 12-6 **Suggestions for delivering stuttering treatment to adolescents.**

- Improve the adolescent's knowledge of stuttering, including what causes it and how it is treated
- Teach cognitive and self-instructional strategies that promote the adolescent's awareness of and responsibility for treatment outcomes
- Introduce relaxation strategies to promote awareness and use of relaxation techniques
- Use mental imagery in which the adolescent pictures himself or herself in different speaking situations, communicating fluently
- Model the use of positive self-talk and the use of positive language when describing self
- Teach positive coping strategies, such as how to express negative emotions and how to recover after stuttering episodes
- Introduce assertiveness training and emphasize alternative means of asserting oneself, such as art, exercise, and writing
- Identify social support systems available to the adolescent, including friends, teachers, and family members

Sources: Based on Blood (1995); Daly, Simon, and Burnett-Stolnack (1995).

a word or phrase, providing a gentle entrance into speaking. *Soft contact* describes the use of gentle and soft movement of the articulators, including their contact with one another (e.g., a soft touch of the tongue to the teeth when producing the first sound in "to"). With *continuous airflow* the airflow continues across phrases and words, decreasing the stops and starts of normal airflow for speech. These and other techniques are used to increase the adolescent's production of fluent speech and elimination of disfluencies.

Treatment for Adults

Treatment of stuttering in adults utilizes both stuttering modification and fluency shaping approaches or an integration of the two. For the adult who may have experienced stuttering for years, treatment emphasizes the following:

1. *Knowledge about stuttering:* Treatment helps adults understand and confront the disorder of stuttering. They can examine their own core and secondary features and even confront their own stuttering in a mirror or video to develop an intimate catalog of their own behaviors.
2. *Reduction of negative feelings:* Treatment helps adults reduce their fear, embarrassment, and discomfort with stuttering. They are guided to view their stuttering with interest and curiosity, to discuss stuttering openly and honestly, and to resist word and situation avoidances.
3. *Fluency building:* Treatment helps adults increase their use of fluency-enhancing strategies and work through moments of stuttering. Strategies to increase fluency include talking at a slower rate and using easy onsets and soft contact. Strategies to help adults work through moments of stuttering—or to stutter more easily—include using cancellations and pull-outs. Treatment helps adults maintain improvements outside the therapy room (Guitar, 1998).

As a complement to these approaches, pharmaceutical intervention is increasingly being explored for stuttering treatment. Several medications used in the treatment of anxiety and depression have been shown to reduce stuttering symptoms, including several selective-serotonin reuptake inhibitors (SSRIs; Costa & Kroll, 2000; Riley et al., 2001). The use of medication to treat stuttering provides a promising and interesting avenue for future research on fluency disorders.

Case Study and Clinical Problem Solving

SPEECH AND LANGUAGE EVALUATION REPORT

New River Speech and Hearing Clinic

Client: Harry Benson
Age: 3 years, 8 months
Parents: Amy and Harold Benson
Referral Source: Parents
File No: 02-08-9982
Date of Birth: 6-15-01
Evaluation Date: 2-28-05

Background and History

Harry was referred to the New River Speech and Hearing Clinic for a speech-language evaluation because of Mrs. Benson's concerns regarding possible stuttering behaviors. Mrs. Benson reported that Harry demonstrates increasing frustration due to difficulties in communicating.

Information regarding Harry's developmental history was obtained in a parent interview conducted on 2-28-05. Mrs. Benson served as the informant. She reported that her pregnancy with Harry was unremarkable. Major developmental milestones were reached within normal limits, including motor (e.g., walked alone at approximately 1 year) and language (e.g., babbled at approximately 5 months). No feeding, swallowing, or other oral-motor problems have been observed. Harry has experienced no notable illnesses with the exception of two instances of high fever and two bouts of influenza. Harry lives at home with his parents (both students at the local university) and has no siblings.

Harry first demonstrated stuttering behaviors in the fall of 2004, which Mrs. Benson attributed to an increase in language skill (at that time Harry began to speak in longer sentences). During the month of December, when Harry's parents were home more regularly and he spent less time with his babysitter, Mrs. Benson reported that Harry's disfluencies disappeared. These behaviors reappeared, however, in January as Harry began to go to his babysitter's house again. Mrs. Benson believes that the day care environment may contribute to his disfluencies, as Harry does not like going to the sitter's house. In the last month, Harry has displayed disfluencies frequently in spontaneous speech, estimated by his mother at about 10% of his words. Harry has demonstrated a great deal of frustration recently regarding his difficulties in communicating, according to his mother. For example, when talking with his grandparents, Harry was very disfluent and unable to communicate, which resulted in his crying and saying, "I can't talk." Mrs. Benson has obtained information on the Internet on how to enhance Harry's communication skills and reported that she and her husband have been organizing "quiet times" at night for Harry to talk with them. She also has been giving him positive feedback regarding his communication attempts (such as "I love to hear you talk").

During the clinical assessment, Harry was somewhat quiet and appeared to be shy. He grew more communicative with the examiner by the end of the session. However, the number of spontaneous utterances was low.

Oral Examination

Examination of Harry's oral-motor mechanism was conducted. Labial structure was unremarkable and within normal limits for function. Dentition and alignment appeared normal. Lingual movement ranges were good. Harry showed no difficulty with volitional oral-motor control.

Voice

Harry's vocal quality appeared to be within normal limits.

Fluency

Core Features: Harry engaged in play with his mother and the examiner for a 45-min period. No disfluencies were observed in imitation or specific rote speaking tasks (e.g., reciting numbers, reciting the alphabet), but disfluencies were observed in conversational routines for 11% of his words. Disfluencies were primarily part-word repetitions (90% of disfluencies) and ranged from no instances per utterance to more than three in a five-word utterance. Some single-syllable whole-word repetitions and sound prolongations were observed, but these occurred with much less frequency than part-word repetitions. When part-word repetitions did occur, no abnormality of the repeated syllable was observed (i.e., no tension, abruptness, or schwa insertion). Harry typically persevered through the repetitions until the target word was produced. During the evaluation, he did not demonstrate an overt awareness of his disfluencies when they occurred.

Secondary Features. No associated motor behaviors were evident. Some facial tension was observed, as well as blinking of the eyes. Harry's mother reported having observed instances of facial grimacing, fist clenching, and feet stamping, none of which were observed at present.

Harry demonstrated some word avoidance during the evaluation (i.e., changing a word). Mrs. Benson reported the following insights concerning Harry's feelings: (1) he often gives up speaking when a disfluency occurs; (2) he frequently shows frustration regarding speech; and (3) he sometimes seems worried or anxious about speech. It is possible that Harry is being teased at day care regarding his speech.

Phonology and Articulation

Speech-sound production was not formally assessed, but sound production appeared age appropriate.

Language

The Preschool Language Scale–3 was administered to examine Harry's expressive and receptive language skills. Results indicated that Harry's language skills were well within normal limits, with a standard score of 118 for auditory comprehension and 111 for expressive communication.

Clinical Impressions/Recommendations

This evaluation provided evidence of stuttering-like disfluencies in Harry's conversational speech. These disfuencies may be resulting in feelings of frustration and perhaps anxiety toward communication. As explained to Mrs. Benson, most typically developing children are disfluent to some extent, and this is particularly true for children of Harry's age. However, observational evidence suggests that Harry's patterns of disfluency may not be normal disfluencies but are characteristic of borderline stuttering. Observations included these: (1) Harry demonstrates part-word repetitions and some prolongations; (2) when repetitions occur at the beginning of words, the number of units repeated is typically more than two units; and (3) he is demonstrating frustration and discomfort with communication. These may be considered warning signs for which ongoing observation is warranted to monitor and enhance Harry's fluency development.

All of the above information was discussed in detail with Mrs. Benson, and options for intervention were discussed, particularly the implementation of environmental modification to improve Harry's fluency in the home. Continuing observation by parents and follow-up assessment and/or consultation with this SLP in 2 or 3 months are recommended. Recommended environmental modification includes the following:

1. Limit situations that make strong communicative demands on Harry
2. Provide lots of listening time (as parents are already doing in the evenings)
3. Provide praise and positive feedback for Harry's communicative attempts
4. Model a slow and even rate of speech for Harry
5. Provide pleasurable speaking/communicative experiences for Harry (e.g., telling stories, singing, making rhymes)
6. Try to reduce time pressures for Harry when he is speaking

Enclosed is a copy of a pamphlet from the Stuttering Foundation of America titled *If Your Child Stutters: Seven Ways to Help*. This pamphlet provides very good additional information to enhance Harry's communication skills.

It was a pleasure meeting Harry and his mother, Mrs. Benson. I hope to be informed of Harry's progress and to see Harry and Mrs. Benson again in several months for a follow-up observation and consultation. If Harry's fluency changes in any way or if there are questions about this report, please feel free to contact me immediately.

Michael Lam, M.Ed., CCC-SLP
Speech-Language Pathologist

CLINICAL PROBLEM SOLVING

1. Harry's evaluation was conducted in a clinical setting. How might the clinical observations have differed if the evaluation had been conducted in Harry's home?
2. The clinician concluded that Harry showed signs of borderline stuttering. How serious is borderline stuttering? How should this information be communicated to Harry's parents?
3. The clinician provided suggestions for environmental modification in the home to improve fluency. In your opinion, what is the likelihood that these suggestions will be followed? What are some other possibilities for home-based activities to improve fluency?
4. The clinician did not recommend a clinic-based treatment program. Why do you think he did not recommend treatment by a clinician in a clinic?

CHAPTER SUMMARY

A fluency disorder occurs when a person's ability to produce speech effortlessly and automatically is significantly compromised by the presence of disfluencies, specifically sound and word repetitions, sound prolongations, and blocks. When these core features persist over time, the individual with a fluency disorder develops secondary features as well, including escape and avoidance behaviors and negative feelings toward speaking, including fear.

The majority of fluency disorders emerge during early childhood and are referred to as developmental fluency disorders or developmental stuttering. Although about 5% of the population has experienced developmental stuttering at some time, only about 1% of the population continues to experience stuttering in adolescence and adulthood. For the others stuttering is resolved either therapeutically or spontaneously. Acquired fluency disorders occur less frequently than developmental fluency disorders but may occur at any time as a result of trauma, disease, or illness.

A prevalent classification system focuses on the symptoms of the disorder, differentiating five levels of disfluency. Normal disfluency is the first level, which describes children whose disfluencies reflect normal processes. Borderline stuttering describes children who show early signs or risk factors of stuttering, namely a higher rate of disfluencies when speaking (more than 10 per 100 words) and the presence of part-word repetitions and sound prolongations. Beginning stuttering is the third level; it describes children who show clear stuttering behaviors, including sound repetitions, sound prolongations, and blocks. Additionally, the beginning stutterer begins to show escape and avoidance behaviors and negative feelings toward moments of stuttering. Intermediate and advanced stuttering are the fourth and fifth levels of fluency disorders, respectively. These describe individuals who may have experienced years of stuttering and who show complex secondary features, including significant negative feelings toward stuttering, such as fear and embarrassment.

Assessment of fluency disorders is the domain of the speech-language pathologist, who carefully studies an individual's speech in a variety of situations to determine the type and number of disfluencies. The SLP also carefully identifies any secondary features, including physical behaviors that signal escape from and avoidance of moments of stuttering, as well as the individual's feelings toward stuttering. When the fluency assessment is completed, the SLP provides an estimate of severity, for which one common metric is the Stuttering Severity Index. Fluency disorders range from very mild to very severe.

Treatment of fluency disorders involves a variety of different evidence-based techniques, most commonly differentiated into those treatments that emphasize stuttering modification and those that emphasize fluency shaping. Stuttering modification focuses on helping the individual work through and modify the moment of stuttering, whereas fluency shaping focuses on reducing disfluencies and promoting overall speaking fluency. Both approaches are useful; selection is usually determined by SLP and client preferences.

KEY TERMS

advanced stuttering, p. 399
avoidance behaviors, p. 403
beginning stuttering, p. 399
between-word disfluency, p. 402
block, p. 390
borderline stuttering, p. 397
circumlocution, p. 404
cluttering, p. 400
core features, p. 390
developmental stuttering, p. 393
disfluency, p. 390
escape behaviors, p. 403
evidence-based practice, p. 418
fluency, p. 390
fluency shaping, p. 420
intermediate stuttering, p. 399
neurogenic stuttering, p. 396
precipitating factors, p. 406
predisposing factors, p. 406
prolongation, p. 390
psychogenic stuttering, p. 396
repetition, p. 390
secondary features, p. 391
situation avoidance, p. 404
sound avoidance, p. 404
stuttering, p. 387
stuttering modification, p. 420
stuttering-like disfluencies, p. 395
within-word disfluency, p. 402
word avoidance, p. 404

ON THE WEB

Check out the Companion Website! On it you will find

- suggested readings
- reflection questions
- a self-study quiz
- discussion of hot topics in fluency disorders
- description of current technological innovations in fluency disorders
- links to additional online resources

Pediatric Hearing Loss

L. A. Pakulski

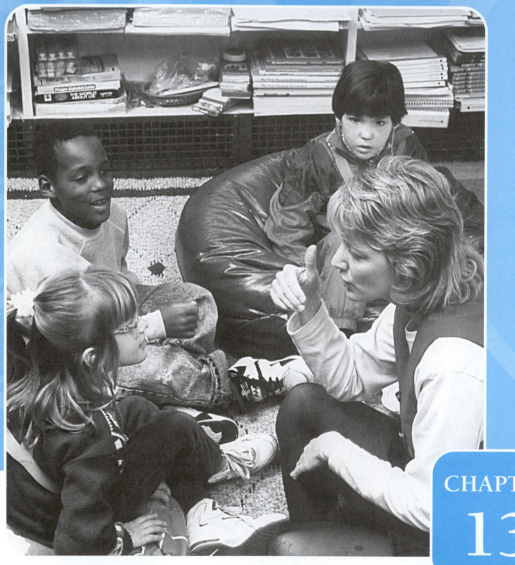

CHAPTER 13

FOCUS QUESTIONS

This chapter answers the following questions:

1. What is pediatric hearing loss?
2. How is pediatric hearing loss classified?
3. What are the defining characteristics of prevalent types of pediatric hearing loss?
4. How is pediatric hearing loss identified?
5. How is pediatric hearing loss treated?
6. What is an auditory processing disorder, and how is it identified and treated?

INTRODUCTION

Deafness is a much worse misfortune [than blindness] for it means the loss of the most vital stimulus—the sound of the voice that brings language, sets thoughts astir, and keeps us in the intellectual company of man. *(Helen Keller, 1933)*

The sense of hearing is a miraculous one. The ear contains the smallest bones in the human body and specialized sensory cells that can process sounds ranging from the drop of a pin to the takeoff of an airplane. The human ear can also perceive minute changes in pitch and loudness, recognize a familiar voice on the telephone, and differentiate among the many sounds at an amusement park. In short, hearing links us to the world around us and is a remarkable capability. When an individual's hearing is diminished or lost because of injury, illness, or even genetics, the results are life altering.

The human auditory system is a complicated mechanism. It is responsible for not only the detection of sounds, but also the categorization and comprehension of sounds. For instance, it distinguishes speech from nonspeech sounds and then enables comprehension of speech within the language centers. Because of these complexities, impairment of the auditory mechanism is also complex, resulting in many types of hearing problems. Consider the elderly person who complains, "I can hear just fine, if only people wouldn't mumble." This individual is able to detect the overall loudness of sound but misses enough auditory cues to make it difficult to understand what others say.

Speech-language pathologists, audiologists, and educators play important roles in diagnosing and treating children with hearing loss. However, to work effectively with these children, these professionals must understand the auditory mechanism and its disorders, the impact of the disorder on children's social and academic selves, and a variety of intervention strategies to promote the child's achievement possibilities.

What Is Pediatric Hearing Loss?

Definition

A pediatric **hearing loss** refers to a condition in which a child or adolescent is unable to detect or distinguish the range of sounds normally available to the human ear. In some

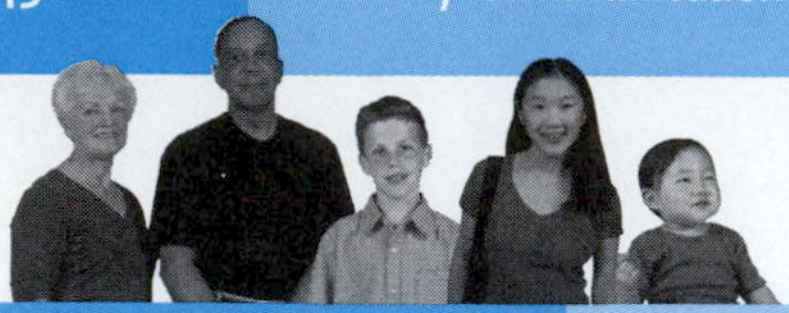

BOX 13-1 Pediatric Hearing Loss: Case Examples

Mesha is a 12-month-old child who was recently diagnosed with profound sensorineural hearing loss. Her father, Michael, also has a significant hearing loss and considers himself Deaf, that is, a member of the Deaf community. Michael was raised in the Deaf community by his parents and grandparents; all of his siblings are deaf, too. Michael's family and friends communicate with American Sign Language (ASL) and with e-mail and instant messaging on the Internet. He feels fortunate to have a full and happy life.

Michael's hearing loss is not as severe as that of his siblings; he attended a mainstream school and learned to speak. However, despite his fine voice and good oral speaking skills, he chooses not to talk in most circumstances; he considers ASL his primary language. Even though he believes he received a better education than his siblings, who attended a residential school for the deaf, Michael does not want Mesha to grow up conflicted between a hearing and a deaf world. He believes that she should have a strong identity as a Deaf person. Michael's wife, Debra, agrees. Although she does not have a hearing loss, Debra embraces the Deaf community and shares her husband's conviction that Mesha should be raised with her Deaf culture first. Until Mesha was born, Debra did not feel accepted by Michael's family since she herself is not deaf. However, after having a daughter who is deaf, Debra feels that she is becoming a part of the community.

At 12 months Mesha is producing a few words in sign and actively communicates with her family. Michael and Debra have decided not to get hearing aids for Mesha. For the time being, they are satisfied that she is a well-adjusted child who interacts with her family and is learning new words every day.

Internet research

1. How large is the Deaf community in the United States?
2. How does the Deaf community view amplification devices, such as hearing aids and cochlear implants?
3. As a native user of ASL, what kind of educational programs will be available for Mesha through the U. S. public school system?

Brainstorm and discussion

1. If you were an interventionist working with Mesha and her parents, would you endorse their decision? Why or why not?
2. What challenges face children who are raised in the Deaf versus the hearing community?

Jack is a 30-month-old child with one younger sister. Although Jack's physical development was typical and age appropriate, he has not yet started talking and does not always seem to listen. At 18 months of age, his mother, Kate, reported her concerns to the pediatrician. (Since Jack had passed the infant hearing screening, there was little concern about a permanent hearing loss.) Upon inspection of Jack's ears, the pediatrician found bilateral middle ear infections. Although Jack had not shown any outward signs of infection, other than a cold and a runny nose, the pediatrician indicated that the middle ear infection was rather severe and that Jack's auditory responses would be inconsistent, possibly causing a delay in his speech and language. Jack's pediatrician recommended that the middle ear problem be cleared up through medical means and then an audiometric evaluation be conducted to ensure that Jack's hearing had returned to normal.

Jack was started on a course of medication that lasted for nearly 6 months as the bouts of ear infection continued. When he reached 2 years of age, Kate's concerns with his delayed speech and language led her to consult a speech-language pathologist. Following the evaluation, the speech-language pathologist recommended a comprehensive audiological evaluation, which found Jack to have a moderately severe mixed hearing loss at age 30 months.

Internet research

1. What are some common treatments for middle ear infection?
2. What effect does chronic middle ear infection have on the development of speech, language, audition, and other communication skills?
3. Why is the incidence of middle ear infection on the rise?

Brainstorm and discussion

1. In your opinion, what is Jack's prognosis for achieving normal speech and language milestones in the next few years?
2. Why wasn't Jack's hearing evaluated as soon as his mother noted a delay in his communication skills?
3. How might Jack's future be different if his mixed hearing loss had been identified earlier? How much difference do you think the delay in identification will make?

Lilly is a healthy 12-year-old child with a congenital, profound sensorineural hearing loss secondary to a syndrome that also affects the electrical system of her heart. However, in the first few years of life, all seemed normal for Lilly with the exception of delays in speech and language development. Despite the concerns of Lilly's mother, Lisa, the pediatrician would not approve a referral for a hearing evaluation during Lilly's first 2 years, taking a wait-and-see attitude because Lilly's position as the youngest of three children is often associated with slower communication development (according to the pediatrician).

At 3 years of age, Lilly began having seizures. Despite extensive medical testing, a cause was not established. However, while in the waiting room during one of the medical appointments, Lisa found an article about an unusual disorder that caused both deafness and seizures—Jervell and Lange-Nielsen syndrome. Lisa persuaded the pediatrician to make a referral to a cardiologist, who identified the syndrome. At age 3 Lilly was diagnosed with profound hearing loss and Jervell and Lange-Nielsen syndrome.

Although the audiologist tried to persuade Lilly's parents to begin sign language because of the severity of the hearing loss and the delay in diagnosis, Lisa and her husband, Rick, were determined that Lilly would learn to listen and speak like her family members and friends. Lisa and Rick studied Lilly's disorder, the impact of the hearing loss, and the concerns about speech and language development. They consulted with nationally recognized professionals and decided to use an auditory-verbal approach, to homeschool Lilly with their other children, and to have her receive a cochlear implant at age 5. At age 12 Lilly is a well-adjusted, articulate young lady who performs in the ballet and children's theater, reads and writes above grade level, and looks forward to her role in advocating for other children with hearing loss.

Internet research

1. How common is Jervell and Lange-Nielsen syndrome?
2. At what age is this syndrome typically diagnosed?
3. What are the advantages and disadvantages of cochlear implantation?

Brainstorm and discussion

1. What role can parents of children with hearing loss play in advocating for the needs of individuals with hearing loss?
2. What factors likely contributed to Lilly's positive outcome?

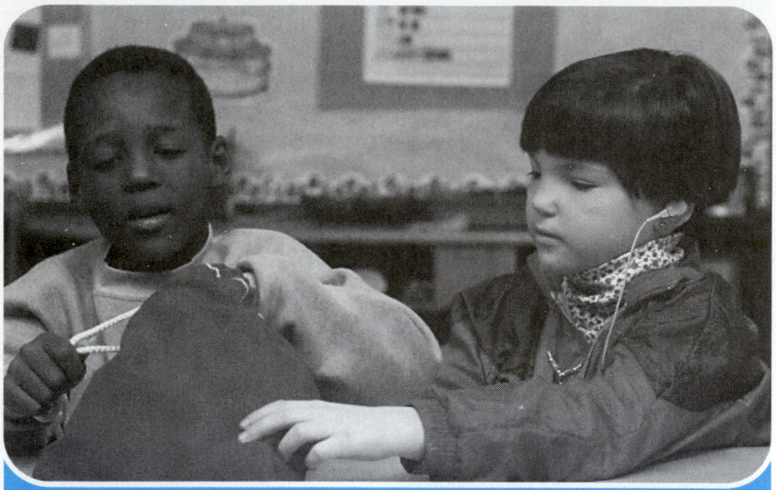

Hearing loss that occurs before a child has developed language is called a prelingual hearing loss.

cases children are born unable to hear at typical levels. In other cases children's hearing acuity is lost sometime after birth because of an illness, injury, or trauma. Chapter 3 described how the perception and processing of auditory information moves from the outer to the middle to the inner ear and then along the auditory nerve to the processing centers of the brain. Accordingly, a hearing loss can result from damage to the structures of the outer, middle, or inner ear and occasionally the auditory nerve. Hearing losses resulting from damage to the processing centers of the brain are called **auditory processing disorders** (APD) and are discussed in the final section of this chapter.

Hearing loss among children is highly variable. First, there is variability in the location of damage to the hearing structures. Hearing loss resulting from damage to the outer or middle ear is different from the loss resulting from damage to the inner ear. Second, because humans have two ears, hearing loss varies in whether it affects both ears, called a *bilateral* hearing loss, or whether it affects only one ear, called a *unilateral* hearing loss. Third, hearing loss varies considerably in the extent to which hearing acuity is impacted. Some children exhibit slight or minimal loss, whereas others have a profound loss, in which hearing is not functionally available as a sense.

Hearing loss also varies in how long it is present—that is, its *chronicity.* A short-term hearing loss is present for only a brief period of time, as it is with children who have infections of the middle ear that are resolved in a week or two. A fluctuating hearing loss is essentially a short-term hearing loss that reappears periodically. A permanent hearing loss is a condition that is not going away, and a progressive hearing loss is a condition that grows worse over time. In addition, hearing loss in children varies in its timing. Hearing loss may be present at birth—a **congenital hearing loss**. Other hearing loss occurs soon after birth but before a child has developed language—a **prelingual hearing loss**, which also includes all types of congenital loss. Hearing loss that develops after birth is an acquired hearing loss, and if it occurs in later childhood or adolescence after language skills are well established, it is considered a **postlingual hearing loss**.

Terminology

Many terms are used to describe hearing loss and the persons affected by this condition. A hearing loss is often called *hearing impairment, hearing disorder, deafness,* or being *hard of hearing.* In this chapter we use the term *hearing loss* to emphasize the decrease in hearing acuity that is the hallmark of this condition. Terms such as *hearing impairment* and *hearing disorder* imply abnormality of the auditory system or hearing function and indicate the impact of the loss on a person's life. However, not all cases of hearing loss result in disability or disordered functioning. With early identification a child may have a hearing loss but may not exhibit impaired abilities. Thus, the term *hearing loss* is preferred because it focuses solely on the physical condition that is present and carries no connotation of handicap.

When describing people with hearing loss, it is appropriate to refer to them as having hearing loss or being **hard of hearing**. **Deaf** is also acceptable but is typically reserved for those persons whose hearing loss is severe. *Deafness* is commonly thought of as a complete loss of hearing, but even those with profound hearing loss retain some amount of residual hearing, making true deafness—that is, the inability to hear at all—extremely rare. *Deaf* with a capital *D* denotes a member of the **Deaf community**. Those individuals whose hearing loss is severe but who do not identify with the Deaf community use the term *deaf* with a lowercase *d*.

Prevalence and Incidence

The reported prevalence of hearing loss among children varies significantly, depending on the criteria used to identify the loss. Some reports include only profound loss, whereas others include all types of hearing loss, even minimal and temporary losses. The rates also vary according to the age group of children studied. Historically, statistics showed only 1 or 2 children per 1,000 as born with significant hearing loss. However, universal newborn screening programs are identifying more children as exhibiting significant loss at birth, indicating that children have been previously underidentified. The early hearing detection and intervention (EDHI) program found 5 to 6 infants per 1,000 children as born with hearing loss (Center for Disease Control and Prevention, 2001). This apparent discrepancy is most likely due to previous classification of hearing loss as acquired when it was actually congenital.

Although relatively few children of school age exhibit severe or profound permanent hearing loss—estimated at about 1–2% of students—a surprisingly large number of students exhibit hearing loss that is serious enough to impact their educational achievement. Estimates from research conducted in the last 2 decades suggest that about 8% of school children have a hearing loss that is educationally significant (American Speech-Language-Hearing Association [ASHA], 2005a). The term *educationally significant* refers to a hearing loss that is serious enough to impact a child's ability to perform well educationally. About one third of these students also exhibit additional disabilities, which increase their educational risk (ASHA, 2005a). Currently, in American schools about 70,000 students between the ages of 6 and 21 receive specific educational services solely for hearing loss or deafness (U.S. Department of Education, 2002).

There are several reasons for the high rates of hearing loss among school children (ASHA, 2005a). First, these prevalence estimates include cases of acquired hearing loss attributable to middle ear infections; current estimates suggest that 35% of children experience ongoing middle ear infections throughout childhood (ASHA, 2005a), which typically result in intermittent hearing loss that is mild to moderate. Second, the hearing apparatus is a delicate yet complex set of structures that can be negatively impacted through a host of causes. Prevalence estimates include cases of congenital hearing loss resulting from prenatal genetic influences (i.e., heredity, genetic syndromes), prenatal or perinatal injuries (e.g., birth trauma, fetal alcohol exposure), and peri- or postnatal illnesses (e.g., meningitis, measles). Identification methods are constantly improving so that hearing loss resulting from these many causes can be more readily identified.

Impact

Given the integrative relationships among hearing, speech, language, and communication, hearing loss in children varies considerably in the extent to which it impacts these areas of development. In many ways the impact on communication is the major handicapping influence of hearing loss. If communication is not affected, hearing loss may have little or no impact on a child's life and should not be seen as a disability. This is true, for instance, of children who are born congenitally deaf, are reared to speak American Sign Language (ASL) as their first language, and have a community in which to use this native language. On the other hand, if communication ability is compromised and children with hearing loss do not develop a native language in a timely manner, hearing loss may have a significant effect on a child's life, including the ability to develop relationships with parents and peers, to succeed academically, and to be involved with extracurricular activities. In such cases hearing loss may exert a handicapping influence on broad areas of development.

What is particularly important in determining the impact of hearing loss is how a family responds to the loss and when the loss is identified. If hearing loss is identified early and the child's family responds proactively and intensively, the hearing loss may have little if any adverse impact on the child's life, even if the loss is severe. Consider Ashley, the 9-year-old-girl with severe hearing loss who is featured on the accompanying CD-ROM. Because of early intervention, the effects of her hearing loss on her life at home and school are minimal, if not nonexistent. On the other hand, if a hearing loss is not identified and a family is not able to respond proactively, the impact on the child's life can be profound, even if the hearing loss is mild or moderate.

Integration into the Community

When a significant hearing loss is identified early in a child's life, preferably at birth through newborn hearing screening, parents must make a series of important decisions about their child's identity and place in the community; they must choose a communication mode and orientation. Communication mode refers to how the child will communicate—the two common alternatives being speech and sign. Orientation refers to whether the child with hearing loss will be a member of the oral community or the Deaf community. These decisions are not easy for the family of a newborn but are potentially the most important they will make.

More than 80% of children with hearing loss are born to parents with normal hearing. A study conducted by Gallaudet Research Institute (2001) of 6,907 hard-of-hearing children ranging in age from 1 to 18 years showed that for 5,877 of the children both parents were hearing; only 4% of the children had two deaf or hard-of-hearing parents. Not surprisingly, then, many parents of children with hearing loss do not link their families with the Deaf community because they themselves are part of the hearing society. Of children and youth who are deaf or hard of hearing, only 26% have family members who regularly sign; 69% have family members who do not sign (Gallaudet Research Institute, 2001). Parents with normal hearing often focus on integrating their children into the mainstream oral community. Many of these children learn to listen and speak with the use of assistive technology, such as hearing aids, and require considerable intervention to meet the goal of integration.

Discussion Point: *Consider the case of Mesha in Box 13-1, whose parents are Deaf. Identify specific ways in which Mesha's socialization and education will be influenced by her parents' membership in the Deaf community.*

On the other hand, some parents whose children are identified as deaf or profoundly hard of hearing may choose to support their children's entry into the Deaf community. This is most likely for children with hearing loss who are born to parents already in the Deaf community, which views deafness as central to its identity. Membership in the Deaf community is contingent on many factors. First, it is a choice to align oneself with the Deaf community; the choice is typically influenced by family identity and shared experiences and ideas. Second, there must be a common language or communication mode, usually ASL. Membership in the community implies an appreciation of the history, folklore, and traditions of the community and an active role in the group's activities.

Communication Development

Discussion Point: *What are some explanations for the difficulty in identifying hearing problems in infants and toddlers?*

Critical to the healthy development of a child with hearing loss are early identification and intervention—preferably before 6 months of age (Yoshinaga-Itano, Sedey, Coulter, & Mehl, 1998). Consequently, most states have initiated infant assessment programs to identify children with hearing loss at birth. However, the current age of identification of children with significant congenital hearing loss continues to be around 2 years of age nationally.

When early identification does not occur or when intervention efforts are either fragmented or ineffective in communication development (whether oral or manual), hearing loss will likely result in delayed receptive and expressive speech and language development. These delays may range from mild to profound and are likely to have further deleterious

TABLE 13-1 The degree of hearing loss and possible impacts

Degree of Hearing Impairment in dB HL	Potential Impact		
	Speech and Language	Education	Social-Emotional Adjustment
Normal hearing −10 to +15	In the presence of background noise, may have difficulty discriminating speech	None	None
Minimal 16 to 25	May have difficulty detecting faint and distant speech, listening in a noisy room, and detecting word-sound distinctions (e.g., verb tenses, plural forms, possessives, etc.)	May miss 10% of classroom instruction; may appear inattentive or uninterested; may be more fatigued because of increased listening effort	If missing fast pace or subtleties of peer conversation, may act awkward or uninterested or respond inappropriately; may behave immaturely
Mild 26 to 40	Depending on degree of loss, may miss 25–50% of speech signal, including many consonants necessary for intelligibility; will find language development and articulation affected	May appear to daydream or listen only when interested; likely to be more fatigued or irritable	May impact self-concept and cause confusion as speech is increasingly unclear; may feel stress and uneasiness and perceive a lack of ability to succeed
Moderate 41 to 55	Without amplification will miss 75% or more of speech signal; likely to have delayed syntax, limited vocabulary, imperfect speech production, and voice quality issues	Will have difficulty with receptive and expressive language, reading, spelling, and other school concepts; will miss most of classroom instruction presented orally	Will lack socialization with peers, leading to isolation and loneliness; may be judged/judge self as incompetent learner
Moderately severe 56 to 70	Will miss up to 100% of speech signal; will have marked difficulty in both one-on-one and group conversations; will show delayed language and syntax and reduced voice quality and speech intelligibility; may be 75% unintelligible in speech	Will not be able to keep up with oral instruction and will fall behind academically, probably in all subjects	Will have difficulty with social behaviors; may experience a sense of frustration and rejection; poor self-concept
Severe 71 to 90 and profound 91+	Without amplification may not develop speech and/or language; if acquired condition, may lose preexisting skills	Without intervention, will not be able to participate in typical academic setting	Without spoken or manual language, will not be able to communicate with others, leading to severe isolation and possible social and emotional problems
Unilateral loss (mild or worse)	May have difficulty hearing faint or distant speech, localizing sounds, and understanding speech in poor listening conditions	May miss important oral instructions or descriptions (particularly in noise), leading to incomplete concept development or misunderstanding	May be more distractible, frustrated, dependent; less attentive and less confident

Source: Based on Flexer (1994).

impact on the child's cognitive development, academic achievement, self-concept, and social-emotional well-being (Yoshinaga-Itano, 2003). In turn, any or all of these are likely to have a negative impact on vocational choices and the child's long-term occupational achievements. The relationship between the severity of hearing loss and psychosocial and educational concerns is depicted in Table 13-1.

FIGURE 13-1 An illustration of comprehension difficulties due to figurative language.

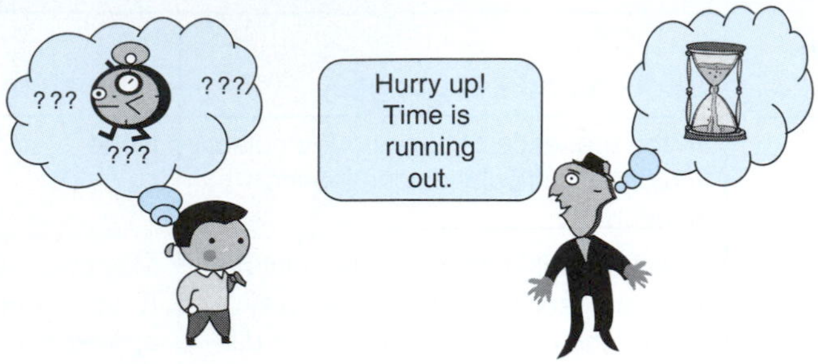

The speech and language delay associated with hearing loss can include difficulties in (1) vocabulary (semantics), (2) grammar (syntax), (3) communicative intent and interaction style (pragmatics), (4) and speech intelligibility (phonology). In the area of vocabulary, children with hearing loss typically learn concrete words like *red, car, four,* and *push* since they can be matched to an object or action. However, function words like *an* or *the* and abstract concepts such as *think* or *earlier* are very difficult for these children to grasp. Additionally, words or phrases with multiple or subtle meanings can be confusing (see Figure 13-1), because these tend to require a well-developed vocabulary. In the area of grammar, the use of grammatical morphemes—such as the past tense *-ed,* the plural *-s,* the possessive *'s,* and the present progressive *-ing*—all may be delayed in development. These markers tend to be particularly difficult to hear in spoken language; they are not stressed in a word and/or occur at the end of a word, which is spoken with less intensity and loudness. Consequently, children with hearing loss may not understand or use common structures that broaden and enhance word use and grammatical development.

In the area of pragmatics, certain aspects of conversation are difficult for children with hearing loss. They may miss out on subtle aspects of communication in group settings and have difficulties following the use of figurative language, such as idioms and humor. Delays in language development can also impact a child's ability to negotiate with peers, initiate communicative acts with others, and navigate the structured turn-taking of conversations.

Finally, phonology is often impacted when a child exhibits moderate to more severe hearing loss. If a child cannot hear the sounds of speech adequately, the natural development of accurate production of those sounds does not occur (Ling, 2001), affecting both nouns and consonants. For children with significant hearing loss, as many as 80% of spoken words may be unintelligible (Tye-Murray, 2000). Other aspects of speech production are also affected—resonance characteristics, causing hyponasality; fluency characteristics, resulting in slow speaking rate; and prosodic characteristics, producing a monotonic and arhythmic speech (Tye-Murray, 2000).

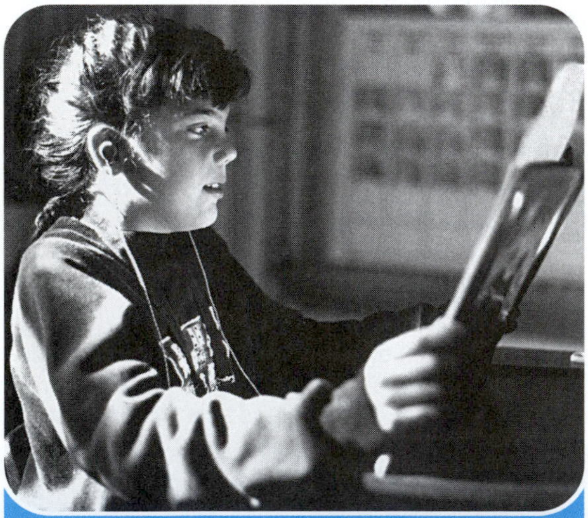

Without proactive intervention, children who have a severe to profound hearing loss often do not achieve reading and writing skills beyond a third-grade level.

Academic achievement for children with hearing loss is challenging on many levels, particularly reading and mathematical concepts (Allen, 1986; Berg, 2001; Bess, Dodd-Murphy, & Parker, 1998). As children progress through school, the gaps between children with typical hearing and those with hearing loss tend to widen, particularly when appropriate and intensive early intervention is not in place. Without appropriate management, children with bilateral mild to moderate hearing loss achieve, on the average, one to four grade levels less than their peers with normal hearing (ASHA, 2000a). A unilateral hearing loss causes similar academic concerns.

How Is Pediatric Hearing Loss Classified?

Hearing loss in children and adolescents is typically classified according to its etiology, its manifestation and impact, and its severity.

Etiology

Hearing loss results from many different causes. In characterizing the etiology of hearing loss, experts identify the genetic or environmental cause, the age of onset, and the type of loss.

Genetic or Environmental Cause

Genetic and environmental factors that can result in hearing loss are numerous, although in many cases the specific cause is unknown (Martin & Greer Clark, 2002). The high-risk register identifies conditions present in infants that signal an elevated risk of hearing loss (see Figure 13-2).

When congenital loss is present, about 50% of the cases result from genetic causes, in which hearing loss is transmitted genetically from parents to their offspring. With *autosomal dominant hearing loss,* one parent has a hearing loss and is a carrier of a dominant gene for hearing loss, which is passed on to the child (ASHA, 2005a). The child then has a 50% chance of having a genetic-linked hearing loss. With *autosomal recessive hearing loss,* both parents carry a recessive trait for hearing loss, but neither exhibits hearing loss. Their offspring has a 25% chance of congenital hearing loss, which might be unexpected by the parents.

Children can also experience congenital hearing loss due to infection, injury, or illness in the prenatal, perinatal, or 28-day postnatal period. Possible prenatal causes include maternal

FIGURE 13-2 **The high-risk register: Indicators of elevated risk of hearing loss in infancy.**

- Family history of congenital hearing loss
- Congenital infection linked to hearing loss (e.g., herpes, rubella)
- Craniofacial anomaly affecting the ear
- Low birth weight
- Ototoxic medications
- Bacterial meningitis and other infectious diseases associated with hearing loss (e.g., measles)
- Low Apgar scores at birth
- Mechanical ventilation for 10 days or longer
- Presence of syndrome associated with hearing loss (e.g., Down syndrome)
- Head trauma during or soon after birth

Sources: Based on Joint Committee on Infant Hearing (1991); Martin (1994).

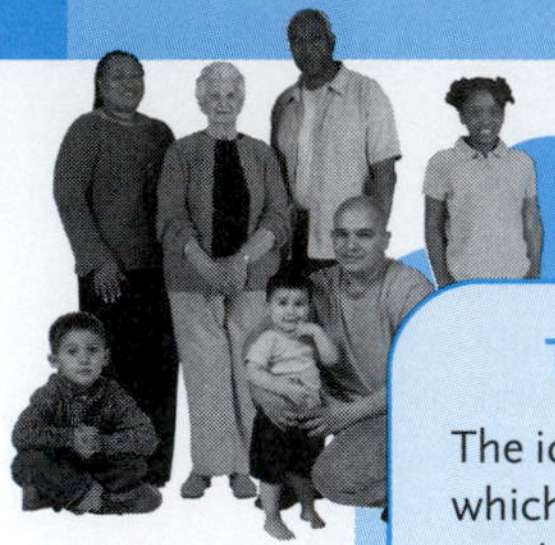

BOX 13-2 Multicultural Focus

The Culture of the Deaf Community

The identity of the Deaf community is centered on shared attitudes and a common language, which in the United States is American Sign Language (ASL). The Deaf community does not reside in its own geographical space but shares a social community based on a shared set of beliefs. The members of the Deaf community are as diverse as those belonging to the larger society and have formed a community for many of the same reasons—primarily, the desire for the companionship of others with similar psychological and social needs (Scheetz, 2001).

A common belief of the Deaf community is that deafness is an attribute rather than a deficiency, in contrast to the perspective of the more mainstream society, in which deafness is seen as a disability that should be corrected/treated (Scheetz, 2001). For the Deaf community, deafness is akin to left-handedness. Being unable to hear need not present any disadvantage to a person, just as being left-handed need not be disabling.

The Deaf community of the United States has many of the same cultural materials that other communities have:

- Deaf magazines, such as *Deaf Life*
- Deaf newspapers, such as *SIGNews*
- Deaf schools, such as the Atlanta Area School for the Deaf
- Deaf universities, such as Gallaudet University
- Deaf recreational clubs, such as Seattle's Greater Seattle Club for the Deaf
- Deaf sports organizations, such as the American Deaf Volleyball Association
- Deaf theatrical groups, such as Cleveland's Signstage Theatre
- Deaf churches, such as the Calvary Baptist Deaf Church in Auburn, Washington
- Deaf film festivals, such as Amsterdam's International Deaf Film Festival

Parents who are not part of the Deaf community but whose children are deaf must consider this reality carefully and decide whether they can see their children as members of the Deaf community. Do they want their children to develop ASL as a native language and align themselves with that community? Or will they raise their children to be truly bilingual and bicultural, fully integrated into the Deaf community but functioning equally well in the larger society? Is this possible? An alternative is to raise their children as hearing children, whose hearing loss will be corrected and/or treated through medical means and other intervention.

For Discussion

How should parents go about deciding whether they and their children should embrace the Deaf community culture?

Both Mesha's and Lilly's parents had to make these difficult decisions. Read more about their perspectives in Box 13-1. How would you rate their decisions?

Companion Website

To answer these questions online, go to the Multicultural Focus module in chapter 13 of the Companion Website.

diabetes, cytomegalovirus, rubella, herpes, syphilis, and taxoplasmosis. Perinatal causes include anoxia (i.e., lack of oxygen to the brain), head trauma, and hyperbilirubinemia (i.e., excessive bile pigments in the blood). Further, in the first 28 days after birth, children who receive ototoxic medications for any reason may experience damage to the ear. Unfortunately, this is a side-effect of some medicines for which the alternative, including death, is clearly worse than loss of hearing. In addition, some children are born with specific physical deformities, like malformation of the outer or middle ear, or with syndromes, like Down syndrome, that make hearing loss probable (Martin, 1994).

Beyond these physical or biological causes, the environment can occasionally induce a child's hearing loss. Although less common than biologically based loss, exposure to noise in the environment can result in a noise-induced hearing loss, which can range from mild to profound. Noise exposure from ventilation systems and other medical equipment in the neonatal intensive care unit (NICU) can cause permanent hearing loss in children who stay in the NICU for a long period of time. Sudden exposure to loud noise, such as a gunshot close to the ear, can also permanently damage the ear, as can barotrauma, a sudden change in air pressure.

Discussion Point: *Compare and contrast the causes of hearing loss for the three children described in Box 13-1.*

Age of Onset

The age of onset for hearing loss is typically differentiated into developmental or acquired. Developmental loss is present at birth; acquired loss occurs sometime after birth. Experts also differentiate between prelingual and postlingual loss, with prelingual loss occurring before language is acquired and postlingual loss occurring after language is acquired. There is no consistent age that separates prelingual from postlingual loss. However, the more time a child has had to develop language and speech through oral means before a hearing loss occurs, the more likely it is that oral communication can be conserved (Martin, 1994).

Type of Loss

Type of loss identifies the auditory structures that are affected. In considering the pathway of sound from the outer ear to the brain, we must differentiate between two sets of mechanisms that transport the sound. The outer ear and middle ear are considered *conductive* mechanisms, whereas the cochlea and auditory nerve are considered *sensorineural* mechanisms. Three types of loss are possible, based on the extent to which these mechanisms are involved.

- **Conductive hearing loss** is caused by damage to the outer or middle ear, with the inner ear and cochlea intact.
- **Sensorineural hearing loss** is caused by damage to the cochlea or the auditory nerve, with the outer and middle ear intact.
- **Mixed hearing loss** is caused by damage to both the conductive and sensorineural mechanisms.

In classifying the hearing loss of a given individual, experts consider all of these sources of information—cause of loss, age of onset, and type of loss. Consider Ashley from the companion CD-ROM. Ashley is a 9-year-old girl with a moderate to severe hearing loss. Ashley has a congenital (prelingual) mixed loss; the sensorineural component resulted from an unknown cause, whereas the conductive aspect resulted from chronic infections of the middle ear cavity.

Manifestation

Hearing loss is also classified according to the aspects of audition that are impacted, that is, how the disorder is manifested. Some children with hearing loss experience loss of hearing acuity, referring to the precision of hearing at different levels of loudness. Loss of hearing acuity can range from slight to profound in one or both ears; it results in sounds being softer or less audible. You can experience the impact of such a loss by turning down the radio until it is only slightly audible or by putting cotton in your ears. The individual with a loss of hearing acuity strains to hear what others hear without straining.

More problematic than a loss in acuity is a decrease in auditory comprehension of spoken language and speech perception, which can accompany hearing loss. Whereas a number of technologies, such as hearing aids, can increase sound intensity, or volume, to make up for a decrease in acuity, a loss of speech perception is more difficult to manage. A child who experiences loss of acuity can turn up the television temporarily or use a hearing aid when conversing with friends. When a loss of auditory comprehension and speech perception occurs, as it may with sensorineural loss, a child must compensate in many ways, such as paying attention to visual cues or requesting written notes.

Severity

Hearing loss is also classified according to its severity, using the decibel (dB) system. **Decibels**, which are the standard unit of sound intensity, represent the differences in loudness available to human hearing, from the threshold of sound at 0 dB (the drop of a pin) to the threshold of pain at about 140 dB (a fire alarm close to your ear). The prevailing approach to hearing loss is to identify the **threshold**, or earliest point, at which a person can begin to hear, that is, the *threshold of hearing*. For normal hearing this threshold is between –10 and +15 dB. The threshold of hearing becomes higher as hearing loss becomes more severe:

- 16 to 25 dB: Minimal hearing loss
- 26 to 40 dB: Mild hearing loss
- 41 to 55 dB: Moderate hearing loss
- 56 to 70 dB: Moderately severe hearing loss
- 71 to 90 dB: Severe hearing loss
- 91 dB or higher: Profound hearing loss

Estimates from the Gallaudet Research Institute (2001) show that hearing loss among children and youth runs the full range of severity. Recent data on children from birth through 18 years who are considered deaf or hard of hearing show these rates of occurrence:

- 15% with minimal hearing loss
- 11% with mild hearing loss
- 12% with moderate hearing loss
- 12% with moderately severe hearing loss
- 17% with severe hearing loss
- 33% with profound hearing loss

Typically, hearing loss is not described in percentages of loss, even though you may occasionally see references such as "Joey has a 15% hearing loss in the right ear." Experts caution against using percentiles to describe hearing loss, because the decibel system is not amenable to this type of interpretation. The decibel system is a logarithmic system, in which the relationship between units is not linear, and the scale increases exponentially. Thus, the difference between 15 dB and 30 dB is not the same as the difference between 70 dB and 85 dB in magnitude; as the decibel level increases, the difference between decibels increases exponentially. Because percentage rankings imply an equal difference between units, they do not do a good job of characterizing hearing loss. To say that Henry has a 15% hearing loss and Tisha has a 40% hearing loss is basically meaningless, given the logarithmic nature of decibels.

FIGURE 13-3 Audiogram depicting average range of speech energy and levels of hearing impairment in dB HL.

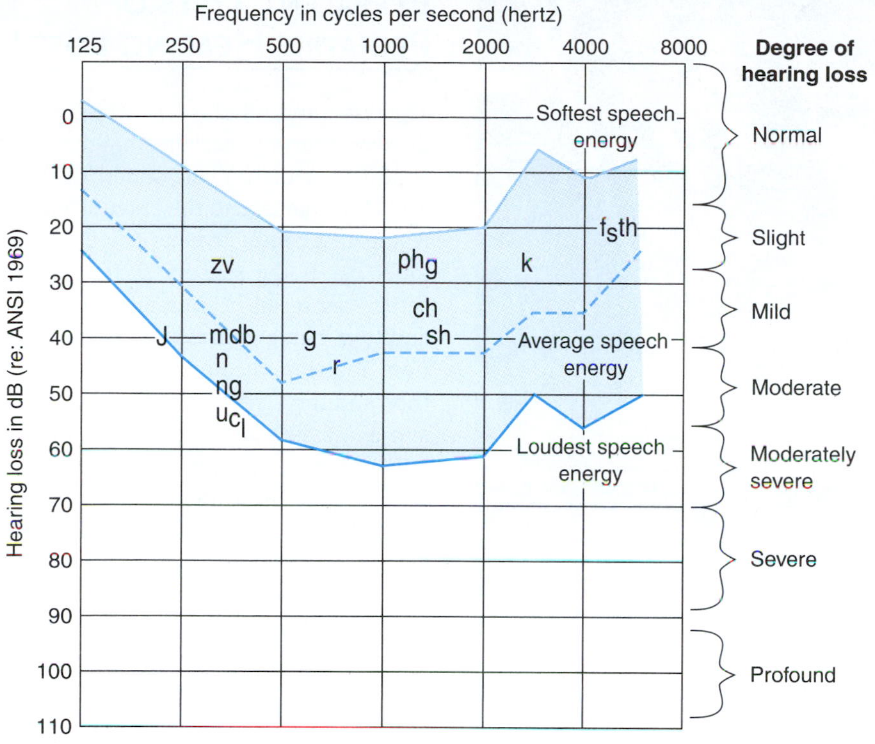

Source: From *Hearing in Children* (4th ed.) by J. Northern and M. Downs, 1991, Baltimore: Williams & Wilkins. Copyright 1991 by Williams & Wilkins. Reprinted with permission.

Hearing level in decibels is plotted on a graph called an *audiogram,* as shown in Figure 13-3. The y-axis denotes decibels and loudness perception for the range of −10 dB to 110 dB, which is the normal range of human hearing from just audible to painfully loud. The threshold of hearing is plotted on the x-axis in hertz (Hz) along the frequency range of human hearing, from very low (125 Hz) to very high (8000 Hz). The audiogram presented in Figure 13-3 shows where different speech sounds are located perceptually for the dimensions of pitch (i.e., frequency) and loudness.

The severity of hearing loss can vary across the frequency range. For example, a child with bilateral hearing damage from noise exposure may have normal hearing (threshold between −10 dB and 15 dB) for all of the frequencies except 4000 Hz and 8000 Hz, at which the threshold is 40 dB, indicating a high frequency hearing loss. A child with persistent bilateral middle ear infections may have depressed hearing thresholds (about 30 dB to 40 dB) across all frequencies from 125 Hz to 8000 Hz.

It is important to note that the level of severity in decibels does not necessarily correspond to the severity of impairment. A slight hearing loss does not imply a slight problem, nor does a profound hearing loss indicate a complete loss of sound. In fact, the severity of a loss does not necessarily correspond with its manifestation. We must differentiate between the concepts of *loss,* which is an objective term used to describe hearing status, and *disability,* which is a subjective term describing the impact of the loss on a person's life. Someone with a mild hearing loss may have a significant disability, whereas someone with a severe loss may have virtually no disability.

Discussion Point: *To understand the difference between hearing loss and hearing disability, compare and contrast the ways in which a mild hearing loss might affect the owner of a pesticide company versus a 9-1-1 dispatcher.*

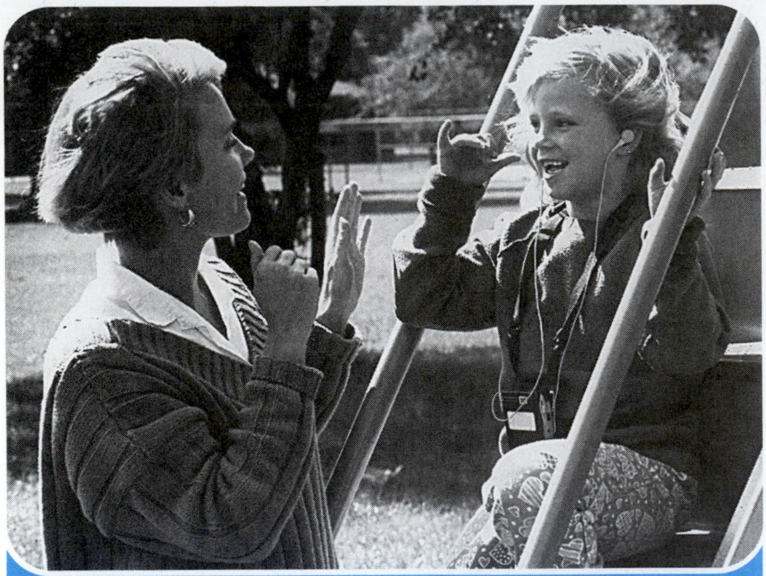

Hearing loss and hearing disability are two different concepts. A child with a profound hearing loss may have no disability, given high-quality exposure to a language system.

What Are the Defining Characteristics of Prevalent Types of Pediatric Hearing Loss?

The outer and middle ear make up the conductive hearing mechanism—that is, they conduct, or deliver, the sound to the inner ear. Thus, damage to the outer or middle ear results in a conductive hearing disorder. The inner ear is the sensory system where the actual "sense" of hearing is located, and the auditory nerve represents the neural portion. Together, the inner ear, or cochlea, and the auditory nerve make up the sensorineural hearing mechanism. Damage to either of these systems is collectively termed sensorineural hearing loss. A mixed hearing loss occurs if both conductive and sensorineural loss occur simultaneously.

Identifying a child's hearing loss as conductive, sensorineural, or mixed is one of the most prevalent ways of classifying pediatric hearing loss. Here we consider the defining characteristics of each type of loss, as well as common causes and risk factors.

Conductive Hearing Loss

Defining Characteristics

When sound is not conducted efficiently through the outer and/or middle ear, the result is an attenuation, or reduction, of the sound heard. This attenuation of sound is the defining characteristic of a conductive hearing loss. You can readily experience a temporary conductive hearing loss by putting your index fingers into your ears (not too far, please!). A conversation in the near distance can still be heard, but the loudness of the conversation is reduced.

Children who have a conductive hearing loss, whether it is temporary or persistent, experience this attenuation of loudness. When a conductive hearing loss is present, children often report that their ears feel plugged or full. This sense of fullness makes sounds around a person appear softer but exaggerates the sense of loudness of the individual's own voice or the noise of chewing crunchy foods. You can try yet another simulation by plugging your ears while eating some chips or other crunchy foods. The reason your voice seems so loud is because of **bone conduction**, which is the transmittal of sound vibrations along the bones of the skull.

***Discussion Point:** Replicate a slight temporary conductive hearing loss by wearing earplugs for a few hours. In what ways does this conductive hearing loss impact your daily living activities?*

Conductive hearing loss generally causes a slight to moderate loss of hearing in one or both ears. The impact is not severe because some sounds still travel to the auditory processing system of the brain via bone conduction. As long as the cochlea is functioning, it will carry some sound information to the brain. However, the loudness of the sound is attenuated, and thus some auditory information may be lost. Conductive hearing loss is typically amenable to medical or surgical intervention and therefore is often a temporary loss given that it is identified and treated.

Causes and Risk Factors

Children frequently experience conductive hearing loss, which in many cases can be reversed. Cerumen (i.e., ear wax) blockage is a common cause. Because it is unwise to clean the ear canal with cotton swabs and many children have narrow ear canals, wax buildup can occur frequently and block sound transmission. Foreign objects inappropriately put into ear canals or inflammation of the ear canal (e.g., swimmer's ear) can also block the transmission of sounds to cause conductive hearing loss.

In addition, malformations of the outer and middle ear can cause conductive hearing loss. Sometimes children are born with a malformed or absent external auditory canal or a congenital blockage of the ear canal so that there is no opening through which sound waves can travel. And some types of oral-facial anomalies result in underdeveloped or missing ossicles (malleus, incus, or stapes) so that they do not work together to transmit sound waves through the middle ear.

The most common cause of conductive hearing loss in children is middle ear dysfunction caused by **otitis media**, which results from a viral or bacterial infection of the middle ear space. Some estimates indicate that at least 50% of children experience otitis media, (ASHA, 2005a), which may be an underestimation since some ear infections have no symptoms. Typically, otitis media progresses in the following way: First, the child has an infectious organism in the pharyngeal area, which makes its way into the middle ear space via the eustachian tube. The mechanism is likely a sneeze or a nose-blow (Martin, 1994). Second, a eustachian tube dysfunction results in a buildup of negative pressure behind the eardrum. Third, fluid builds up in the middle ear space, which may or may not be infected. Here, pus can accumulate, and the mucosal lining of the middle ear cavity can swell. Fourth, the fluid and pressure eventually perforate the tympanic membrane. Most young children do not show outward signs until the problem has developed into a fluid-filled middle ear or a perforated tympanic membrane, both of which cause significant hearing loss.

With intervention this progression of events can be halted. For instance, the bacterial infection can be brought under control with antibiotics. Also, pressure-equalizing (PE) tubes can be inserted through the eardrum to equalize the pressure building up in the inflamed middle ear and to release any fluids. Careful monitoring of infection and skilled intervention to decrease the impact on hearing and communication are critical to the well-being of children.

Otitis media is common among children because of several factors. First, from a biological

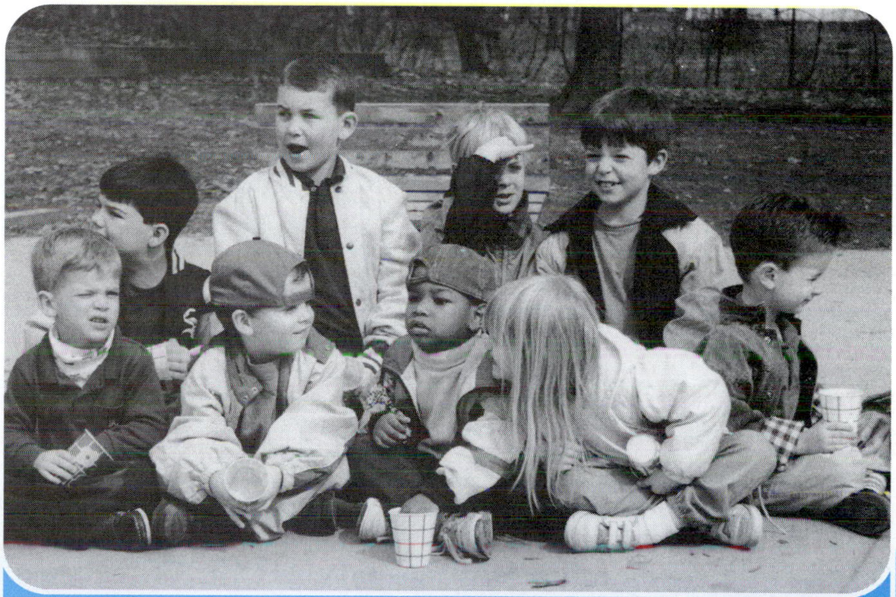

Exposure to a large number of children in early child-care settings elevates children's risk of chronic ear infections.

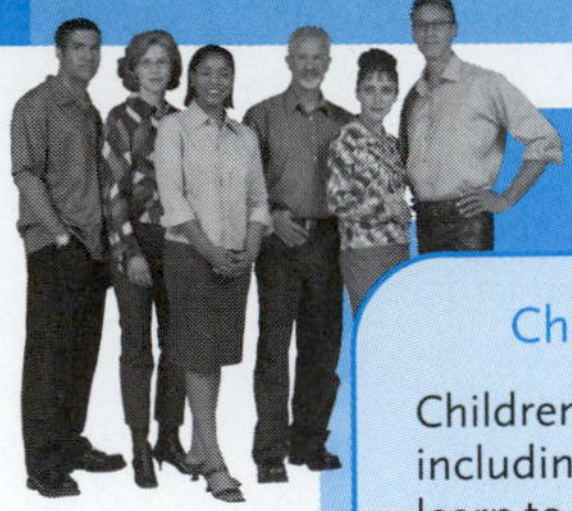

BOX 13-3 Ecological Contexts

Children with Hearing Loss at Home, at School, and in the Community

Children with significant hearing loss may need to rely on manual means to communicate, including sign language. Children whose parents do not know manual communication must learn to use sign systems. Often, parents become interpreters for their children since they are most apt to understand their children and are sensitive to their needs. However, this role can be both burdensome and inconvenient for parents, especially as children grow older. And children may become frustrated, angry, or sad in trying to get their daily needs met, not wanting to rely on their parents to mediate their communication with others. In social situations, these children are likely to experience isolation and loneliness if they cannot find peers with whom they can exchange ideas and thoughts.

Academic situations can also be troublesome. Parents may choose to have their children mainstreamed in regular education, they may select a special program for children who are hearing impaired or who have special needs, or they may send their children to residential schools for the deaf and hard of hearing. Each of these choices has ramifications, particularly if the academic setting does not provide the appropriate support.

For Discussion

Lilly's parents in Box 13-1 decided against mainstream education and used homeschooling for Lilly. What are the advantages and disadvantages of homeschooling for a child with hearing loss?

How might a different educational choice have influenced Lilly's identity, communication abilities, and academic success?

Companion Website

To answer these questions online, go to the Ecological Contexts module in chapter 13 of the Companion Website.

standpoint, the angle and short length of the eustachian tube in young children make it easier for organisms to enter and move through the tube. With age the tube will take on more of an *S*-shape, but in children it is relatively straight and short. Second, from an environmental standpoint, some allergens, such as cigarette smoke, seem to make children more susceptible to otitis media (Martin, 1994). Third, some evidence points to the fact that group child care may serve as a significant risk factor (Froom & Culpepper, 1991).

Young children who attend early child-care programs do experience greater rates of otitis media than do children who are cared for at home. Estimates show that children under the age of 2 who attend day care are three times more likely to have a history of otitis media than are children not attending day care. With the number of single-parent households on the rise, as well as the number of homes in which both parents work outside the home, more children are attending child-care programs today; current statistics show that about 50% of young children are cared for outside the home (Children's Defense Fund, 2000). However, it is not care outside the home that seems to be the defining variable; rather, it is the number of children with whom a given child interacts. Thus, children who attend large-population child-care centers face greater risk of otitis media than do children attending centers with fewer children (Marx, Osguthorpe, & Parsons, 1995).

Sensorineural Hearing Loss

Defining Characteristics

Sensorineural hearing loss is the most common type of hearing loss; it results from damage to the cochlea or the auditory nerve that travels from the cochlea to the brain. The presence of a sensorineural hearing loss can cause a slight to profound loss of hearing in one or both ears. Even though sensorineural disorders are thought of as a decrease in overall loudness, they are also associated with a decrease in speech perception and a decreased ability to distinguish speech from background noise. Thus, not only is loudness affected, but also the clarity of what is heard. Some children also experience ringing in the ears (i.e., tinnitus) and reduced tolerance of loud sounds. Sensorineural loss can be treated effectively with amplification or other types of intervention, but hearing cannot usually be restored.

Causes and Risk Factors

Most often, sensorineural hearing loss is present at birth as a congenital hearing loss. The most influential factors include maternal health during pregnancy, the birth process, the child's health at birth, hereditary factors, exposure to medications that are toxic to the ear, and disease. The following present the greatest risk:

1. Serious illness, drug use, or other problems of the mother during pregnancy
2. In-utero infections, including CMV, herpes, toxoplasmosis, syphilis, and rubella
3. Complicated birth process or poor infant health, including hyperbilirubinemia, oxygen deprivation, low birth weight, or trauma
4. Family history of permanent childhood hearing loss
5. Noise exposure, including exposure to mechanical ventilation
6. Syndrome associated with hearing loss or cranio-facial anomaly
7. Recurrent or persistent otitis media with effusion (i.e., fluid) for at least 3 months (Martin & Greer Clark, 2002)

Data from the Gallaudet Research Institute's annual survey of deaf and hard-of-hearing children and youth provide useful information about the leading causes of sensorineural hearing loss, ranging in severity from minimal to profound. The 1999–2000 survey interviewed over 43,000 deaf and hard-of-hearing children and youth, ranging in age from birth to young adulthood. For 51% of the children, the cause of hearing loss was unknown; among the remaining 49%, the leading causes of deafness and hearing loss included these:

- Genetics and heredity (20% of children surveyed)
- Meningitis (6%)
- Otitis media (5.5%)
- Consequences of prematurity (5%)
- Pregnancy complications other than maternal illness (4%)
- Maternal illness during pregnancy (CMV, rubella; 3%)
- Other infections (2%)
- Birth trauma (1.5%)
- Ototoxic medications (1.4%)
- Trauma after birth (1%)

Mixed Hearing Loss

When both conductive and sensorineural loss exist, the loss is termed *mixed*. For example, a child with a congenital sensorineural hearing loss may also acquire a conductive hearing loss from a bout of chronic otitis media or because of cerumen buildup. Thus, a mixed hearing loss typically includes a permanent reduction of sound (the sensorineural component) as well as additional temporary loss of hearing from the conductive component.

How Is Pediatric Hearing Loss Identified?

Assessment for hearing loss in pediatric populations requires a multitiered approach, as illustrated in Figure 13-4, to include both identification and ongoing monitoring. Identification of a hearing loss often begins with a routine screening, such as an infant hearing screening conducted in the hospital immediately after birth. Once a hearing loss is identified, ongoing monitoring is essential to track changes over time and to monitor the effects of specific interventions.

The Assessment Process

Referral

Early diagnosis of hearing impairment (EDHI) programs are present in most states; their goal is to detect hearing loss at birth, while the infant is still in the hospital. Infants who do not pass EDHI screenings are referred by their pediatricians to an audiologist for follow-up testing.

In the toddler and preschool years, children who exhibit developmental delays in communication, have a hereditary predisposition to hearing loss, or develop diseases or disorders that impact the auditory mechanism should be referred for a hearing screening or evaluation. Typically, the referral is made by the pediatrician or speech-language pathologist. Additionally, children with risk factors for hearing loss should receive regular audiologic monitoring. If no specific risk factors are present, children are typically evaluated for hearing acuity in kindergarten, first through third grades, and then again in seventh and eleventh grades.

Screening

Screening generally falls into two categories, depending on the child's age. Infant hearing screenings, also called newborn hearing screenings, are completed at birth and involve specialized testing that is typically completed before a newborn leaves the hospital. Older children are screened using conventional methods, involving an audiometer, headphones,

FIGURE 13-4 The assessment process.

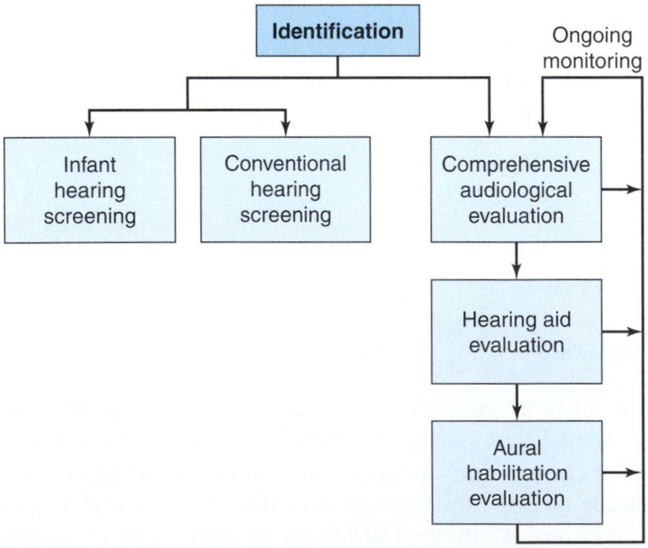

and tones presented to both ears. If a child does not pass a screening, a comprehensive audiological evaluation is scheduled. Depending on the suspected cause of loss (e.g., birth anomaly or disease), medical evaluation may also be warranted.

Infant Screening. Infant screening includes objective tests that do not require a response from the infant. There are two commonly used measures, each of which is administered relatively quickly while the infant sleeps, causing little or no discomfort. **Otoacoustic emissions** (OAEs) are a measure of cochlear function (specifically, the functioning of the outer hair cells) and are considered a good indicator of hearing acuity. **Evoked auditory potentials** (EAPs) measure the electrical response of the auditory system to a sound stimulus. Audiologists or trained personnel under their supervision provide infant screenings.

Conventional Hearing Screening. Conventional screenings require a child to respond when a soft tone is heard. Any screening that requires a response on the part of the child is called behavioral testing. Soft level tones are introduced into each ear using an audiometer at three test frequencies, typically 1000, 2000 and 4000 Hz. The examiner determines the child's ability to detect each frequency in each ear at the threshold of 20 dB. The examiner may allow younger children to respond in the form of a play activity (e.g., dropping a block into a box) or by raising their hand. Speech-language pathologists, audiologists, and other supervised, trained personnel provide conventional hearing screenings for children 3 years and older, but only audiologists can screen younger children. Children who fail to respond to a tone at any frequency in either ear are considered to have failed the screening and need to be rescreened within 2 weeks or referred for a comprehensive audiological evaluation (Martin, 1994).

Comprehensive Audiological Evaluation

A comprehensive audiological evaluation assesses the type and degree (i.e., severity) of hearing loss, speech discrimination and auditory perception abilities in quiet and in noisy conditions, and any other concerns (e.g., loudness tolerance level). The evaluation also provides information about the cause of any loss. When a comprehensive evaluation indicates a significant hearing loss, a hearing aid evaluation is often conducted if it is in line with family preferences. The hearing aid evaluation involves assessment for and fitting of amplification or other assistive technology. The major tools of the evaluation include (1) case history and interview, (2) other interviews and observation, (3) otoscopic examination, (4) audiometry, and (5) objective measures. Pediatric audiologists also assess related family and child needs—such as social or emotional concerns, educational problems, and speech/language functioning—to inform their assessment and to determine the need for referral to other professionals.

Case History and Interview. As a first step in the comprehensive audiological evaluation, the parent or primary caregiver completes a case history form and a case interview with the clinician. The case history and interview are important in uncovering further concerns or behaviors related to the auditory problems. Combined, the case history and interview help the clinician determine the primary reason for referral, family background, health and developmental history, communication history, and other important concerns.

Other Interviews and Observation. Interviews are inexpensive and useful ways to obtain parental input about a child's auditory and communicative behaviors and to gather input from other professionals who work with the child, such as a speech-language pathologist, special or general educator, or early interventionist. Observations can be used to understand a child's strengths and needs in many different contexts, including the clinic, home, classroom, and various community settings.

TABLE 13-2 Listening instruments for evaluating children

Questionnaire	Purpose	Target Population	Completed by Whom
Early Listening Function (ELF) by Anderson (2001)	Evaluates listening in home environment	Infants and toddlers with/without amplification	Parent (may include early interventionist)
Children's Home Inventory for Listening Difficulties (CHILD) by Anderson & Smaldino (2001)	Evaluates child's auditory access to dynamics of family communication	3–12 years with mild, fluctuating, or unilateral hearing loss	Parent/child
Auditory Behavior in Everyday Life (ABEL) by Purdy, Moran, Chard, & Hodgson (2002)	Evaluates auditory behavior in everyday life	4–14 years with mild–profound hearing loss	Parents
Children's Abbreviated Profile of Hearing Aid Benefit (CA-PHAB) by Kopun & Stelmachowitz (1998)	Evaluates benefits of amplification across settings	Older than 9 years with any degree of hearing loss	Parent or child (2 versions)
Listening Inventories for Education (LIFE): Student Appraisal or Teacher Appraisal by Anderson & Smaldino (1998)	Evaluates classroom listening	School-aged children with any degree of hearing loss	Teacher or child (2 versions)
Screening Instrument for Targeting Educational Risk (SIFTER) and Preschool SIFTER by Anderson (1989), Anderson & Matkin (1996), Anderson & Smaldino (2001)	Evaluates classroom listening	3 years to kindergarten or school-aged (two versions) with any degree of hearing loss	Teacher

Source: From "A Parent Questionnaire to Evaluate Children's Auditory Behavior in Everyday Life (ABEL)" by S. C. Purdy, D. R. Farringon, C. A. Moran, L. L. Chard, and S. Hodgson, 2002, *American Journal of Audiology, 11,* pp. 72–82. Copyright 2002 by ASHA. Adapted with permission.

A variety of tools are available to the pediatric audiologist. Table 13-2 identifies some questionnaires for gathering information and structuring interviews about listening activities, amplification possibilities, and classroom contexts. One of these instruments, Auditory Behavior in Everyday Life (ABEL; Purdy, Moran, Chard, & Hodgson, 2002) is shown in Figure 13-5. This brief questionnaire, completed by parents, provides useful information concerning children's auditory behaviors in everyday activities with family members and peers.

The audiologist is likely to supplement interview data with direct observations of the child's listening behaviors. For instance, after administration of parent and teacher questionnaires, a school-based audiologist would observe the following in the child's classroom:

- Listening demands in the classroom and curriculum
- Teacher and student speaking behaviors
- Level of noise in classroom

For the student being assessed, the audiologist would document oral and aural behaviors (e.g., responses to the teacher, asking questions) as well as social-communicative behaviors (e.g., turn-taking with peers, voice use).

Otoscopic Examination. An otoscope is a lighted magnifying device used to evaluate the structures of the outer and middle ear. With an otoscope the audiologist can inspect the external auditory canal and the tympanic membrane. The purpose of the **otoscopic examination** is to detect any abnormalities in these structures, as well as to ensure a clear external auditory canal prior to testing. The otoscopic examination is an important tool for studying the characteristics of the tympanic membrane; it will reveal whether there is negative pressure

FIGURE 13-5 The Auditory Behavior in Everyday Life (ABEL) parent questionnaire.

Auditory Behavior in Everyday Life (ABEL)
by S. C. Purdy, C. A. Moran, L L. Chard, S.-A. Hodgson

Child's name: _________ Completed by: _________ Date: _________

Instructions: We would like to know how you feel about your child's auditory development. Please circle the number beside each item that best describes your child's behavior during the past week.

0 Never **1 Hardly ever** **2 Occasionally** **3 About half the time**
4 Frequently **5 Almost always** **6 Always**

1. Initiates spoken conversations with familiar people.	0	1	2	3	4	5	6
2. Says a person's name to gain their attention.	0	1	2	3	4	5	6
3. Says "please" or "thank you" without being reminded.	0	1	2	3	4	5	6
4. Responds verbally to greeting from familiar people.	0	1	2	3	4	5	6
5. Initiates spoken conversations with unfamiliar people.	0	1	2	3	4	5	6
6. Takes turns in conversations.	0	1	2	3	4	5	6
7. Answers telephone appropriately.	0	1	2	3	4	5	6
8. Responds to own name spoken in the same room.	0	1	2	3	4	5	6
9. Talks using a normal voice level.	0	1	2	3	4	5	6
10. Asks for help in situations where it is needed.	0	1	2	3	4	5	6
11. Makes inappropriate vocal noises.	0	1	2	3	4	5	6
12. Shows interest in spoken conversations around him/her.	0	1	2	3	4	5	6
13. Responds verbally to greeting from unfamiliar person(s).	0	1	2	3	4	5	6
14. Says the names of siblings, family members, classmates.	0	1	2	3	4	5	6
15. Responds to a door bell or knock.	0	1	2	3	4	5	6
16. Will whisper a personal message.	0	1	2	3	4	5	6
17. Quietens activity when asked to.	0	1	2	3	4	5	6
18. Asks about sounds heard around him/her (e.g., planes, trucks, animals).	0	1	2	3	4	5	6
19. Knows when making loud sounds (e.g., slamming doors, stomping feet).	0	1	2	3	4	5	6
20. Ignores telephone ringing.	0	1	2	3	4	5	6
21. Plays cooperatively in a small group without adult supervision.	0	1	2	3	4	5	6
22. Sings.	0	1	2	3	4	5	6
23. Knows when hearing aids are not working.	0	1	2	3	4	5	6
24. Experiments with newly discovered sounds.	0	1	2	3	4	5	6

Source: From "A Parent Questionnaire to Evaluate Children's Auditory Behavior in Everyday Life (ABEL)" by S. C. Purdy, D. R. Farringon, C. A. Moran, L. L. Chard, and S. Hodgson, 2002, *American Journal of Audiology, 11,* pp. 72–82. Copyright 2002 by ASHA. Reprinted with permission.

behind the membrane (the membrane would be retracted), whether the middle ear is inflamed (the membrane would appear red), and whether there is fluid in the middle ear chamber (the line of fluid might be discernible through the transparent membrane).

Audiometry. **Audiometry**, also called pure-tone testing, provides objective information about hearing acuity. Audiometric testing is a behavioral measure because it relies on a child's cooperation and participation. Typically, children repeat words and respond to tones (e.g., by pushing a button or raising a hand). When preschool or older children are tested, toys and visual displays are used to reinforce responses. This is called play audiometry, since the child is engaged in what appears to be a game. For example, a child might be taught to put colorful pegs in a peg board each time a sound is heard. While the child enjoys the game, the audiologist is able to gain valuable auditory information from the child's responses.

FIGURE 13-6 Air (A) and bone (B) conduction pathways.

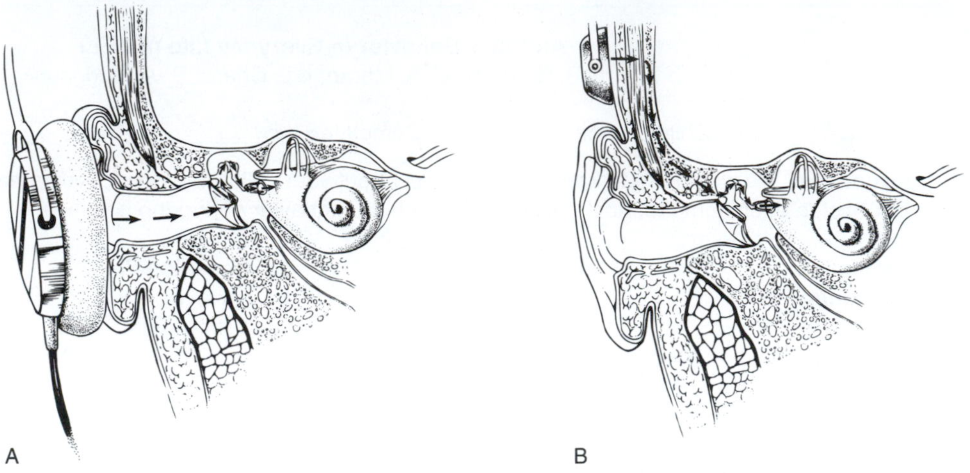

Audiometric testing is completed in a specialized test room or a sound-treated booth that is designed to minimize interference from background noise. The audiometer produces pure-tone sounds in a range of frequencies (from 125 Hz to 8000 Hz) and a range of intensities from soft to loud (−10 dB to 110 dB). The sounds, or pure tones, can be delivered through a variety of transducers, including earphones placed over the ears or into the ear canals, loudspeakers, or a small vibratory device placed on the mastoid bone behind the ear. When the pure-tone sounds are delivered through earphones or loudspeakers, air conduction of sounds is being tested. **Air conduction** is the way most sounds are delivered to the cochlea and auditory pathway; the sound waves pass along the auditory canal and then, as mechanical energy, through the middle ear space. Air conduction testing provides information about hearing acuity, particularly the functioning of the outer and middle ear. Air conduction testing is illustrated in part A of Figure 13-6.

Pure-tone sounds can also be delivered directly to the inner ear by transmitting sound vibrations across the mastoid bone. In this case the audiologist places vibratory devices that look like headphones against the bones right behind the ears. (See part B in Figure 13-6.) This form of testing is called bone conduction; it provides information on the functioning of the cochlea and auditory nerve. The audiologist can then compare results from the bone conduction and the air conduction testing to help determine the type of hearing loss. For instance, an individual may exhibit a significant hearing loss at low frequencies with air conduction testing but not with bone conduction testing, suggesting that the cochlea and auditory nerve are functioning but the outer and middle ear pathways are not.

As described earlier, the audiologist plots hearing acuity on a graph called an *audiogram.* You may recall that the softest level at which a person can detect a pure-tone sound is called a *threshold,* and it is measured in decibels from −10 dB to 120 dB hearing level (HL). Unlike other units of measurement, 0 dB HL does not represent an absence of sound but rather the threshold of hearing. The audiologist measures an individual's threshold of hearing on a range of frequencies between 250 Hz and 8000 Hz. As shown in Figure 13-7, the audiogram maps hearing for the frequency range (perceived as pitch) from very low (250 Hz) to very high (8000 Hz) and the intensity range (perceived as loudness) from very soft (−10 dB HL) to very loud (110 dB HL). A person's hearing acuity, or threshold, is recorded for each frequency. The shaded portion of the audiogram represents the average region for speech sound energy. When a child's hearing is below the shaded region, many key speech sounds will not be naturally audible. This audiogram

FIGURE 13-7 **Deciphering an audiogram.**

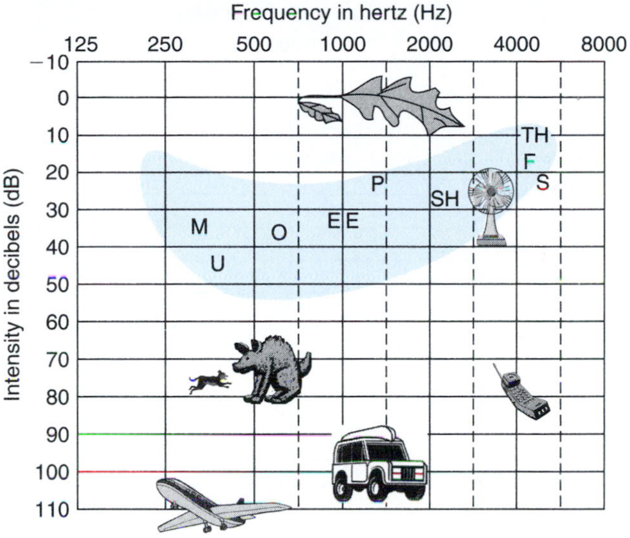

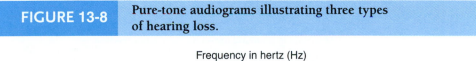

Source: From "Understanding Your Audiogram" by A. S. Mehr, 2005, Reston, VA: American Academy of Audiology. Retrieved January 10, 2005, from http://www.audiology.org/consumer/guides/uya.php Reprinted with permission.

also shows several sounds with which most readers are familiar (e.g., a leaf falling, a phone ringing), and the frequency intensity levels for some speech sounds (e.g., M, O).

Sample audiograms illustrating the three types of hearing loss—conductive, sensorineural, and mixed—are shown in Figure 13-8. On the first audiogram (A), showing a conductive hearing loss, note the normal bone conduction thresholds (representing the functioning of the cochlea and the auditory nerve) and the diminished air conduction thresholds (representing an abnormality in the outer or middle ear). The difference between these two thresholds is called

FIGURE 13-8 **Pure-tone audiograms illustrating three types of hearing loss.**

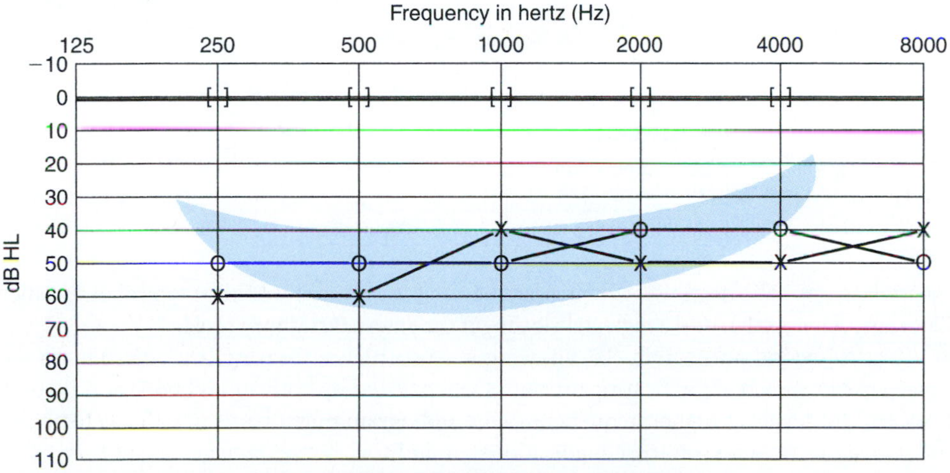

A. Mild conductive hearing impairment

FIGURE 13-8 *Continued*

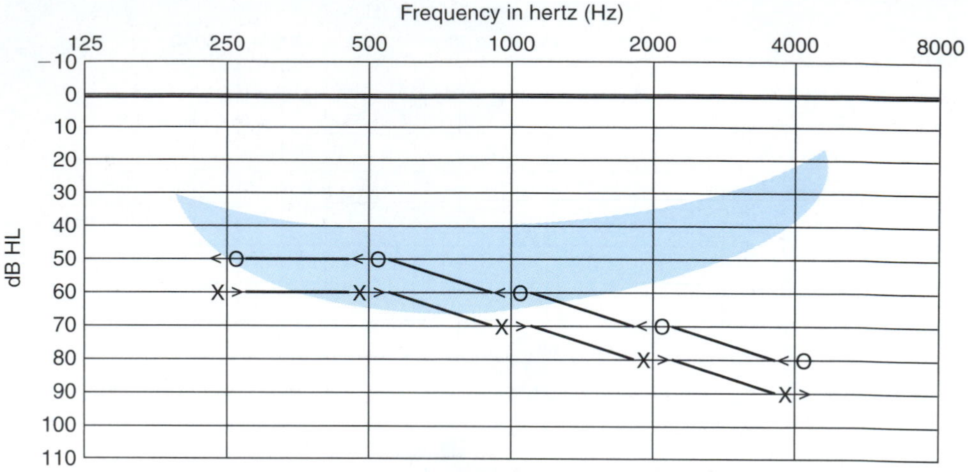

B. Moderate to severe sensorineural hearing impairment

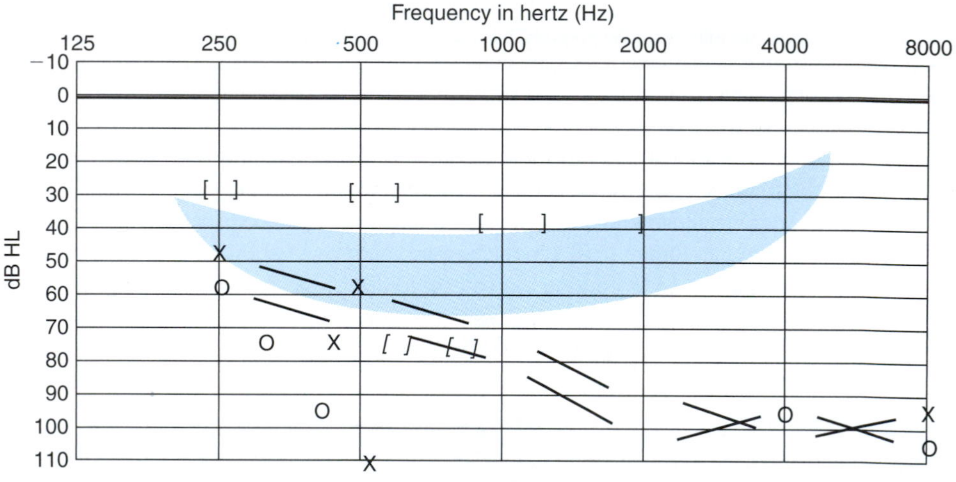

C. Moderate to profound mixed hearing impairment

Audiometric Symbols

	Right ear	Left ear
Air conduction	O	X
Bone conduction	< [	>]
Unaided Aided	Soundfield	

the *air-bone gap*. The hearing loss represented on this audiogram would be typical of cerumen blockage, otitis media, or a congenital closure of the external auditory canal.

In the second audiogram (B), showing a sensorineural hearing loss, there is no air-bone gap but a decrease in hearing threshold when tested by both air and bone conduction. Loss is more severe at higher frequencies. This audiogram might be seen with a genetic disorder, long-term use of ototoxic medications, or auditory nerve damage.

A mixed hearing loss, as shown in the third audiogram (C), occurs when both sensorineural and conductive problems are present. Consequently, both air and bone conduction thresholds are diminished and an air-bone gap is present. The air-bone gap occurs because air conduction testing detects both the conductive and sensorineural components of the mixed loss, whereas bone conduction testing detects only the sensory component.

An audiologist uses speech audiometry as a companion to pure-tone testing to study an individual's hearing responses to speech. In this case an audiometer delivers a speech signal via a microphone, either live speech or a recording. A child's ability to discriminate words in the presence of background noise or other adverse listening conditions can also be evaluated. It is important to understand that hearing acuity and speech perception may not be directly related. For example, a child may have poor speech perception even when hearing loss is minimal. Conversely, many children with profound hearing loss have good speech perception when the speech signal is audible through hearing aids or a cochlear implant.

Discussion Point: *Figure 13-8 shows a mixed hearing loss. What are some possible causes of a mixed hearing loss?*

Objective Measures. The audiologist can use a set of objective measures to evaluate middle ear function, auditory acuity, and the integrity of the auditory system. Objective tests require expensive equipment and extensive training, but they can be completed on infants and children of all ages and do not require a child to respond. In fact, the infant or child is typically asleep during testing.

- *Immittance.* **Immittance** describes the acoustic flow of energy through the middle ear space; *admittance* is the forward flow of energy, and *impedance* is the oppositional energy against the flow. These two forces are tested by studying the vibratory movements of the tympanic membrane. Thus, immittance testing evaluates middle ear function. The audiologist uses several different tools, including **tympanometry**, which examines tympanic membrane movement, or vibration, and graphs the results on a tympanogram. Children with conductive hearing loss—perhaps from wax blockage, otitis media, or perforated eardrums—will have abnormal tympanograms. When a sensorineural hearing loss is present, the tympanogram should be normal.
- *Otoacoustic emissions.* Otoacoustic emissions (OAEs) are a relatively new form of objective testing; they provide an inexpensive, noninvasive, and relatively quick screening or diagnostic tool. The audiologist introduces a series of tones into the ear canal, using insert-style earphones, and records the responses of the auditory system. These responses are called *otoacoustic emissions*. The sensory cells of the cochlea produce an audible byproduct, like an echo, in response to sounds; these can be detected and recorded in the ear canal. The audiologist studies OAEs for children who have no evidence of middle ear dysfunction, which would interfere with the delivery of the sound stimulus to the cochlea. When the cochlea is impaired, the OAEs are abnormal or absent.
- *Evoked auditory potentials.* Evoked auditory potentials (EAPs) are another type of effective, objective test. EAPs test the auditory nervous system's electrical response to sound stimulation. Although EAPs do not directly assess hearing acuity, the results provide information about the integrity of the auditory pathway. The audiologist measures EAPs by delivering tones or clicks to the ears through headphones. Electrodes attached to the head then record electrical activity in the brain as a result of the auditory stimuli. The audiologist graphs the results to study the integrity of the auditory pathway.

Hearing Aid Evaluation

An audiologist who identifies a hearing loss in a child works with the child and the child's family to determine the most appropriate avenue for habilitation. For children with permanent hearing loss and a family desiring an oral orientation, a **hearing aid** will likely be considered. Hearing aid evaluations are used to fit and monitor the use of hearing aids, cochlear implants, and other assistive listening devices. The hearing aid assessment uses several important approaches, including probe microphone measurement and electroacoustic evaluation.

Probe Microphone Measurement. **Probe microphone measurement**, or real ear testing, is an objective, computerized method of measuring hearing aid function in a child's ear. The audiologist places a small probe in the ear canal, along with the hearing aid. A computer generates a series of sounds and measures the output of the hearing aid near the tympanic membrane. Probe microphone measures take into account the individual characteristics of the ear canal as well as the hearing loss.

Sophisticated hearing aid programs are available that consider age, hearing loss, and type of hearing aid and prescribe an appropriate amount of amplification. Comparing the hearing aid output with the computer-generated prescription provides information about whether the hearing aid is meeting the prescribed target. If it is not, changes can be made on the hearing aid, and the effects will be immediately observed. Probe microphone measurement is a critical step in ensuring that children are not over- or underamplified.

Discussion Point: *What problems might arise for a child who is over- or underamplified?*

Electroacoustic Evaluation. Electroacoustic testing electronically verifies the sound properties of a hearing aid. Audiologists use electroacoustic evaluation to choose an appropriate hearing aid for a child and verify that the hearing aid is working properly. Testing is completed in a specially designed box that eliminates outside noise and interfaces with a computer capable of generating and measuring a wide range of sounds. The audiologist studies three key features of the hearing aid:

- Gain: amount of amplification
- Output: intensity of sound the hearing aid can produce at full volume
- Frequency response: the pitch range amplified by the hearing aid

Electroacoustic evaluation is a quick, easy way to determine whether an aid is working properly.

The Importance of Accurate Diagnosis

Hearing loss is an invisible disorder; there is typically no outward physical sign that a problem exists. This complicates the identification and treatment of hearing loss among children of all ages, as the case studies of Jack and Lilly (Box 13-1) illustrate. Too often, children's hearing loss is not diagnosed until after it has exerted a deleterious impact on communication development.

Among this nation's schoolchildren, the number who have unidentified hearing loss is significant (ASHA, 2005). Implementation of newborn hearing screening programs is a necessary and important step to reduce that rate among infants. Among older children, including those of preschool or elementary age, screening programs can fail to identify children who are experiencing ongoing conductive and sensorineural loss, particularly in group screening programs, in which audiometers can easily become uncalibrated. It is important that educators and other professionals who work with children remain vigilant in detecting signs of hearing loss in children.

As important as it is that children with hearing loss are identified, professionals must also take care not to mistake other conditions for hearing loss. The misdiagnosis of a hearing loss is certainly possible, given the difficulty of ensuring that children's responses to audiometric tasks truly represent auditory performance. Children might respond inconsistently, attempt to fake a loss, or simply not cooperate in hearing screening or assessment. These possibilities underscore the importance of a comprehensive test battery that includes reliability checks and objective measures. Not only would a misdiagnosis lead to inappropriate treatment, but it could also harm the child if unnecessary amplification is provided; damage to the cochlear sensory cells can result from overamplification. In addition, it is possible that a child could be mistakenly diagnosed as having a hearing impairment when another condition is present, such as autism. In such a situation the child would not receive the needed intervention.

BOX 13-4 Spotlight on Research

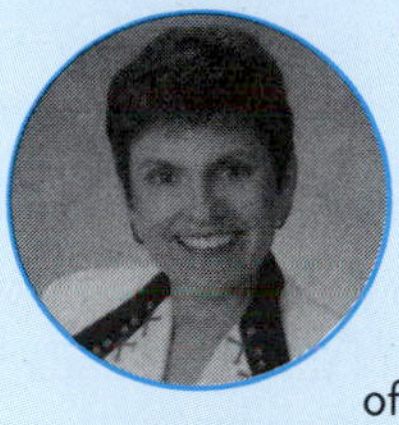

Carol Flexer, Ph.D., CCC-A, FAAA
Distinguished Professor of Audiology
The University of Akron

Carol Flexer has been at the University of Akron for 23 years; she is a professor of audiology in the School of Speech-Language Pathology and Audiology. Dr. Flexer directs and supervises the pediatric diagnostic teaching clinic at the University of Akron and codirects the auditory-verbal (A-V) early intervention clinic. Dr. Flexer's research is applied and collaborative in nature and focuses on two main areas: outcome studies of auditory-verbal intervention and the use of classroom soundfield systems.

Whenever a treatment is offered—whether that treatment is therapeutic, like auditory-verbal intervention, or technological, like soundfield systems—the value of that treatment must be investigated. To that end, Dr. Flexer has conducted a series of studies with colleagues that investigates (1) the benefits of soundfield systems, particularly for literacy development, (2) the outcome of auditory-verbal intervention for children with significant hearing loss, and (3) the outcome for children who receive services at the University of Akron's auditory-verbal early intervention clinic.

Dr. Flexer's research provides evidence that soundfield systems improve literacy development and that literacy has a strong auditory basis. Outcome studies of auditory-verbal graduates from the university's clinic and other A-V programs indicate that students reach important goals, including mainstreamed education using auditory and spoken communication skills and adult postsecondary and work opportunities consistent with those of hearing peers.

Dr. Flexer conducts much of her research in real-life settings, asking questions that are directly related to clinical practice in the field: Is the treatment working? Are the intended outcomes actually achieved? Can we justify continuing the treatment or the use of the technology? For her research and advocacy for children with hearing loss, Dr. Flexer received the Volta Award, the most prestigious award conferred by the Alexander Graham Bell Association for the Deaf and Hard of Hearing.

BOX 13-5 Spotlight on Practice

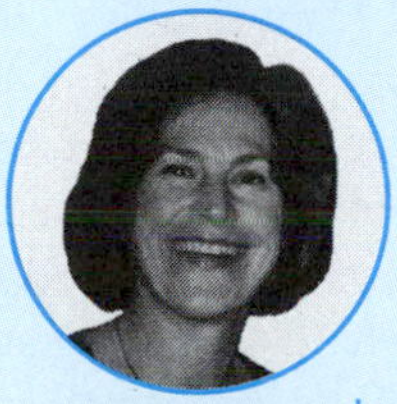

Nancy Caleffe-Schenck, M.Ed., CCC-A, CED, Cert. FAAA
Audiologist, Teacher of the Deaf, and Auditory-Verbal Therapist®
Director, Auditory-Verbal Services, Inc., Evergreen, CO

"Nancy, where are you?"

"Up here, Mom."

"Please tell me where 'here' is," her mom echoed back.

After developing hearing loss from otosclerosis and Meniere's disease, Nancy's mom wore two huge body hearing aids that boomed sound into her ears. Listening through hearing aids was challenging for her mom, so Nancy learned at an early age some practical strategies for helping. Her dad, who had lost much of his hearing at a young age from spinal meningitis, did not wear hearing aids until Nancy was studying audiology in graduate school. Noisy restaurants, weddings, and lively discussions at family meals were venues for Nancy's first practicum in aural habilitation. Her parents were her first and greatest teachers in more ways than she could have imagined as a young girl. From them she learned persistence, courage, and the critical importance of a positive attitude in overcoming the challenges of hearing loss.

Nancy founded Auditory-Verbal Services, Inc., in 1985 and continues there in private practice today with local and out-of-state adults and children of all ages. She also lectures around the world on intervention for hearing loss—in South Africa, Hungary, Taiwan, Brazil, Scotland, Australia—and conducts training for professionals. She publishes on topics such as a hierarchy for listening, children's literature, play, partnerships with parents, and cochlear implants. She coauthored, with Doreen Pollack and Donald Goldberg, the third edition of *Educational Audiology for the Limited Hearing Infant and Preschooler*, the most widely used textbook in auditory-verbal training programs. She is a founding board member of Auditory-Verbal International and has chaired the professional education or certification committees during her 13 years on the board.

From Nancy's perspective, the future is bright because of continued advances in cochlear implant technology, computer and Internet possibilities, and increased training for professionals and students. Children and adults who are deaf will be presented with a widening array of opportunities to learn spoken language through listening.

How Is Pediatric Hearing Loss Treated?

Communication Choices

The overarching goal of all interventions for pediatric hearing loss is the development of healthy, socially and emotionally balanced individuals who are able to integrate fully into society and lead productive lives. Achieving this goal often is dependent on the extent to which these children can form meaningful, sensitive relationships. And that capability relates to their own sense of identity and the way they relate to the world that surrounds them (Scheetz, 2001). Consideration of self-concept, or identity, is particularly relevant in discussions of children who are deaf or hard of hearing, for the parents of these children will need to choose whether to embrace the Deaf community or the mainstream oral community. Even though the Deaf community functions within the larger mainstream oral community, the general approach to life may differ significantly for members of this community.

To understand the importance of parental orientation, we must understand that children are not *taught* speech and language. Rather, they learn the language in which they are immersed through incidental learning and exposure. Children with significant prelingual hearing loss whose parents use oral language will not develop speech and language spontaneously. In fact, to develop speech and language orally, these children will need significant and intensive amounts of intervention. On the other hand, children who are deaf or hard of hearing (and even those with normal hearing) who are raised in a home using a manual language (e.g., American Sign Language) will learn to communicate in that language as effortlessly as a hearing child reared in a home with spoken language.

For children born with a significant hearing loss, families need to make several very important decisions regarding communication choices. For some families the choice will be to maximize their children's hearing so they can learn to speak and listen. Other families may choose to communicate primarily through sign language, focusing on building their children's competence in a manual system. But families are not limited to these two choices; there is a wide continuum from which to choose, as shown in Figure 13-9. Many families will not choose a strict orientation (i.e., ASL or spoken English) but will use a combination of approaches called *total communication,* employing a variety of techniques to support the speech, language, and hearing of their children. Of the children who are hard of hearing or deaf, 49% use both speech and sign, whereas 44% use speech only and 6% use sign only (Gallaudet Research Institute, 2001). Nearly 50% of the children who are deaf or hard of hearing attend regular schools with hearing children, receiving their education fully mainstreamed in the regular education setting. The other half attend school in a self-contained program for children with hearing loss and other disabilities or a residential school or center.

Discussion Point: *For two parents who are hard of hearing and users of American Sign Language, what would be some pros and cons of raising their hearing infant to use ASL versus spoken language?*

Amplification and Listening Devices

Many children with mild to severe hearing loss are fitted with amplification devices; data from the Gallaudet Research Institute (2001) show that 63% of students and youth with hearing loss use hearing aids for instructional purposes. Amplification devices include hearing aids and other assistive listening devices, as well as surgically implanted devices called cochlear implants. None of these devices restore hearing, but they do make sounds accessible to a child's auditory system.

Hearing Aids

Hearing aids are available in many styles and electronic configurations. Children are typically fitted with behind-the-ear hearing aids (BTEs) rather than the in-the-ear aids

FIGURE 13-9 A continuum of communication choices.

American Sign Language (ASL)	< A mixture of language features representing manual and/or spoken languages with various syntactical structures from ASL and English >						Spoken English
	Pidgin signed English (PSE)	Manually coded English	Seeing Essential English and Signing Exact English	Cued speech	Aural/oral	Auditory-verbal	
Manual	Manual	Manual or combined	Manual or combined	Combined	Oral, visual and auditory cues	Oral and auditory cues	Oral
Distinct grammatical language	Mixture of syntax features from ASL & English	ASL signs produced using English syntax	English words signed, may include word endings	Phonemically based, uses physical gestures to enhance speech reading	Spoken English learned with residual hearing; supplemented with visual cues	Spoken English learned using residual hearing	Distinct grammatical language

Source: From "Auditory-Verbal Therapy for Children with Hearing Loss" by M. Harrison, June 1999, presented at Listening to Learn: Partnering Families and Professionals to Teach Children with Hearing Loss, Celebrate the Power Conference, Department of Special Education, Eastern Michigan University, Ypsilanti, MI. Adapted with permission.

that adults prefer for their small size and cosmetic appeal. As shown in Figure 13-10, BTEs are coupled to the ear with an earmold that fits into the outer portion of the ear and attaches to the aid with a connecting tube. Earmolds are custom-made of silicone or similar materials for each child. The earmolds, tubing, and hearing aid all help to shape the sound as it enters the ear. BTEs offer several distinct advantages for children: They are sturdy, and the earmold is more flexible and damage resistant than an in-the-ear style aid. BTEs also have longer battery life (2–3 weeks) and can accommodate more options because they are relatively large; they can be fitted with tamper-resistant battery doors and volume controls, as well as specialized components that couple with other assistive listening devices.

Hearing aids have improved greatly in recent years because of technological advances. Historically, hearing aid users complained of volume control issues and poor speech perception in noise. These were legitimate complaints of the older analog models, which could amplify sound but were not well configured to an individual's

FIGURE 13-10 A behind-the-ear hearing aid.

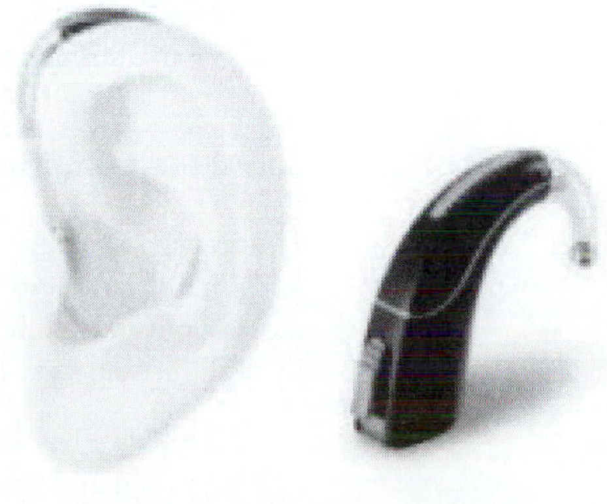

Source: Photo courtesy of Phonak.

specific type of hearing loss. New innovations, including digital processing and multiple-microphone technology, help to maximize hearing in many difficult listening conditions.

Assistive Listening Devices

Many devices can be used in lieu of hearing aids or in conjunction with personal amplification. Assistive listening devices (ALDs) are designed to improve a person's ability to hear in difficult listening situations, such as background noise or distance, both of which are common conditions in classrooms. Sometimes ALDs are used to enhance the amplification of personal hearing aids; at other times ALDs are used instead of hearing aids.

The most common ALD used by children is an **FM system**, which is a personal amplification system that can be used independently or with hearing aids. FM systems are used both in noisy situations and with distant speakers or signals. FM technology relies on radio waves to send a signal from the microphone/transmitter of the speaker to the listener's device (the receiver). The receiver can be an ear-level device or a desktop speaker. In a classroom a child might be provided a personal FM system to amplify the teacher's voice during instruction.

A similar type of system is the soundfield system, which is a type of public address system. Soundfield amplification distributes enhanced sound across an entire room, again using wireless FM microphones. In this case the soundfield surrounds the classroom space. These wireless listening systems are beneficial not only to the child with a hearing loss but often to all of the children in the classroom. However, they are susceptible to interference from other electronic equipment, such as cellular phones.

Cochlear Implants

A **cochlear implant** is a surgically implanted device that provides direct electrical stimulation to the auditory nerve; it is appropriate for children who have severe to profound sensorineural hearing loss. The cochlear implant delivers sound directly to the auditory nerve via an array of electrodes that are surgically implanted in the turns of the cochlea. The implant relies on an external microphone, a speech-processing device, and a transmitter to deliver the sound signals to the internal device. Cochlear implants require extensive testing prior to approval for surgery; factors considered include a child's overall health, chronological age, hearing age, severity of hearing loss, speech perception, spoken language skill, and family expectations and support.

Cochlear implants restore access to sound as soon as they are activated. However, hearing sensitivity alone does not ensure understanding of speech and language. Early implantation and long-term intervention to support speech and language development can maximize the benefit. Other implantable devices are in various stages of use and/or investigation, including middle ear and brain stem devices.

Aural Habilitation

Hearing loss among children and adolescents requires individualized intervention, called **aural habilitation**, to achieve fluent communication in a manual and/or oral modality. Audiologists must carefully design treatment strategies that account for differences in hearing ability and learning style. Aural habilitation typically involves the following set of activities:

- Reception and comprehension of language
- Speech and voice production
- Auditory training

- Speech reading and visual cues
- Communication strategies
- Education and counseling
- Family/caregiver participation
- Follow-up service (ASHA, 1997)

Three general best-practice principles are commonly used for all children: ensuring an appropriate listening environment, maximizing audition, and supporting listening development.

Ensuring an Appropriate Listening Environment

Children with hearing loss require listening environments that are sensitive to their hearing needs. An appropriate listening environment requires that auditory distractions be minimized; turning off an unwatched television, decreasing radio volume, and running a dishwasher at night all help to alleviate background noise at home. School classrooms may also have sources of unnecessary sounds that add to the overall background noise, and modifications should be made. Typical and inexpensive solutions include placing carpet or rugs on the floor, putting cut tennis balls on the bottoms of chairs (if they are sitting on hard floors), hanging window treatments, and placing absorbent materials on the walls, such as tapestries, banners, and even egg cartons. FM technology should also be considered.

Maximizing Audition

Maximizing audition for a child with hearing loss is imperative but is often overlooked as an essential aspect of habilitation. Digital hearing aids, FM systems and soundfield systems, and even cochlear implants are beneficial but must be appropriately fitted, programmed, and properly maintained. Maximizing audition involves more than simply using good equipment; it requires attention to the details of audition.

A pediatric audiologist begins the process with state-of-the-art fitting methods, utilizing every decibel of hearing available to a child and continually striving for improvement. Once the potential for maximum audition is in place, children's hearing devices must be checked on a daily basis. Each day a parent should check the instruments with a listening *stethoset* (a device used to listen to another person's hearing instrument); a visual inspection for damage, moisture buildup, or wax blockage; and a battery check. This check is best done each evening, since battery energy can store up temporarily overnight and provide inaccurate results in the morning. As children grow older, they can take on both the visual inspection and the battery check.

Discussion Point: *In what ways might the daily regimen of caring for hearing aids impact on a child's life at home and at school?*

Additionally, a child's use of a hearing aid should be tested regularly with a listening check, which determines whether the child can hear sounds across the speech spectrum and at a distance. The child listens to a variety of sounds—including /oo/, /ah/, /ee/, /s/, /sh/, /m/, and /r/, which represent the important frequency range for speech perception (Ling, 2001). A parent or teacher presents these sounds at varying distances to determine the maximum distance at which the speaker is still audible without the aid of an FM system—commonly referred to as the circle of hearing.

Further, adults who interact with children with hearing loss should enhance the acoustic signal to provide more audible cues during interactions. This is known as *acoustic highlighting* and includes a variety of techniques:

- A slower rate
- Nearness to the listener

- Increased pitch and rhythm
- Increased repetition and redundancy
- Shorter sentences
- Emphasis on key words
- Emphasis on unstressed function words (i.e., pronouns, articles, verb tense markers, prepositions)
- Emphasis on end of sentence (Simser, 1995)

Over time, these techniques can be reduced as the child's audition improves.

Supporting the Continuum of Listening Development

Aural habilitation typically features a range of activities to improve auditory detection, discrimination, identification, and comprehension (see Figure 13-11). Detection tasks, such as differentiating a speech sound from a nonspeech sound, are easier than comprehension tasks, such as listening to familiar phrases. A clinician supports a child's development of listening skills by gradually increasing the auditory demands of tasks and providing the amount of support needed for the child to be successful. The clinician might give visual cues

FIGURE 13-11 A hierarchy of listening development.

Detection	• Noise and nonspeech sounds • Speech sounds with reinforcement • Speech sounds without reinforcement • Response to own name

Discrimination	• Two or more items differing in suprasegmental (i.e., pitch, stress) features
	  • Linguistic ("moo" vs. "go", "car" vs. "pencil")
	  • Nonlinguistic (joyful voice vs. angry voice, male voice vs. female voice, child voice vs. adult voice)

Identification	• Three or more items differing in segmental features
	  • Single-syllable words varying in vowel and consonant content
	  • Words in which vowel is constant and consonant varies in manner, place, and voicing
	  • Two or more elements varied in a phrase

Comprehension	• Familiar phrases • Simple and complex directions • Sequence of directions and events in a story • Coversation with cues (e.g., picture context or familiar story) • Connected discourse • Different settings (in quiet, then noise) • Onomatopoeic words

Source: From "Learning Through Listening: A Hierarchy" by C. Edwards and W. Estabrooks, 1994, in W. Estabrooks (Ed.), *Auditory-Verbal Therapy for Parents and Professionals* (p. 58), Washington, DC: Alexander Graham Bell Association for the Deaf. Copyright 1994 by Alexander Graham Bell Association for the Deaf. Adapted with permission.

(e.g., pictures or gestures) or use a technique called auditory sandwiching. An auditory sandwich involves saying the word, signing or providing a visual cue, and then saying the word again (e.g., say "apple," sign apple, say "apple"). The clinician is coupling visual cues with auditory cues and over time will reduce the visual cues.

Intervention Principles

Infants, Toddlers, and Preschoolers

When first identified with hearing loss, infants and young children have different intervention needs from those of older children. Because they are learning language, treatment focuses on facilitating natural developmental sequences and promoting acquisition of functional communication. The guiding principles for providing aural habilitation to infants, toddlers, and preschoolers are consistent with the principles of other forms of intervention for children of this age, including early intervention, parental involvement, naturalistic environments, social interaction, and functional outcomes.

Early Intervention. Early intervention is the single most important factor in determining long-term achievement for children with hearing loss. Implementing intervention before 6 months of age is optimal. Even though clinicians do not provide conventional therapy for an infant, they do provide hearing aids or other listening devices and guide parents' use of natural and developmentally appropriate interactions to encourage communication development.

Parental Involvement. Parents who understand natural developmental sequences and use that information to creatively expose their children to language and learning opportunities are the most important change agent in children's developmental achievements. Parents also monitor services to ensure carryover and coordination among professionals; they are the advocates and the negotiators on whom their children depend.

Naturalistic Environments. Intervention for children with hearing loss is most effective when it engages them in those environments in which they must use their skills. Naturalistic environments include the home and the classroom. And although children may be seen for intervention in therapy contexts, the room should be child friendly, with activities centered on the floor or on child-sized furniture. Working across multiple environments also provides valuable information about the child's ability to generalize skills from one environment to the next, and multiple exposure to key concepts in multiple environments reinforces the child's experiences and learning.

Social Interaction. Generally, children are social by nature. Communication facilitates social interaction, and in turn, social interaction creates opportunities for communication development. Supporting the development of children with hearing loss within authentic social interactions is considered an essential best practice. It is not uncommon that a child and one or both parents learn sign language but that other family members and friends do not, leaving the child unable to communicate effectively and independently with other family and friends and inhibiting social engagement and interaction. A clinician works closely with the child's family to enhance the child's opportunity and potential for socially embedded communication experiences.

Functional Outcomes. The average age of identification of children with congenital hearing loss is about 2 years of age. If a 2-year-old child has little or no language, frustration and related behavioral problems are likely. Thus, it is imperative that intervention ensure functional communication and provide the child a means to communicate in everyday contexts, whether with words, signs, or gestures. As communication skills improve, functional communication targets become more sophisticated but no less important.

School-Age Children

School-age children diagnosed with an acquired hearing loss or an undetected congenital loss have established audition, speech, and language skills. Although their communication skills may be delayed or disordered, school-age children with hearing loss have a foundation from which to begin intervention. However, increasing levels of academic complexity and social sophistication continually challenge these children; frequently, they find themselves interested in activities and experiences that relate to their peers but lack the communication skills to effectively participate. Professionals and families must be mindful of the intervention principles that guide service provision to school-age children: an effective means of communication, self-advocacy, and literacy.

An Effective Means of Communication. Children with severe to profound hearing loss often struggle with communication, and some fail to develop a fluent and effective means of communicating with people across different environments. Instead, they may flounder between inadequate oral and sign skills. By the time a child reaches school age, an effective means of communication must be established.

If a child is an inadequate oral communicator, parents must consider enhancing communication with sign language or seek ways to improve audition. A child who is taught sign language must have the support of family (and friends to the extent possible), or the child must be given other opportunities (e.g., cochlear implant) to maximize hearing and improve oral communication skills. Further, families should foster the development of relationships with peers who share the same language (e.g., ASL) if children are not naturally involved in activities or experiences with other children with whom they can communicate.

Self-Advocacy. Children with hearing loss often have special needs with respect to communication, particularly outside the home. They may need to request clarification, assistance, or special consideration. In class, students may require that instructions be repeated or written down, or they may need the assistance of an interpreter. Participation in a sporting event may require assistance with technology to enable the athlete to hear the coach from a distance. In a restaurant or noisy cafeteria, students may benefit from moving to a small table away from the kitchen. Children who are able and willing to seek support and assistance develop into confident adults who are able to have their needs met through effective communication.

Literacy. Literacy includes more than reading and writing; it also includes literate thought, or the ability to think critically and reflectively and to use language to solve problems and reason (Paul, 1998). Literate thought, as well as reading and writing, requires the acquisition of a solid language foundation (whether oral or manual) at the earliest age possible; literacy skills will enhance and extend this early foundation (Paul, 1998). Because children with hearing loss too often exhibit weaknesses in their language base, literacy is often compromised. School-age children must be given consistent and intensive supports to achieve literacy and literate thought. Audiologists, speech-language pathologists, reading specialists, and special educators must work together.

What Is Auditory Processing Disorder, and How Is It Identified and Treated?

An auditory processing disorder (APD) is a type of hearing loss that adversely affects an individual's processing, or interpretation, of auditory messages. An individual with APD has problems in one or more of the following aspects of auditory processing:

1. Sound localization and lateralization with both ears
2. Auditory discrimination (i.e., hearing the differences between different sounds)
3. Recognition of patterns of sound
4. Differentiation of the temporal aspects of sound
5. Reduced auditory performance when the message is incomplete or competing acoustic signals are present (ASHA, 1996; Schow, Seikel, Chermak, & Berent, 2000)

Auditory processing disorders are not typically accompanied by a loss of hearing acuity. Rather, these reflect difficulty processing specific elements of the auditory signal, such as timing or patterns.

Terms used to describe auditory processing disorders in children include *central auditory processing disorder* (CAPD), *central deafness, auditory perception deficit,* and *auditory comprehension disorder.* The terms *auditory processing disorder* and *central auditory processing disorder* indicate that the disorder is in the auditory center of the brain, not in the peripheral auditory system that includes the ear and the auditory nerve. Thus, the problem lies in deciphering a message as opposed to hearing it.

Defining Characteristics

APD is a neurological problem in which a child has difficulty interpreting and processing auditory information, even though hearing acuity is intact. Thus, the child exhibits no apparent problems with the outer, middle, or inner ear functions or structures; the problem resides in the areas of the brain that process auditory information. Although the child may have some subtle auditory difficulties, the processing of auditory information tends to be particularly degraded in the presence of background noise or other distractions (Martin & Greer Clark, 2002). Children with auditory processing problems exhibit academic and communicative difficulties, including inability to follow complex verbal directions, poor performance on verbally instructed tasks, spelling and reading deficits, and inability to engage in classroom discussion. Some of the most common indicators of APD include the following:

- Behaves as if a hearing loss is present although it is not
- Shows problems following complex, multistep directions
- Exhibits difficulties with reading and spelling performance
- Reveals degraded listening and audition in noisy environments or with competing auditory stimuli
- Appears to seek out visual cues from the environment (e.g., from other children)
- Has a history of fluctuating hearing loss, including middle ear infections
- Has difficulty staying on task, finishing assignments, and working independently (Bellis, 1996)

Although children with auditory processing disorders exhibit many of the negative impacts experienced by children with more general hearing loss, there are numerous differences.

Since auditory processing disorders do not cause a loss of hearing acuity, children with APD typically demonstrate little difficulty with speech production. However, their vocabulary development, pragmatics, listening, and academic achievement may be affected. In addition, amplification through hearing aids is not an option for children with APD.

Causes and Risk Factors

Scientists do not fully understand the underlying processes of the auditory processing mechanisms or the ways they malfunction to result in communication disorders. Consequently, the specific cause of APD is often unknown. In children APD is sometimes associated with other disorders, including dyslexia, attention deficit disorder, autism spectrum disorder, specific language impairment, and developmental delay (National Institute for Deafness and Other Communication Disorders, 2003).

Assessment

The auditory processing centers of the brain form a complex system. There is currently no gold standard for identifying the presence of an auditory processing disorder, although an audiologist does have a set of tools to study auditory processing capabilities. Because these often involve asking the individual to listen carefully and respond behaviorally to auditory stimuli for a long period of time in a soundproof booth, auditory processing assessment is not recommended for children under 7 years of age (Bellis, 1996). The assessment tasks examine sensitivity to the temporal ordering of sounds, ability to listen to sounds when they are degraded or have other sounds competing, and ability to listen to different stimuli in both ears simultaneously. The audiologist also uses observation and interview to determine how the child functions in different listening environments, such as the classroom. Typically, additional professionals are involved with auditory processing evaluation—special educators, speech-language pathologists, and neuropsychologists.

Discussion Point: *A comprehensive auditory processing assessment should include a speech and language evaluation. What might the speech and language evaluation uncover that would not be discovered in an assessment by an audiologist alone?*

Treatment Approaches

Currently, treatment for APD focuses on treating the symptoms of the disorder. The most common symptoms cluster into four areas of concern: behavior, such as problems listening and attending; literacy, such as problems with phonological awareness, reading, and spelling; linguistic ability, such as vocabulary and pragmatics; and organization, such as difficulties with planning responses and tasks (Bellis, 1996).

Audiologists work directly with teachers and speech-language pathologists to provide treatment that involves three main approaches: environmental modification, remediation activities, and compensatory strategies (Bellis, 1996). Environmental modification changes the learning environment so that it provides highly redundant and better-quality auditory information. Common techniques include notetakers, frequent checks for clarification, assistive listening devices, and preferential seating. Remediation activities focus on alleviating the disorder by improving auditory processing abilities. The clinician engages the child in structured activities designed to stimulate various aspects of the auditory processing system, such as training in the temporal organization of sounds. Compensatory strategies teach the child to be proactive as a listener and a communicator and to use strategies that improve both roles. The child is helped to learn when communication breakdowns occur and to implement approaches that resolve these breakdowns.

Case Study and Clinical Problem Solving

INTERIM DIAGNOSTIC REPORT: SUMMARY

Client: Andy Duvall
Evaluation Date: 6/3/05
Date of Birth: 11/18/98
Age: 6 years, 6 months

Overview

Andy was seen for an interim assessment to update progress and review goals. His mother and speech-language pathologist report good progress with significant receptive and expressive language growth and improved speech intelligibility. He still has problems with functional communication.

Pertinent History

Andy has a history of congenital bilateral profound sensorineural hearing loss. Hearing screening was completed at age 2 years, followed by a full evaluation and hearing aid fitting by 26 months. Etiology of the hearing loss is unknown. Andy has bilateral Phonak Claro digital behind-the-ear hearing aids, which he wears during all waking hours. He also frequently uses a personal FM system. Andy's speech, language, and auditory skills are severely delayed. He and his family know sign language; however, Andy has oriented himself as an oral communicator and uses signs only on occasion to facilitate communication. Andy's mother, Jenna, reported that she and Andy's father are usually able to understand him; however, the extended family and friends often have difficulty. Andy currently attends first grade in a mainstream classroom. He uses an FM system and has a part-time itinerant teacher. Andy's father is employed full-time as a psychiatric nurse, and his mother is a full-time graduate student in speech-language pathology. He has an 8-year-old brother who is typically developing. Andy is a healthy, energetic child. He has a positive history of chronic otitis media. He had pressure equalization tubes placed last spring. The right tube is out, but the left tube remains in place.

Diagnostic Results and Impressions

Hearing Evaluation

Otoscopic examination and tympanometry revealed normal middle ear function. The flat response for the left ear was consistent with a pressure-equalizing tube in place. Pure-tone results revealed a severe to profound sensorineural hearing loss between 250 Hz and 4000 Hz with no response present at higher test frequencies. Speech discrimination is poor at 40% (right ear), 56% (left ear), and 44% (aided) accuracy at 5–15 dB sensation level. Otoacoustic emissions are absent, which is consistent with a cochlear (sensory) loss.

Aided Evaluation

Andy consistently responds to vowel and nasal speech sounds ("oo," "ee," "ah," and "m") up to 3 feet but has difficulty with "s" and "sh" even at close distance. Impressions were taken for new earmolds in an effort to improve aided benefit. The Speech Perception Instructional Curriculum and Evaluation for children with cochlear implants and hearing aids (SPICE) was also administered. Andy used his FM system during this evaluation to maximize audition. Andy's suprasegmental perception is good when stimuli differ in duration, stress, and/or intonation. He can discriminate among 3 stimuli. On vowel and consonant perception, Andy can discriminate 3–4 words with high levels of contrast. Andy cannot readily discriminate connected speech without significant prompting or support.

Language

Assessment of language skills was conducted via informal observation, language sample, and Clinical Evaluation of Language Fundamentals–Preschool (CELF-P). Andy demonstrated a mean length of utterance (MLU) of 4.0, which places him in Brown's Stage IV. Andy demonstrates use of questions, negatives, articles, past irregular, and some auxiliaries. Andy's standard scores on the CELF-P for receptive and expressive language skills were 67 and 65, respectively (percentile rank of 1).

Speech

Informal observation showed Andy's speech to be about 50% intelligible; errors were primarily sound substitutions and deletions. Three processes were identified (stopping, deaffrication, and cluster reduction) as occurring more than 40% of the time, which detract from intelligibility.

Conclusions

Andy is a pleasant and energetic child who cooperated during the evaluation. He demonstrates age-appropriate developmental skills and no evidence of cognitive delays. Andy exhibits severely delayed communication skills related to his severe-to-profound sensorineural hearing loss. Audition is not maximized at present time; new earmolds need to be fitted, and his FM system is intermittent. Expressively, Andy displayed difficulty with articulation of many sounds that should be mastered at his present age. He also exhibited phonological processes that should be suppressed by the age of 6. Given Andy's family's interest in increasing his success as an oral communicator, it is imperative that he continues in intensive therapy and maximizes audition. With implementation of appropriate treatment, he has a good prognosis for improvement of speech intelligibility based on his age, family support, and motivation to communicate.

Recommendations

1. Continue enrollment in individualized speech, language, and aural habilitation therapy for two 50-minute sessions per week.
2. Have new earmolds fitted and amplification adjusted to maximize audition.
3. Provide Andy's parents and teachers with materials and strategies to implement across settings.

Joy Simon, M.A., CCC-SLP, C-AVT

CLINICAL PROBLEM SOLVING

1. Andy's school teacher was not interviewed. What might the clinician have learned by interviewing his teachers?
2. What other professionals should be involved with Andy's treatment plan?
3. The speech-language pathologist indicated a good prognosis for Andy. What factors led her to this judgment? What factors influence his prognosis?

CHAPTER SUMMARY

Hearing loss is a complex problem that has the potential to impact children's lives dramatically. Children's communication skills and academic achievement influence their identity and course in life. Deafness in particular is unique because it involves a separate community with its own language and values for those who choose to embrace it.

Hearing loss covers a broad spectrum of problems. The loss may be temporary, permanent, or fluctuating. It can vary in degree from slight to profound, and it can affect one or both ears. The loss can affect hearing acuity, comprehension, and speech perception, all of which influence development of functional communication and cognition.

Parents, teachers, physicians, or other professionals may make the initial referral for a hearing loss. Screening tests are often used to establish the underlying problem. Depending on the nature of the problem, an audiologist develops a comprehensive test battery. Audiometry and immittance are used to determine the type and degree of hearing loss. Audiologists use a separate, four-factored test battery for children with auditory processing problems. If a hearing loss exists, parents are counseled regarding communication options. If families choose to have their child use spoken language, the audiologist determines the need for amplification and assesses aural habilitation needs. An aural habilitation evaluation requires an interdisciplinary team to evaluate speech, language, cognition, and other factors such as social-emotional concerns.

Once an intervention plan is developed, the clinician initiates therapy and works with other professionals to maximize the child's communicative success. Aural habilitation includes targets for development/remediation and strategies to achieve those targets and may take place across contexts. Intervention principles are geared toward the individual child and family. With early and appropriate identification and intervention, children can learn to listen and speak.

KEY TERMS

air conduction, p. 450
audiometry, p. 449
auditory processing disorders, p. 432
aural habilitation, p. 458
bone conduction, p. 442
cochlear implant, p. 458
conductive hearing loss, p. 439
congenital hearing loss, p. 432
deaf/Deaf, p. 432
Deaf community, p. 433
decibels, p. 440
evoked auditory potentials, p. 447
FM system, p. 458
hard of hearing, p. 432
hearing aid, p. 453
hearing loss, p. 429
immittance, p. 453
mixed hearing loss, p. 439
otitis media, p. 443
otoacoustic emissions, p. 447
otoscopic examination, p. 448
postlingual hearing loss, p. 432
prelingual hearing loss, p. 432
probe microphone measurement, p. 454
sensorineural hearing loss, p. 439
threshold, p. 440
tympanometry, p. 453

ON THE WEB

Check out the Companion Website! On it you will find

- suggested readings
- reflection questions
- a self-study quiz
- links to additional online resources, including current technologies in communication sciences and disorders

Hearing Loss in Adults

L. A. Pakulski

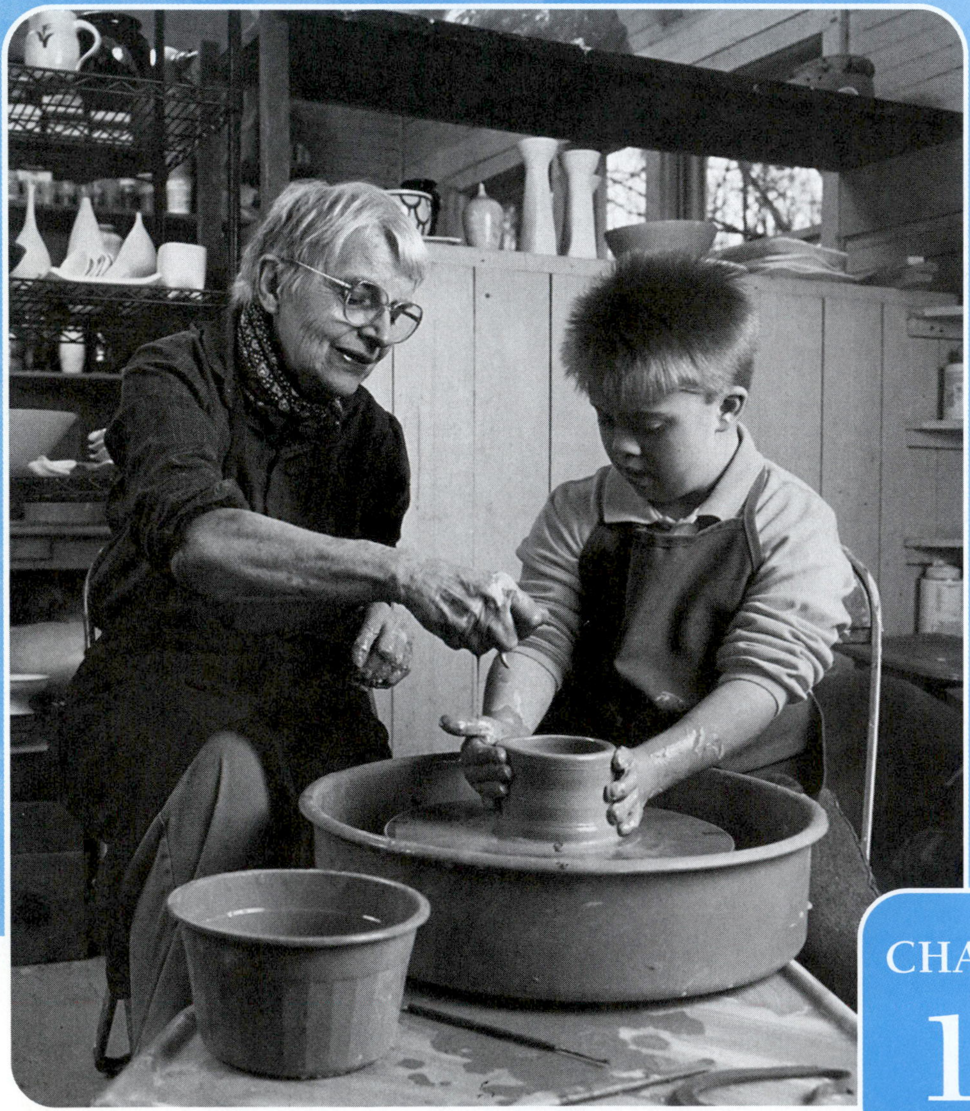

CHAPTER 14

FOCUS QUESTIONS

This chapter answers the following questions:

1. What is hearing loss in adults?
2. How is adult hearing loss classified?
3. What are the defining characteristics of prevalent types of adult hearing loss?
4. How is adult hearing loss identified?
5. How is adult hearing loss treated?

INTRODUCTION

Mr. Jones picks up the telephone, listens for a moment, and asks, "You're trying to save the nation?" "No, sir," the voice responds, "I said I'm trying to get some information!" Mr. Jones hangs up in frustration, still not understanding what the call was all about. This brief snippet provides a glimpse into the life of an adult with a moderate hearing loss. Mr. Jones himself is not aware of the loss, nor are any of his family members or friends, although his wife occasionally wonders if her husband is losing his hearing. Consequently, despite the fact that Mr. Jones experiences daily difficulties in his communication with others, he has yet to receive any assistance. His condition remains undiscovered.

As Mr. Jones' experiences illustrate, hearing loss in adults is called an invisible disability because there are often no outward signs of diminished hearing. And because hearing loss in adults often emerges gradually with age, the symptoms of hearing loss may be mistaken for other conditions, such as cognitive decline or psychological issues like irritability or depression. Nonetheless, hearing loss among adults can have detrimental effects on an individual's social-emotional, psychological, and physical well-being (e.g., Kirkwood, 1999; Radcliffe, 1998). Beyond the personal cost, untreated or mismanaged hearing loss costs the U.S. economy billions of dollars annually. However, these costs need not occur; hearing loss can be treated through a wide array of technologies and interventions.

Approximately 28 million Americans have hearing loss, representing about 10% of the population (National Institute on Deafness and Other Communication Disorders, 2005). Estimates also show that well over one fourth of the adult population will experience a hearing loss sometime in their lifetime (Cruikshanks et al., 1998). In fact, it is nearly guaranteed that individuals who are fortunate enough to live a long life will experience a significant decline in hearing; epidemiological studies show that 90% of persons over age 80 have hearing loss (Cruikshanks et al., 1998). Thus, it is not surprising that hearing loss ranks third among common health complaints of older adults, with only hypertension and arthritis ranking higher (Adams & Benson, 1991).

In the next decade the number of adults living with hearing loss will increase substantially, as 78 million of the "rockin' and rollin' Baby Boomers" reach an advanced age (Garstecki & Erler, 1995). Fortunately, these individuals will have numerous technologies and interventions available to help compensate for their hearing loss. However, less than 22% of those who might benefit from intervention receive services; estimates suggest that "22 million Americans do not use hearing aids to compensate for their hearing loss" (American Speech-Language Hearing Association [ASHA], 2004a; Kochkin, 1993, 1999).

Adults often resist seeking intervention for hearing loss for several reasons: (1) a perception that the hearing loss is not severe enough, (2) the costs associated with treatment, and (3) negative images associated with hearing aids (Erler & Garstecki, 2002; Kirkwood, 1999). Additionally, because hearing screenings occur rarely during routine medical visits (Newman & Sandridge, 2004), physicians on the front line miss important opportunities to identify hearing loss among their patients and to refer them for proactive interventions. Fortunately, when appropriate intervention does occur, adults can learn to live well with hearing loss with little or no negative impact on daily life (e.g., Backenroth & Ahlner, 2000; Bridges & Bentler, 1998; Lewis, et al., 2003).

This chapter considers hearing loss among the adult population. Although adults between the ages of 21 and 65 experience hearing loss, the elderly comprise the largest percentage of the population with hearing loss. This chapter reintroduces and builds on many concepts introduced in chapter 13. Consequently, you are encouraged to study these two chapters in the order in which they occur in this text.

What Is Adult Hearing Loss?

Definition

Discussion Point: *Consider Kristina, Lenny, and Jimmy in Box 14-1. To what extent does each of these individuals exhibit a hearing handicap in addition to a hearing loss?*

Hearing loss is a "deviation or change for the worse in either auditory structure or auditory function" that differs significantly from normal (American Speech-Language-Hearing Association [ASHA], 1981, p. 293). When this deviation impacts a person negatively, it is considered a hearing handicap or a hearing impairment, suggesting the disadvantage to an individual's daily living routines, including communication (ASHA, 1981).

A hearing loss results from change in the outer, middle, or inner ear or the auditory nerve to the brain. When the disorder affects the outer or middle ear, it is a conductive disorder. Sensorineural loss results from outer or inner hair cell damage in the cochlea or damage to the auditory nerve, which travels from the cochlea to the brain (Killion & Niquette, 2000). Among adults sensorineural hearing loss is most common; it is the cochlea and the auditory nerve that are most readily affected by aging, noise exposure, illness, disease, and injury. You probably recall from chapter 13 that among children conductive hearing loss is most prevalent, because of the high rates of middle ear infections in early childhood. Among adults conductive problems occur relatively infrequently.

Cochlear damage results in a loss of sensitivity to sound, or a decrease in hearing acuity. Consequently, a person experiences difficulty hearing soft sounds (e.g., a bird chirping) and understanding soft speech (e.g., a spouse speaking from another room). The change in hearing sensitivity also affects people's perception of loud sounds. Specifically, they may experience a reduced tolerance for loud sounds, termed *recruitment*. **Recruitment** makes it difficult for a person with hearing loss to tolerate common loud sounds, such as the increase in volume of a typical television commercial or a crying baby. Many adults with hearing loss also experience another auditory phenomenon called *tinnitus*. **Tinnitus** is described as a ringing, roaring, buzzing, or hissing sound in one or both ears. It may be occasional or frequent, intermittent or continuous. Tinnitus may be a result of damage to the ears (e.g., excessive noise exposure), or it may be related to high blood pressure, stress, fatigue, excessive caffeine, or other physical concerns.

Damage to the cochlea can also result in a decrease in clarity of speech perception, especially in noise. Such a decrease is different from a decrease in audibility or acuity, as shown in Figure 14-1. Hearing loss and loss of speech clarity due to inner hair cell damage are termed **signal-to-noise ratio (SNR) loss**. SNR loss is a relatively new concept that explains why some people complain that they can hear just fine if people wouldn't mumble or if there wasn't so much background noise. This type of loss is based on the relationship of a signal (e.g., the voice of a friend in the room) to the noise in the environment (e.g., a fan and a television). In general, signals become more difficult to discern as noise levels increase, a concept referred to as the signal-to-noise ratio. However, individuals with SNR loss experience difficulty even when the signal-to-noise ratio is relatively low. They require a greater signal intensity than other people require.

Although rare, sensorineural hearing loss can also result from damage to the eighth cranial nerve, the auditory nerve, referred to as *neural loss*. Loss of or damage to neurons along the auditory pathway causes a loss of hearing acuity and a loss of clarity.

In defining adult hearing loss of a sensorineural type, it is important to consider the impact of the loss on both hearing acuity and hearing clarity. Even though the symptoms often cooccur, the loss of clarity is actually independent of hearing acuity (Killion & Niquette, 2000). Loss of hearing acuity can be readily improved by amplifying sound, as with a hearing aid. Loss of clarity due to inner hair cell or neural damage, on the other hand, results in a reduction in or degradation of the flow of auditory information to the

Discussion Point: *SNR loss causes a reduction in clarity, especially in noise. How does this differ from a loss of acuity?*

FIGURE 14-1 **A visual analogy of normal hearing, loss of clarity, and loss of acuity.**

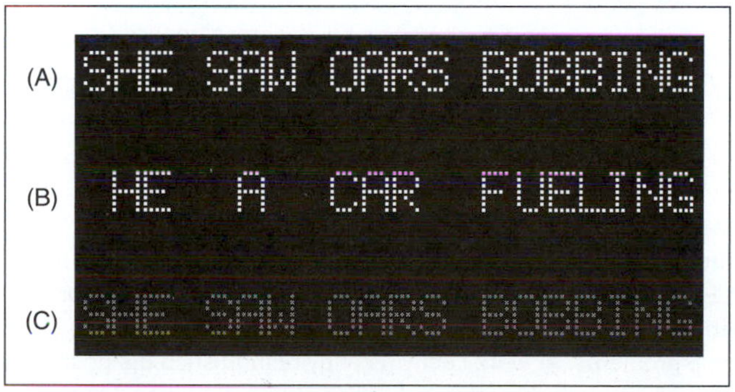

Note: Imagine an electronic sign in which each light bulb has its own wire that delivers the electrical current. Each bulb represents an inner hair cell, and each wire represents a neuron. When a bulb is out, it can be because of the bulb itself (inner hair cell damage) or a cut wire (neuron damage).

A: All lights are lit normally; thus all components are functioning properly.

B: Approximately 35% of the bulbs are burned out, leading to interpretation of the original message as "HE A CAR FUELING." This illustrates a loss of clarity. If additional damage occurs, it may be impossible to interpret any of the message, even if the remaining bulbs are very bright.

C: The lights are all working, but they are quite dim. This corresponds to a loss of acuity due to outer hair cell damage. The message may be difficult to read, but amplification can make up for the loss of sensitivity.

Source: From "What Can the Pure-Tone Audiogram Tell Us About a Patient's SNR Loss?" by M. C. Killion and P. A. Niguette, 2000, *Hearing Journal*, *53*, pp. 46–53. Copyright 2000 by Lippincott Williams & Wilkins. Adapted with permission.

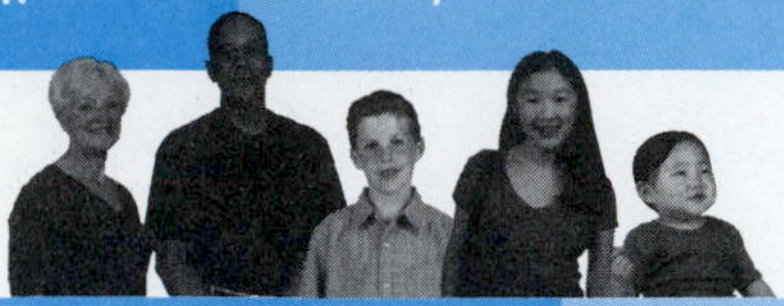

BOX 14-1 Hearing Loss in Early and Later Adulthood: Case Examples

Kristina, age 22, is a single mother of an 8-month-old daughter. Kristina has a hearing loss that was first identified when she was in high school. She tried hearing aids briefly at that time but was not satisfied and discontinued use. Recently, she started taking college courses and working part-time at a convenience store. Her hearing loss interferes with her ability to hear her daughter, understand her instructors in the classroom, and communicate with customers. Kristina shared her concerns with her physician, who recommended a hearing evaluation.

Kristina saw a student intern at the university, who conducted a comprehensive hearing evaluation. The results showed a moderately severe high-frequency sensorineural hearing loss in both ears. An aural rehabilitation assessment was also completed and found that Kristina is an adequate speech/lip reader. Based on self-perception surveys, it appears that Kristina has a perception of significant handicap related to her hearing loss. A conversational observation, completed with her mother as communication partner, revealed many communication breakdowns, inadequate use of repair strategies, inappropriate topic shifts, and an imbalance in conversational turn-taking.

Audiometric and aural rehabilitation findings were explained to Kristina. The intern recommended that she reconsider hearing aids and undergo a hearing aid assessment and trial program with digital amplification that can be programmed to match her current hearing loss contour. An aural rehabilitation program was also suggested to counter the negative consequences of Kristina's untreated hearing loss.

Internet research

1. What laws protect the rights of employees with hearing loss? What changes might her employer have to make to accommodate Kristina's loss?
2. What sources of funding are available for lower income persons to cover the cost of hearing aids? How much does a digital hearing aid typically cost?

Brainstorm and discussion

1. In what ways will amplification impact Kristina's communication with her daughter?
2. What are some possible explanations for Kristina's limited use of hearing aids in the past? Why might she be more likely to use amplification now?

Lenny, age 53, is an ironworker who has experienced a gradual decrease in hearing in both ears. He has a history of industrial noise exposure, including an acoustic trauma from an explosion close to his right ear. Currently, he has a moderate sensorineural hearing loss in the 3000–6000 Hz range in both ears. Lenny and his wife perceive his hearing problems as a significant handicap. He and his family experience communicative problems in the home and, as a result, have diminished their conversations, leading to relationship problems. At work Lenny recently relinquished his position as foreman because he cannot communicate effectively with his employees, particularly on the two-way radios. He stopped attending church, movies, and many social events because of his inability to effectively communicate. Although amplification and aural rehabilitation were recommended during a recent hearing assessment, Lenny is reluctant to follow this course of treatment because of financial constraints.

Internet research

1. If a person such as Lenny experiences work-related hearing loss, what recourse does he have from his employer?
2. What can be done to prevent hearing loss in the workplace?
3. If third party payers do not cover hearing aids and related services and a client cannot afford them, what other possible funding sources or options are available?

Brainstorm and discussion

1. What are some activities that Lenny and his family could practice to promote better communication?
2. What are some approaches Lenny's wife might use to support Lenny's pursuit of intervention?

Jimmy, age 81, is a retired engineer in Nebraska. For more than 30 years, he has successfully worn behind-the-ear (BTE) hearing aids for a bilateral moderate-to-severe sensorineural hearing loss. He lives with his wife in a rural area about 25 minutes away from the audiologist's office. Because he has experienced some vision problems and can no longer drive, his wife, who is younger and in good health, drives him to appointments and is responsible for many of his other care needs.

Jimmy has recently experienced a series of problems related to his hearing and hearing aids. First, he was unable to hear in his right ear. A visit to the audiologist uncovered a plugged right earmold as a result of cerumen buildup in that ear. The audiologist removed the cerumen and reminded Jimmy about how to check and clean his earmolds. Because of his limited vision, Jimmy had difficulty detecting the wax in the earmold, so the audiologist suggested that his wife learn to assist in caring for the hearing aids. She declined.

Approximately 1 month later, Jimmy returned, complaining that his hearing aids were not functioning. This time Jimmy was using his 15-year-old hearing aids rather than his newer ones. Jimmy was confused but thought perhaps he had mistakenly switched them while cleaning them since he keeps all the aids in one cigar box. He was instructed to try the newer digital aids when he got home. Unfortunately, Jimmy was unable to distinguish the new from the old hearing aids and made another appointment, cigar box in hand, to have the audiologist help him identify the appropriate hearing aids and check them. The newer aids were found, checked, and refitted. The older aids were then placed in a separate box to avoid future confusion.

A few weeks later, Jimmy made another appointment because his wife was complaining that he was not paying attention to or hearing her consistently. At that appointment it was determined that the batteries were placed in the hearing aids upside down. Again, Jimmy was reminded of proper care procedures, and his wife again declined to assist him. However, this time the audiologist enlisted a friendly neighbor of Jimmy's who was willing to help him care for his hearing aids. The neighbor was given instructions and notes on hearing aid care and troubleshooting. Finally, Jimmy's hearing aid problems diminished, and he no longer had to make the frequent, long trips to the audiologist's office for minor concerns.

Internet research

1. How many audiologists practice in Nebraska?
2. What support services are available for people like Jimmy's wife, who are frustrated by a significant other's diminished capacity?

Brainstorm and discussion

1. To care for themselves, adults with diminished capacity must rely on others to assist them. For people without a helpful neighbor, what are some support options?
2. What are some other approaches that might have been used to support Jimmy and his hearing needs?

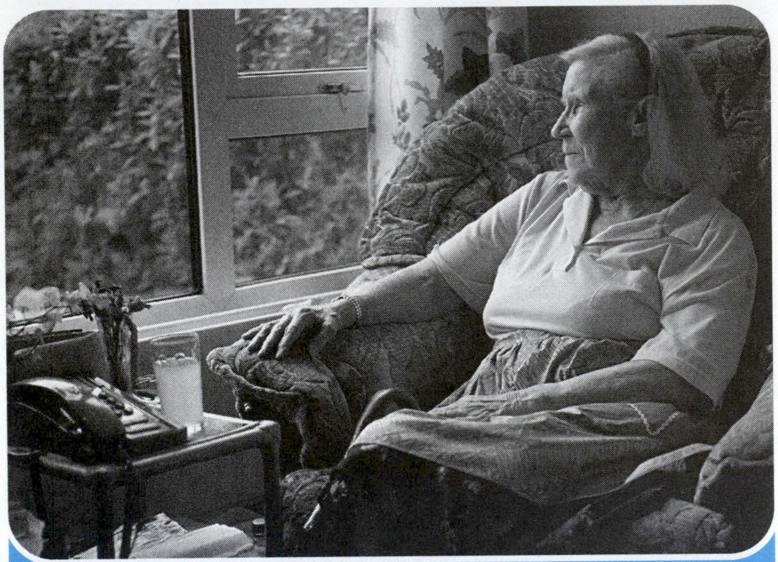

Significant others may limit their conversations with family members with hearing loss, given the challenges of communicating effectively.

brain (Killion & Niquette, 2000), which cannot be remedied with amplification alone, but requires an improved signal-to-noise ratio. The presence of either recruitment or SNR loss is a particularly important consideration in choosing the appropriate amplification device to ensure that sounds are perceived as clearly and comfortably as possible in both quiet and noisy conditions.

Social-Emotional, Psychological, and Physical Impact

Hearing loss goes undetected and/or untreated in more than 75% of adults with hearing loss (Newman & Sandridge, 2004). When left untreated, hearing loss—particularly the sensorineural variety, which impacts hearing acuity and clarity—can have devastating effects on an individual's social-emotional and psychological well-being, physical health, lifestyle, and educational and vocational choices. Sometimes, people are aware of a hearing loss and make changes in their own lifestyles rather than admit the loss and seek intervention; others are unaware of their loss, and it goes undetected by medical professionals and family members, too. Regardless, hearing loss can impact life in many ways. Consider Jorges, an elderly grandfather who decides to quit attending family functions because "no one is interested in what an old man has to say" and he's tired of sitting alone at gatherings with no one to talk to. In reality, after years of increasingly difficult communication because of his poor hearing ability, Jorges' family has stopped taking the time to converse with him in group settings. Contrast Jorges' experience with that of Mr. Johnson on the companion CD-ROM. Mr. Johnson's hearing loss from noise exposure has little effect on his life because of his use of hearing aids and participation in habilitation programs.

What is particularly striking about hearing loss in the adult population is that its effects can be significant even when the hearing loss is minimal, as with a unilateral loss or a mild bilateral loss (Newman, Hug, Jacobson, & Sandridge, 1997). In a major survey commissioned by the National Council on Aging (NCOA), researchers found that people who do not appropriately manage their hearing loss report significantly higher rates of these problems:

- Depression (e.g., fatigue, insomnia, thinking a lot about death)
- Anger and frustration (likely to get annoyed and irritated easily)
- Paranoia (believing they are blamed for something that is not their fault)
- Denial of the severity and extent of hearing-related problems
- Feelings of loss of control
- Pretending to understand others when they do not
- Violating the rules of communication (e.g., interrupting a speaker or inappropriately shifting topics) (Kirkwood, 1999)

Unmanaged hearing loss directly impacts interpersonal relationships with family members, coworkers, and friends. Adults with untreated hearing loss and their spouses suffer in both their social and their family roles and report more negativity and arguments in their relationships, often leading to crises (Armero, 2001; Radcliffe, 1998).

Discussion Point: *Many individuals seek treatment for hearing loss when the problem reaches a crisis stage. What example of a crisis might propel an adult to seek treatment for a hearing loss?*

However, untreated hearing loss results in significant lifestyle limitations that go far beyond socialization. This is particularly true for individuals who have had ongoing hearing loss since early childhood that has been untreated or treated with fragmented approaches. The reading abilities and educational outcomes of adults who are congenitally hearing impaired are staggeringly low; studies show the average reading ability at a fourth-grade level (Gallaudet University Center for Assessment and Demographic Study, 1998). Labor force participation is also lower for people with hearing loss (Mohr et al., 2000), and they show less involvement in community activities, such as volunteering. Hearing loss also influences retirement decisions; more people with hearing loss retire early (i.e., between the ages of 51 and 61) than do their typical hearing peers (Mohr et al., 2000). And more retired people with hearing loss report that poor health led to their retirement.

Estimates suggest that untreated hearing loss costs the U.S. economy billions of dollars in lost productivity and medical care. People with hearing loss in the workforce earn only about 50–70% of the income of their hearing peers, reducing their earnings by up to $500,000 in a lifetime (Mohr et al., 2000). The costs of economic-induced hearing loss are also considerable, specifically **noise-induced hearing loss** caused by exposure to occupational noise. As the second most common cause of sensorineural hearing loss among adults, noise-induced hearing loss costs the American economy greatly in unemployment and disability benefits (Daniell, Fulton-Kehoe, Smith-Weller, & Franklin, 1998).

Discussion Point: *If the impact of hearing loss is so far reaching, why is there such a stigma attached to hearing loss and hearing aid use?*

Terminology

As introduced in chapter 13, the term *hearing loss* is an objective one that refers specifically to a decrease in hearing acuity or clarity as a malfunction of the hearing mechanisms. The terms *handicap, disability,* and *impairment* reference the impact of hearing loss on an individual's daily living activities.

Hearing loss that occurs as a result of aging is called **presbycusis**. The noise-induced hearing loss just discussed is acquired from exposure to noise, often through occupational conditions (e.g., machinery operation) or recreational activities (e.g., gun use). *Nerve loss* is a term often used incorrectly to describe sensorineural hearing loss, which *can* be caused by neuron damage but is far more often the result of damage to the hair cells of the cochlea.

Prevalence and Incidence

Hearing loss is the third most prevalent chronic condition in the older population (Yueh, Shapiro, MacLean, & Shekelle, 2003). Approximately 10% of the population, or 28 million Americans, have hearing loss, and this number is expected to increase significantly over the next decades, particularly for people of advanced age (Garstecki & Erler, 1995). The incidence of acquired hearing loss increases dramatically with age, as shown in Figure 14-2. In contrast to the number of persons exhibiting hearing loss, the number of adults receiving treatment or intervention for hearing loss is much lower, estimated at about 25% of adults with hearing loss, as shown in Figure 14-3.

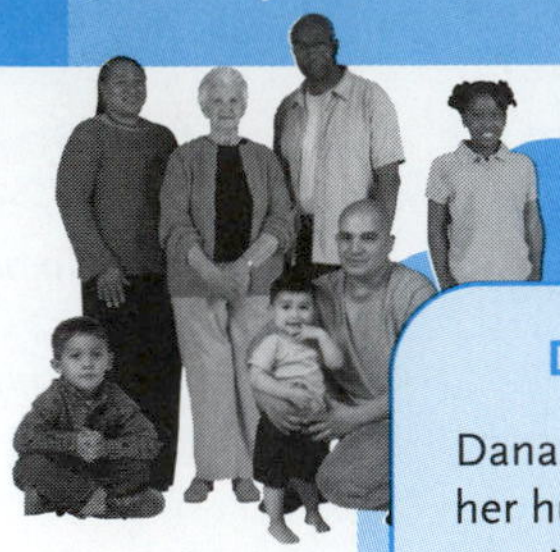

BOX 14-2 Multicultural Focus

Deafness and Culture

Dana, age 30, has had a profound hearing loss since birth. She is a wife and mother. Although her husband also has hearing loss, their children are all hearing. Dana is also a person who considers herself bilingual/bicultural.

Dana's mother contracted German measles while she was pregnant with Dana, causing Dana's hearing loss, which was identified early. Dana's mother, a speech-language pathologist, wanted Dana to learn to talk. Consequently, hearing aids were fitted, and she was enrolled in intervention as a toddler. For the most part, Dana's speech and language developed typically, and she attended public school, growing into an independent, articulate young woman.

When Dana was ready to enter college, her father suggested that she attend Gallaudet University rather than the state university. Dana's father believed that she should learn about her Deaf heritage. Although reluctant, Dana agreed.

Gallaudet University is known for its strong Deaf community and pride in its culture. It is promoted as the only university that brings together deaf, hard-of-hearing, and hearing students and faculty with a commitment to sign communication. At Gallaudet there is a shared belief that hearing loss is not a disability that requires intervention. Rather, the focus is on preserving and promoting the psychosocial integrity of people who are deaf and hard of hearing through acceptance, education, and celebration of their differences.

As Dana became acclimated to the culture of Gallaudet, she immersed herself in her studies, learned American Sign Language, and started orienting herself as a person who is Deaf rather than as a person with a hearing disability. With many friends who were Deaf, Dana straddled the deaf and hearing worlds, functioning successfully in both. She also worked diligently to change what she viewed as society's misconceptions, prejudices, and discrimination against people who are deaf or hard of hearing.

After graduating and starting her family, Dana began to hear about the benefits of cochlear implantation. As an oral communicator, she knew there could be tremendous benefits. However, she was concerned about the message she would be conveying, that she was attempting to fix her deafness. While she privately began obtaining information about cochlear implants, she also tuned in to the viewpoints of her friends in the Deaf community. She realized that a decision to get a cochlear implant would likely alienate her from many of her friends.

After a lengthy struggle, Dana decided to go through with the implant, but she kept it a secret. After activation, Dana was thrilled with her new access to sound, but she remained ambivalent about telling others. As people began to notice the implant (despite her new, longer hair style), reactions varied. Some people respected her right to make the decision for herself and even took interest in the benefits she received. However, a few friends thought her decision was a betrayal of all that they valued.

For Discussion

What aspects of Deaf culture would differ most from the mainstream hearing culture?

Why would Dana's friends view cochlear implants as a betrayal? How real do you find this scenario?

Companion Website

To answer these questions online, go to the Multicultural Focus module in chapter 14 of the Companion Website.

FIGURE 14-2 The age groups of adult Americans with hearing loss.

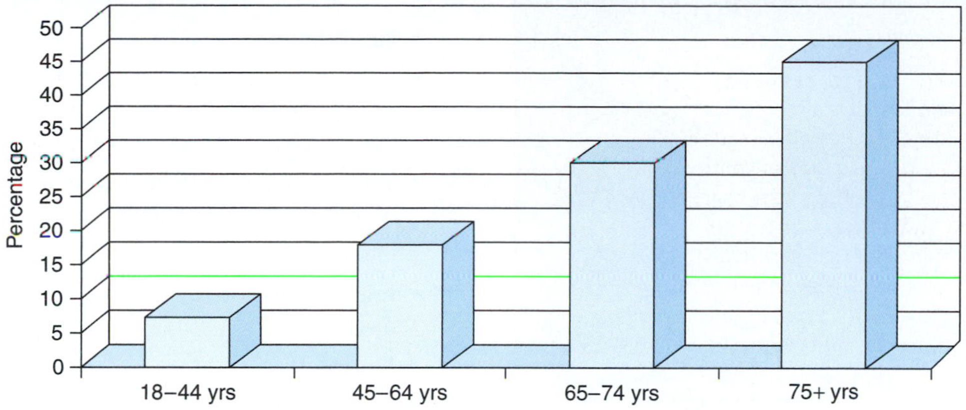

Source: Data from National Health Interview Survey (2002).

How Is Adult Hearing Loss Classified?

Hearing loss in the adult population is classified in terms of etiology, manifestation, and severity.

Etiology

Identifying the cause of adult hearing loss is a common way to classify the different types of loss. Etiology identifies the area of the auditory pathway or brain that is affected (e.g., outer ear, middle ear, cochlea, auditory nerve). A conductive loss places the site of breakdown in the outer ear or middle ear. A sensorineural loss occurs from a breakdown either of the outer or inner hair cells of the cochlea or of the auditory nerve.

As discussed in chapter 13, hearing loss can be congenital or acquired. Among the adult population with hearing loss, most often the loss is acquired sometime during the course of adulthood, either from a sudden event, such as a tumor of the auditory nerve, or

FIGURE 14-3 Estimated percentages of responses to hearing loss among adults.

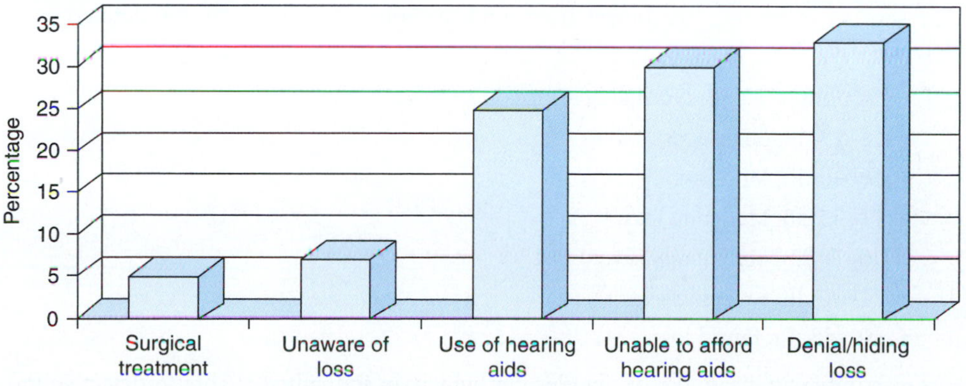

Source: Data from Society for Neuroscience (2004).

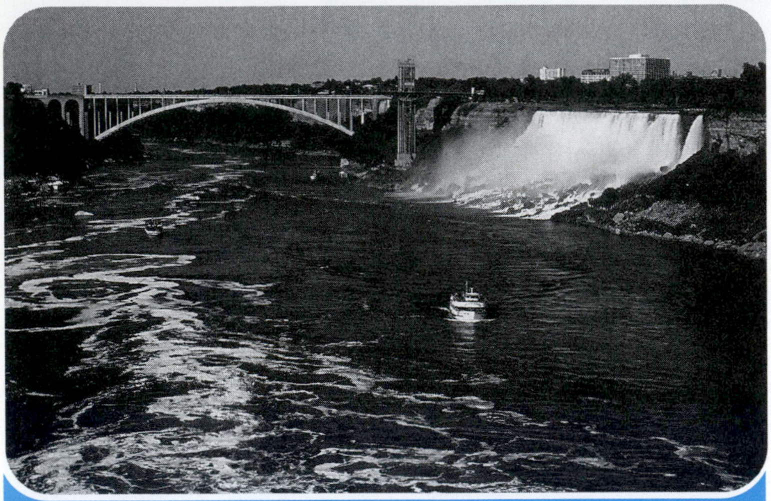

From the observation decks the roar of Niagara Falls is about 80 dB and thus would be inaudible to persons with profound hearing loss.

from a gradual process, such as illness or disease. The most common causes include the following:

- Head trauma
- Barotrauma (excessive change in atmospheric pressure that cannot be matched by ear pressure changes)
- Tumor (e.g., acoustic neuroma, a tumor on the auditory nerve)
- Ototoxic drugs
- Infection/disease (e.g., Meniere's disease)
- Illness
- Noise exposure/damage
- Aging

The last two are the most prevalent causes of adult acquired hearing loss.

Manifestation

Hearing loss is also classified according to the aspects of audition that are affected, or the ways the disorder is manifested. This approach considers whether the loss impacts acuity and audibility of sounds alone or whether comprehension of spoken language and speech perception (i.e., clarity) are affected as well. A change in hearing acuity is the most commonly recognized manifestation of hearing loss; a decrease in hearing acuity results in sounds being softer or less audible, a symptom familiar to many whose grandparents may have asked them to "speak a little louder." More problematic, however, is an SNR loss, resulting in a decrease in comprehension of spoken language and speech clarity. With an SNR loss the speech signal itself is compromised and degraded. Whereas sound intensity (i.e., volume) can be increased to make up for a decrease in acuity, a loss of clarity is more complicated to treat. Commonly experienced problems resulting from loss of both acuity and clarity are provided in Figure 14-4.

Severity

Discussion Point: *Consider the cases of Kristina, Lenny, and Jimmy in Box 14-1. Identify the cause of hearing loss for each of these individuals. Which causes could have been prevented?*

The severity of hearing loss ranges from mild to profound and is typically defined using decibels (dB):

- −10 dB to 15 dB: Normal hearing
- 16–25 dB: Slight loss
- 26–40 dB: Mild loss
- 41–55 dB: Moderate loss
- 56–70 dB: Moderately severe loss
- 71–90 dB: Severe loss
- >91 dB: Profound loss

These numbers indicate the decibel level at which an individual is able to detect sound. Thus, an individual with normal hearing detects sounds when they are between −10 dB

FIGURE 14-4 Commonly reported problems of adults with hearing loss and of their significant others.

Problems of adults with hearing loss

- Environmental challenges
  - Sounds in background noise
  - Conversations in the dark or poor lighting
  - Sounds at a distance or in another room
  - Speech or music in the automobile
  - Large group situations
  - Rooms with poor acoustics
  - Conversations outdoors (particularly in noisy places or on windy days)
  - Telephone and cellular phone conversations
  - Voices on television, radio, or film
- Speaker challenges
  - Conversations with multiple speakers
  - Unfamiliar speaker or a foreign accent
  - Unfamiliar topic (e.g., medical explanation)
  - Speaker who looks away or provides poor facial cues (e.g., covering face with veil, beard, or hand)
  - Speaking without getting attention of listener
  - Misinterpreting listener's failure to understand
- Listener challenges
  - Isolation
  - Trying to concentrate, even when fatigued
  - Loss of spontaneity and/or intimacy

Problems of significant others

- Speaking challenges
  - Remembering to get listener's attention, speak clearly, and face the listener
  - Reducing conversational frequency/duration
- Interpersonal challenges
  - Not being able to determine when listener understands
  - Variability in listener's ability to understand
  - Finding creative ways to make listener understand
  - Having to repeat a lot
  - Responding when listener doesn't understand another speaker
  - Failure of listener to pay attention
  - Attempting to get listener to understand in emergency situations
  - Minimizing frustration
  - Being patient, even when fatigued
  - Having to act as an interpreter
  - Not being able to enjoy certain activities (e.g., traveling, theater)
  - Isolation imposed by significant other
  - Loss of spontaneity and/or intimacy
- Other challenges
  - Television or radio volume too loud

Source: From *Living with Hearing Loss Workbook* by S. Trychin, 2002, Erie, PA: Author. Copyright 2002 by S. Trychin. Adapted with permission.

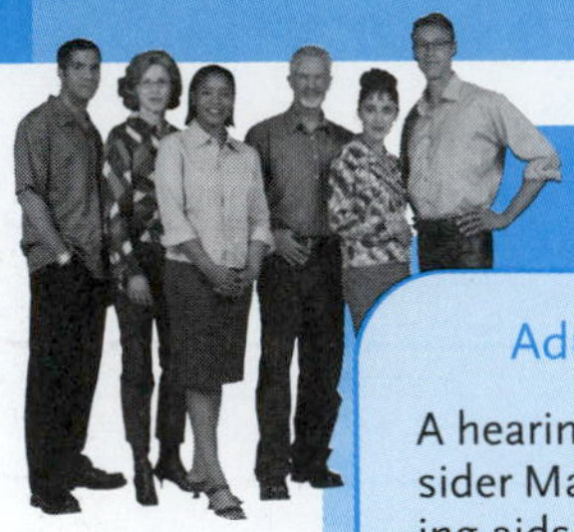

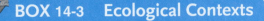

BOX 14-3 Ecological Contexts

Adults with Hearing Loss at Home and in the Community

A hearing loss can have a dramatic impact on life at home and in the community. Let's consider Max, a retired farmer with a moderate-to-severe hearing loss who will not consider hearing aids. On a daily basis, Max struggles. Even though he no longer needs an alarm clock in the morning, Max can't hear the doorbell, smoke detector, oven buzzer, and other household sounds. His wife must handle all the telephone calls because he doesn't usually hear the phone ring and can't understand very well, even with the amplified phone his children gave him for his birthday. In order to hear the radio, he must turn the volume up much higher than his wife prefers. They now sit in different rooms to watch their evening TV programs.

When neighbors drive by, Max can't hear their friendly car horn beeps. And with his diminished vision, it's unsafe for him to take walks or ride his bicycle along the road because he can't discern when traffic is approaching. Driving is also problematic. When Max is with his wife, they can't agree on a radio volume. And when driving alone, he can't hear the sirens or car horns alerting him to a potential problem. Further, when Max sees his physicians, his wife does all the talking and must later interpret the doctor's orders for him. Similarly, when they visit the bank, post office, or other places of business, Max must rely on her to handle all of the affairs.

Max's family life is greatly affected by his hearing problems. His wife is frustrated by their inability to communicate effectively and effortlessly. She also doesn't like her new role as interpreter and misses the intimacy they used to share in quiet conversations. In addition, the soft voices of Max's grandchildren aren't discernible, especially when they're on their way to pet the horses or chase the kittens. At the dinner table, Max feels left out when his family gives up trying to repeat everything. And he can't hear their performances in school plays or the church choir. In fact, he rarely attends church any longer since he can't understand the priest.

Once a social and active person, Max's leisure activities with friends are remarkably different now. His acquaintances wonder about his diminished capacity to carry on an intelligent conversation or attend to the topic of conversation. Conversation is often awkward. Max no longer attends the weekly breakfast with his golfing buddies because understanding in the noisy restaurant is impossible. His golf game is still good, but he can't communicate with the others in his foursome unless he's talking to them one on one within arm's reach. Max no longer attends movies or the theater with his wife and friends. At the football game the cheering bothers his friend, who wears hearing aids, but not Max. However, Max can't follow the game very well since he's unable to hear the announcer. He rarely attends the local Lion's Club meetings anymore since he no longer can follow the speakers or participate effectively in the meetings. In short, Max's life is completely altered by his untreated hearing loss. But it is not Max alone who suffers; his relationships and activities with his family and friends are also changed.

For Discussion

What community supports might be available to assist Max and his wife in these challenges?

Why will Max not seek the help available to him through numerous technologies?

Companion Website

To answer these questions online, go to the Ecological Contexts module in chapter 14 of the Companion Website.

and 15 dB. By contrast, a person who does not detect sounds until they are at about 30 dB has a mild loss.

It might be helpful to consider the decibel levels of various environmental sounds (Van Bergeijk, Pierce, & David, 1960):

- 10 dB: Rustle of leaves
- 20 dB: Whisper at 20 feet
- 30 dB: Quiet street with no traffic
- 40 dB: Night noises in a city

- 50 dB: A car engine 10 feet away
- 60 dB: The interior of a department store
- 70 dB: Busy traffic on a city street
- 80 dB: Niagara Falls

Using these reference points, consider the experiences of a person with a mild or moderate hearing loss. In everyday living numerous sensory experiences would be missed, and conversations with friends and family members would likely be impaired unless some communication enhancements are used.

What Are the Defining Characteristics of Prevalent Types of Hearing Loss?

Conductive Hearing Loss

Defining Characteristics

Conductive hearing loss is less common in adults than it is among children. As described in chapter 13, it occurs when sound is not conducted efficiently through the outer and/or middle ear, resulting in an attenuation of the sound. Conductive hearing loss results in a sense of fullness or plugged ears and generally causes a slight to moderate loss of hearing in one or both ears. Conductive hearing loss is typically amenable to medical or surgical intervention and therefore is often a temporary loss.

Causes and Risk Factors

A common cause of conductive loss in adulthood is cerumen blockage, particularly due to the use of cotton swabs. Even though many people use cotton swabs to keep their ears clean, their use is actually detrimental. The human ear produces cerumen as a protective agent to keep objects out of the ear canal and to keep it lubricated and healthy. When swabs are pushed into the ear, they serve as a plunger, removing some wax while pushing other wax deep into the ear canal. When significant wax builds up, sound transmission is blocked. Wax pushed into the ear canal near the tympanic membrane can become hard and stiff and difficult to remove, necessitating its removal by an audiologist. Attempting to remove cerumen that is deep in the ear canal makes the tympanic membrane vulnerable to rupture.

Foreign objects inappropriately put into the ear canals or inflammation of the ear canal can also block the transmission of sound, causing conductive hearing loss. One elderly woman who suffered from Alzheimer's disease mistakenly placed her hearing aid battery in her ear canal rather than in the hearing aid. It was not discovered for several months, by which time it had turned into a serious infection and had to be removed surgically.

Adults also experience otitis media, although it occurs far less frequently than it does with children because of structural changes in the ear mechanism (e.g., the lengthening and curving of the Eustachian tube) and an improved immune system, which allows adults to resist chronic infections. Adults who have allergies, sinus-related problems, and a childhood history of chronic otitis media are at greatest risk for adult bouts of otitis media. As with children, otitis media needs to be treated thoroughly and well to minimize its impact on the middle ear structures and hearing acuity.

Damage to the outer and middle ear structures can also cause conductive hearing loss. For example, individuals who suffer head trauma in an automobile accident may experience perforation of the eardrum or disarticulation (i.e., dislocation) of the ossicles. Sometimes trauma is self-induced, as it was with a college student who fell asleep and jammed her pencil into her ear, perforating the tympanic membrane. Accidents like this are very painful but can be repaired surgically in most cases. *Myringoplasty* is a medical intervention in which tissue is grafted onto the tympanic membrane to repair perforations. With clean tears the membrane can often heal itself.

Another cause of adult-onset conductive hearing loss is **otosclerosis**, a condition in which abnormal bone growth develops around the ossicles (especially the stapes). That bone growth impedes the movement of the stapes, compromising the transmission of sound energy along the ossicular chain to the footplate of the stapes, which transmits energy to the cochlea through the oval window. The bone growth can also invade the inner ear. Otosclerosis is relatively common, affecting approximately 1 of 100 adults in the United States, with the incidence in women approximately twice that in men (Martin & Greer Clark, 2002). There is a strong genetic link in the risk for this disease, and it seems to be aggravated by hormonal changes in pregnancy or menopause. Although otosclerosis can be treated surgically—often through a *stapedectomy,* in which the diseased bone is replaced with a prosthesis—a significant, long-term conductive hearing loss is common.

Sensorineural Hearing Loss

Defining Characteristics

Sensorineural hearing loss is the most common type of hearing loss in adulthood, resulting most often from damage to the outer or inner hair cells of the cochlea. Whereas outer hair cell damage often results in difficulty with hearing acuity, inner hair cell damage results in a more complicated problem—SNR loss. SNR loss, which also occurs with auditory nerve damage, results in both a decrease in acuity and a loss of clarity, especially in noise. Depending on the location of damage, people may experience recruitment and/or tinnitus as well. Sensorineural loss can be treated effectively with amplification or other types of intervention, but hearing cannot usually be restored.

Causes and Risk Factors

There are many causes of sensorineural hearing loss, the most frequent being presbycusis and noise exposure. Presbycusis is a degeneration of the inner ear and other auditory structures as a result of the normal aging process. It is a progressive loss that begins in early adulthood but may not be noticeable until the fifth or sixth decade of life. Figure 14-5 illustrates

FIGURE 14-5 **Expected hearing level decreases for aging men and women.**

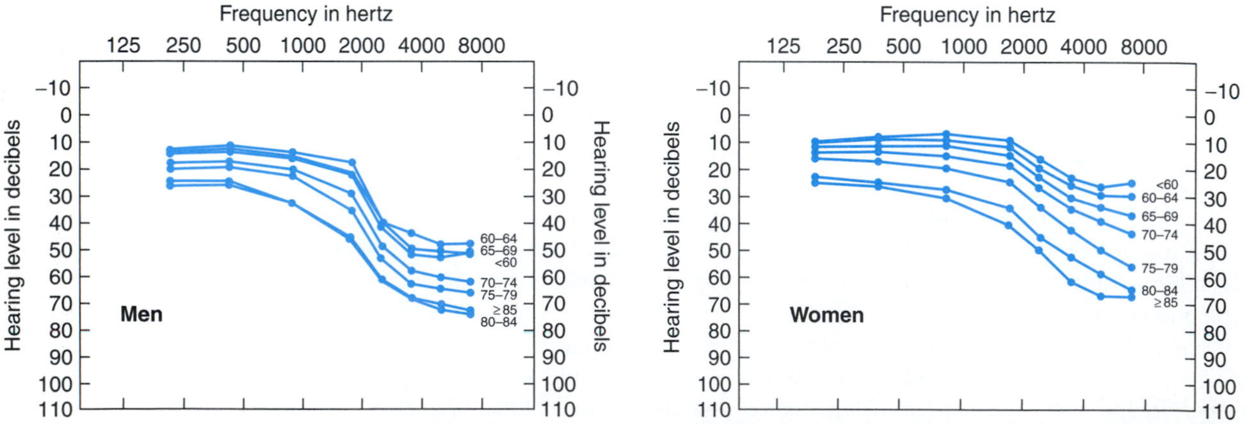

Source: From *Geriatric audiology* by B. E. Weinstein, 2000, New York: Thieme. Copyright 2000 by Thieme. Reprinted with permission.

expected hearing levels by decade, considering only aging factors. Presbycusic losses result in a decrease in the high frequency range and may be accompanied by SNR loss, tinnitus, and recruitment; these losses are more prevalent and severe in men. Some individuals are genetically predisposed to presbycusis and may be more susceptible to these changes. Thus, a parent with age-related hearing loss increases the risk of a son or daughter having age-related hearing loss (Gates, Couropmitree, & Myers, 1999). Other risk factors include disease or illness (e.g., diabetes), cardiac problems and high blood pressure, noise exposure, and certain medications.

Noise-induced hearing loss results from exposure to damaging levels of noise. Noise exposure can be in the form of industrial or construction noise, music, gunfire, or other sounds greater than 85 dB. Some common activities with very high noise levels include taking an aerobics class (78–106 dB), playing in an orchestra (87–98 dB), running a power mower (107 dB), spending time in a club or a bar (110 dB), listening to stereo headphones (110 dB), or attending a rock concert (130 dB; Peck, 1997; Wilson & Herbstein, 2003). A single exposure to noises at these levels may not be enough to result in permanent damage, because the hair cells of the cochlea are able to self-repair within a relatively short period of time. If you have had a temporary hearing loss due to a loud noise (e.g., a rock concert), you have experienced this self-repair. However, with ongoing exposure the self-repair mechanisms of the cochlea become overwhelmed or unable to compensate, as several well-known musicians (e.g., The Who's Pete Townsend) have learned the hard way. The alarming rates of noise-induced hearing loss due to occupational conditions have resulted in numerous hearing conservation programs in American industries with high noise levels, such as mining, lawn care, the airline industry, machine-repair shops, and construction. An estimated 30 million Americans experience excessive noise in their workplace, and efforts are underway to enhance hearing screening and protection.

Discussion Point: *Lenny, described in Box 14-1, has a noise-induced hearing loss, which is a preventable type of loss. What might a prevention program for noise-induced hearing loss look like?*

Like presbycusis, noise-induced hearing loss appears to have a strong genetic link. Animal studies indicate that the gene that influences presbycusic loss can also influence susceptibility to noise-induced hearing loss (Tremblay & Cunningham, 2002). Other influencing factors include (1) the intensity of the noise, (2) the length of exposure, (3) use of hearing protection, (4) recovery time between exposures, and (5) other forms of damage to the cochlea. Table 14-1 illustrates the relationship between intensity level and hours of safe exposure.

TABLE 14-1 The relationship between the intensity level of noise and the hours of safe exposure

Noise Level (dB)	Hours of Safe Exposure: Without Hearing Protection	Hours of Safe Exposure: With 15 dB Hearing Protection
90	8	Unlimited
95	4	Unlimited
100	2	Unlimited
105	1	8
110	½	4
115	¼	2
120	0	1
125 or greater	0	0

Source: Data from Occupational Safety and Health Administration (OSHA) (1992).

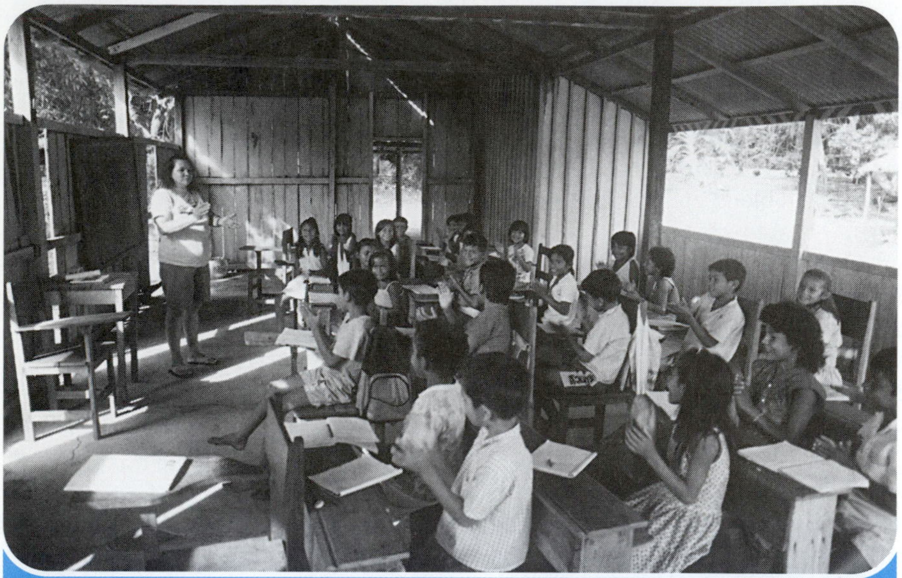

Antimalarial treatment can cause hearing loss, but it can also save one's life by preventing malaria.

Ototoxicity is another common cause of inner ear damage and sensorineural hearing loss. An ototoxic drug is one that negatively affects the hearing mechanism, such as certain antibiotics (e.g., streptomycin and neomycin), aspirin (salicylates) in large quantities, diuretics (e.g., Lasix), and chemotherapy drugs (e.g., cisplatin). Damage may be temporary, but it is more often permanent, particularly when the medication is used for a long period of time at high dosages. Drugs that are known to be ototoxic are often administered because of their lifesaving affects. For instance, the drug quinine is used to prevent malaria, although it has a clear ototoxic effect. For people who travel frequently to malarial regions, the impact on hearing may be an unfortunate but necessary trade-off for protection from the potentially life-threatening malaria. Occasionally, a substitute, nonototoxic drug can be given when testing indicates signs of damage to the outer hair cells, which are particularly susceptible to ototoxic agents. When ototoxic drugs are used, hearing should be carefully monitored.

Many diseases and infections can also cause sensorineural hearing loss, including Meniere's disease and labyrinthitis, cerebral-vascular disease, diabetes, tuberculosis, kidney disease, autoimmune diseases, HIV, and other sexually transmitted diseases, including herpes. **Meniere's disease** and **labyrinthitis** affect the labyrinth of the inner ear in both the vestibular and cochlear mechanisms. The vestibule of the inner ear controls balance functions, whereas the cochlea mediates hearing. When both the vestibule and the cochlea are damaged, as occurs in these two disorders, the symptoms include hearing loss, vertigo (i.e., dizziness), and tinnitus. Labyrinthitis is a short-term infection that is treated medically; Meniere's disease is a long-term disorder caused by an overproduction or underabsorption of endolymph, a fluid that circulates in the inner ear, resulting in a progressive hearing loss. Between 3 million and 5 million cases are present in the United States (American Academy of Otolaryngology—Head and Neck Surgery, 2004). Meniere's disease typically strikes between 20 and 50 years of age, affecting men and women equally.

An additional illness that can result in sensorineural hearing loss is meningitis, which is also one of the leading causes of acquired postnatal hearing loss, accounting for about 6% of cases (Gallaudet Research Institute, 2001). Meningitis is an inflammation of the meninges, a layer of tissues that encase the brain. Meningitis occurs from both viral and bacterial agents; it is not spread by casual contact but is spread through close or prolonged physical contact between two people. Those who care for people with bacterial meningitis must take special care, including antibiotic treatment, not to contract the illness themselves. Symptoms include a rapid-onset high fever, vomiting, extreme weakness, spots on the body, and painful, achy joints.

Finally, tumors, particularly along the auditory nerve, can cause sensorineural hearing loss, primarily because of the space they occupy. Described as acoustic neuromas, tumors can be hard to identify and are usually noticed first by a decrease in hearing in one ear, followed by a feeling of fullness or pressure. Surgical removal of the tumor can result in a complete loss of hearing and facial paralysis. Although surgeons try hard to preserve hearing in the removal of acoustic neuromas, their immediate goal is always to remove the tumor and preserve the patient's life. The most efficient route to removal is through the ear directly, which can damage much of the ear and result in a significant unilateral loss.

Mixed Hearing Loss

Defining Characteristics, Causes, and Risk Factors

When people with a sensorineural hearing loss experience a bout of otitis media or a buildup of cerumen, the concomitant loss is termed a mixed hearing loss. It is a combination of a permanent reduction of sound (i.e., the sensorineural component) and temporary loss of hearing from a conductive component.

How Is Hearing Loss Identified?

The Assessment Process

Assessment of hearing loss in adults can be initiated with an audiometric screening, but it more often begins with a complete hearing evaluation. Generally, assessment tools fall into three categories: (1) observation and self-assessment, (2) conventional audiometry, and (3) objective measurement. Screenings can include questionnaires completed by the individual and/or a significant other and observations about communication in various environments/situations. Screenings also include measurement of auditory system response to sounds through conventional audiometry and/or objective measures (e.g., otoacoustic emissions).

A comprehensive audiometric test battery is described in chapter 13; it includes conventional audiometry as well as objective measures, such as otoacoustic emissions (OAEs) and evoked auditory potentials (EAPs). Adults and their significant others can also provide substantial information through self-assessment instruments. Assessment should determine hearing acuity (or degree of loss), the type of loss (e.g., outer versus inner hair cell damage) and likely cause, and speech perception ability in quiet and noise (e.g., presence of SNR loss). If there are specific medical concerns, such as acoustic neuroma or otosclerosis, testing of auditory system integrity (e.g., EAP, OAEs) should also be completed.

Once a hearing loss is diagnosed, assessment for hearing aids should follow, as described in chapter 13:

- Conventional audiometry in a sound-treated room to determine functional improvement in the aided condition for tones and for speech perception
- Electroacoustic testing
- Probe microphone or real-ear assessment

The audiologist also conducts an aural habilitation assessment to develop a comprehensive and appropriate intervention plan. That assessment includes careful evaluation of the following:

- The individual's background, including health status, stage of life, and audiological expectations

- Identification of audiologic concerns
- Conversational skills, including appropriateness of topic shifts or balance of turn-taking
- Use and effectiveness of communication strategies, such as lip-reading, using gestures, and asking for clarification
- Status of any current assistive technologies, including hearing aids or cochlear implants
- Degree and areas of perceived handicap, such as problems communicating with spouse or in public forums
- Educational/vocational goals and challenges
- Specific lifestyle concerns, such as family issues, hobbies, and recreational activities

Discussion Point: *Consider the case of Lenny in Box 14-1. To what extent would auditory rehabilitation be useful for him? What might it entail?*

The Importance of Accurate Diagnosis

Hearing loss among adults often has no outward signs. Since it frequently has a gradual onset, the affected person may not be aware that a problem exists or may be unaware of its severity. Nevertheless, the negative consequences of untreated or mismanaged hearing loss can be devastating and far reaching, impacting general well-being, lifestyle, and interpersonal relationships, as well as economic livelihood. The importance of accurate diagnosis is underscored by the improved quality of life for those who obtain appropriate intervention. Specifically, hearing aid use, and to a lesser extent aural rehabilitation, results in improved personal well-being, enhanced interpersonal relationships, higher productivity, and greater success (Backenroth & Ahlner, 2000; Bridges & Bentler, 1998; Kirkwood, 1999; Lewis et al., 2003). However, an inaccurate diagnosis can lead to inappropriate hearing aid fitting, which can lead to additional loss of hearing if the hearing aid's output is too intense for the individual's hearing level.

Discussion Point: *Consider some possible explanations for a misdiagnosis of a hearing loss when hearing is, in fact, intact.*

BOX 14-4 Spotlight on Research

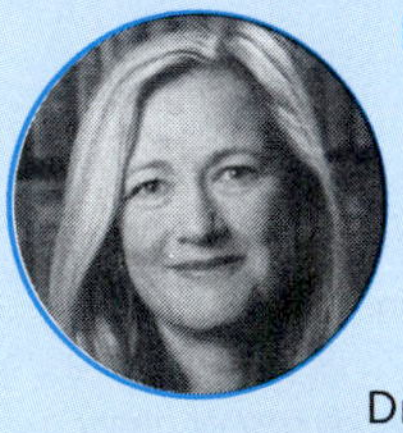

Nancy Tye-Murray
Senior Research Scientist and Professor
Washington University School of Medicine, St. Louis

Dr. Tye-Murray began her career at the University of Iowa Hospitals. There, she started the children's cochlear implant project and developed aural rehabilitation procedures for adults who use cochlear implants. She was one of the first researchers to develop computerized interactive speech-reading and communication-strategy training programs for the purpose of aural rehabilitation. She then served as the director of research of the Central Institute for the Deaf in St. Louis, where she oversaw both the Center for the Biology of Hearing and Deafness and the Center for Childhood Deafness and Adult Aural Rehabilitation. Under her leadership, the department became a major center for hair cell regeneration research and applied aural rehabilitation studies.

Tye-Murray's current research targets both ends of the lifespan. She is working on several projects concerning older adults, including the use of psychosocial therapy and aural rehabilitation for adult cochlear implant users and their frequent communication partners. She also works with Susan Jerger at the University of Texas at Dallas to assess how young children with normal hearing and those with hearing loss process spoken words. In addition to writing and presenting extensively in the field of hearing loss, Tye-Murray is also the mother of two daughters and enjoys writing fiction in her spare time. Her first novel, *The Crib Experiments,* is soon to be published.

BOX 14-5 Spotlight on Practice

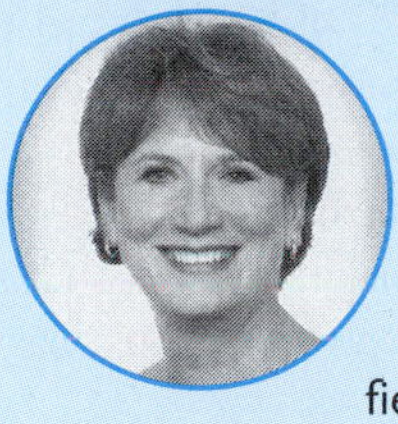

Joyce Johnson, M.S., CCC-A, FAAA
Owner/Audiologist
Kenwood Hearing Center,
Toledo, OH

Joyce Kinker Johnson has been in the field of audiology for 30 years. After graduating from Bowling Green State University, she was director of audiology for the Toledo Otolaryngology Group for 20 years. During this time, she created the first hearing aid dispensing practice managed by an audiologist in the state of Ohio.

Joyce first became interested in the field of audiology in high school, when she helped care for a child who was deaf. She babysat for this child and took him to therapy two times per week. It became, and still is, her belief that children who are deaf can learn to talk and have the right to learn to talk. She has actively promoted the oral approach for children who are deaf.

In 1993 Joyce, along with her colleague Diann Harrison, created Kenwood Hearing Center, a private practice in audiology. Their practice has grown to three offices, allowing the audiologists there to better serve the needs of the hearing impaired population of northwest Ohio.

Joyce is an expert in the diagnosis of hearing loss in both adults and children and in the fitting and programming of all levels of hearing aid technology, including the most advanced digital signal processing. Joyce is licensed by the State of Ohio and is certified by and a member of the American Speech-Language-Hearing Association. She is a fellow of the American Academy of Audiology and a member of the Academy of Dispensing Audiologists and Self-Help for the Hard-of-Hearing.

How Is Hearing Loss Treated?

Research shows that the human auditory system, including the brain systems that support audition, remains plastic throughout life, suggesting that the auditory system can be retrained in its functions (Moore, 1993; Tremblay, 2003). The most effective treatment approach for adult hearing loss is an individualized and comprehensive plan that combines counseling, fitting of amplification devices, and aural rehabilitation (Montgomery & Houston, 2000; Tye-Murray, 1998). Counseling enables an individual to learn how to live life with a hearing loss and not permit it to become a handicap. Counseling also helps family and friends cope with the loss. Amplification devices provide a means to improve hearing acuity and, to some extent, hearing clarity. And aural rehabilitation provides not only an opportunity to learn compensatory approaches to contend with the hearing loss, but also a chance to help the auditory system relearn and improve some of its lost or impaired functions.

Despite the known benefits of such an approach, services are too often limited to basic counseling and hearing aid orientation (Pakulski & Hinkle, 2003; Schow, Balsara, Smedley, & Whitcomb, 1993). Many professionals, particularly those working in private practice and hospital programs, indicate that this gap in service provision is due, at least in part, to the fact that most third-party payers do not reimburse for hearing aids or adult aural rehabilitation services (Pakulski & Hinkle, 2003; Prendergrast & Kelley, 2002). Other explanations include client perceptions that problems are not severe enough to warrant such services, professional concerns about cost-effectiveness and time constraints, and the costs of rehabilitation.

Discussion Point: *Advocates such as ASHA and the American Academy of Audiology (AAA) continually lobby insurance companies and Congress to cover the cost of hearing aid services for adults. Why do you think there is resistance to covering these important services?*

Limitations of Current Approaches

Considering the high cost of untreated hearing loss as well as the negative stigma attached to both hearing loss and hearing aid use (Erler & Garstecki, 2002), professionals must continually seek creative ways to make comprehensive services accessible to clients, increase client satisfaction with those services, and reach more individuals in need of such services. Less than one quarter of all adults with hearing loss get hearing aids, and far fewer participate in aural rehabilitation. It is not surprising then that 40% of hearing aid users report dissatisfaction with their hearing aids (Kochkin, 2002) and more than 15% of people completely reject them following a trial period (Kochkin, 2002; Strom, 2001).

A recent survey of the experiences of 651 hearing aid recipients examined the types of information and services they received from their audiologists (Stika, Ross, & Cuevas, 2002). Most of the recipients received information focused on aspects of the hearing aid:

- Audiogram results (78%)
- Reasons for the specific hearing aid selection (79%)
- Care of the hearing aid (79%)
- Care of the hearing aid battery (67%)
- Hygiene for the hearing aid and earmold (60%)

However, the survey showed that other types of information were neglected. Only 21% of the audiologists involved spouses or other family members in discussions of strategies for coping with hearing loss, only 19% of hearing aid recipients received information about consumer resources and self-help groups for persons with hearing loss, only 17% received information about strategies to improve communication, and only 13% received information about communication strategies for dealing with hearing loss at work (Stika, Ross, & Cuevas, 2002).

Discussion Point: *What might counseling focus on for Kristina, whose case is described in Box 14-1? How important is it that she be provided with counseling as well as amplification?*

Thus, although most professionals provide counseling and **hearing aid orientation**, the scope and focus of those services may not be sufficient. Counseling that focuses on a client's cognitive and emotional response to the hearing loss promotes appropriate expectations for hearing aid use and living well with hearing loss (English, Mendel, Rojeski, & Hornak, 1999). In addition, there are remarkable benefits in interpersonal relationships when the significant others and family members of individuals with hearing loss are included in counseling (Armero, 2001).

Further, the fitting of amplification devices is often limited to hearing aid orientation and evaluation of the instrument. However, many hearing aid users benefit from extended training in use of hearing aids in various situations and settings and in coupling their devices with other forms of technology (e.g., cellular phones or sound systems in theatres). And even short-term training in aural rehabilitation provides benefit to adults with hearing loss and their significant others (Abrams, Hnath-Chisolm, Guerreiro, & Ritterman, 1992). However, many do not receive aural rehabilitation because they do not seek treatment for hearing loss in general or they do not understand the potential of rehabilitating the auditory system.

Amplification and Assistive Listening Devices

Hearing Aids and FM Systems

For most adults who seek treatment for hearing loss, hearing aids are the intervention of choice to improve access to auditory information and increase communication effectiveness (Weinstein, 2000). Modern technology provides many solutions, depending on the etiology, severity, and manifestations of the hearing loss. Hearing aids are available with a wide range of processing abilities, ranging from analog to completely digital. Hearing instruments for adults also vary in size and cosmetic appeal, as illustrated in Figure 14-6. Although most hearing instruments are custom fitted, there are disposable devices that can be used for emergency situations, such as when a hearing aid is being repaired. Consequently, prices range from a few hundred dollars to several thousand dollars. Such a wide array of possibilities can be overwhelming for the consumer without the proper assistance and support of professionals.

Individuals whose hearing loss is caused by damage to the outer hair cells of the cochlea or who have a long-term conductive hearing loss have many choices in instrumentation, since their primary concern is a loss of sensitivity and hearing acuity. When the hearing loss is related to inner hair cell damage or neural damage, resulting in SNR loss, there are two problems to solve: acuity and clarity. The acuity can be remedied quite well with appropriate hearing aids, but the remaining SNR loss cannot be solved with amplification alone (Killion & Christensen, 1998; Killion & Niquette, 2000). Especially if it is moderate to severe or profound, an SNR loss requires an improvement in the signal-to-noise ratio in order to improve the clarity of speech in noise.

Technological advances have provided several methods of improving SNR for adults. Some adults couple their hearing aids to FM systems that require a speaker to use a small wireless transmitter/microphone, which sends the speech signal to a compact FM receiver. This technology provides remarkable improvement in the SNR of listening situations. For meetings or small groups, FM transmitters are available in the form of a conference microphone, which can be placed in the center of a table. However, this equipment is not suitable for all situations, such as group settings with multiple speakers or with people moving around.

An alternative to FM systems is hearing aid microphone technology. Directional microphones have long been used on hearing aids to focus reception on the pathway directly in front of the instrument. An omnidirectional microphone detects sounds all around the instrument. A good directional microphone improves the SNR sufficiently for a mild to moderate loss of clarity, but individuals whose SNR loss is more severe require an array of microphones (i.e., multiple microphone technology) to compensate for their loss of clarity (Killion & Niquette, 2000).

Assistive Listening Devices

Assistive listening devices (ALDs) include a variety of technologies—telephone amplifiers, strobe-light doorbells, amplified or lighted fire alarms, and vibrating alarm clocks. All of these provide important options for safety, lifestyle, and vocational choices. Nonetheless, ALDs are

FIGURE 14-6 **Hearing aid styles for adults.**

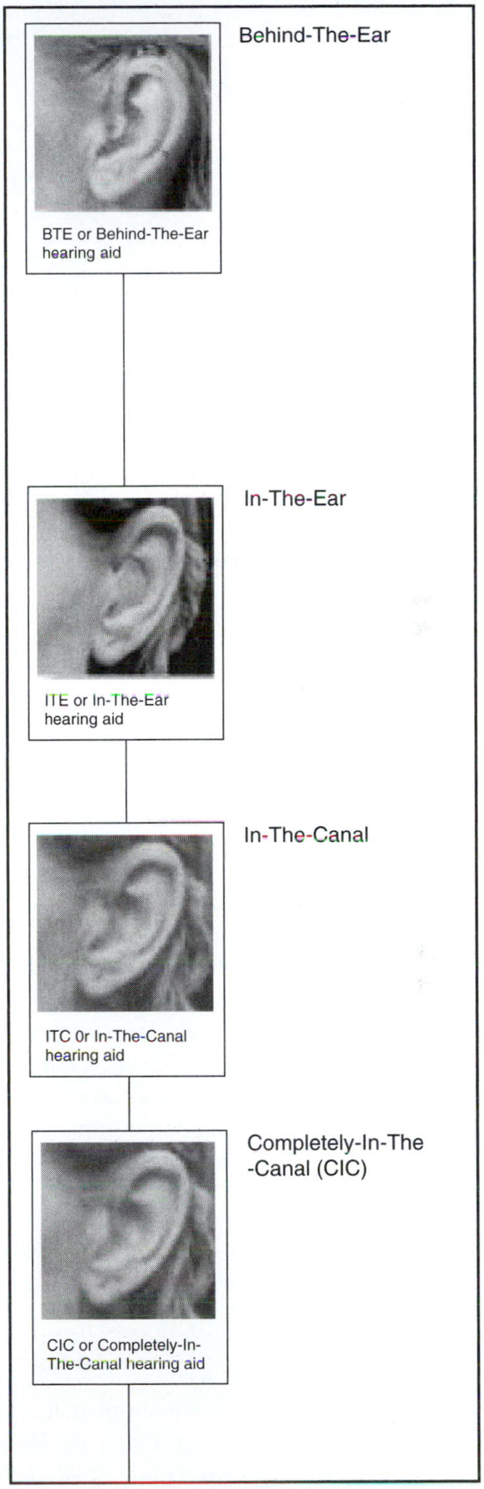

Source: Photos courtesy of the Hearing Planet.

FIGURE 14-7 Anatomy of the cochlear implant.

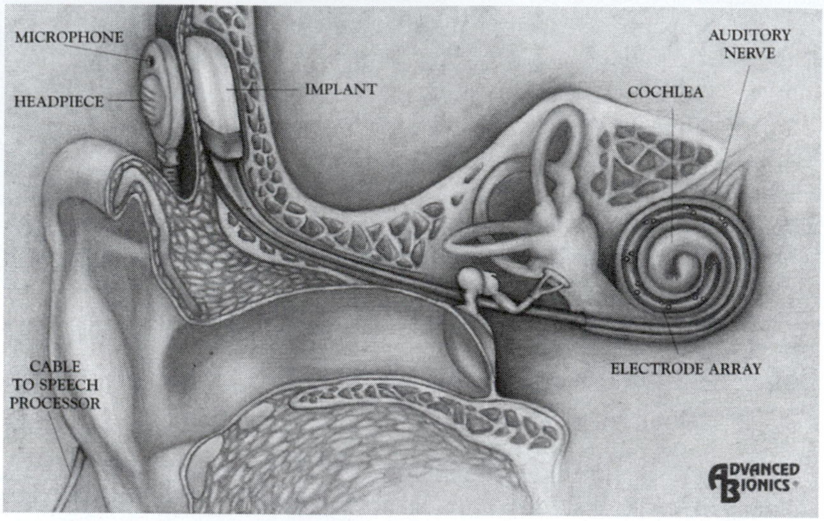

Source: Photo courtesy of Clarion.

Discussion Point: *People do not typically wear hearing aids to bed at night. What circumstances might arise while someone is asleep that would call for the use of ALDs?*

not widely used, primarily because of cost. Hearing aids are a significant purchase, and many users believe that the hearing aids alone should handle most situations. Consequently, situation-specific ALDs, which may be helpful, are considered an unnecessary luxury. Awareness of these devices and their availability are other factors. Many audiologists do not dispense ALDs.

Cochlear Implants and Other Implantable Devices

Recent years have seen dramatic scientific advances in the restoration of hearing following a sensorineural loss. Individuals with severe and profound loss now have access to surgically implantable devices, including cochlear implants and middle ear and brain stem implants, which are designed to restore function to damaged areas of the auditory system. A cochlear implant involves the implantation of a device in the cochlea, as well as use of an external sound processor (see Figure 14-7) to capture sounds from the environment. Such implants are widely used but may be controversial for some adults, as in the case of Dana in Box 14-2.

Not all adults with significant hearing loss are candidates for cochlear implants. Those who desire implantation must go through an extensive evaluation to determine their candidacy. Adults considered optimal candidates for implantation have these characteristics:

- Postlingual deafness with severe to profound loss
- Marginal or no speech-perception benefit from hearing aids
- Good health with no physical abnormalities that will compromise implantation
- Access to optimal education and habilitation services following implementation (National Institutes of Health [NIH], 1995)

The implantation procedure is generally quite safe, although any surgical procedure carries some risk. The rate of complication is about 5%, less than other implantation procedures (e.g., placement of a defibrillator; NIH, 1995). Major complications that are possible, albeit rare, include failure of the device, migration of the device from the site of original placement, and facial palsy resulting from surgical damage to the facial nerve.

Since cochlear implants restore access to sound, adults who have used their sense of hearing to listen and speak prior to their loss can receive great benefit. However, the sound, or sensations, received via the cochlear implant are markedly different from the acoustical sounds to which most listeners are accustomed. Consequently, adults require aural rehabilitation to learn to listen again and to interpret the information provided by the cochlear implant.

Discussion Point: *In Dana's case (Box 14-2), some friends viewed her cochlear implantation as a betrayal. What are some reasons for the Deaf community's resistance to cochlear implantation?*

Aural Rehabilitation

Living Well with Hearing Loss

There are a multitude of treatment strategies that can be used to meet the unique needs of adults with hearing loss. All strategies are aimed at preventing hearing loss from diminishing the quality of life, particularly for individuals whose hearing loss has gone undetected or untreated. When hearing loss interferes with perception of self-worth and ability to function appropriately in daily life, a diminished sense of personal well-being negatively affects interpersonal relationships, resulting in concomitant problems such as loss of intimacy and strained interactions. Individual counseling focuses on issues of self-perception, understanding hearing loss and its manifestations, and learning how to live well with hearing loss. Some of the strategies addressed in counseling are presented in Figure 14-8.

Group counseling is a useful tool to examine **communication breakdowns** and the ways they affect relationships. People converse dozens of times each day with family, friends, colleagues, service providers, even strangers. And conversation occurs in every imaginable situation and listening environment, many of which are not conducive to good communication. For instance, people may say hello as they pass in a stairwell and then

FIGURE 14-8 **Strategies for living well with hearing loss.**

Environment
- Optimize visual cues with good lighting.
- Reduce extraneous background noise (e.g., television in the background).
- Minimize distance between speaker and listener (e.g., don't try to converse in different rooms).
- Determine best location for listening in important settings.

Communication style
- Take responsibility for communication needs (e.g., request that TV be turned off during conversation).
- Ask for assistance when needed (e.g., Will you please look at me when you speak?).
- Do not bluff.
- Be patient.
- Take interest in the speaker and concentrate on the conversation.

Expectations
- Be realistic. Hearing aids do not restore hearing; they make sounds accessible.
- Some listening situations are difficult for everyone, including those with good hearing.
- Relearning to listen takes time. Think of it as retraining the brain now that the ears can hear.
- Seek professional help when problems arise.
- Use hearing aids consistently, every day, not just for special occasions.

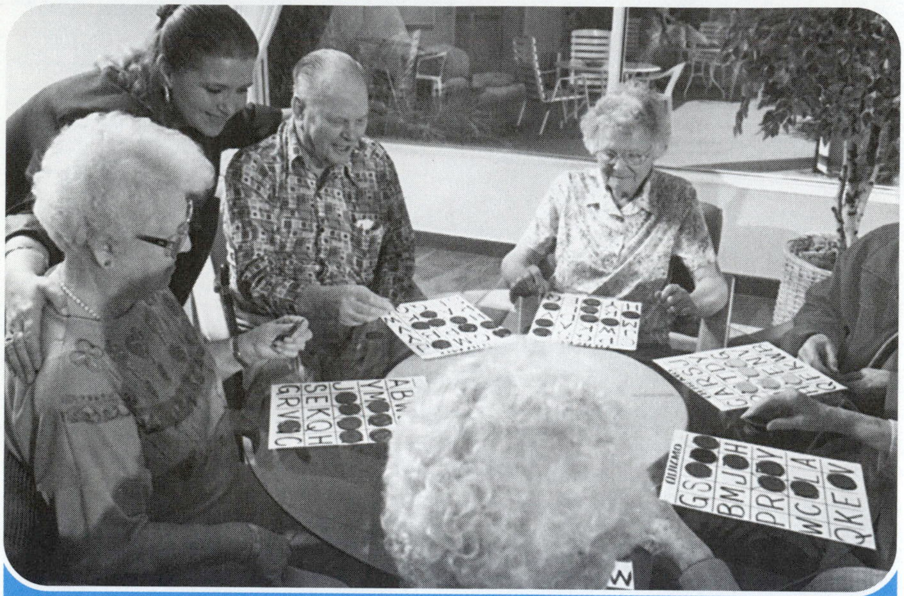

Group counseling can provide people with hearing loss the opportunity to identify and discuss reasons for communication breakdowns.

continue the conversation as one continues to climb up and the other down. For people with hearing loss, these daily conversations on the run can be impossible to manage and often produce misunderstandings or hurt feelings. Imagine that Jill has a hearing loss and passes her neighbor in a busy grocery store. Without stopping to chat, Jill mindlessly asks, "How are you?" Her neighbor, having just found out that her mother is gravely ill, replies, "Not great—it's been a difficult week for us." But Jill hears only "great" and replies, "Glad to hear it."

When information is missed, those with hearing loss have to decide how to handle the situation. Should they bluff? If not, frequently asking a communication partner to repeat can become irritating. Is there a solution? Some adults with hearing loss end up either saying nothing or dominating the conversation. Group counseling can bring together clients and family members/significant others to explore troublesome communication patterns, establish realistic expectations, and learn ways that everyone involved can contribute to improving communication interaction.

Discussion Point: *Communication breakdowns occur for everyone at some time. What are some strategies you use to repair breakdowns during communicative interactions?*

Goals of Aural Rehabilitation

The overarching goal of aural rehabilitation is to improve the fluency and effectiveness of communication, which is key to quality of life. Specific targets include (1) evaluating communication partners' roles in conversation, (2) determining whether social rules are broken (e.g., with inappropriate topic shifts), and (3) teaching strategies to facilitate communication and repair breakdowns effectively. Such strategies can incorporate a variety of methods—for example, improving use of visual cues or building listening and attention skills. Some communication training strategies are listed in Figure 14-9.

As a function of improving communication, rehabilitation focuses on maintaining (or restoring) an individual's lifestyle and vocation. Age, stage of life, and lifestyle will all strongly influence a treatment approach. For example, a corporate executive will need to listen effectively in a variety of settings and may require ALDs (e.g., conference microphone/FM system) or hearing aids interfacing with a cellular telephone. A retired homemaker who lives alone might benefit from safety/alerting devices, as well as ways to communicate with people outside the home (e.g., amplified telephone or e-mail). Maintaining lifestyle and vocation is also addressed along with protecting hearing from further loss.

Building Treatment Plans

Following diagnosis of hearing loss and evaluation for any treatable medical causes (e.g., otitis media), a hearing aid evaluation and aural rehabilitation assessment are completed

FIGURE 14-9 Communication training strategies.

Strategies for significant others	
	• Do not talk too loudly or abnormally slowly; speak naturally and distinctly • Rephrase rather than repeat • Get a person's attention before starting conversation and emphasize the subject or idea you are speaking about • Do not try to speak from another room or from a distance • Follow rules of conversation (e.g., turn taking, shared ideas, etc.)
Strategies for listeners with hearing loss	
Keys to good listening	• Practice paying attention • Be assertive; admit the presence of hearing impairment and explain how others can be helpful • Do not try to get every word; concentrate on the thread and spirit of the message • Manipulate the environment to facilitate communication • Be prepared; review topics or be familiar with concepts before attending a listening event, such as a movie or a lecture
Using visual cues to enhance listening	• Practice interpreting gestures and facial expressions and pay attention to these cues during conversation • Observe situational cues • Consider linguistic constraints • Practice and use visual recognition of sounds (speech and/or lip reading)

Preventing communication breakdowns	• Follow rules of conversation
	  • Choose topics of importance and interest to conversational partners
	  • Take turns; make sure one person does not do all the talking
	  • Change topics in an orderly fashion
	  • Do not bluff or disregard missed information
	  • Be specific when requesting clarification
	• Stay focused and attentive; choose appropriate moment to get clarification if something is missed
	• Be prepared for difficult situations, such as communicating in the car, at a large gathering, etc. (e.g., use FM system)

Repairing communication breakdowns	• Request clarification or missed information thoughtfully; be specific about what was not clear • Ask for repetition of entire message, a specific aspect, key word, or unclear content • Choose a repair strategy and implement it at an appropriate moment • Be patient and appreciative of partner's efforts

Source: Information on communication breakdowns based on Tye-Murray (1998).

to develop an effective treatment plan. A hearing aid fitting includes counseling regarding expectations as well as orientation to device operation and use. A hearing aid trial period (typically 30 days) is initiated, during which time additional hearing aid evaluations are completed to ensure that the instrument is providing appropriate amplification.

When the appropriateness of the fitting is confirmed, the aural rehabilitation program is initiated. An aural rehabilitation plan takes into account a wide range of concerns related to individual needs. Depending on the severity, length, and type of loss, clients' needs will vary from minimal to extensive rehabilitation. One program incorporates five areas of rehabilitation following the acronym FACES:

- **F**amily/significant other participation
- **A**uditory skill building
- **C**onversation strategies
- **E**ducation and counseling
- **S**peech reading and visual cues (Schow, 2001; Weinstein, 2000)

The participation of family/significant others refers to the ongoing commitment and involvement of family members in the rehabilitation process. Family members should receive training in how to change their communication styles to enhance the audibility of their speech, how to address communication-related relationship issues, and how to support the individual with hearing loss in use of amplification devices.

Auditory skill building concerns the ability of the person with hearing loss to relearn how to listen. For cochlear implant users, auditory skill building may need to start with basic sound detection (e.g., whether the radio is on or off), discrimination (e.g., attending to the stress or length of an utterance), and identification (e.g., identifying a spoken phrase). Individuals who receive implants soon after the loss of hearing and whose language skills were good prior to the loss will likely progress well through this rehabilitation process. For new hearing aid users, problems are often situational—listening in noise or comprehending spoken language from a distance. Consequently, auditory skill building for them may focus on use of instrumentation or accommodations to improve the audibility of sounds (e.g., interfacing with a telephone at work or using an FM system at church or in the theater).

Conversational strategies address issues related to maintaining conversational fluency—facilitating conversation and repairing communication breakdowns. Examples of both facilitative and repair strategies are provided in Figure 14-10. Teaching these strategies through

FIGURE 14-10 Strategies for maintaining conversational fluency.

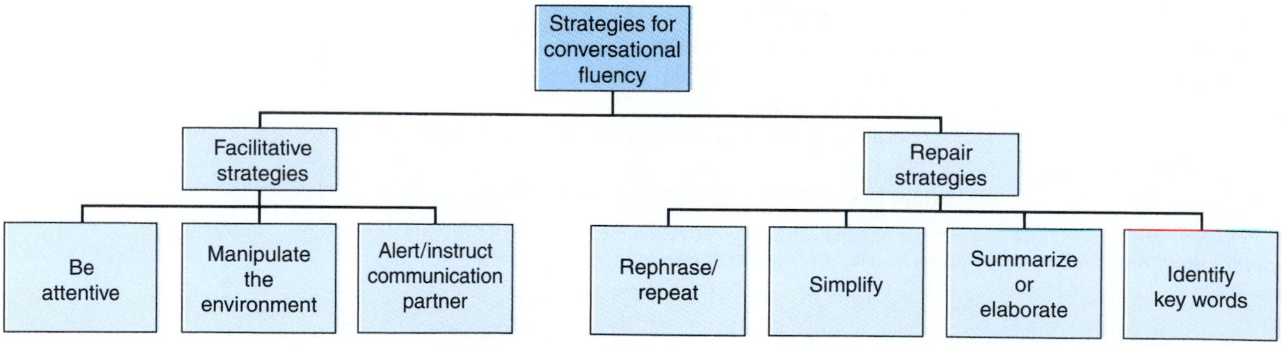

example and practice is effective and may involve group therapy so that individuals can apply specific strategies in interactions with others. For example, Karen might ask Susan, "Did you borrow my yellow cardigan last week?" Susan might hear something about borrow but not understand the message. If she says, "What?" or "I didn't hear you," Karen will have to repeat the entire phrase. Instead, Susan should determine which key words she understood and then simplify her request: "I didn't get that. You asked if I borrowed what?"

In turn, Karen can learn strategies for giving clearer messages. She can use repetition and simpler phrasing: "My sweater, did you borrow my sweater?" Thus, analyzing a conversation provides invaluable information that can be used to discuss and train communication partners in the elements of shared conversation with persons with hearing loss. Through practice and attention to what is heard and not heard, miscommunication and frustration are less likely, and individuals with hearing loss can improve their communication participation and their fluency.

Also important are education and counseling at the time of hearing aid fitting; they can significantly reduce the self-perception of a hearing handicap (Abrams et al., 1992; Taylor & Jurma, 1999), a perception that often leads to rejection of hearing aids or high rates of infrequent use and dissatisfaction (Armero, 2001). Other important aspects that should be addressed include these:

- Function, use, and maintenance of hearing aids/related devices
- An understanding of hearing loss and the impact on communication
- Realistic expectations of instrumentation
- Social, emotional, and psychological underpinnings of hearing loss

Despite the known benefits of counseling, many professionals have received little training in counseling and psychology (Armero, 2001) and have difficulty with the emotions of personal and relationship counseling. Nonetheless, significant others share in the handicapping effect of hearing loss, experiencing a reduced quality of life, embarrassment in public communication situations, and social withdrawal (Armero, 2001). The impact of hearing loss is considerable and extends far beyond the client.

A treatment plan should also include speech and lip reading and other visual cues, useful tools in interpreting messages. Given minimal instruction, people can learn to read sounds and words as they are formed and use this skill to help fill in missing parts of conversation in difficult listening situations. However, some subtle auditory cues that provide information about emotion or meaning may not be audible, even with hearing aids, or accessible to speech reading. For example, a wife may question her husband with hearing loss: "You're going to wear *that*?" with heavy emphasis on the final word. Her husband would miss the subtle auditory cue but, if he was able to detect nonverbal cues like facial expression, could still determine that his wife was not thrilled with his selection. Aural rehabilitation provides an individual with a range of tools for effective communication.

Early Identification and Intervention

Early identification is just as important for adults with hearing loss as it is for children. Adult-onset hearing loss typically manifests itself as a gradual decrease in hearing acuity, often in the higher frequencies, as well as a possible loss of clarity. Consequently, people first notice that they do not seem to understand as well as they used to or they miss some sounds. Yet the auditory system still functions, and individuals learn to make-do with the hearing they have, sometimes relying on visual or other cues to help decipher messages.

When prompted by a family member or a physician to get a hearing assessment or a hearing aid, the common response is that the problem is not "that bad." This situation is complicated by the fact that only about 16% of senior citizens receive a hearing screening as part of their routine physical (Kochkin, 2002).

As people experience a gradual decrease in auditory acuity and clarity, they become increasingly accustomed to a more quiet world. The auditory system is relied on less and less, especially as individuals make significant changes in lifestyle to avoid difficult situations. Much like a muscle that is not exerted for a long period of time, the auditory system becomes unaccustomed to deciphering speech or managing noise. People who avoid hearing aids and treatment for many years often find it difficult, if not impossible, to adjust to amplification. However, early identification of adult hearing loss, combined with appropriate amplification, allows the auditory system to maintain function and continue its auditory capability. Timely intervention maximizes the chance of maintaining good listening skills.

Healthy People 2010, an initiative of the U.S. Department of Health and Human Services (USDHHS), focuses on health promotion for the American people and seeks to increase the number of referrals primary care physicians make for hearing evaluations. Healthy People 2010 recommends frequent hearing screenings for anyone over age 50 (USDHHS, 2000). Physicians can identify individuals who should receive audiological screenings by asking a few pointed questions that focus on whether hearing difficulties are impacting life (Newman & Sandridge, 2004).

One quick, easy, and no-cost tool is the Hearing Handicap Inventory for the Elderly—Screening Version (Ventry & Weinstein, 1982), which provides 10 questions a physician or other professional can ask to determine whether a hearing loss exists. Examples of questions include these:

- Does a hearing problem cause you to attend religious services less often than you would like?
- Does a hearing problem cause you to have arguments with family members?
- Does a hearing problem cause you difficulty when listening to TV or radio?

The items on the inventory identify ways in which a person's life might be impacted by a hearing loss. Scores can range from 0 to 40; a score of 10 or higher warrants a referral for an audiological evaluation. Tools like this, which can be administered in minutes, are important in increasing the identification of hearing loss among the adult population and improving access to services.

Case Study and Clinical Problem Solving

DIAGNOSTIC REPORT: SUMMARY

Client: Emily Jackson
Evaluation Date: 6/6/05
Date of Birth: 4/20/23
Age: 82 years
Referral Source: Self

Pertinent History

Mrs. Jackson is a retired physical education teacher, who also worked in a factory in her early twenties. She is in good physical condition with the exception of some arthritis and low blood pressure. Over the past several weeks she has noticed a decrease in her right ear hearing and can no longer hear on the telephone in that ear. She reports occasional tinnitus of a buzzing nature. Mrs. Jackson recently experienced bouts of dizziness and a feeling of fullness on the right side of her head. She is concerned that a head cold may have affected her hearing. Mrs. Jackson lives with her husband. She has children and grandchildren with whom they interact regularly. She is also active in her church, participates in a water aerobics class, and tutors at the local elementary school. Cerumen removal was completed prior to today's visit, and her head cold is reportedly gone, with the exception of the right-sided fullness feeling and dizziness.

Test Results

Hearing Evaluation

Otoscopic examination and tympanometry revealed normal middle ear function with no evidence of cerumen today. Pure-tone testing revealed a slight high-frequency sensorineural hearing loss, worse at 4000 Hz, and good word discrimination in the left ear. These findings are consistent with noise exposure. Right ear testing revealed a moderate to moderately severe sensorineural hearing loss with poor word discrimination. Stapedial reflexes were abnormal in the right ipsilateral and left contralateral pathways and found right side reflex decay, suggesting a possible auditory nerve lesion. Additional testing was completed to rule out a retrocochlear lesion.

Otoacoustic Emissions

OAEs are present and essentially normal in both ears, with a slight reduction in response in the 4000 Hz region, suggestive of noise-induced outer hair cell damage. The presence of OAEs in the right ear despite the significant sensorineural hearing loss suggests that etiology is of a neural origin.

Evoked Auditory Potentials

EAPs were recorded at suprathreshold levels in each ear in response to broadband clicks. Normal latency and waveform morphology was noted in the left ear; responses were abnormal in the right ear. EAP Wave V thresholds were noted at 25 dBnHL in the left ear and 75 dBnHL in the right ear.

Conclusions

Mrs. Jackson's pure-tone testing, word discrimination ability, SISI, stapedial reflex threshold and decay, and OAE and EAP results all suggest the presence of a retrocochlear lesion.

Recommendations

1. Immediate consult with ear, nose, and throat (ENT) physician.
2. Return for further evaluation following medical consult/treatment for monitoring purposes.
3. Initiate treatment plan once medical concerns have been alleviated.

CLINICAL PROBLEM SOLVING

1. If Mrs. Jackson had ignored the initial signs of hearing loss, what might have been the consequences?
2. Mrs. Jackson is an active woman, participating in an exercise class, church activities, and volunteering. How might her hearing loss impact her communicative ability in these situations? What problems might arise?
3. What other professionals should be involved in Mrs. Jackson's care?

CHAPTER SUMMARY

At this time about 10% of the population experiences hearing loss. However, the incidence of hearing loss is expected to increase dramatically as Baby Boomers reach advanced age after years of loud music in addition to work-related and environmental noise exposure. Considering the incredible advances in technology, the likelihood of successful rehabilitation is greater than ever. Yet research continues to show that, as a whole, people with hearing loss are reluctant to seek treatment. In fact, fewer than 25% of those with significant hearing loss are hearing aid users. Failure to seek initial treatment stems from financial concerns as well as denial of the severity and extent of the problem.

Individuals who do seek treatment have mediocre success because many delay intervention until the problem reaches alarming severity and also fail to participate in comprehensive aural rehabilitation programs. Professionals report that the gap in service provision can be attributed to their inability to convince potential clients of the benefits of aural rehabilitation, coupled with a lack of third-party reimbursement.

Although most adults with hearing problems function in a hearing society as individuals who are hearing impaired, a small percentage of adults who are deaf or hard of hearing align themselves with the Deaf community. Members of the Deaf community do not view their deafness as a loss that needs to be remediated. They seek to preserve and promote the integrity of the Deaf community.

Research consistently shows that individuals with hearing loss who do not seek treatment (especially those who function in the hearing world and then experience a deterioration in their hearing) suffer significant reductions in quality of life. In fact, the cost of untreated or mismanaged hearing loss is enormous on both the personal and societal levels.

Audiologists and speech-language pathologists have the tools to provide intervention to those who seek it. Amplification and other assistive devices, coupled with comprehensive aural rehabilitation programs, are highly effective in improving access to auditory information as well as countering the negative impact of hearing loss. Professionals are challenged to reach potential clients early and convince them to avail themselves of services.

KEY TERMS

communication breakdowns, p. 491
hearing aid orientation, p. 488
labyrinthitis, p. 484
Meniere's disease, p. 484
noise-induced hearing loss, p. 475
otosclerosis, p. 482
ototoxicity, p. 484
presbycusis, p. 475
recruitment, p. 470
signal-to-noise ratio (SNR) loss, p. 471
tinnitus, p. 470

ON THE WEB

Check out the Companion Website! On it you will find

- suggested readings
- reflection questions
- a self-study quiz
- links to additional online resources, including current technologies in communication sciences and disorders

Complex Communication Needs and AAC

J. M. King

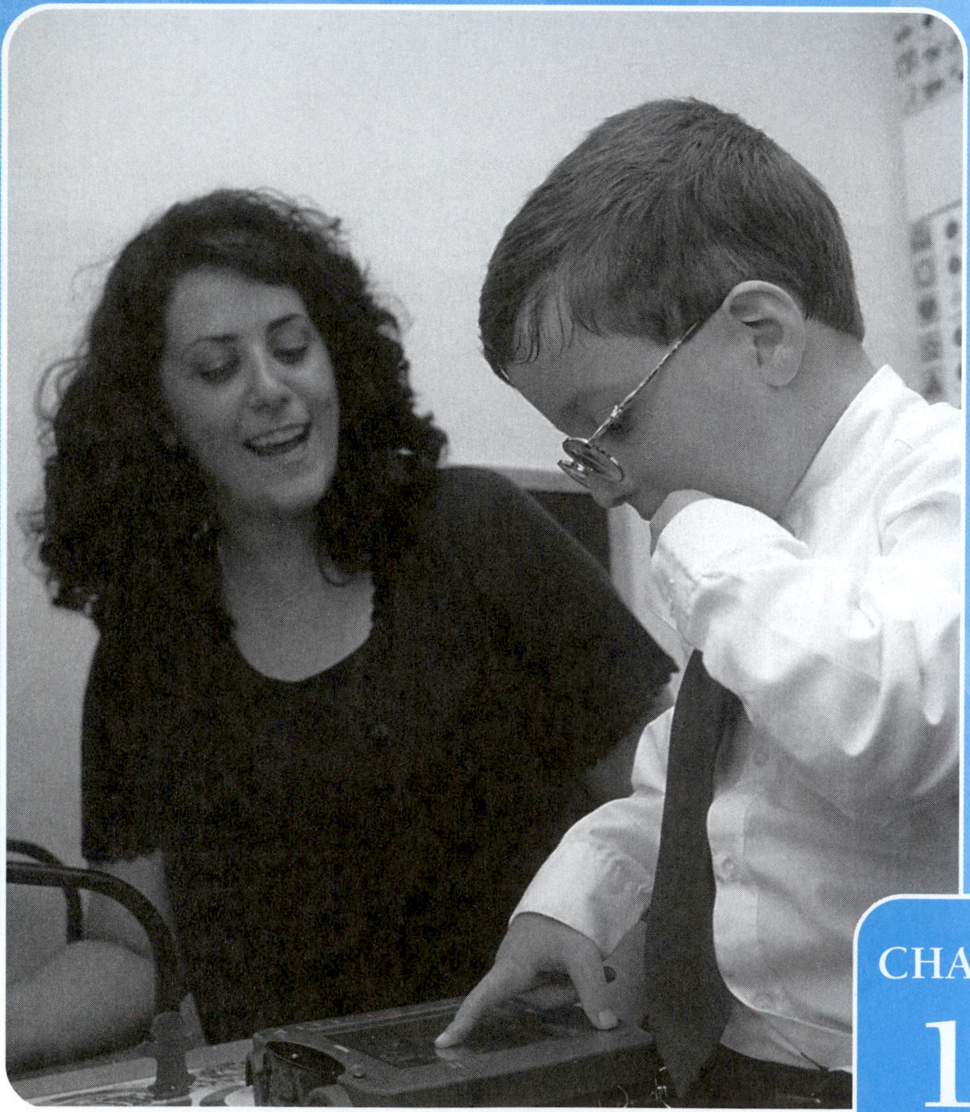

CHAPTER 15

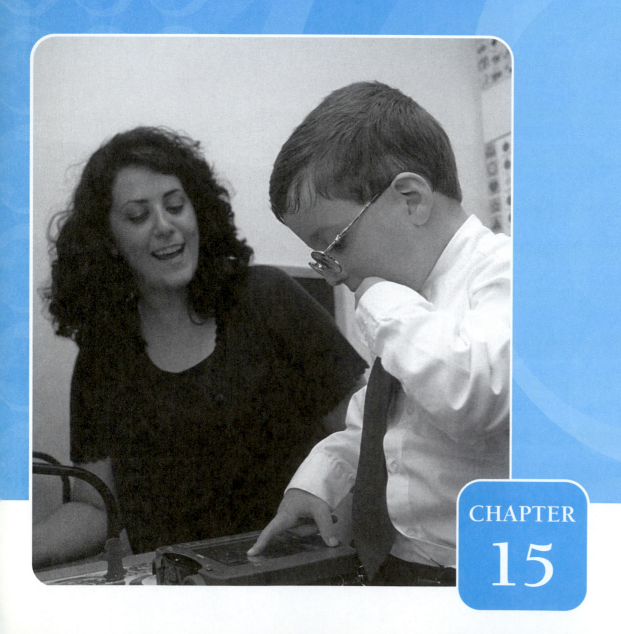

FOCUS QUESTIONS

This chapter answers the following questions:

1. What are complex communication needs?
2. What is AAC?
3. How is AAC classified?
4. What are the defining characteristics of common causes of complex communication needs?
5. How are complex communication needs and AAC systems identified?
6. How are complex communication needs treated with AAC?

INTRODUCTION

Communication is a basic need, and a basic right of all human beings. *(National Joint Committee for the Communication Needs of Persons with Severe Disabilities, 1992)*

Many people take the power of communication for granted. How many times have you thought about how you use your speech and language skills to greet a friend, order food, negotiate a transaction, or express your feelings? Imagine what it would be like if one day people did not understand your speech or you could use only eye blinks to express your thoughts. This is an everyday reality for many children and adults with complex communication needs. **Complex communication needs** result from significant speech, language, motor, and/or cognitive impairments that prevent individuals from communicating in conventional ways. Fortunately, numerous possibilities are now available to meet these needs and help these individuals participate more fully in society. The tools used to promote communication for persons who cannot communicate conventionally are called **augmentative and alternative communication** (AAC); these tools augment existing abilities or provide an alternative means to communicate. Speech-language pathologists, special educators, audiologists, physical therapists, and other health and educational professionals who specialize in this area of practice are called AAC specialists.

AAC is an area of clinical practice that attempts to compensate, either temporarily or permanently, for communication deficits (ASHA, 1991). AAC utilizes symbols, aids, strategies, and techniques to supplement current ways of communicating or, in some cases, to teach alternative ways of communicating. For instance, an individual who loses hearing in late adolescence might learn to use sign language to augment other means for communication, such as gesturing and writing. A child with cerebral palsy who cannot coordinate the precise motor movements needed for speech might use an electronic communication board to produce words and phrases as an alternative to speaking. Professionals who work in this area assess the need for AAC and provide treatment to improve the effectiveness of communication in a variety of settings and with many different communication partners.

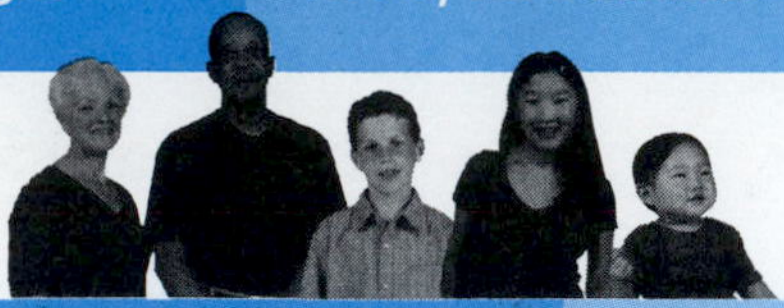

BOX 15-1 Complex Communication Needs and AAC: Case Examples

Sara is a 3-year-old twin who was born 6 weeks prematurely. She has a diagnosis of athetoid cerebral palsy, severe dysarthria, and a mild–moderate receptive and expressive language delay. Sara has significant gross and fine motor impairments because of her cerebral palsy. She communicates with gestures (eye gaze, reaching, pointing), vocalizations, and facial expressions but has no formal symbolic means of communicating at this time. At home she uses her voice to gain attention from and to protest to her parents, older brother, and twin sister, Susan, who has no documented disabilities. Sara also communicates with grandparents, aunts and uncles, and several older cousins at family gatherings. At school she communicates with her teacher and the teacher's aide but does not currently communicate with other children because they do not know how to recognize and respond to her communication behaviors.

Recently, Sara's mother observed her looking out the window, watching neighbor children pulling dolls in a wagon. When she asked Sara what she was doing, Sara gazed at the children, reached/pointed toward them, looked back at her mom, and then smiled. Sara's mother believes Sara comprehends much of what is said to her and has the potential to express much more than she is able to right now. Sara's mother wants to learn about what kind of help is available so she can communicate with her daughter.

Internet research

1. What is the rate of premature births in the United States? How often do children born prematurely exhibit developmental disabilities like Sara's?
2. What kind of preschool programs are available to children like Sara, who exhibit complex communication needs?

Brainstorm and discussion

1. What information could the AAC team learn from Sara's twin sister, Susan, during an AAC assessment?
2. What are some possible AAC options for Sara that could be used at home and at preschool to facilitate communication?

Jan is a 14-year-old young woman in the eighth grade with a moderate intellectual disability and speech and language impairment. Because Jan is in an inclusive school, she receives support in the regular classroom from specialists (e.g., a speech-language pathologist and a special educator) and remains in general education for all her classes. Jan communicates with gestures, speech, and facial expressions. She successfully communicates with her family and several other familiar communication partners who have learned what her gestures mean and can understand her speech. However, Jan has difficulty communicating at school with her teachers and other students and will rarely initiate with students in her classes. Jan has recently expressed an interest in joining the bowling club at school, and Jan's mother is concerned that she will have difficulty communicating with people who do not know her very well. Jan's current speech-language pathologist (SLP) has started developing a communication book, but Jan has not used it at school, although her mother says she uses it occasionally at home. Jan's school SLP referred her to the school district's assistive technology team for a comprehensive AAC assessment.

What Are Complex Communication Needs?

Definition

Complex communication needs exist when individuals cannot meet their daily communication needs through their current method(s) of communication. These complex communication needs result from a "wide range of physical, sensory, and environmental causes which restrict/limit their ability to participate independently in society" (Balandin, 2002, p. 2). To maximize participation in society, these individuals benefit from alternative and augmentative ways to communicate. For example, if a 9-year-old girl has the desire to call her

Internet research

1. Is it common for students with an intellectual disability to be fully included in their schools?
2. What proportion of people with an intellectual disability have complex communication needs?

Brainstorm and discussion

1. What benefits might Jan realize if she participates in a comprehensive AAC assessment?
2. What barriers might prevent Jan from participating in bowling or other activities at school?

Steve is a 28-year-old man who had a brain stem stroke 3 years ago, which resulted in a form of locked-in syndrome. He has profound dysarthria with no functional speech output but some control over his vocalizations and his eye movements. He has severe motor impairment of his limbs and trunk and uses an electric wheelchair for mobility. He has limited control of the muscles to move his head and neck.

Steve currently communicates using eye gaze, an eye gaze board, and a head pointer mounted to a headband to select keys on the keyboard. He communicates with his family, friends, paid attendants, and medical caregivers using either eye gaze or his eye gaze board. He is dependent on familiar partners to communicate with unfamiliar partners. Steve is interested in getting an AAC system to help him be more independent when communicating. Prior to his stroke, Steve owned and worked in an auto repair garage; his hobbies included computers, motorcycles, and race cars. Steve is currently managing his auto repair garage and attending college, majoring in computer information systems.

Internet research

1. What is locked-in syndrome? Is it common?
2. What are some risk factors and causes of strokes?
3. Are strokes common in young adults?

Brainstorm and discussion

1. How might Steve's previous interest in computers help in exploring AAC options?
2. What features would be important for Steve in an AAC system?

friend to come over to play but her speech is not intelligible over the telephone, she has an unmet communication need—that is, using the telephone. This unmet need is considered a complex communication need because many factors must be considered to make the communicative exchange happen successfully—the child's capacity to communicate, the reasons she wants to communicate, the capacities and needs of the listener, and the modality through which communication occurs.

Complex communication needs are as varied as individuals are unique and can occur in any form of communication (i.e., listening, speaking, writing, gesturing), in any environment (e.g., school, home, community), and with a variety of **communication partners** (e.g., parent, spouse, friend, stranger). Additionally, complex communication needs can occur

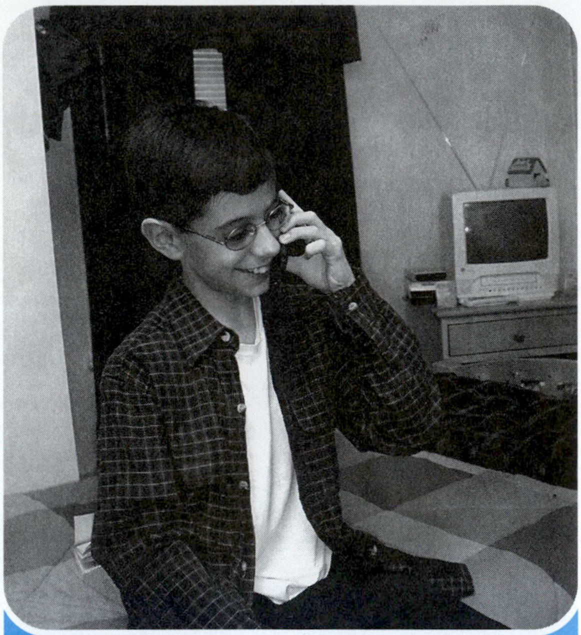

An unmet communication need is present if a young child is unable to call a friend on the telephone to invite him over to play.

when an individual is not able to use communication for all of its purposes, which are described in Table 15-1. The purposes of communication presented in Table 15-1 vary in their focus, duration, and predictability.

Purposes of Communication

Needs and Wants. One purpose of communication is expressing needs and wants. Within moments of birth, infants communicate for this very basic purpose. In communicating **needs and wants**, an individual is able to regulate the behavior of another person to obtain something—either a desired object or a desired action (Light, 1988). The content of the message is very important in relaying needs and wants. For example, a young boy pointing to the kitchen cupboard to indicate that he is hungry hopes that his communication partner, his father, will open the cupboard and remove some food for him to eat. In this example how the communication is conveyed (i.e., by pointing) is just as important as the message, which in this case is poorly represented in the child's communicative act. Communication for this purpose is usually brief in duration and predictable.

Information Transfer. We also communicate to give and to receive information—that is, **information transfer**. The information being conveyed may be novel and unknown to the recipient, posing special challenges for someone with complex communication needs. Communication for this purpose may be lengthy and unpredictable in its content. Consider an individual who does not speak conventionally being stopped by a hearing person who asks for directions to a local restaurant. The individual who does not speak conventionally may have a difficult time transferring this information. Communication partners may be familiar or unfamiliar to the person with complex

TABLE 15-1 The purposes of communication interactions

Purpose	Description
Needs and wants	Goal: regulate behaviors of others Focus: desired action or object Duration: limited Predictability: very predictable
Information transfer	Goal: share information with others Focus: shared information Duration: lengthy Predictability: not predictable
Social closeness	Goal: establish and maintain relationships with others Focus: interpersonal relationship Duration: lengthy Predictability: ranges from very to not predictable
Social etiquette	Goal: engage in social conventions Focus: social conventions (e.g., being polite, greeting) Duration: limited Predictability: very predictable

Source: Based on Light (1988).

communication needs. Giving directions, ordering food in a restaurant, giving medical personnel details of an illness, telling about the day's activities—these are all examples of the need to communicate specific information in a message with varied communication partners.

Social Closeness. **Social closeness** is another reason people interact and communicate with one another. Human beings are social creatures, and as such we strive to establish, develop, and maintain interpersonal relationships (Light, 1988). Individuals who have difficulty communicating may need intervention to assist them in finding ways to promote social closeness with their communication partners. One way people establish and maintain closeness is to share stories about their lives. Have you ever discovered that you had a similar experience to another person after hearing that person's story about childhood? Did you feel closer to the other person after learning about the common experience? Enabling persons with complex communication needs to tell their own stories of who they are and how their experiences have shaped their lives is an important focus of intervention. Communication for this purpose may be lengthy and unpredictable in its focus.

Social Etiquette. Another purpose of communication is **social etiquette**, which has to do with being polite and conforming to the social conventions of one's culture. In mainstream North American society examples include introducing oneself to someone new, saying hello and goodbye in phone conversations, and not interrupting others during conversations. Communication for this purpose is often brief in duration and highly predictable. Of course, what is considered a social nicety in one cultural community may not be so in another, and part of being an effective communicator is learning and using the communicative approaches that are appropriate in a given community. For individuals with complex communication needs, learning and/or using communication in a socially appropriate way can pose a special challenge. In social situations the content of the message may not be as important as meeting the expectations of both familiar and unfamiliar communication partners.

Terminology

The International Society of Augmentative and Alternative Communication (ISAAC) recently adopted the term *complex communication needs* to replace previously used terms, such as *severe communication disorders* or *severe communication impairments* (Balandin, 2002). The term *complex communication needs* emphasizes the importance of speech, language, and/or cognitive abilities for a person's participation in society. It also emphasizes the complexity of communication—how it varies as a function of different contexts, participants, and modalities. And a focus on needs emphasizes the individual's use of communication as a tool of personal expression.

Prevalence and Incidence

Successful communication is a challenge for many children and adults, but estimates vary on how many people have complex communication needs or challenges meeting their daily communication needs. Beukelman and Ansel (1995) estimate that about 8 to 12 of every 1,000 Americans are unable to meet their daily communication needs, and the American Speech-Language-Hearing Association estimates that 2 million Americans currently have complex communication needs (ASHA, 1987).

What Is AAC?

AAC is a set of procedures and processes through which an individual's expressive and receptive communication skills are maximized for functional and effective communication (ASHA, 2002a). AAC uses symbols to supplement or replace natural speech and/or writing. A **symbol** is something that stands for something else. For instance, a child might point to

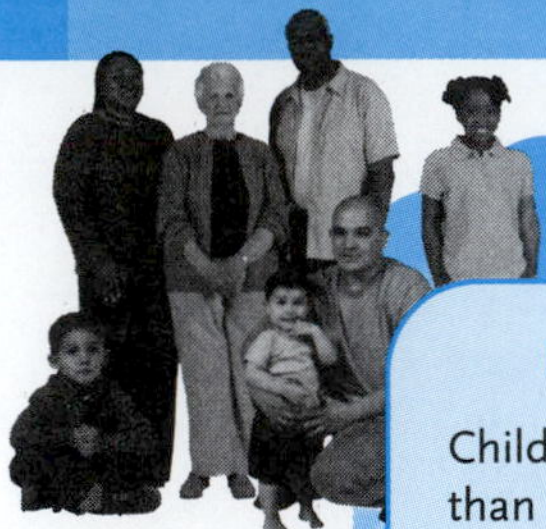

BOX 15-2 Multicultural Focus

Multiculturalism and AAC

Children and adults who use AAC belong to many different cultural groups, sometimes more than one culture at the same time. Culture is "a lens through which individuals see themselves in relation to others and to the world" (Soto, Blake Huer, & Taylor, 1997, p. 406). For AAC intervention to be successful, the members of an AAC team must understand the values, beliefs, behaviors, and communication styles of each identified culture of the person with complex communication needs. AAC service providers also need to be aware of their own cultural beliefs and practices and the ways those might influence their clinical practice (Soto et al., 1997).

People with complex communication needs, their families, and other communication partners from diverse cultural groups may also have diverse linguistic backgrounds. Some may be monolingual, and others may be bilingual or multilingual. In addition, the language used at home may differ from that used at school or in the community, posing special challenges to the individual with complex communication needs:

> Individuals who use AAC who come from diverse cultural and linguistic backgrounds face additional demands in developing communicative competence because they must learn receptive and expressive skills in the language spoken by their family as well as receptive and expressive skills in the language of the broader social community (e.g., educational system, business community). (Light, 2003, p. 9)

When designing an AAC intervention plan, service providers must respect culturally appropriate rules for social interaction and social participation (Soto et al., 1997). People with bilingual/bicultural communication needs require different systems to meet the unique needs of each language and culture. A bicultural AAC system allows the individual to function and participate in both cultures.

For Discussion

How would an AAC intervention plan be different for someone using a bicultural AAC system versus someone using a monocultural AAC system? What are some advantages to a bicultural AAC system?

What are some examples of a bicultural system of AAC?

Companion Website

To answer these questions online, go to the Multicultural Focus module in chapter 15 of the Companion Website.

a line drawing of a glass to indicate the need for a glass of water. That line drawing is a symbol used to replace the spoken word *drink.*

AAC also refers to the field of clinical, educational, and research practice in which individuals with complex communication needs are provided with supplements or alternatives to enhance communication. AAC strives to improve, temporarily or permanently, the communication skills of individuals with little or no functional speech and/or writing through the use of symbols to represent their communication intents (ASHA, 2002).

Effective communication is **multimodal**; that is, people use a combination of communication modalities to meet their intended communication goals. They may speak and listen, read and write, or use sign language, all of which are language-based modalities. Communicators also use modalities that are not language based, including gestures, facial expressions, vocal inflection, speaker proximity, posture, and eye gaze. Many of us use gestures and facial expressions along with speech when communicating in face-to-face interactions.

FIGURE 15-1 AAC system components.

Symbol	Something used to represent an object, action, concept, or idea
Aid	An assistive device used to augment communication modes or provide another method of communication
Strategy	A method used to enhance communication performance
Technique	A method used to select or access messages

The nature of AAC is also multimodal. As the term *augmentative and alternative communication* suggests, meeting complex communication needs may involve augmenting (i.e., supplementing) current communication modes and/or providing an alternative form of communication (e.g., a picture communication board or a computer-based voice output communication system). Some people with complex communication needs may benefit from both augmentative and alternative forms of communication.

How Is AAC Classified?

AAC is a system, meaning that it has many parts that are integrated to form a whole. An **AAC system** is an integrated group of components—symbols, aids, strategies, and techniques—used by individuals to enhance communication. The system supplements any gestural, spoken, and/or written communication modalities the individual already uses (ASHA, 1991), and each AAC system is individualized to meet the unique communication needs of that one person. As shown in Figure 15-1, an AAC system has four elements (ASHA, 1991).

Symbol

Each AAC system contains symbols, which stand for something else (Vanderheiden & Yoder, 1986); they can be acoustic, graphic, manual, and/or tactile. Symbols are also classified as aided or unaided (ASHA, 2002a).

Acoustic Symbols. Acoustic symbols are sounds or tones processed in the auditory system to interpret meaning. What meaning does the ring of a doorbell have? When you press the wrong key on your computer and it beeps, what does that mean? An example of an acoustic symbol set used in AAC systems is the Morse code system (see Figure 15-2). In Morse code the different sounds represent letters, which can be used to program a computer-based AAC system.

FIGURE 15-2 Morse code symbols.

A	.−	N	−.
B	−...	O	−−−
C	−.−.	P	.−−.
D	−..	Q	−−.−
E	.	R	.−.
F	..−.	S	...
G	−−.	T	−
H	....	U	..−
I	..	V	...−
J	.−−−	W	.−−
K	−.−	X	−..−
L	.−..	Y	−.−−
M	−−	Z	−−..

FIGURE 15-3 Graphic symbols in the form of line drawings on a communication board.

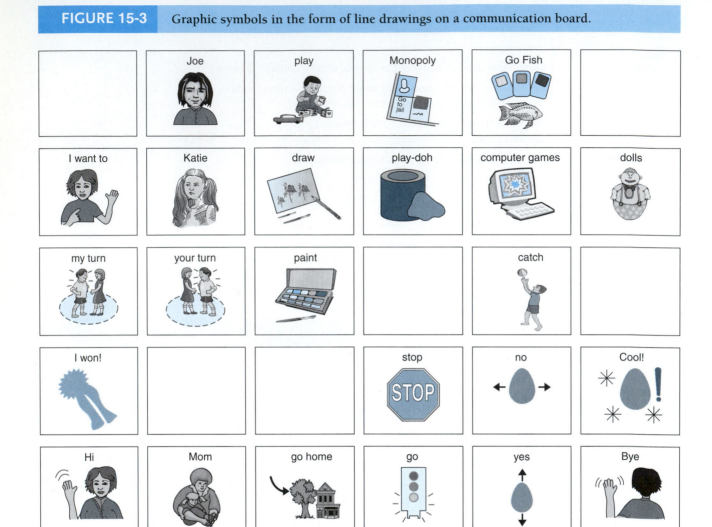

Source: Illustrations courtesy of Boardmaker™ (Mayer-Johnson, Inc.).

Graphic Symbols. Graphic symbols are printed symbols that are usually represented on paper, boards, and/or computer screens. Commonly used graphic symbols in AAC systems include photographs, line drawings, and orthographic characters, such as alphabet letters on a keyboard. Figure 15-3 shows one set of graphic symbols commonly used. These line drawings, coupled with written words, come from Mayer-Johnson's Boardmaker™ system.

Manual Symbols. Manual symbols are produced using the body; examples include gestures, sign language, and facial expressions. Figure 15-4 shows two manual symbols from American Sign Language (ASL).

Tactile Symbols. Tactile symbols are physically manipulated. A well-known example of a tactile symbol system is the Braille alphabet, used by individuals with visual impairment to access written language for reading. Tactile symbols are also used by people with complex communication needs. For instance, an early childhood special educator might use a cracker or a yogurt container to represent snack time in his classroom. A child obtains the meaning of the symbol from the physical properties of the object.

Discussion Point: *Symbols are prevalent everywhere. What type of symbols do you use each day? What type of symbols does Jan use in Box 15-1?*

FIGURE 15-4 Signs for *mother* (left) and *father* (right) in American Sign Language.

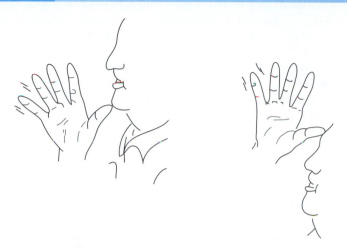

Variations in the Use of Symbols

Symbols are used to represent objects, actions, concepts, and ideas. However, the way in which various AAC systems use symbols to promote communication can vary. For instance, in some AAC systems symbols are used alone, whereas in other systems symbols are combined with one another. As an example, a child might point to two Boardmaker™ symbols in succession to communicate "I don't want to go home" (i.e., *no* + *go home*). Many AAC systems permit use of symbols alone or in combination. For instance, in sign language, an individual can successfully communicate hunger using a single sign (*eat*) or can add additional signs to communicate hunger for a particular food (e.g., *eat* + *potato chips*). AAC symbol systems also vary in other ways.

Static and Dynamic Symbol Systems. **Static** symbols do not require movement or change to understand their meaning—for example, a photograph or an illustration. An AAC system using static symbols might be one in which a child points to photos in a book to request specific family members. In contrast, **dynamic** symbols require movement or change to understand their meaning (ASHA, 2002a). Gestures are one example of a dynamic symbol system—think of the gestures to signal *come here* or *go away.* Some electronic devices used as AAC systems feature an animated graphic system in which different symbols are expressed dynamically.

Iconic and Opaque Symbol Systems. Symbols also vary in their iconicity and opaqueness. **Iconicity** is the degree to which symbols visually resemble what they refer to. A symbol that is **opaque** has little resemblance to what it represents, whereas an iconic symbol is very transparent (ASHA, 2002a). Figure 15-5 shows two symbols for *carrot.* The opaque symbol on the left comes from a symbol system called Blissymbols. Developed and maintained by the nonprofit organization Blissymbolics Communication International (BCI), this system contains more than 3,000 symbols, many of which are relatively opaque. The system was designed specifically for children and adults with significant disabilities who are nonspeaking (BCI, 2005).

FIGURE 15-5 An opaque (A) and an iconic (B) symbol for *carrot.*

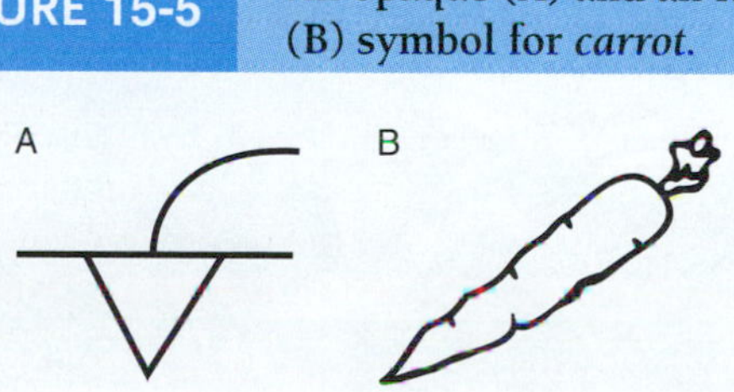

Source: (A) From Online Blissword Dictionary (http://www.blisswords.co.uk). Reprinted with permission. (B) From *Picture Communication Symbols* by Mayer-Johnson, 1995, Solana Beach, CA: Mayer-Johnson. Reprinted with permission.

The symbol on the right, which is iconic, comes from a symbolic system titled Boardmaker™, developed and marketed by Mayer-Johnson, Inc. Boardmaker™ is a set of more than 3,000 picture-communication symbols that are widely used in the design of individual AAC systems. Many of the picture-communication symbols used in Boardmaker™ are iconic, although more opaque symbols are needed for abstract or complex concepts, as in the symbol for "cool" in Figure 15-3.

Some AAC systems are built to use only iconic symbols—for example, a picture board with line drawings representing specific actions, such as an apple for *eat lunch* and a sun for *go outside*). Other AAC systems are very opaque, to the extent that those who do not know the system are unable to understand what is being communicated. However, even within one system, the symbols may vary in their iconicity. In sign language, for instance, the sign for *drink* is very transparent, produced by moving a cupped hand toward the mouth. And the sign for *think* uses the index finger tapped against the forehead. But other signs—such as those for *dream, cracker,* and *mother*—are relatively opaque.

Discussion Point: *Consider the pros and cons of AAC systems comprised entirely of iconic or opaque symbols.*

Aided and Unaided. Symbol systems are also classified as aided or unaided. An **aided** symbol requires a device or accessory that is external to the body to transmit a message. Typing a message, drawing a picture, or pointing to photographs—these are all examples of aided systems. **Unaided** symbols require only one's body—for example, speaking, gesturing, vocalizing, and signing (Fuller, Lloyd, & Stratton, 1997).

Aid

Many AAC systems are aided; the term **aid** refers to a type of assistive device that supplements or replaces natural speech and/or writing. Aids can augment language comprehension as well, as when a teacher uses an amplifier and microphone in the classroom to help a child whose comprehension is compromised by background noise. Aids used to supplement and replace speech can be **electronic**, such as voice output communication aids (VOCAs). The term *assistive technology* (AT) is also used to describe assistive aids that promote communication, as well as other aspects of well-being, such as physical or motor performance. Figure 15-6 presents six different kinds of commonly used VOCAs.

An aid does not have to be electronic. For instance, a very young child might have a communication book with photographs depicting a variety of activities (e.g., reading a book, playing outside, using the restroom, eating lunch). The child communicates by pointing to photographs (ASHA, 2002a). This, too, is an aid—a supplement to communication.

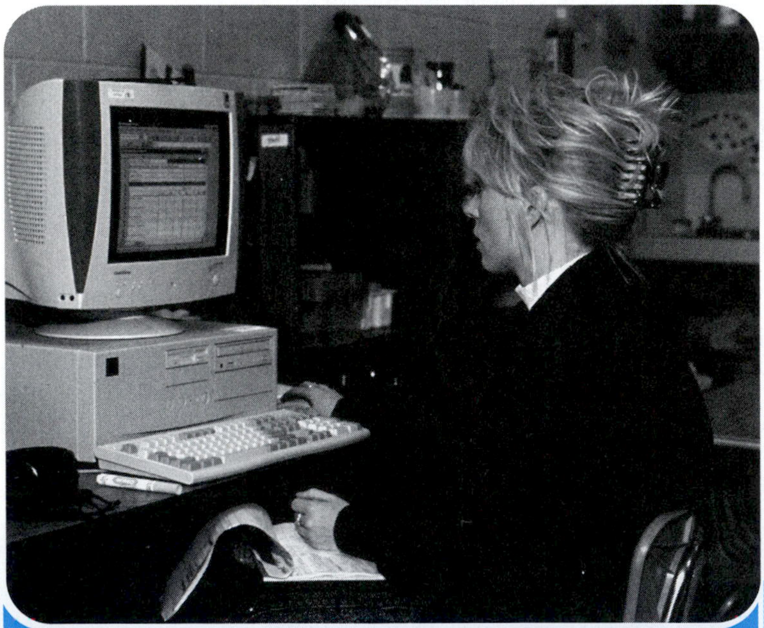

An aided system requires a tool external to the body, such as a computer.

FIGURE 15-6 Examples of electronic VOCAs.

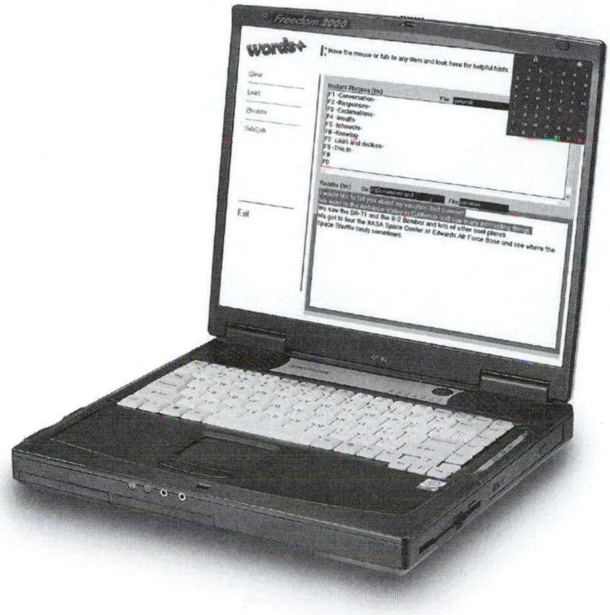

a. Freedom 2000 Toughbook™

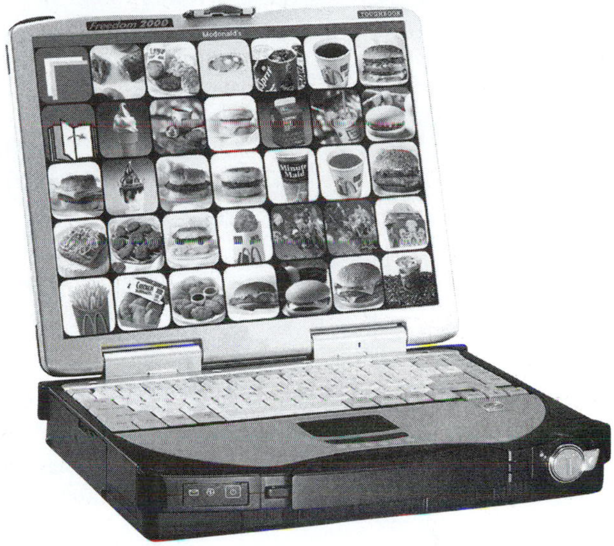

b. Freedom 2000 Extreme™

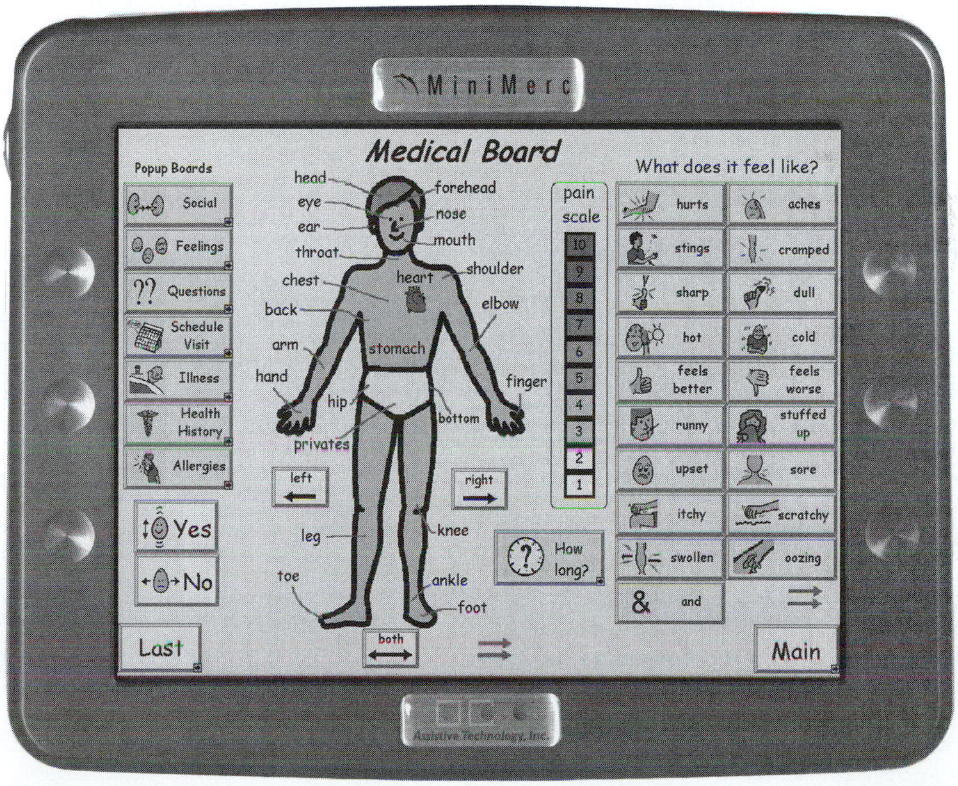

c. MiniMerc™

FIGURE 15-6 *(continued)*

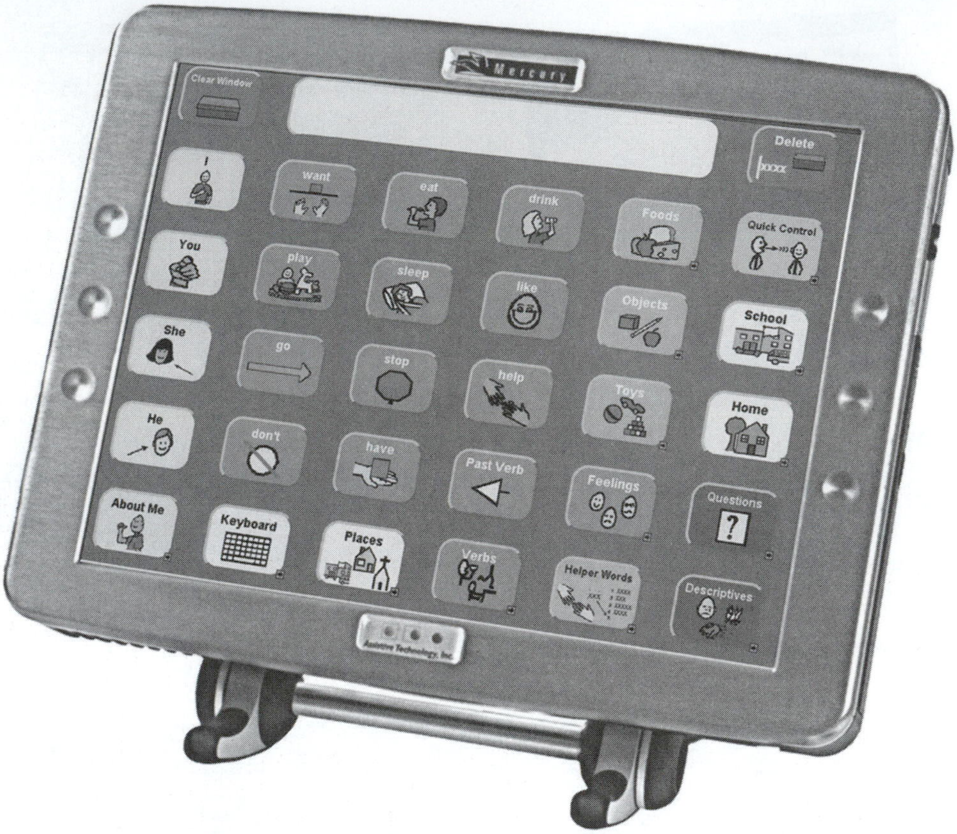

d. Mercury II™

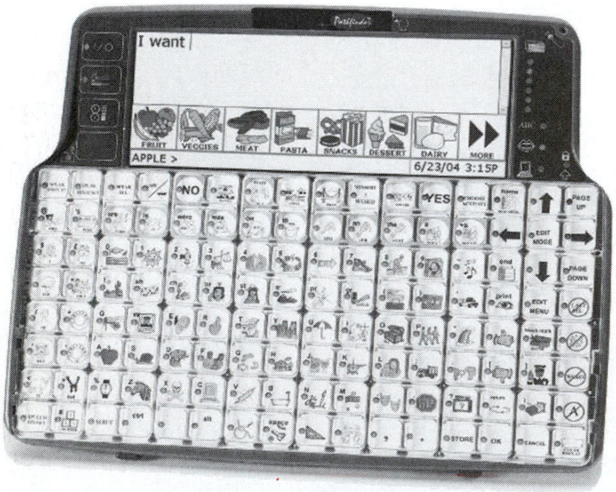

e. Pathfinder Plus™

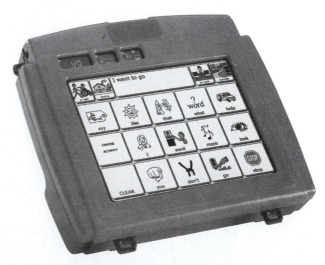

f. SpringBoard Plus™

Source: Photos courtesy of (a & b) Words+, Inc.; (c & d) Assistive Technology, Inc.; and (e & f) Prentke Romich Company.

Strategy

Strategies are also part of an AAC system. A **strategy** is the process or method that an individual employs to improve or enhance communication (ASHA, 2002a). Examples of AAC system strategies include setting the topic before initiating a conversation, using software that predicts letters or words in order to eliminate keystrokes, and having an index card available for unfamiliar communication partners to explain how the individual communicates. A strategy is, in essence, how the AAC is used (the symbol and the aid) to promote communication performance. Much of AAC intervention is promoting an individual's use of strategies.

Technique

Technique refers to the way in which messages are transmitted—that is, how an individual selects or accesses messages on a display. Displays contain the symbols in an AAC system; they can be fixed or dynamic. A **fixed display** remains the same before and after a symbol is selected. For example, a picture of a TV on a picture communication board remains the same and does not change. **Dynamic displays** are visual and change after a symbol is selected (ASHA, 2002a). A dynamic display usually involves a computer screen presenting a visual message, typically either letters or pictures. As symbols are selected, the screen changes automatically to a set of programmed symbols (Beukelman & Mirenda, 1998). Dynamic displays are available in several commercially available AAC systems. They are also used in many ATM machines and electronic payment systems in stores. For instance, the display of an ATM machine changes in response to input (e.g., "To continue in English, press 1; to continue in Spanish, press 2") to feature a set of programmed symbols.

Technique also refers to how individuals access their AAC systems—with either direct or indirect selection (Dowden & Cook, 2002). **Direct selection** is a direct motor act that is not dependent on time (Dowden & Cook, 2002); there are four types (Beukelman & Mirenda, 1998). The first type is physical pressure, or depression; individuals select symbols using a controlled body movement to depress a key or apply sufficient pressure for activation to occur. This body movement can involve a body part, such as a finger, or an instrument attached to the body, such as a stick mounted to a headband. The second type of direct selection is physical contact. With this technique the individual needs only to have physical contact with the AAC system, such as touching a finger to a symbol or a word on a communication board.

The third type of direct selection technique is pointing without contact, as shown in Figure 15-7. One example is eye pointing, in which an individual looks at an item long enough for a communication partner to assess the person's intent (Beukelman & Mirenda, 1998). After a severe spinal cord injury, an individual might use eye pointing to select an activity on a communication board (e.g., watching television or reading a book). Eye pointing can also use a light beam attached to a headband to

FIGURE 15-7 An eye gaze board.

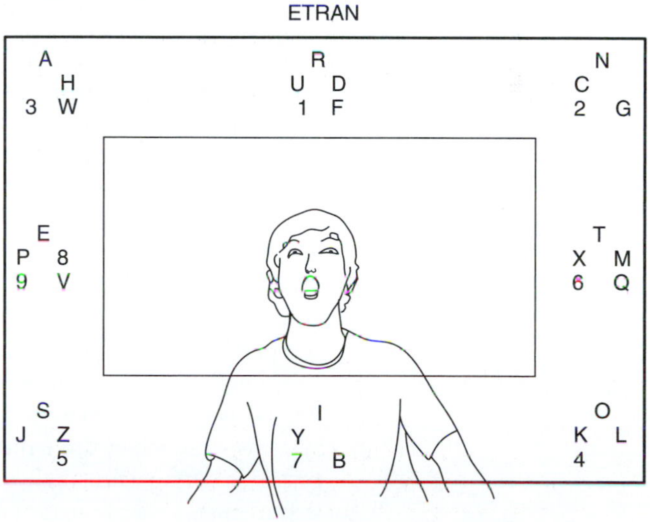

Source: From *Augmentative Communication: An Introduction* by S. W. Blackstone, 1986, Rockville, MD: American Speech-Language-Hearing Association. Copyright 1986 by ASHA. Reprinted with permission.

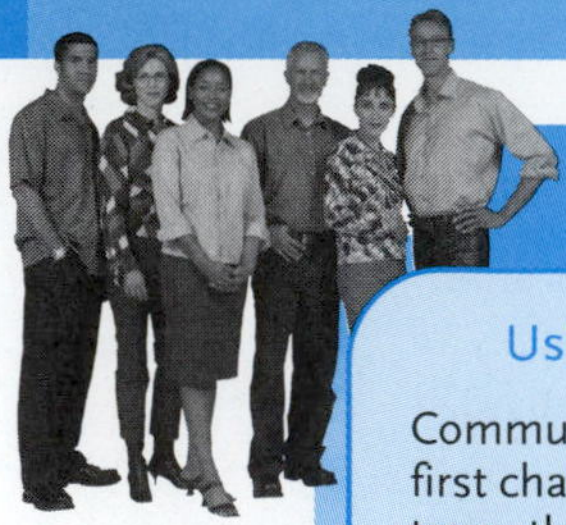

BOX 15-3 Ecological Contexts

Using AAC to Communicate in the Community

Communicating in the community can be a challenge even for competent AAC users. As a first challenge, consider the issue of access. Some people who use AAC have lightweight systems they can carry in a case or attach to a beltlike apparatus. But the system must be portable enough not to interfere with ambulation yet still accessible for communication when needed. Others may mount their AAC systems on a wheelchair or attach them to a tray on the wheelchair. The challenge may come when they need to control their electric wheelchair and cannot access their AAC system at the same time. Such factors need to be addressed during an AAC assessment and intervention program so that the person using an AAC system can access it in any environment.

Another potential challenge has to do with adjusting the features of an AAC system to meet the demands of each situation. For example, voice output communication systems (VOCAs) may be difficult to understand in noisy environments; visual displays may be difficult to see outside. Weather can also be a barrier. VOCAs are electronic and will be damaged if exposed to moisture. AAC intervention plans must include training for all environments and conditions.

Another situation that can be challenging is communicating with unfamiliar partners. Communication modalities that may be successful with familiar communication partners (e.g., gestures, facial expressions) may not be successful with unfamiliar communication partners. When communicating with people they do not know well, AAC users may need to rely on more formal modes of communication, such as communication books, VOCAs, and writing. AAC training should focus on not only learning to use all the different modalities to communicate successfully but also determining when and how to use different modes of communication.

For Discussion

What are some additional challenges to using AAC in the community?

What types of approaches might a therapist use to prepare an AAC user for various communication challenges in the community?

Companion Website

To answer these questions online, go to the Ecological Contexts module in chapter 15 of the Companion Website.

point to desired selections. Some computer systems allow eye pointing with an infrared light-emitting diode to type on keyboards or to activate certain images. For instance, a toddler who cannot speak because of severe muscular impairment might use eye pointing to activate songs on a computer screen.

Discussion Point: *Steve in Box 15-1 uses eye pointing to select messages from his eye gaze board. Should he be a candidate for using speech or voice input to access an AAC system? Explain.*

The fourth direct selection technique is speech or voice input. Some AAC systems can be accessed by speech or voice input to activate messages and functions. Some cell phones come with voice activation for hands-free calling, an example of a system accessed by voice input. Some computers are also equipped with this technology, so that saying "Computer turn on" accomplishes that feat. This same technology is used by companies—when we're asked to "Say 1 for English or 2 for Spanish" when calling, for instance.

Individuals with severe motor and/or sensory impairments can also access their AAC systems with one of three **indirect selection** techniques (Dowden & Cook, 2002). The first is scanning with single or dual switches. With **scanning**, a selection set of symbols is presented in a predetermined configuration by either a communication device or a communication partner (Beukelman & Mirenda, 1998). For instance, an electronic device might highlight pictures in a linear format following a preset, one-at-a-time order. The individual waits until the desired symbol is presented and then signals his or her choice using eye gaze, eye blinks, head nods, or switch activation. Because of the time needed for the device to scan through items, the number of possible symbols should be kept low, typically 15 or fewer. Figure 15-8 shows a communication board attached to a switch. As the board scans the letters, the individual hits the attached switch when the desired symbol is lighted.

The second indirect technique is directed scanning, which is the use of multiple switches or a joystick interface to move a cursor to a specified target location (Dowden & Cook, 2002). This approach is considered a hybrid of typical scanning. An individual uses a joystick or other type of switch to select a scanning direction and then makes a selection. Directed scanning provides a more efficient approach to communication than regular scanning and is used by people who have the motor control needed for coordination.

FIGURE 15-8 **Scanning with a single switch.**

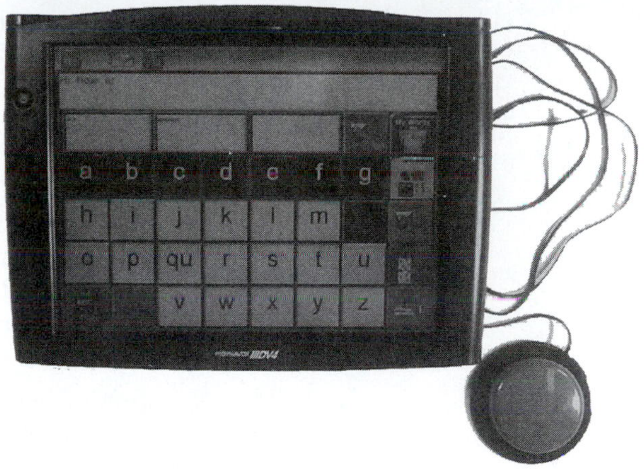

Source: Photo courtesy of AbleNet, Inc., and Dynavoc Systems, LLC.

The third type of indirect selection is **coded access**, which requires an individual to use a sequence of movements to select a symbol from a set (Dowden & Cook, 2002). Morse code is an example of coded access that many individuals with complex communication needs have used successfully to access their AAC systems. It can be inputted to an AAC system with switches.

Discussion Point: *Motor and sensory skills often determine which technique is best for accessing communication symbols and messages. What AAC technique does Sara in Box 15-1 use? What about Jan?*

What Are the Defining Characteristics of Common Causes of Complex Communication Needs?

Complex communication needs can result from developmental or acquired disabilities. Common developmental disabilities include intellectual disability, cerebral palsy, autism, and childhood apraxia of speech. Disabilities acquired later in life may come from trauma, illness, or a degenerative disease.

Intellectual Disability

The American Association on Mental Retardation (2002) defines an **intellectual disability** (also known as mental retardation) as significant limitations in both intellectual functioning and adaptive behavior, as expressed in conceptual, social, and practical adaptive skills. Some children and adults with severe or profound intellectual disabilities may not be able to communicate at all using speech; thus, AAC presents the only option for communicating. Consider Jane, a 42-year-old woman with a profound cognitive disability. She works 5 days a week (3 hours per day) placing caps on pens in a factory. She communicates that she is finished with a set of pens by hitting a switch, which signals her supervisor to bring her more pens. AAC interventions can improve communication opportunities in natural environments for many individuals with intellectual disabilities (Beukelman & Mirenda, 1998).

Cerebral Palsy

Cerebral palsy is a neuromotor impairment resulting from trauma or damage to the developing child before, during, or soon after birth (McDonald, 1987). The impact on a child's ability to communicate ranges from little or no impact to a complete inability to use speech at all. Children and adults with cerebral palsy may use AAC to meet the complex communication needs resulting from speech, language, cognitive, and/or sensory (i.e., vision, hearing) impairments. The type of AAC selected is based on the individual's communication needs as well as motor and cognitive abilities.

Autism

Autism is a developmental disability characterized by impaired social interaction and communication and by restricted, repetitive, and stereotypical patterns of behavior and interest (APA, 1994). Children and adults with autism are likely to have communication difficulties, which may result in complex communication needs. Beukelman and Mirenda (1998) state that early intervention is critical for individuals with autism. AAC approaches can facilitate the development of speech, augment current modes of communication, and/or provide alternative means of communication.

One well-known augmentative communication device for individuals with autism is the picture exchange communication system (PECS; Bondy & Frost, 1994). PECS is a structured teaching approach that features the use of pictures and is used with children (or adults) who are communicating for functional purposes. The approach begins by teaching the children to initiate communication by exchanging a picture for a desired item (e.g., a piece of candy, a favorite toy). The children gradually develop the skill to link pictures to more complex ideas (e.g., *I want + toy*) and to communicate for many different purposes, such as commenting on actions in the environment. Several studies have shown the benefits of PECS in enhancing the communication skills of children with autism. In addition, this approach is low cost, can be used in a variety of contexts, and requires few specialized materials (Charlop-Christy, Carpenter, Le, LeBlanc, & Kellet, 2002; Frea, Arnold, & Vittimberga, 2001; Kravitz, Kamps, Kemmerer, & Potucek, 2002).

Childhood Apraxia of Speech

Childhood apraxia of speech (CAS) is a neurologically based disorder in which the planning and/or execution of articulatory movements for speech production is impaired (Jakielski & Davis, 1995). The impact of CAS on the intelligibility of speech can range from mild to severe, with some children unintelligible even to those with whom they are very familiar, including parents. Some children with severe or profound CAS use AAC to help meet their communication needs as they work to improve their speech intelligibility. Although some parents may be concerned that the use of an AAC system may inhibit their children's speech development, this is typically not the case. This speech disorder is described in chapter 6.

Traumatic Brain Injury

Traumatic brain injury (TBI) is an acquired injury to the brain, caused by a traumatic event (e.g., head hitting the pavement at high speed after falling off a motorcycle or head hitting the windshield of an automobile in a car accident). The brain damage from a TBI can result in motor speech disorders (dysarthria and/or apraxia) and cognitive-linguistic impairments, as described in chapter 8. If the impairment is severe, the person with a TBI may benefit from AAC, which can improve communication during all phases of recovery. Early in recovery, AAC provides a means for consistent responses—for instance, pointing to a picture of water to identify the desire for a drink. Some people progress to normal speech following TBI, using AAC as a temporary solution to an inability to communicate effectively or efficiently. Other individuals never achieve oral speech again, especially if the brain injury is severe. For them AAC is used to improve the quality of life and allow them to communicate again with a variety of partners (Carlisle Ladtkow & Culp, 1992).

Stroke

A **stroke** occurs when a blood clot blocks a blood vessel or artery or when a blood vessel breaks, resulting in an interruption of blood flow to an area of the brain (National Stroke Association, 2005). Strokes can occur in the brain or in the brain stem. Depending on where the damage occurs, a person may have motor speech, language, sensory, and/or cognitive impairment. Language expression and comprehension are frequently impacted by left-hemisphere strokes, although language use is also impacted by frontal-lobe and right-hemisphere strokes. For people with severe impairments, AAC can improve functional and effective communication and increase their participation in society.

Discussion Point: *Brain stem strokes can result in locked-in syndrome, in which a person is completely paralyzed except for limited eye movement and possible eye blinks. Does Steve in Box 15-1 have a complete or incomplete form of locked-in syndrome? How do you know?*

Degenerative Diseases

Degenerative diseases can result in the loss of motor, language, cognitive, and/or sensory functioning. In many cases this loss is progressive and becomes more severe over time. People with degenerative diseases often lose their ability to meet their daily communication needs independently and may become isolated from society.

One degenerative disease that may result in complex communication needs is **amyotrophic lateral sclerosis** (ALS). Also known as Lou Gehrig's disease, ALS is "a relentlessly and rapidly progressive disease" (Mathy, Yorkston, & Gutmann, 2000, p. 186). People with ALS may experience a deterioration of speech skills, resulting in unintelligible speech (i.e., dysarthria), and/or poor respiratory functioning, resulting in mechanical ventilation. AAC services can help these individuals meet their complex communication needs. Communication is a particularly important goal of therapy for these individuals, as language and intellect remain intact even while speech control rapidly deteriorates.

Parkinsons disease (PD) is a slowly progressive disease of the basal ganglia in the central nervous system. Complex communication needs usually stem from dysarthria, a motor speech disorder discussed in chapter 6. If the dysarthria becomes severe, a person with PD may have difficulty initiating voicing and will produce short rushes of poorly articulated speech (Yorkston, Miller, & Strand, 1995). Thus, people with PD may benefit from AAC to augment their speech.

Primary progressive aphasia (PPA) is another degenerative disease; it can result in a gradual loss of language functioning over 5 to 10 years, eventually becoming severe or profound (Weintraub, Rubin, & Mesulam, 1990). This loss is isolated in the initial stages, as memory and other cognitive functions tend to be spared, allowing a person with PPA to continue many activities of daily living until the late stages of the disease. AAC can help meet the communication needs of people with PPA by using proactive management, which focuses on anticipating needs and teaching strategies to maintain communication competence (Rogers, King, & Alarcon, 2000).

How Are Complex Communication Needs and AAC Systems Identified?

The Assessment Team

A **multidisciplinary team** of professionals conducts the AAC assessment. Possible team members include individuals with complex communication needs, parents, teachers, speech-language pathologists, physical therapists, occupational therapists, rehabilitation engineers, social workers, psychologists, vocational counselors, nurses, and doctors. Typically, one professional serves as the team leader; often the speech-language pathologist leads the team and coordinates the assessment process.

Discussion Point: *AAC team members represent a diverse group of professionals. What important information do you think each of the team members brings to the assessment?*

The Assessment Process

AAC teams work in schools, clinics, and hospitals: assessments occur in all of these settings and in other environments in which people communicate (e.g., home or work site). But regardless of the setting, the assessment process is similar.

Referral

A referral for an AAC assessment can be made by anyone who identifies unmet communication needs in a person. Common referral sources include parents, speech-language pathologists, teachers, counselors, and nurses. After a referral is made, a member of the AAC team contacts the identified person and his or her communication partners to schedule a comprehensive AAC assessment.

Comprehensive Assessment

The purpose of a **comprehensive AAC assessment** is to "identify why an individual's level of participation in a particular activity might be restricted due to his/her lack of access to an effective means of communication" (ASHA, 2002, p. 421). Thus, the focus of the AAC team is to identify unmet communication needs from a functional perspective. The team carefully studies four aspects of the individual's communication, as shown in Figure 15-9:

1. Needs
2. Skills
3. Partners
4. Environments

Identification of Communication Needs. The AAC team must identify the communication needs of the individual and determine which are not being met (Beukelman & Mirenda, 1998). Each AAC assessment begins with a case history to gather background information about the individual's communication development, current methods of communicating, medical history, the history of any treatment for a communication impairment, and pertinent family information. The team then interviews the individual and key communication partners and may also observe a range of natural environments, such as home, school, and work. The team focuses on how to enable the individual to interact with family, friends, acquaintances, and others in order to improve the person's quality of life.

Discussion Point: *Who do you think would be the best informant regarding the current communication abilities and needs of Sara, Jan, and Steve in Box 15-1? Why?*

FIGURE 15-9 An AAC assessment profile.

Communication needs	Determine what specific ideas, thoughts, concepts, and messages the person needs to communicate
Communication skills	Determine strengths and present level of performance in speech, language, cognition, and overall communication
Communication partners	Determine the person's communication partners in all daily living routines
Communication environments	Determine all the environments in which the person does and will communicate

In addition, the team must determine the extent to which the individual is participating in all of the communication activities of age-matched peers. To identify participation patterns and communication needs, the team initially conducts an activity inventory, which examines the range and type of everyday activities characteristic of same-age peers (Beukelman & Mirenda, 1998). The team must then determine whether the individual is participating in the same activities. If there is a discrepancy, the team must determine what barriers are preventing participation.

The team looks specifically for the presence of opportunity and access barriers in the community. **Opportunity barriers** are imposed by other people and prevent an individual's participation in communication activities, as summarized in Table 15-2. An example of an opportunity barrier is a school policy that places children with complex communication needs in segregated classrooms so that they have little time to communicate with peers. **Access barriers** can also prevent participation in communication activities, but they stem from the capabilities, attitudes, and resources of the person using AAC (Beukelman & Mirenda, 1998). For instance, an individual with AAC might resist participating in community activities because of his or her own attitude about how other people will perceive the use of AAC.

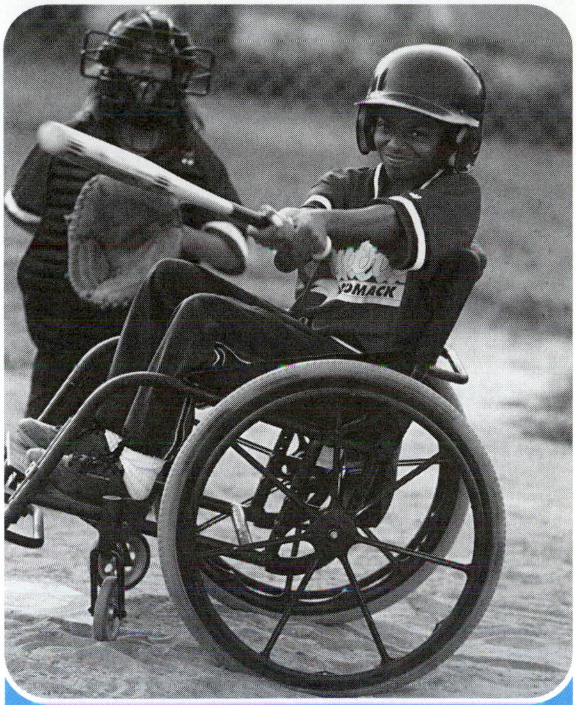

An activity inventory examines the range and types of activities engaged in by same-age peers.

Identification of Communication Skills. The assessment team identifies the individual's current level of communication skills using a variety of formal and informal assessment tools. One

TABLE 15-2 Opportunity barriers to participation in communication activities

Barrier	Example
Policy: Regulations that prevent participation	Some school districts do not allow students to use their AAC systems outside school.
Practice: Procedures or routines that are commonplace and prevent participation	Some school districts have students share AAC systems because they do not have enough systems for everyone to have one.
Attitude: A belief or perspective that prevents participation	People who hold negative attitudes toward others with disabilities may not allow opportunities for communication.
Knowledge: A lack of information that prevents participation	School personnel may not understand technology and may not wish to learn how to facilitate communication with someone using an AAC system.
Skill: A lack of technical and communicative support that prevents participation	Communication partners may not demonstrate adequate skills to facilitate communication interactions.

Source: From *Augmentative and Alternative Communication: Management of Severe Communication Disorders in Children and Adults* by D. R. Beukelman and P. Mirenda, 1998, Baltimore: Brookes. Copyright 1998 by Brookes. Adapted with permission.

Discussion Point: *What communication needs did you identify for Sara, Jan, and Steve in Box 15-1? What communication activities might they be restricted from participating in, given their current methods of communicating?*

important assessment tool in achieving this information is titled *Social Networks* (Blackstone & Hunt Berg, 2003), which seeks information from important communication partners about varied topics:

- The skills and abilities of the individual
- Modes of expression used by the individual
- Symbols, selection techniques, and strategies the individual uses to communicate
- Topics of conversation the individual would choose to communicate about

The team also assesses oral motor skills, hearing acuity, receptive and expressive language skills, speech production, cognitive skills, and overall communication skills. Many of the tools used by the AAC team are described in chapter 6 and chapter 7. The goal is to determine communication strengths and challenges.

For the individual with complex communication needs, professionals must be prepared to adapt test materials to significant motor, speech, cognitive, and language limitations. For instance, a child with cerebral palsy may not be able to point to pictures to show comprehension of vocabulary words; thus, tests that require pointing need to be modified for this child, and standardized tests that do not permit deviations from standard test protocols may be inappropriate. Of concern to the team is how to validly represent an individual's capabilities when significant limitations are present. Consider how challenging it might be to accurately represent the language comprehension abilities of a child with severe autism who does not interact with others at all. AAC team members must be especially knowledgeable about different tests and measures when significant motor, speech, cognitive, and language limitations are present.

***Discussion Point:** Consider the case of Sara in Box 15-1. How do you think tests could be adapted to assess her language comprehension?*

Complementing the communication assessment is an examination of an individual's visual and motor abilities, important considerations in selecting AAC systems. Some systems require an individual to select messages or keys or activate switches with precise motor movements. An adult with very limited motor capabilities, perhaps in advanced stages of Parkinson's disease, might not have the motor functions to coordinate use of a complex VOCA. And knowledge of visual acuity is needed to determine what type, size, and array of symbols can be used in an AAC system. Typically, the occupational and physical therapists on the AAC team complete the vision and motor assessments.

Identification of Communication Partners and Communication Environments. An important part of an AAC assessment is the identification of communication partners. One paradigm often used is circles of communication partners (CCP) (Blackstone, 1999; Falvey, Forest, Pearpoint, & Rosenberg, 1994). CCP consists of five concentric circles with the person with complex communication needs in the center. The first circle includes the person's lifelong communication partners. The second circle includes close friends and relatives; the third, acquaintances. The fourth circle is for paid workers, and the fifth, for unfamiliar partners. Blackstone (1999) recommends using CCP as part of an AAC assessment for three purposes:

1. To identify communication partners
2. To gather information about communication partners, identifying those who understand the individual's AAC system and those who will need training to understand it
3. To determine what communication methods are used with which partners (e.g., speech with familiar partners and AAC methods with unfamiliar partners)

***Discussion Point:** Draw CCPs for Sara, Jan, and Steve in Box 15-1, based on the information provided. Which circle has the most partners? Why do you think that is the case?*

The team must also identify **communication environments** in which the person currently participates and those in which the person wishes to participate. Environments in which people communicate vary with factors such as age, culture, health, occupation, hobbies, and interests. Consider the environments in which you communicate often and the ways these have changed in recent years. For many people with complex communication needs, barriers prevent them from communicating in certain environments.

Recommendations

Once the comprehensive assessment is completed, the AAC team makes certain recommendations.

An AAC System to Meet Communication Needs. The team collaborates to identify the specific features of an AAC system that will meet an individual's identified communication needs, increase participation in desired activities, and improve communication competence. The team also identifies the best positioning of the individual for AAC system use and the optimal placement of a switch, if appropriate. In determining the specific symbols, aids, strategies, and/or techniques, the team must consider the preferences of the individual and the communication partners.

Consider the real case of a 12-year-old adolescent with complex communication needs following the surgical removal of a tumor in the left hemisphere. One possible unaided approach considered by the team was a manual communication system, namely Signed Exact English (SEE). However, the family did not want to use SEE or any other system that would require others to learn the system in order to interact with the child. They preferred a VOCA, which would transmit spoken English. As this example shows, the AAC team considers family values and preferences in identifying an appropriate AAC system (ASHA, 2002a).

Ultimately, the team recommends a specific AAC system tailored to the individual's needs and strengths and also recommends training for the individual and all relevant communication partners in system function and use. It is common practice to recommend a trial period of days or months to ensure that the new system meets the complex communication needs of the individual.

Funding for the System. The AAC team will also likely provide some guidance on funding. Although some AAC systems may be relatively inexpensive, such as the PECS approach described earlier, others are quite expensive, costing between $4,000 and $8,000 (Assistive Technology Funding & Systems Change Project, 1999). Historically, some individuals, including both the elderly and the young, have had a difficult time affording the recommended systems.

Medicare, one possible funding agent for the elderly, long considered speech-generating devices (SGDs) to be convenience items and thus did not fund their purchase or use. However, Medicare policies have changed in recent years to include coverage of some SGDs as durable medical equipment (AAC Rehabilitation Engineering Research Center [AAC RERC], 2005). This change occurred, in part, because of a series of legal appeals that awarded coverage to people for AAC devices (Assistive Technology Funding & Systems Change Project, 1999):

- Emlyn J. (California, August 1993): A 70-year-old man received benefits to cover a computer and supplies used to communicate after a stroke.
- Richard A. (Idaho, May 1997): A 69-year-old man received benefits to cover a Canon communicator, used to communicate after a stroke.
- Celia C. (New York, September 1998): A 79-year-old woman received benefits to cover a Lightwriter, used to communicate after she developed ALS.

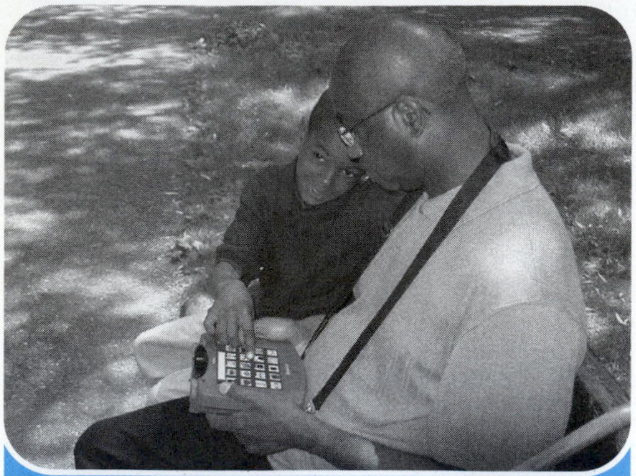

Medicare may cover an AAC system when it is needed to meet physical and medical needs.

Thus, Medicare may cover the cost of SGDs for individuals whose physicians prescribe them and whose speech-language pathologists recommend them to meet daily communication needs. For coverage to occur, a certified speech-language pathologist must conduct a thorough communication assessment, evaluating daily communication needs and abilities as well as identifying why an SGD is needed, clarifying why natural speech and low-tech solutions are not being used, and identifying the functional communication goals to be met with the SGD (AAC RERC, 2005). These are possible goals (AAC RERC, 2005):

1. Meeting physical needs (e.g., advocating for self, giving directions to caregivers)
2. Meeting community and family needs (e.g., communicating with family members by telephone, participating in family decision making)
3. Meeting medical and health-related needs (e.g., giving information on medical status, requesting prescriptions)

BOX 15-4 Spotlight on Research

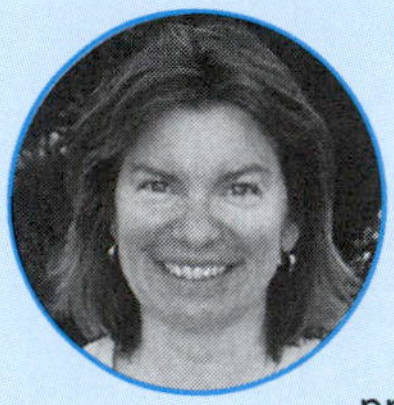

Mary Hunt-Berg, Ph.D., CCC-SLP
Research Program Director
The Bridge School,
Hillsborough, CA

Dr. Mary Hunt-Berg is the research program director at the Bridge School in Hillsborough, California. The Bridge School is a nonprofit organization that serves the educational and clinical needs of individuals with complex communication needs who use AAC. At the Bridge School students have access to a wide range of assistive technologies and intensive services to support their communication skill development and their access to the educational curriculum. For example, students explore the use of voice output communication devices, power mobility devices, computer-supported instructional approaches, and various environmental control devices.

Several unique features make the Bridge School an optimal setting for a range of AAC research activities. The school serves a maximum of 14 students at any given time. Each of two classrooms is staffed by an educational team that includes a full-time teacher, a full-time SLP, and several instructional assistants. This staff-to-student ratio allows for detailed and ongoing assessment and documentation of student performance for educational planning. Additionally, the Bridge School is considered a transitional placement: students attend for an average of 2 to 3 years before returning to their respective school districts to continue their education. Some students enter as preschoolers whereas others begin in late elementary grades. Once students transition from the Bridge School, their new educational team is supported by Bridge School staff as needed. And because the Bridge School remains in regular contact with most former students and families, its research team is able to measure the long-term outcomes of students who have received intensive AAC intervention.

To guide her research efforts, Dr. Hunt-Berg draws on over 20 years of AAC experience working in various public schools and in private practice. As a clinician it was often necessary for her to look for clinical guidance to the research of related fields, such as child language development, early intervention, gesture and sign language development, and linguistics. However, individuals who use AAC raise important theoretical questions for researchers in related fields. For example, when a child cannot use natural speech to communicate, do familiar developmental milestones occur in predictable ways? Any theory of language development must account for the wide variety of developmental paths taken by individuals with complex communication needs who use AAC. Hopefully, careful documentation of the developing communication abilities of students at the Bridge School, as well as the interventions they received, will inform these kinds of discussions.

BOX 15-5 Spotlight on Practice

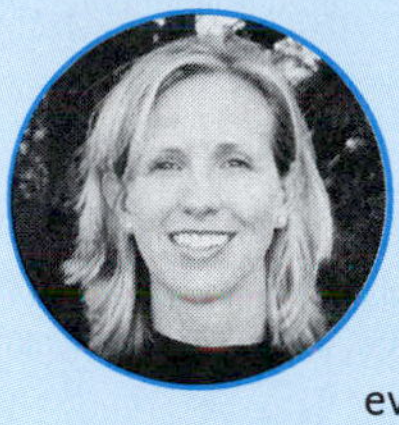

Naomi Murphy, M.S., CCC-SLP
Speech-Language Pathologist
Private Practice, San Francisco

The challenges and learning opportunities that drew me to the field of speech-language pathology are most evident in my work with children who use augmentative and alternative communication (AAC). AAC is a changing and advancing field. New technologies are constantly being developed, and research is uncovering better, more effective ways to serve people who use AAC. Keeping up with that research and mastering the ever-changing technology are sometimes challenging, but the opportunity to help a child communicate more effectively makes the work very rewarding.

Because people who use AAC often work with a large team, I end up working with occupational therapists, physical therapists, special education teachers, general education teachers, assistive technology specialists, adaptive physical education teachers, and specialists for the visually impaired. Collaboration with these professionals not only provides a more rounded view of the student but also allows me to learn about other fields. In addition, it provides an opportunity to troubleshoot questions and obstacles that I encounter in working with a student.

The skills and experiences that have served me best include my AAC coursework in graduate school, a good foundation in early language development, a willingness to learn about new technologies and research, and an ability to collaborate and work as a team member. I have also been extremely fortunate to have a knowledgeable and accessible mentor who has helped me gain confidence in this field. Access to someone with experience in the field of AAC is invaluable. If you are interested in working with people who use AAC, I would suggest that you seek out programs that offer coursework in AAC and professionals who work with people who use AAC. And I would stress the importance of understanding early language development because it is the basis of many AAC interventions.

There are many rewards in working with people who use AAC. For me the greatest reward is helping a child communicate in a new way or with a new person. Watching children react when they are able to tell a joke or seeing their pride when they are able to communicate with someone new is an exciting experience.

When Medicare is not available, AAC users have sought financial coverage through private agencies and third-party insurance payers and, for school-age children, through the public school system. As part of the 1997 authorization of the Individuals with Disabilities Education Act (IDEA), an AAC can be identified in a student's individualized education program (IEP), thus requiring the school to provide the AAC. However, the school can insist that the student leave the AAC at school or share it with other students. A number of consumer guides are available to lead individuals through the funding process for AAC systems.

How Are Complex Communication Needs Treated?

The long-term goal of treatment for people with complex communication needs is to maximize effective and successful communication between individuals who use AAC and their communication partners (ASHA, 2002a). For anyone with complex communication needs, access to AAC treatment is a right, not a privilege; and for children in U.S. public schools, intervention for significant communication difficulties is legislated through the Individuals with Disabilities Education Act.

__Discussion Point:__ Researcher David Wilkins (2003) of the Max Planck Institute for Psycholinguistics has said, "There are no impaired communicators, only impaired conversations." To what extent do you agree or disagree with this statement and why?

An AAC intervention is conducted in real-world and authentic contexts and is "organized to match the individual's needs and capabilities for today while building future capabilities for tomorrow" (Beukelman & Mirenda, 1998, p. 147). The AAC team plans a treatment program that will achieve three purposes: (1) meet unmet communication needs, (2) increase communication competence, and (3) increase participation in society.

Meeting Unmet Communication Needs

Once the team identifies unmet communication needs, short-term treatment goals are developed to enable the individual to meet these needs. For example, an unmet communication need for a student in an elementary school might be greeting friends within the classroom, and a treatment goal might be to use his AAC to greet friends. Specific activities are then designed to help the AAC user achieve the treatment goal—perhaps selecting vocabulary and identifying specific messages to convey, selecting symbols to represent vocabulary and messages, encoding messages, and developing approaches to increase the rate of communication delivery (ASHA, 2002a).

Discussion Point: *Consider the case of Jan in Box 15-1. What are some of her unmet communication needs, and what are some specific approaches to meeting those through AAC?*

In developing a treatment plan, the team must address each unmet communication need and determine which aspect of an AAC system will meet that need. And as treatment progresses through specific activities, the AAC team must carefully monitor the effectiveness of treatment in meeting the unmet needs. The team must also identify a method of modifying the AAC system as communication abilities and needs change and as new technologies arise (ASHA, 2002a).

Improving Communication Competence

The process of working toward **communication competence** requires significant time and effort (Light, 2003). Many factors impact the attainment of communication competence—factors that are both intrinsic and extrinsic to an AAC user (Light, 2003). The intrinsic factors include the person's knowledge, judgment, skills, motivation to improve, attitude toward AAC, confidence, and resilience (Light, 2003). Extrinsic factors include the communication demands of interactions and the environment. Factors in the environment can support or hinder communicative competence.

In helping a person gain communication competence, the AAC team considers the level of support needed or the level of independence the person has when communicating. The level of support ranges along a continuum (Blackston & Hunt Berg, 2003; Dowden, 1999) from emerging communication to context-dependent communication to independent communication. These three descriptors describe what an individual is able to do communicatively at a given point in time but should never be used to define an individual's potential for communication (Dowden, 1999).

Emerging Communication. Individuals at the point of **emerging communication** have no reliable method of symbolic expression and are limited to nonsymbolic methods of communicating, such as facial expressions, physical movements, or vocalizations (Blackstone & Hunt Berg, 2003). The term *emerging communication* is often used to describe the presymbolic behaviors of infants, which others interpret as communicative, such as vocalizations and babbles, vegetative sounds like burps and coughs, and gross gestures. The term is also appropriate for the nonsymbolic behaviors of individuals with complex communication needs. AAC intervention often focuses on three goals (Blackstone & Hunt Berg, 2003):

1. *Establishing reliable symbolic expression.* This goal focuses on using a physical, verbal, or vocal communicative behavior consistently to represent an action, person, or object, such as pointing to a cup or a picture of a cup consistently to identify thirst.
2. *Increasing opportunities for communication with many different partners.* This goal focuses on increasing the number of communicative partners with whom an

individual interacts—for example, initiating a greeting to students in a classroom when previously the child greeted only the teacher.

3. *Moving communication beyond the immediate context.* This goal focuses on using communication to consider events and actions removed from the here and now, both past and future and beyond the immediate physical space. The child might describe a meal from the day before, an activity planned for the next day, or a person who is out of the room.

Context-Dependent Communication. Individuals at the point of **context-dependent communication** have reliable symbolic communication but communicate in only a few contexts or with only a few partners. Thus, communication seems to be stuck to, or dependent on, a specific context. Such communication limits are usually due to strategies that require partner familiarity or a vocabulary that is limited to a highly specific context (Blackstone & Hunt Berg, 2003). AAC intervention focuses on "increasing access to vocabulary, increasing the use of AAC strategies, decreasing dependence on others, and most importantly, developing language and literacy skills to maximize communication independence" (Blackstone & Hunt Berg, 2003, p. 16).

Independent Communication. Individuals at the point of **independent communication** are usually literate and interact with both familiar and unfamiliar communication partners in a variety of communication environments. Because independent communicators can usually program their own AAC systems, intervention focuses on improving their competence with the operational features of the AAC systems, increasing the number of communication options available (e.g., using e-mail or the telephone), increasing the rate of communication, and improving competence in social situations with unfamiliar communication partners (Blackstone & Hunt Berg, 2003).

Discussion Point: *What level of communication would be the focus of intervention for Steve in Box 15-1? How about for Jan or Sara?*

Communication Partners. The definition of *communication* emphasizes the importance of there being both a sender and a receiver—in other words, a communicative partnership. For AAC treatment to be successful, one or more communication partners must be involved with the AAC user. Thus, an important part of treatment is helping communication partners develop positive and efficacious perspectives toward the use of AAC. A good conversation partner shows patience and an interest in and comfort with different methods of communication. The partner must also make an effort to understand impaired speech, interpret signs and gestures, be comfortable with silence, and admit any lack of understanding (Blackstone, 1999). Communication partners can benefit from explicit training to help them facilitate and support the use of AAC.

Increasing Participation in Society

Effective and successful communication is more than meeting communication needs and being competent. Communication is truly successful when an individual with complex communication needs can participate in any desired aspect of society. Any barrier to effective communication needs to be addressed in treatment to allow complete participation in all social and communication roles.

The AAC team specifically considers the social roles of the person with complex communication needs, seeking to increase the person's participation in society. **Social roles** are the roles each person has in society—the different hats people wear. Some roles may change over a lifetime; others remain constant. A current social role for you may be that of student, but this role will likely change in the future. Importantly, social roles determine communication demands (Light, 2003); each social role has corresponding

FIGURE 15-10 Examples of social roles and communication roles.

Social roles:	Communication roles:
daughter/son	listener
mother/father	director
student	advisor
employee/employer	reader
friend	storyteller
consumer	questioner

communication roles that must be met. A student's communication roles include such things as communicating with teachers and classmates orally, corresponding in writing with teachers and classmates using e-mail, preparing written papers and tests, and so forth.

Given a variety of social roles, the number of communication roles may be considerable. Consider a 14-year-old who is a student, a son, a brother, a friend, and a scorekeeper for his soccer team. Each of these social roles has expected communication roles: The student needs to be a listener, responder, reader, and writer. At home the brother needs to be an advisor to his younger siblings, and the son needs to be a listener and a negotiator with his parents. Figure 15-10 shows other examples of social roles and communication roles.

Discussion Point: *Identify the social and communication roles of Jan in Box 15-1. What changes might occur if she develops a more effective way of communicating and can participate in more environments?*

The individual with complex communication needs and other members of the AAC team must identify current and desired social and communication roles. Treatment should then focus explicitly on the skills necessary to meet the communication demands of each role so that the person can participate fully in society.

Case Study and Clinical Problem Solving

DIAGNOSTIC REPORT: Hocking Valley Community Hospital AAC Team Report

Client: Scott Smith
Evaluation Date: 10-3-05
Date of Report: 10-6-05
Date of Birth: 09-01-60
Age: 45 years

Background

Scott Smith, a 45-year-old male, was referred for an AAC assessment by his vocational rehabilitation counselor, Jim Ho. Mr. Smith is seeking employment skills training with the goal of obtaining gainful employment. Mr. Ho has concerns about Mr. Smith's communication skills and how they may affect his employment options. Mr. Ho and Anna Smith, Scott's mother, accompanied him to the assessment session.

According to Mr. Smith and his mother, Mr. Smith has spastic cerebral palsy. Mr. Smith has lived with his parents until recently, when he moved to the Hocking Valley Center for Independent Living. He currently has three caregivers who help him with his personal care, cooking, and cleaning. Unfortunately, there is a high turnover rate for caregivers, and Mr. Smith is constantly training new people. There are 10 other people who have apartments in the center. Mr. Smith communicates with most of the other residents on a daily basis. He also has a sister who lives in the same town.

Mr. Smith participated in special education services in his local school district from kindergarten through high school. He also received physical, occupational, and speech-language therapy off and on throughout his school career. Mr. Smith and his mother report that he has difficulty with reading and currently signs his name with an *X*, but fully understands what others say. However, many people do not understand Mr. Smith when he talks. Mr. Smith also reports using gestures, facial expressions, and a photo communication book when he communicates with unfamiliar communication partners. His communication book contains 10 photos of places he often frequents; an introduction card with his name, address, and description of why it is difficult for him to speak; and two pages of photos of family members.

Assessment Findings

Speech

Mr. Smith's speech is characterized by imprecise consonant production. His speech rate is slow. Speech intelligibility was assessed using the Sentence Intelligibility Test (Yorkston, Beukelman, & Tice, 1996). Mr. Smith is 25% intelligible when producing sentences. He is intelligible to an unfamiliar listener in a face-to-face interaction approximately 50% of the time. Mr. Smith's mother reports that familiar listeners understand Mr. Smith's speech approximately 75% of the time in face-to-face interactions but only 25% of the time over the telephone. Mr. Smith has a moderate spastic dysarthria.

Vision

With glasses Mr. Smith's vision is corrected to 20/20. He accurately identified half-inch symbols with 100% accuracy.

Physical

Mr. Smith has spastic quadriplegia. He currently uses a battery-powered wheelchair for mobility. He uses his right index finger to point to photos in his communication book and to access keys on a keyboard with 100% accuracy.

Language and Cognition

Mr. Smith answered complex yes/no questions with 100% accuracy and followed 3–4-step spoken directions with 100% accuracy. He identified picture symbols from an array of 60 with 100% accuracy. Reading is not functional for Mr. Smith at this time. He can write an *X* for his signature but does not spell any words. Language and cognitive skills are functional for use of an AAC system.

Communication Needs

Mr. Smith currently communicates one-to-one and in small-group situations. He communicates at home, at the job-training facility, and in the community. Mr. Smith has many communication partners, including his family, caregivers, residents at the Center for Independent Living, colleagues at the job-training facility, and people in the community. Mr. Smith needs to communicate basic care messages to his caregivers; communicate with potential employers, other employees, and unfamiliar communication partners; express opinions; and choose activities. He currently communicates with facial expressions, gestures, speech, and a photo communication book. Mr. Smith expressed difficulty communicating new information to unfamiliar communication partners and using the telephone to make appointments and talk to friends. He is concerned that people might not understand him in a new work environment. Mr. Smith is dependent on his family and caregivers to convey new information to unfamiliar communication partners and to make all his phone calls.

AAC System

Mr. Smith tried several AAC systems during the evaluation session. He learned operational features and recalled stored vocabulary represented with line-drawing symbols after minimal instruction. He learned to navigate between screens using a dynamic display with minimal cues. Each screen had 30 half-inch line-drawing symbols. Using his right index finger, Mr. Smith accurately selected target symbols and activated communication messages independently. A synthetic speech synthesizer produced each communication message that Mr. Smith selected. Mr. Smith, his mother, and his vocational counselor reported understanding the messages produced by the speech synthesizer. Mr. Smith practiced using the AAC system to make a phone call, to ask for more work at a potential job, and to ask his friends what they thought about the current national election.

Based on the AAC system assessment, Mr. Smith demonstrates the potential to use an AAC system with a dynamic display, 30 half-inch line-drawing symbols per screen, a synthetic speech synthesizer, and preprogrammed vocabulary. He will require a wheelchair mount to attach the AAC system to his wheelchair to allow him access to the system at all times.

Recommendations

1. Purchase of an AAC system that uses an electronic voice output communication aid with the following features:
   - Half-inch line-drawing graphic symbols
   - Dynamic display
   - Direct selection
   - Synthesized speech output
2. Wheelchair mount for the system

3. Training for Mr. Smith and his communication partners in implementing the AAC system; team working to meet his communication needs, increase communication competence, and ensure his participation in his desired communication and social roles.

CLINICAL PROBLEM SOLVING

1. How might the recommendations be different if Mr. Smith's literacy skills had been better developed?
2. Who are Mr. Smith's main communication partners? Why is it important to know who his partners are?
3. In what new activities or environments do you think Mr. Smith might participate with the recommended AAC system?

CHAPTER SUMMARY

Millions of Americans have complex communication needs; that is, they have difficulty meeting their daily communication needs with their current methods of communicating. Children and adults with speech, language, sensory, and/or cognitive impairments are at risk of having complex communication needs. The most common causes of these speech, language, sensory, and/or cognitive impairments include intellectual disability, cerebral palsy, autism, childhood apraxia of speech, traumatic brain injury, stroke, and degenerative diseases.

The clinical approach of AAC addresses the complex communication needs of individuals. The goal is to maximize functional and effective communication via multiple modalities. An AAC system may help some people gain communicative competence. An AAC system includes a symbol, an aid, a strategy, and a technique. An AAC team evaluates the individual to determine what specific components will best meet identified needs. An AAC approach to treatment focuses on meeting individual communication needs, improving communication competence, and increasing participation in social and communication roles.

KEY TERMS

AAC system, p. 507
access barriers, p. 519
aid, p. 510
aided, p. 510
amyotrophic lateral sclerosis, p. 517
augmentative and alternative communication, p. 501
autism, p. 516
cerebral palsy, p. 515
childhood apraxia of speech, p. 516
coded access, p. 515
communication competence, p. 524
communication environments, p. 520
communication partners, p. 503
communication roles, p. 526
complex communication needs, p. 501
comprehensive AAC assessment, p. 518
context-dependent communication, p. 525
direct selection, p. 513
dynamic, p. 509
dynamic display, p. 513
electronic, p. 510
emerging communication, p. 524
fixed display, p. 513
iconicity, p. 509
independent communication, p. 525
indirect selection, p. 514
information transfer, p. 504
intellectual disability, p. 515
multidisciplinary team, p. 517
multimodal, p. 506
needs/wants, p. 504
opaque, p. 509
opportunity barriers, p. 519
Parkinson's disease, p. 517

primary progressive aphasia, p. 517
scanning, p. 514
social closeness, p. 505
social etiquette, p. 505
social roles, p. 525
static, p. 509
strategy, p. 513
stroke, p. 517
symbol, p. 505
technique, p. 513
traumatic brain injury, p. 516
unaided, p. 510

ON THE WEB

Check out the Companion Website! On it you will find

- suggested readings
- reflection questions
- self-study quiz
- links to online resources

References

AAC Rehabilitation Engineering Research Center. (2005). *Medicare funding of AAC technology*. Retrieved January 10, 2005, from http://www.aac-rerc.com

Abbs, J. H., Gracco, V. L., & Cole, K. J. (1984). Control of multimovement coordination: Sensorimotor mechanisms in speech motor programming. *Journal of Motor Behavior, 16*(2), 195–231.

Abitol, J. (1995). *Atlas of laser voice surgery.* San Diego, CA: Singular.

Abrams, A., Hnath-Chisolm, T., Guerrerio, S., & Ritterman, S. (1992). The effects of intervention strategy on self perception of hearing handicap. *Ear and Hearing, 13,* 371–377.

Adams, P., & Benson, V. (1991). Current estimates from the National Health Interview Survey, National Center for Health Statistics. *Vital Health Statistics 1991, 10,* 184.

Adams, S. G. (1997). Hypokinetic dysarthria in Parkinson's disease. In M. R. McNeil (Ed.), *Clinical management of sensorimotor speech disorders* (pp. 261–285). New York: Thieme.

Adamson, L. B., & Chance, S. E. (1998). Coordinating attention to people, objects, and language. In A. M. Wetherby, S. F. Warren, & J. Reichle (Eds.), *Transitions in prelinguistic communication.* Baltimore: Paul H. Brookes.

Addy, D. A., Golinkoff, R. M., Sootsman, J. L., Pence, K., Pulverman, R. G., Salkind, S., & Hirsh-Pasek, K. (2003, June). *Understanding /ing/: Sensitivity to grammatical morphemes precedes their production.* Paper presented at the Jean Piaget Society. Chicago.

Allen, T. E. (1986). Patterns of academic achievement among hearing impaired students: 1974 and 1983. In A. N. Schildroth & M. A. Karchmer (Eds.), *Deaf children in America* (pp. 161–202). San Diego, CA: College-Hill Press.

Ambrose, N. G., Cox, N., & Yairi, E. (1997). The genetic basis of persistence and recovery in stuttering. *Journal of Speech, Language, and Hearing Research, 40,* 567–580.

Ambrose, N. G., & Yairi, E. (1999). Normative disfluency data for early childhood stuttering. *Journal of Speech, Language, and Hearing Research, 42,* 895–909.

Ambrose, N. G., Yairi, E., & Cox, N. (1993). Genetic aspects of early childhood stuttering. *Journal of Speech and Hearing Research, 36,* 701–706.

American Academy of Otolaryngology—Head and Neck Surgery. (2004). *Meniere's disease.* Retrieved February 11, 2004, from http://www.entnet.org/healthinfo/balance/meniere.cfm

American Association on Mental Retardation. (2002). *Mental retardation: Definition, classification, and systems of supports* (10th ed.). Washington, DC: Author.

American Association on Mental Retardation. (2002). *The AAMR definition of mental retardation.* Retrieved September 22, 2003 from http://www.aamr. org/Policies/faq_mental_retardation.shtml

American Diabetes Association. (1996). *National diabetes fact sheet.* Washington, DC: Author.

American Psychiatric Association. (1994). *Diagnostic and statistical manual of mental disorders* (4th ed.). Washington, DC: Author.

American Speech-Language-Hearing Association. (1981). On the definition of hearing handicap. *ASHA, 23,* 293–297.

American Speech-Language-Hearing Association. (1987). Developed by the National Association for Hearing and Speech Action under agreement with the American Speech-Language-Hearing Association as part of Contract No. 300-85-0139, U.S. Department of Education, *Augmentative Communication for Consumers,* 3.

American Speech-Language-Hearing Association. (1991). Report: Augmentative and alternative communication. *ASHA, 33* (Suppl. 5), 9–12.

American Speech-Language-Hearing Association. (1993). Definitions of communication disorders and variations. *ASHA, 35* (Suppl. 10), 40–41.

American Speech-Language Hearing Association. (1996). Central auditory processing: Current status of research and implications for clinical practice. *American Journal of Audiology, 5*(2), 41–54.

American Speech-Language Hearing Association. (1997). *Preferred practice patterns for the profession of audiology* (pp. 43–46). Rockville, MD: Author.

American Speech-Language-Hearing Association. (1998). *National outcomes measurement system.* Rockville, MD: Author.

American Speech-Language-Hearing Association. (2000a). Asking your audiologist about preventing and identifying hearing loss through audiologic screening and audiology services, *Audiology Information Series, 1,* 1–4.

American Speech-Language-Hearing Association. (2000b). Clinical indicators for instrumental assessment of dysphagia (guidelines). *ASHA Desk Reference, 3,* 225–233.

American Speech-Language-Hearing Association. (2001). *Scope of practice in speech-language pathology*. Rockville, MD: Author.

American Speech-Language-Hearing Association. (2002a). Augmentative and alternative communication knowledge and skills for service delivery. *ASHA Supplement, 22,* 97–106.

American Speech-Language-Hearing Association. (2002b). Background information and criteria for the registration of speech-language pathology assistants. In *ASHA 2002 Desk Reference* (vol. 1, pp. 289–291).

American Speech-Language-Hearing Association. (2002c, April 16). Roles of speech-language pathologists in swallowing and feeding disorders: Position statement. *ASHA Leader,* 7 (Suppl. 22), 73.

American Speech-Language-Hearing Association. (2002d, October 8). SLPs in health care settings: Survey results. *ASHA Leader, 7,* 8.

American Speech-Language-Hearing Association. (2002e). 2002 *Omnibus survey salary report: Annual salaries.* Rockville, MD: Author.

American Speech-Language-Hearing Association. (2003a). *Aphasia.* Retrieved from http://www.asha.org/speech/disabilities/Aphasia.info.cfm

American Speech-Language-Hearing Association. (2003b). *Communication facts: Incidence and prevalence of communication disorders and hearing loss in children— 2002 edition.* Retrieved from http://professional.asha.org/resources/factsheets/children.cfm

American Speech-Language-Hearing Association. (2003c). *Compendium of exemplary practices by colleges and universities in the recruitment, retention and career transition of communication sciences and disorders (CSD) professionals.* Retrieved December 10, 2003, from http://asha.org/about/leadership-projects/multicultural/diversity-fi/compendium.htm

American Speech-Language-Hearing Association. (2003d). *How does your child hear and talk?* [Brochure]. Retrieved October 1, 2004, from http://www.asha.org/public/speech/development

American Speech-Language-Hearing Association. (2003e). *Indicators of the need for speech-language pathologists; audiologists; and speech, language, and hearing scientists.* Retrieved from http://professional.asha.org/careers/employment_indicators.cfm

American Speech-Language-Hearing Association. (2003f). *Minority student recruitment, retention, and career transition practices: A review of the literature.* Retrieved December 10, 2003, from http:llasha.org/about/leadership-projects/multicultural/diversity-fi/litreview.htm

American Speech-Language-Hearing Association. (2004a). *Hearing aids for adults.* Retrieved February 11, 2004, from http//www.asha.org/public/hearing/treatment/adult_aid.htm

American Speech-Language-Hearing Association. (2004b). Knowledge and skills needed by speech-language pathologists performing videofluoroscopic swallowing studies. *ASHA Suppl. 24.*

American Speech-Language-Hearing Association. (2004c). *Scope of practice in audiology.* Rockville, MD: Author.

American Speech-Language-Hearing Association. (2004d). Speech-language pathologists training and supervising other professionals in the delivery of services to individuals with swallowing and feeding disorders: Technical report. *ASHA Suppl. 24.*

American Speech-Language-Hearing Association. (2005a). *Causes of hearing loss in children.* Retrieved January 5, 2005, from http://www.asha.org/public/hearing/disorders/causes.htm

American Speech-Language-Hearing Association. (2005b). Roles and responsibilities of speech-language pathologists in the neonatal intensive care unit [Guidelines]. Retrieved from http://www.asha.org

Anderson, K. (1989). *Screening instrument for targeting educational risk (SIFTER).* Austin, TX: Pro-Ed.

Anderson, K. (2001). *Early listening function: Discovery tool for parents and caregivers of infants and toddlers.* Retrieved October 1, 2003, from http://www.phonak.com/index.cfm?article_id=7281

Anderson, K., & Matkin, N. (1996). *Screening instrument for targeting educational risk in preschool children (age 3–kindergarten) (Preschool SIFTER).* Tampa, FL: Educational Audiology Association.

Anderson, K., & Smaldino, J. (1998). *Listening inventory for education: An efficacy tool.* Tampa, FL: Educational Audiology Association.

Anderson, K., & Smaldino, J. (2001). Children's home inventory for listening difficulties (CHILD). Retrieved October 1, 2003, from http://www.phonak.com/index.cfm?article_id=7281

Anderson, T. K., & Felsenfeld, S. (2003). A thematic analysis of late recovery from stuttering. *American Journal of Speech-Language Pathology, 12,* 243–253.

Andrews, G., Morris-Yates, A., Howie, P., & Martin, N. (1991). Genetic factors in stuttering confirmed. *Archives of General Psychiatry, 48,* 1034–1035.

Andrews, M. L., & Summers, A. C. (2002). *Voice treatment for children and adolescents* (2nd ed.). San Diego, CA: Singular.

Aram, D. M. (1988). Language sequalae of unilateral brain lesions in children. In F. Plum (Ed.), *Language, communication and the brain* (pp. 171–198). New York: Raven Press.

Aram, D. M., Morris, R., & Hall, N. E. (1993). Clinical and research congruence in identifying children with specific language impairment. *Journal of Speech and Hearing Research, 36,* 580–591.

Armero, O. (2001). Effects of denied hearing impairment on the significant other. *Hearing Journal, 54,* 44–47.

Arndt, J., & Healey, E. C. (2001). Concomitant disorders in school-age children who stutter. *Language, Speech, and Hearing Services in Schools, 32,* 68–78.

Aronson, A. E. (1990). *Clinical voice disorders: An interdisciplinary approach.* New York: Thieme.

Arvedson, J. C., & Rogers, B. T. (1993). Pediatric swallowing and feeding disorders. *Journal of Medical Speech-Language Pathology, 1, 203–221.*

Arvedson, J. C., & Rogers, B. T. (1997). Swallowing and feeding in the pediatric patient. In A. L. Perlman & K. S. Schulze-Delrieu (Eds.), *Deglutition and its disorders: Anatomy, physiology, clinical diagnosis, and management* (pp. 419–448). San Diego, CA: Singular.

Assistive Technology Funding & Systems Change Project (1999). *Medicaire, managed care, and AAC devices.* Washington, DC: United Cerebral Palsy Association.

August, D., & Hakuta, K. (Eds.). (1997). *Improving schooling for language-minority children.* Washington DC: National Academy Press.

Autism Society of America (2000). *Advocate, 33*(1), 3.

Avent, J. R. (1997). Group treatment in aphasia using cooperative learning methods. *Journal of Medical Speech-Language Pathology, 5*(1), 9–26.

Awan, S. H. (2001). *The voice of diagnostic protocol: A practical guide to the diagnosis of voice disorders.* Gaithersburg, MD: Aspen.

Awan, S. N., & Mueller, P. B. (1996). Speaking fundamental frequency characteristics of white, African American, and Hispanic kindergarteners. *Journal of Speech and Hearing Research, 39,* 573–577.

Babbitt, R. L., Hoch, T. A., & Coe, D. A. (1994). Behavioral feeding disorders. In D. N. Tuchman & R. S. Walter (Eds.), *Disorders of feeding and swallowing in infants and children* (pp. 77–95). San Diego, CA: Singular.

Backenroth, G. A., & Ahlner, B. H. (2000). Quality of life of hearing-impaired persons who have participated in audiological rehabilitation counselling. *International Journal for the Advancement of Counselling, 22,* 225–240.

Balandin, S. (2002). Message from the president. *The ISAAC Bulletin, 67(2),* 2.

Ballard, K. J. (2001). Response generalization in apraxia of speech treatments: Taking another look. *Journal of Communication Disorders, 34,* 3–20.

Ballard, K. J., Granier, J. P., & Robin, D. A. (2000). Understanding the nature of apraxia of speech: theory, analysis, and treatment. *Aphasiology, 14*(10), 969–995.

Ballard, K. J., & Thompson, C. K. (1999). Treatment and generalization of complex sentence production in agrammatism. *Journal of Speech Language and Hearing Research, 42,* 690–707.

Bankson, N., & Bernthal, J. (1990). *Quick Screen of Phonology.* Chicago: Riverside Press.

Barlow, S. M. (1999). *Handbook of clinical speech physiology.* San Diego, CA: Singular.

Bashir, A. S., Conte, B. M., & Heerde, S. M. (1998). Language and school success: Collaborative challenges and choices. In D. D. Merritt & B. Culatta (Eds.), *Language intervention in the classroom* (pp. 1–36). San Diego, CA: Singular.

Bashir, A. S., & Scavuzzo, A. (1992). Children with language disorders: Natural history and academic success. *Journal of Learning Disabilities, 25,* 53–65.

Basso, A., Marangolo, P., Piras, F., & Galluzzi, C. (2001). Acquisition of new "words" in normal subjects: A suggestion for the treatment of anomia. *Brain and Language, 77,* 45–59.

Bates, E., Camaioni, L., & Volterra, V. (1975). The acquisition of performatives prior to speech. *Merrill-Palmer Quarterly, 21,* 205–226.

Battle, D. (2002). Communication disorders in a multicultural society. In D. E. Battle (Ed.), *Communication disorders in multicultural populations* (pp. 3–32). Woburn, MA: Butterworth-Heinemann.

Bauman-Waengler, J. (2004). *Articulatory and phonological impairments: A clinical focus* (2nd ed.). Boston: Allyn & Bacon.

Bavelier, D., & Neville, H. J. (2002). Cross-modal plasticity: Where and how? *Nature reviews: Neuroscience, 3,* 443–452.

Bayles, K. A., & Kim, E. S. (2003). Improving functioning of individuals with Alzheimer's disease: Emergence of behavioral interventions. *Journal of Communication Disorders, 36*(5), 327–343.

Bayles, K. A., & Tomoeda, C. K. (1993). *Arizona battery for communication disorders of dementia.* Tucson, AZ: Canyonlands Publishing.

Bayles, K. A., & Tomoeda, C. K. (1995). *The ABCs of dementia* (2nd ed.). Tucson, AZ: Canyonlands Publishing.

Bays, C. L. (2001). Quality of life of stroke survivors: A research synthesis. *Journal of Neuroscience Nursing, 33,* 310–322.

Beitchman, J., Hood, J., Rochon, J., Peterson, M., Mantini, T., & Majumdar, S. (1989). Empirical classification of speech/language impairment in children: I. Identification of speech/language categories. *Journal of the American Academy of Child and Adolescent Psychiatry, 28,* 112–117.

Bellis, T. (1996). *Assessment and management of central auditory processing disorders in the educational setting: From science to practice.* San Diego, CA: Singular.

Benjamin, B., & Croxson, G. (1987). Vocal nodules in children. *Annals of Otology, Rhinology, and Laryngology, 96,* 530–533.

Bennett, T., Zhang, C., & Hojnar, L. (1998). Facilitating the full participation of culturally diverse families in the IFSP/IEP process. *Infant-Toddler Intervention, 8,* 227–249.

Bereiter, C. & Engelmann, S. (1966). *Teaching disadvantaged children in the preschool.* Upper Saddle River, NJ: Prentice Hall.

Berg, F. (2001). Educational management of children who are hearing impaired. In R. H. Hull (Ed.), *Aural rehabilitation: Serving children and adults* (pp. 169–185). San Diego, CA: Singular.

Bergbom-Engberg, E., & Haljamae, H. (1989). Assessment of patients' experience of discomforts during respirator therapy. *Critical Care Medicine, 17,* 1068–1071.

Berhane, R., & Dietz, W. G. (1999). Clinical assessment of growth. In D. B. Kessler & P. Dawson (Eds.), *Failure to thrive and pediatric undernutrition: A transdisciplinary approach* (pp. 195–214). Baltimore: Paul H. Brookes.

Bernstein Ratner, N. (1997). Stuttering: A psycholinguistic perspective. In R. Curlee & G. Siegel (Eds.), *Nature and treatment of stuttering: New directions* (2nd ed., pp. 97–127). Boston: Allyn & Bacon.

Bernthal, J. E., & Bankson, N. W. (2004). *Articulation and phonological disorders* (5th ed.). Boston: Allyn & Bacon.

Bess, F. H., Dodd-Murphy, J., & Parker, R. A. (1998). Children with minimal sensorineural hearing loss: Prevalence, educational performance, and functional status. *Ear and Hearing, 19,* 339–354.

Best, W., Herbert, R., Hickin, J., Osborne, F., & Howard, D. (2002). Phonological and orthographic facilitation of word-retrieval in aphasia: Immediate and delayed effects. *Aphasiology, 16,* 151–168.

Best practice: Evidence-based practice information sheets for health professionals. (2000). *Identification and nursing management of dysphagia in adults with neurological impairment, 4*(2), 1–6.

Beukelman, D. R., & Ansel, B. M. (1995). Research priorities in augmentative and alternative communication. *Augmentative and Alternative Communication, 11,* 131–134.

Beukelman, D. R., & Mirenda, P. (1998). Augmentative and alternative communication: Management of severe communication disorders in children and adults. Baltimore: Paul H. Brookes.

Beukelman, D. R., & Yorkston, K. M. (1991). Traumatic brain injury changes the way we live. In D. R. Beukelman & K. M. Yorkston (Eds.), *Communication disorders following traumatic brain injury: Management of cognitive, language, and motor impairments* (pp. 1–14). Austin, TX: Pro-Ed.

Bhatnagar, S. C., & Andy, O. J. (1995). *Neuroscience for the study of communicative disorders.* Baltimore: Williams & Wilkins.

Bickerton, D. (1995). *Language and human behavior.* Seattle: University of Washington Press.

Bird, M. R., Woodward, M. C., Gibson, E. M., Phyland, D., & Fonda, D. (1994). Asymptomatic swallowing disorders in elderly patients with Parkinson's disease: A description of findings on clinical examination and videofluoroscopy in sixteen patients. *Age and Ageing, 23,* 251–254.

Bishop, D. V., & Edmundson, A. (1987). Language-impaired 4-year-olds: Distinguishing transient from persistent impairment. *Journal of Speech and Hearing Disorders, 52,* 156–173.

Bishop, J., Huether, C. A., Torfs, C., Lorey, F., & Deddens, J. (1997). Epidemiologic study of Down syndrome in a racially diverse California population, 1989–1991. *American Journal of Epidemiology, 145,* 134–147.

Black, M. M., Cureton, P. L., & Berenson-Howard, J. (1999). Behavior problems in feeding: Individual, family, and cultural influences. In D. B. Kessler & P. Dawson (Eds.), *Failure to thrive and pediatric undernutrition: A transdisciplinary approach* (pp. 151–172). Baltimore: Paul H. Brookes.

Blackstone, S. (1999). Communication partners. *Augmentative Communication News, 12* (1–2), 1–16.

Blackstone, S. W., & Hunt Berg, M. (2003). *Social networks: A communication inventory for individuals with complex communication needs and their communication partners.* Monterey, CA: Augmentative Communication, Inc.

Bleile, K. (2002). Evaluating articulation and phonological disorders when the clock is running. *American Journal of Speech-Language Pathology, 11,* 243–249.

Blissymbolics Communication International (2005). http://www.blissymbolics.org/blissinternet.shtml

Blitzer, A., & Brin, M. F. (1992). The dystonic larynx. *The Journal of Voice, 6,* 294–297.

Blonsky, E., Logemann, J., & Boshes, B. (1975). Comparison of speech and swallowing function in patients with tremor disorders and in normal geriatric patients: A cinefluorographic study. *Journal of Gerontology, 30,* 299–305.

Blood, G. W. (1994). Efficacy of a computer-assisted voice treatment protocol. *American Journal of Speech-Language Pathology, 3, 57–66.*

Blood, G. W. (1995). POWER: Relapse management with adolescents who stutter. *Language, Speech, and Hearing Services in Schools, 26,* 169–179.

Blood, G. W., Blood, I. M., Bennett, S., Simpson, K. C., & Susman, E. J. (1994). Subjective anxiety measurements and cortisol responses in adults who stutter. *Journal of Speech and Hearing Research, 37,* 760–768.

Blood, G. W., Thomas, E. A., Ridenour, J. S., Qualls, C. D., & Hammer, C. S. (2002). Job stress in speech-language pathologists working in rural, suburban, and rural schools: Social support and frequency of interactions. *Contemporary Issues in Communication Science and Disorders, 29,* 132–140.

Bloodstein, G. (1995). *A handbook on stuttering* (5th ed.). San Diego, CA: Singular.

Bloodstein, O. (1987). *A handbook on stuttering.* Chicago: National Easter Seal Society.

Bobrick, B. (1995). *Knotted tongues: Stuttering in history and the quest for a cure.* New York: Simon & Schuster.

Boersma, P., & Weenink, D. (2004). PRAAT. [Computer software]. University of Amsterdam: Authors.

Bollinger, R. L., Musson, N. D., & Holland, A. L. (1993). A study of group communication intervention with chronically aphasic persons. *Aphasiology, 7,* 301–313.

Bondy, A., & Frost, L. (1994). The picture exchange communication system. *Focus on Autistic Behavior, 9,* 1–19.

Borden, G. J., Harris, K. S., & Raphael, L. J. (1994). *Speech science primer: Physiology, acoustics, and perception of speech* (3rd ed.). Baltimore, MD: Williams & Wilkins.

Bortfeld, H., Rathbun, K., Morgan, J., & Golinkoff, R. (2003). What's in a name? Highly familiar items anchor infants' segmentation of fluent speech. In B. Beachley, A. Brown, & F. Conlin (Eds.), *BUCLD 27: Proceedings of the 27th annual Boston University Conference on Language Development.* Somerville, MA: Cascadilla Press.

Botting, N., Faragher, B., Simkin, Z., Knox, E., & Conti-Ramsden, G. (2001). Predicting pathways of specific language impairment: What predicts good and poor outcome? *Journal of Child Psychology and Psychiatry, 42,* 1013–1020.

Boudreau, D. M., & Hedberg, N. L. (1999). A comparison of early literacy skills in children with specific language impairment and their typically developing peers. *American Journal of Speech-Language Pathology, 8,* 249–260.

Bowerman, M., & Choi, S. (2003). Space under construction: Language-specific spatial categorization in first language acquisition. In D. Gentner & S. Goldin-Meadow (Eds.), *Language in mind: Advances in the study of language and thought* (pp. 387–428). Cambridge, MA: MIT Press.

Boyer, L., & Mainzer, R. W. (2003). Who's teaching students with disabilities? A profile of characteristics, licensure status, and feelings of preparedness. *Teaching Exceptional Children, 35*(6), 8–11.

Brackenbury, T., & Fey, M. E. (2003). Quick incidental learning in 4-year-olds: Identification and generalization. *Journal of Speech, Language, and Hearing Research, 46,* 313–327.

Brain Briefings. (1995, January). *Neuron migration and brain disorders.* Retrieved December 12, 2003, from http://web.sfn.org/content/Publications/BrainBriefings/

Brainard, M. S., & Doupe, A. J. (2000). Auditory feedback in learning and maintenance of vocal behavior. *Nature reviews: Neuroscience, 1,* 31–40.

Bray, M. A., Kehle, T. J., Lawless, K. A., & Theodore, L. A. (2003). The relationship of self-efficacy and depression to stuttering. *American Journal of Speech-Language Pathology, 12,* 425–431.

Bridges, J., & Bentler, R. (1998). Relating hearing aid use to well-being among older adults. *Hearing Journal, 51,* 39–44.

Brin, M. F., Fahn, S., Blitzer, A., Ramig, L. O., & Stewart, C. (1992). *Movement disorders of the larynx.* In A. Blitzer, M. F. Brin, C. T. Sasaki, S. Fahn, & K. S. Harris (Eds.), *Neurological disorders of the larynx.* New York: Thieme Medical.

Brodnitz, F. S. (1988). *Keep your voice healthy* (2nd ed.). Austin, TX: Pro-Ed.

Broen, P. A., & Moller, K. T. (1993). Early phonological development and the child with cleft palate. In K. T. Mollerr & C. D. Starr (Eds.), *Cleft palate: Interdisciplinary issues and treatment* (pp. 219–249). Austin, TX: Pro-Ed.

Brooke, M., Uomoto, J. M., McLean, A., & Fraser, R. T. (1991). Rehabilitation of persons with traumatic brain injury: A continuum of care. In D. R. Beukelman & K. M. Yorkston (Eds.), *Communication disorders following traumatic brain injury: Management of cognitive, language, and motor impairments* (pp. 15–46). Austin, TX: Pro-Ed.

Brookshire, R. H. (2003). *Introduction to neurogenic communication disorders* (6th ed.). St. Louis, MO: Mosby.

Browman, C. P., & Goldstein, L. (1990). Gestural specification using dynamically-defined articulatory structures. *Journal of Phonetics, 18,* 299–320.

Browman, C. P., & Goldstein, L. (1997). The gestural phonology model. In W. Hulstijn, H. F. M. Peters, & P. H. H. M. van Lieshout (Eds.), *Speech production: Motor control, brain research and fluency disorders* (chap. 4, pp. 57–71). Amsterdam: Elsevier.

Brown, R. (1973). *A first language: The early stages* (pp. 57–71). Cambridge, MA: Harvard University Press.

Bruns, J., Hauser, W. A. (2003). The epidemiology of traumatic brain injury: A review. *Epilepsia, 44*(10), 2–10.

Bryan, K. L. (1989). *The right hemisphere language battery.* Leicester, GB: Far Communications.

Buchholz, D. W., & Robbins, J. (1997). Neurological diseases affecting oropharyngeal swallowing. In A. L. Perlman & K. Schulze-Delrieu (Eds.), *Deglutition and its disorders* (pp. 319–342). San Diego, CA: Singular.

Budd, K. S., McGraw, T. E., Farbisc, R., Murphy, T. B., Hawkins, D., Heilman, N., Werle, M., & Hochstadt, N. J. (1992). Psychosocial concomitants of children's feeding disorders. *Journal of Pediatric Psychology, 17,* 81–94.

Burris, B., & Harris, E. (1998). Identification of race and sex from palate dimensions. *Journal of Forensic Science, 43,* 959–963.

Busch, C. (1994, October). How is a treatment plan for an aphasic person reviewed in terms of Medicare policy and guidelines? *Neurophysiology and neurogenic speech and language disorders special interest Division 2 newsletter* (pp. 14–17). Rockville, MD: American Speech-Language-Hearing Association.

Bushmann, M., Dobmeyer, S. M., Leeker, L., & Perlmutter, J. S. (1989). Swallowing abnormalities and their response to treatment in Parkinson's disease. *Neurology, 39,* 1309–1314.

Campbell, T. (2003). *Does training non-speech oral movements facilitate speech-sound production in children with motor speech disorders?* Retrieved March 10, 2004, from www.apraxia-kids.org/faqs/responsefromcampbellin.html.

Cann, C. I., Rothman, K. J., & Fried, M. P. (1996). The epidemiology of laryngeal cancer. In M. P. Fried (Ed.), *The larynx: A multidisciplinary approach* (pp. 425–436). St. Louis, MO: Mosby.

Cannito, M. P., Burch, A. R., Watts, C., Rappold, P. W., Hood, S. B., & Sherrard, K. (1997). Disfluency in spasmodic dysphonia: A multivariate analysis. *Journal of Speech, Language, and Hearing Research, 40,* 627–641.

Cannito, M. P., & Marquardt, T. P. (1997). Ataxic dysarthria. In M. R. McNeil (Ed.), *Clinical management of sensorimotor speech disorders* (pp. 217–247). New York: Thieme.

Cao, Y., Vikingstad, E. M., George, K. P., Johnson, A. F., & Welch, K. M. (1999). Cortical language activation in stroke patients recovering from aphasia with functional MRI. *Stroke, 30,* 2331–2340.

Carey, S., & Bartlett, E. (1978). Acquiring a single new word. *Papers and Reports on Child Language Development, 15,* 17–29.

Carlisle Ladtkow, M., & Culp, D. M. (1992). Augmentative communication with traumatic brain injury. In K. M. Yorkston (Ed.), *Augmentative communication in the medical setting.* Tucson, AZ: Communication Skill Builders.

Case, J. L. (1996). *Clinical management of voice disorders* (3rd ed.). Austin, TX: Pro-Ed.

Case, J. L. (2002). *Clinical management of voice disorders* (4th ed.). Austin, TX: Pro-Ed.

Catts, H. W., Fey, M. E., Tomblin, J. B., & Zhang, X. (2002). Longitudinal investigation of reading outcomes in children with language impairment. *Journal of Speech, Language, and Hearing Research, 45,* 1142–1157.

Catts, H. W., Fey, M. E., Zhang, X., & Tomblin, J. (2001). Estimating the risk of future reading difficulties in kindergarten children: A research-based model and its clinical implications. *Language, Speech, and Hearing Services in Schools, 32,* 38–50.

Center for Disease Control and Prevention, Early Hearing Detection and Intervention (EHDI). (2001). *Health communication and follow-through related to early identification of deafness and hearing loss in newborns.* Retrieved September 25, 2003, from http://www.cdc.gov.ncbddd/ehdi/ehdi.htm

Center for the Voice (2004). *Professions at risk for voice disorders.* Retrieved October 1, 2004, from http://www.nyee.edu/cfv-professions.html#about

Chall, J. S. (1996). *Stages of reading development.* Fort Worth, TX: Harcourt Brace.

Champlin, C. A. (2000). Hearing science. In R. B. Gillam, T. P. Marquardt, & F. N. Martin (Eds.), *Communication sciences and disorders: From science to clinical practice.* San Diego, CA: Singular.

Chaney, C. (1998). Preschool language and metalinguistic skills are links to reading success. *Applied Psycholinguistics, 19,* 433–466.

Chapman, K. L., Hardin-Jones, M., & Halter, K. A. (2003). The relationship between early speech and later speech and language performance for children with cleft lip and palate. *Clinical Linguistics and Phonetics, 17,* 173–197.

Chapman, R. S., Seung, H. K., Schwartz, S. E., & Kay-Raining Bird, E. (1998). Language skills of children and adolescents with Down syndrome: II. Production deficits. *Journal of Speech, Language, and Hearing Research, 41,* 861–873.

Chapman, S. B. (1997). Cognitive-communicative abilities in children with closed head injury. *American Journal of Speech-Language Pathology, 6,* 50–58.

Charlop-Christy, M. H., Carpenter, M., Le, L., LeBlanc, L. A., & Kellet, K. (2002). Using the Picture Exchange Communication System (PECS) with children with autism: Assessment of PECS acquisition, speech, social-communicative behavior, and problem behavior. *Journal of Applied Behavior Analysis, 35,* 213–231.

Chatoor, I., Getson, P., Menvielle, E., O'Donnell, R., Rivera, Y., Brasseaux, C., & Mrezck, D. (1997). A feeding scale for research and clinical practice to assess mother-infant interactions in the first three years of life. *Infant Mental Health Journal, 18,* 76–91.

Chermak, G. D., & Musiek, F. E. (1997). *Central auditory processing disorders: New perspectives.* San Diego, CA: Singular.

Cherney, L. R., & Halper, A. S. (1996). Swallowing problems in adults with traumatic brain injury. *Seminars in Neurology, 16,* 349–353.

Children's Defense Fund. (2000). *The state of America's children: Yearbook 2000.* Washington, DC: Author.

Choi, S., McDonough, L., Bowerman, M., & Mandler, J. M. (1999). Early sensitivity to language-specific spatial categories in English and Korean. *Cognitive Development, 14,* 241–268.

Chouinard, J. (2000). Dysphagia in Alzheimer's disease: A review. *The Journal of Nutrition Health and Aging, 4,* 214–217.

Christensen, C. A. (1997). Onset, rhymes, and phonemes in learning to read. *Scientific Studies of Reading, 1,* 341–358.

Churchill, J., Hodson, B., Jones, B., & Novak, R. (1988). Phonological systems of speech-disordered clients with positive/negative histories of otitis media. *Language, Speech, and Hearing Services in Schools, 19,* 100–106.

Clark, H. M., Robin, D. A., McCullagh, G., & Schmidt, R. A. (2001). Motor control in children and adults during a non-speech oral task. *Journal of Speech, Language, and Hearing Research, 44,* 1015–1025.

Clark, H. M., Stierwalt, J. A. G., & Robin, D. A. (2000). Motor speech disorders. In J. B. Tomblin, H. L. Morris, & D. C. Spriestersbach (Eds.), *Diagnosis in speech-language pathology* (pp. 337–352). San Diego, CA: Singular.

Cleave, P. L., & Fey, M. E. (1997). Two approaches to the facilitation of grammar in children with language impairments: Rationale and description. *American Journal of Speech-Language Pathology, 6,* 22–32.

Colangelo, L. A., Logemann, J. A., & Rademaker, A. W. (2000). Tumor size and pretreatment speech and swallowing in patients with resectable tumors. *Archives of Otolaryngology—Head and Neck Surgery, 122,* 653–661.

Conti-Ramsden, G., & Jones, M. (1997). Verb use in specific language impairment. *Journal of Speech, Language, and Hearing Research, 40,* 1298–1413.

Conture, E. G. (1990). *Stuttering* (2nd ed.). Upper Saddle River, NJ: Prentice Hall.

Cooper, W. E., & Klouda, G. V. (1987). Intonation in aphasic and right-hemisphere-damaged patients. In J. H. Ryalls (Ed.), *Phonetic approaches to speech production in aphasia and related disorders* (pp. 59–77). Boston, MA: Little, Brown.

Costa, D., & Kroll, R. (2000). Stuttering: An update for physicians. *Canadian Medical Association Journal, 1621,* 1849–1855.

Council for Exceptional Children. (2001). *CEC knowledge and skill base for all beginning special education teachers of students in individualized general curriculums.* Washington, DC: Author.

Craig, A., Hancock, K., Tran, Y., Craig, M., & Peters, K. (2002). Epidemiology of stuttering in the community across the entire life span. *Journal of Speech, Language, and Hearing Research, 45,* 1097–1105.

Creskoff, N., & Haas, A. (1999). Oral-motor skills and swallowing. In D. B. Kessler & P. Dawson (Eds.), *Failure to thrive and pediatric undernutrition: A transdisciplinary approach* (pp. 309–318). Baltimore: Paul H. Brookes.

Cruikshanks, K. J., Wiley, T. L., Tweed, T. S., Klein, B. E. K., Klein, R., Mares-Perlman, J. A., & Nondahl, D. M. (1998). Prevalence of hearing loss in older adults in Beaver Dam, Wisconsin: The epidemiology of hearing loss study. *American Journal of Epidemiology, 148,* 879–886.

Cunningham, K. F., & McLaughlin, M. (1999). Nutrition. In D. B. Kessler & P. Dawson (Eds.), *Failure to thrive and pediatric undernutrition: A transdisciplinary approach* (pp. 99–120). Baltimore: Paul H. Brookes.

Curenton, S., & Justice, L. M. (2004). Low-income preschoolers' use of decontextualized discourse: Literate language features in spoken narratives. *Language, Speech, and Hearing Services in Schools, 35,* 240–253.

Curlee, R. F., & Yairi, E. (1997). Early intervention with early childhood stuttering: A critical examination of the data. *American Journal of Speech-Language Pathology, 6*(2), 8–18.

Curtis, H., & Barnes, S. (1989). *Biology* (5th ed.). New York: Worth.

Curtis, M. E. (1987). Vocabulary testing and instruction. In M. G. McKeown & M. E. Curtis (Eds.), *The nature of vocabulary acquisition* (pp. 37–51). Hillsdale, NJ: Erlbaum.

Daly, D. A., Simon, C. A., & Burnett-Stolnack, M. (1995). Helping adolescents who stutter focus on fluency. *Language, Speech, and Hearing Services in Schools, 26,* 162–168.

Damasio, A. R. (1981). The nature of aphasia: Signs and syndromes. In M. T. Sarno (Ed.), *Acquired aphasia* (pp. 51–65). New York: Academic Press.

Damasio, A. R. (1995). *Descartes' error: Emotion, reason, and the human brain.* New York: Quill.

Damasio, H. (1981). Cerebral localization of the aphasias. In M. T. Sarno (Ed.), *Acquired aphasia* (p. 29). New York: Academic Press.

Damasio, H. (2001). Neural basis of language disorders. In R. Chapey (Ed.), *Language intervention strategies in aphasia and related neurogenic communication disorders* (pp. 18–36). Baltimore, MD: Lippincott Williams & Wilkins.

Damico, J. (1991). Clinical discourse analysis: A functional approach to language assessment. In C. S. Simon (Ed.), *Communication skills and classroom success* (pp. 125–150). Eau Claire, WI: Thinking Publications.

Daniell, W. E., Fulton-Kehoe, D., Smith-Wellerr, T., & Franklin, G. M. (1998). Occupational hearing loss in Washington state, 1984–1991. Morbidity and associated costs. *American Journal of Industrial Medicine, 33,* 529–536.

Darley, F. L., Aronson, A. E., & Brown, J. R. (1969). Clusters of deviant speech dimension in the dysarthrias. *Journal of Speech and Hearing Research, 12,* 462–496.

Darley, F. L., Aronson, A. E., & Brown, J. R. (1975). *Motor speech disorders.* Philadelphia: Saunders.

Davis, L. F. (1982). Respiration and phonation in cerebral palsy: A developmental model. *Seminars in Speech and Language, 8,* 101–106.

De Michele, A., & Ruth, R. (2003). Newborn hearing screening. *Emedicine.* Retrieved from http://www.emedicine.com/ent/topic576.htm#

Dedhiya, S., & Kong, S. X. (1995). Quality of life: An overview of the concept and measures. *Pharmacy World and Science, 17,* 141–148.

DeVault, K. R. (2002). Presbyesophagus: a reappraisal. *Current Gastroenterology Reports, 4, 193–199.*

Diamond, P. T., Gale, S. D., & Denkhaus, H. K. (2001). Head injuries in skiers: An analysis of injury severity and outcome. *Brain Injury, 15,* 429–434.

DiMeo, J. H., Merritt, D. D., & Culatta, B. (1998). Collaborative partnerships and decision making. In D. D. Merritt & B. Culatta (Eds.), *Language intervention in the classroom* (pp. 37–98). San Diego, CA: Singular.

Ding, R., & Logemann, J. A. (2000). Pneumonia in stroke patients: A retrospective study. *Dysphagia, 15,* 51–57.

Dodd, B., Gillon, G., Oerlemans, M., Russell, T., Syrmis, M., & Wilson, H. (1995). Phonological disorder and the acquisition of literacy. In B. Dodd (Ed.), *Differential diagnosis and treatment of children with speech disorder* (pp. 125–146). London: Whurr.

Dowden, P. A. (1999). Augmentative and alternative communication for children with motor speech disorders. In A. J. Caruso & E. A. Strand (Eds.), *Clinical management of motor speech disorders in children* (pp. 345–383). New York: Thieme Medical.

Dowden, P., & Cook, A. M. (2002). Choosing effective selection techniques for beginning communicators. In J. Reichle, D. R. Beukelman, J. C. Light (Eds.), *Exemplary practices for beginning communicators: Implications for AAC* (pp. 395–431). Baltimore: Paul H. Brookes.

Drumwright, A. (1971). *The Denver Articulation Examination.* Denver, CO: Ladoca Project and Publishing Foundation.

Duffy, J. R. (1995). *Motor speech disorders: Substrates, differential diagnosis, and management.* St. Louis, MO: Mosby.

Duffy, J. R. (2002). Apraxia of speech: Historical overview and clinical manifestations of the acquired and developmental forms. In L. D. Shriberg & T. F. Campbell (Eds.), *Proceedings of the 2002 Childhood Apraxia of Speech Research Symposium* (chap. 1). Carlsbad, CA: The Hendrix Foundation.

Dworkin, J. P., Marunick, M. T., & Krouse, J. H. (2004). Velopharyngeal dysfunction: Speech characteristics, variable etiologies, evaluation techniques, and differential treatments. *Language, Speech, and Hearing Services in Schools, 35,* 333–352.

Edwards, C., & Estabrooks, W. (1994). Learning through listening: A hierarchy. In W. Estabrooks (Ed.), *Auditory-verbal therapy for parents and professionals.* Washington, DC: Alexander Graham Bell Association for the Deaf.

Ehlers, S., & Gillberg, C. (1993). The epidemiology of Asperger syndrome: A total population study. *Journal of Child Psychology and Psychiatry, 34,* 1327–1350.

Ekberg, O., Hamdy, S., Woisard, V., Wuttge-Hannig, A., & Ortega, P. (2002). Social and psychological burden of dysphagia: Its impact on diagnosis and treatment. *Dysphagia, 17,* 139–146.

Elbert, M. (1997). From articulation to phonology: The challenge of change. In B. W. Hodson & M. L. Edwards (Eds.), *Perspectives in applied phonology* (pp. 43–60). Gaithersburg, MD: Aspen Publishers.

Ellis Weismer, S., Murray-Branch, J., & Miller, J. F. (1994). A prospective longitudinal study of language development in late talkers. *Journal of Speech and Hearing Research, 37,* 852–867.

Elman, R. J., & Bernstein-Ellis, E. (1995). What is functional? *American Journal of Speech-Language Pathology, 4,* 115–117.

English, K. E., Mendel, L. L., Rojeski, T., & Hornak, J. (1999). Counseling in audiology, or learning to listen: Pre- and postmeasures from a counseling class in an audiology doctorate program. *American Journal of Audiology, 8,* 34–39.

Erler, S. F., & Garstecki, D. C. (2002). Hearing loss- and hearing aid-related stigma: Perceptions of women with age-normal hearing. *American Journal of Audiology, 11,* 83–91.

Ezell, H. K., & Goldstein, H. (1991). Observational learning of comprehension monitoring skills in children who exhibit mental retardation. *Journal of Speech and Hearing Research, 34,* 141–154.

Ezrati-Vinacour, R., Platzky, R., & Yairi, E. (2001). The young child's awareness of stuttering-like disfluency. *Journal of Speech, Language, and Hearing Research, 44,* 368–380.

Falvey, M., Forest, M., Pearpoint, J., & Rosenberg, R. (1994). *Using the tools: Circles, MAPs and PATH.* Toronto, Canada: Inclusion Press.

Farber, J. G., & Klein, E. R. (1999). Classroom-based assessment of a collaborative intervention program with kindergarten and first-grade students. *Language, Speech, and Hearing Services in Schools, 30,* 83–91.

Fasano, A., Berti, I., Gerarduzzi, T., Not, T., Colletti, R. B., Drago, S., et al. (2003). Prevalence of celiac disease in at-risk and not-at-risk groups in the United States: A large multicenter study. *Archives of Internal Medicine, 163*(3), 286–292.

Felsenfeld, S., McGue, M., & Broen, P. A. (1995). Familial aggregation of phonological disorders: Results from a 28-year follow-up. *Journal of Speech and Hearing Research, 38,* 1091–1107.

Fenson, L., Pethick, S., Renda, C., Cox, J. L., Dale, P. S., & Reznick, J. S. (2000). Short-form versions of the MacArthur Communicative Development Inventories. *Applied Psycholinguistics, 21,* 95–116.

Fey, M. (1986). *Language intervention with young children.* Boston, MA: Allyn & Bacon.

Fey, M. E., Cleave, P. L., Long, S. H., & Hughes, D. L. (1993). Two approaches to facilitation for grammar in children with language impairment: An experimental evaluation. *Journal of Speech and Hearing Research, 36,* 141–157.

Fey, M. E., Cleve, P. L., Ravida, A. I., Long, S. H., Dejmal, A., & Easton, D. (1994). Effects of grammar facilitation on the phonological performance of children with speech and language impairments. *Journal of Speech and Hearing Research, 37,* 594–607.

Fey, M. E., Long, S. H., & Finestack, L. M. (2003). Ten principles of grammar facilitation to children with specific language impairments. *American Journal of Speech-Language Pathology, 12,* 3–15.

Fisher, K. V., Scherer, R. C., Guo, C. G., & Owen, A. S. (1996). Longitudinal phonatory characteristics after botulinum toxin Type A injection. *Journal of Speech and Hearing Research, 39,* 968–980.

Fitch-West, J., & Sands, E. S. (1987). *Bedside evaluation screening test.* Rockville, MD: Aspen.

Flexer, C. (1994). *Facilitating hearing and listening in young children.* San Diego, CA: Singular.

Folkins, J. W. (1985). Issues in speech motor control and their relation to the speech of individuals with cleft palate. *Cleft Palate Journal, 22*(2), 106–122.

Folkins, J. W., & Bleile, K. M. (1990). Taxonomies in biology, phonetics, phonology, and speech motor control. *Journal of Speech and Hearing Disorders, 55,* 596–611.

Folkins, J. W., Moon, J. B., Luschei, E. S., Robin, D. A., Tye-Murray, N., & Moll, K. L. (1995). What can nonspeech tasks tell us about speech motor disabilities? *Journal of Phonetics, 23,* 139–147.

Folstein, M. F., Folstein, S. E., & McHugh, P. R. (1975). "Mini-mental state": A practical method for grading the mental state of patients for the clinician. *Journal of Psychological Research, 12,* 189–198.

Ford, C. N. (1996). Thyroplasty: Indications, techniques, and outcome. In M. P. Fried (Ed.), *The larynx: A multidisciplinary approach* (2nd ed., pp. 243–252). Baltimore: Mosby.

Fox, C. M., Morrison, C. E., Ramig, L. O., & Sapir, S. (2002). Current perspectives on the Lee Silverman voice treatment (LSVT) for individuals with idiopathic Parkinson disease. *American Journal of Speech-Language Pathology, 11,* 111–123.

Fox, C. M., & Ramig, L. O. (1997). Vocal sound pressure level and self-perception of speech and voice of men and women with idiopathic Parkinson disease. *American Journal of Speech-Language Pathology, 6,* 85–94.

Frank, D. A., & Wong, F. (1999). Effects of prenatal exposures to alcohol, tobacco, and other drugs. In D. B. Kessler & P. Dawson (Eds.), *Failure to thrive and pediatric undernutrition: A transdisciplinary approach* (pp. 275–280). Baltimore: Paul H. Brookes.

Frankenburg, W., Dodds, J., Archer, P., Bresnick, B., Maschka, P., Edelman, N., & Shapiro, H. (1990). *Denver II: Screening manual.* Denver, CO: Denver Developmental Materials.

Frattali, C. M., Thompson, C. M., Holland, A. L., Wohl, C. B., & Ferketic, M. M. (1995). *The American Speech-Language-Hearing Association functional assessment of communication skills for adults (ASHA FACS).* Rockville, MD: ASHA.

Frea, W. D., Arnold, C. L., & Vittimberga, G. L. (2001). A demonstration of the effects of augmentative communication on the extreme aggressive behavior of a child with autism within an integrated preschool setting. *Journal of Positive Behavior Interventions, 3,* 194–198.

Fried, M. P., & Lauretano, A. M. (1996). Conservation surgery for glottic carcinoma. In M. P. Fried (Ed.), *The larynx: A multidisciplinary approach* (2nd ed., p. 519–532). Baltimore: Mosby.

Friel-Patti, S., & Finitzo, T. (1990). Language learning in a prospective study of otitis media with effusion in the first two years of life. *Journal of Speech and Hearing Research, 33,* 188–194.

Froom, J., & Culpepper, L. (1991). Otitis media in daycare: A report from the International Primary Care Network. *Journal of Family Practice, 32,* 289–294.

Fudala, J., & Reynolds, W. (2000). *Arizona Articulation Proficiency Scale* (3rd ed.). Los Angeles, CA: Western Psychological Services.

Fujiki, M., Brinton, B., Morgan, M., & Hart, C. H. (1999). Withdrawn and sociable behavior of children with language impairment. *Language, Speech, and Hearing Services in Schools, 30,* 183–195.

Fujiki, M., Brinton, B., & Todd, C. M. (1996). Social skills of children with specific language impairment. *Language, Speech, and Hearing Services in Schools, 27,* 195–201.

Fujiura, G. T., & Yamaki, K. (1997). Analysis of ethnic variations in developmental disability prevalence and household economic status. *Mental Retardation, 35,* 286–294.

Fuller, D. R., Lloyd, L. L., & Stratton, M. M. (1997). Aided AAC symbols. In L. L. Lloyd, D. R. Fuller, & H. H. Arvidson (Eds.), *Augmentative and alternative communication: A handbook of principles and practices* (pp. 48–79). Needham Heights, MA: Allyn & Bacon.

Gallaudet Research Institute. (2001). *Regional and national summary report of data from the 1999–2000 Annual Survey of Deaf and Hard of Hearing Children and Youth.* Washington, DC: Gallaudet University.

Gallaudet University Center for Assessment and Demographic Study. (1998). 30 years of annual surveys of deaf and hard-of-hearing children and youth: A glance over the decades. *American Annals of the Deaf, 142,* 72–76.

Garn-Nunn, P. G., & Lynn, J. M. (2004). *Calvert's descriptive phonetics* (3rd ed.). New York: Thieme.

Garstecki, D. C., & Erler, S. F. (1995). Older women and hearing. *American Journal of Audiology, 4,* 41–46.

Gates, G. A., Couropmitree, N. M., & Myers, R. H. (1999). Genetic associations in age-related hearing thresholds. *Archives of Otolaryngology—Head and Neck Surgery, 125,* 654–659.

Gauer, L. M., Lombardino, L. J., & Leonard, C. M. (1997). Brain morphology in children with specific language impairment. *Journal of Speech, Language, and Hearing Research, 40,* 1272–1284.

Gentner, D., & Goldin-Meadow, S.(2003). *Language in mind: Advances in the study of language and thought.* Cambridge, MA: MIT Press.

Gierut, J. A. (1998). Treatment efficacy: Functional phonological disorders in children. *Journal of Speech, Language, and Hearing Research, 41*(1), S85–S100.

Gierut, J. A. (2001). Complexity in phonological treatment: clinical factors. *Language, Speech, and Hearing Services in Schools, 32,* 229–241.

Gierut, J. A., Morrisette, M. L., Hughes, M. T., & Rowland, S. (1996). Phonological treatment efficacy and developmental norms. *Language, Speech, and Hearing Services in Schools, 27,* 215–230.

Gillam, R. (1999). Computer-assisted language intervention using Fast Forward®: Theoretical and empirical considerations for decision-making. *Language, Speech, and Hearing Services in Schools, 3,* 363–370.

Gillis, R. J. (1996). *Traumatic brain injury rehabilitation for speech-language pathologists.* Boston: Butterworth-Heinemann.

Gillon, G. (2004). *Phonological awareness: From research to practice.* New York: Guilford Press.

Ginsberg, A. J. (1988). Feeding disorders in the developmentally disabled population. In D. C. Russo & J. H. Kedesdy (Eds.), *Behavioral medicine with the developmentally disabled* (pp. 21–41). New York: Plenum.

Girolametto, L., Pearce, P. S., & Weitzman, E. (1996). Interactive focused stimulation for toddlers with expressive vocabulary delays. *Journal of Speech and Hearing Research, 39,* 1274–1283.

Girolametto, L., Weitzman, E., & Greenberg, J. (2000). *Teacher Interaction and Language Rating Scale.* Toronto, ON: The Hanen Centre.

Girolametto, L., Wiigs, M., Smyth, R., Weitzman, E., & Pearce, P. (2001). Children with a history of expressive vocabulary delay: Outcomes at 5 years of age. *American Journal of Speech-Language Pathology, 10,* 358–369.

Goldberg, S. (1993). *Clinical intervention: A philosophy and methodology for clinical practice.* New York: Macmillan.

Goldman, R. M., & Fristoe, M. (2000). *Goldman-Fristoe Test of Articulation–2.* Circle Pines, MN: American Guidance Service.

Goldman, S. L., Hargrave, J., Hillman, R. E., Holmberg, E., & Gress, C. (1996). Stress, anxiety, somatic complaints, and voice use in women with vocal nodules: Preliminary findings. *American Journal of Speech-Language Pathology, 5,* 44–54.

Golinkoff, R. M., & Hirsh-Pasek, K. (1999). *How babies talk: The magic and mystery of language in the first three years of life.* New York: Dutton.

Goodglass, H., & Kaplan, E. (1983). *The assessment of aphasia and related disorders* (2nd ed.). Philadelphia: Lea & Febriger.

Goodman, R., & Yude, C. (1996). IQ and its predictors in childhood hemiplegia. *Developmental Medicine and Child Neurology, 38,* 881–890.

Gottwald, S. R., & Starkweather, C. W. (1995). Fluency intervention for preschoolers and their families in the public schools. *Language, Speech, and Hearing Services in Schools, 26,* 117–126.

Gracco, V. L. (1997). A neuromotor perspective on speech production. In W. Hulstijn, H. F. M. Peters, & P. H. H. M. van Lieshout (Eds.), *Speech production: Motor control, brain research and fluency disorders* (pp. 37–56). Amsterdam: Elsevier.

Gracco, V. L., & Abbs, J. H. (1987). Programming and execution processes of speech movement control: potential neural correlates. In E. Keller & M. Gopnik (Eds.), *Motor and sensory processes of language* (pp. 163–201). Hillsdale, NJ: Lawrence Erlbaum.

Graham, C. G., Conture, E. G., & Schwenk, K. A. (2004, September). *Using the past to predict the future: Pretreatment variables as a predictor of treatment success, a preliminary study.* Presentation at the Rite Care Conference, Vanderbilt University, Nashville, TN.

Gresham, F. M., & Elliott, S. N. (1990). *Social Skills Rating System.* Circle Pines, MN: AGS.

Grice, H. P. (1975). Logic and conversation. In P. Cole & J. Morgan (Eds.), *Syntax and semantics: Speech acts* (vol. 3). New York: Academic Press.

Gruber, F. A. (1999). Probability estimates and paths to consonant normalization in children with speech delay. *Journal of Speech, Language, and Hearing Research, 42,* 448–459.

Grunwell, P. (1987). *Clinical phonology* (2nd ed). Baltimore: Williams & Wilkins.

Guenther, F. H., Hampson, M., & Johnson, D. (1998). A theoretical investigation of reference frames for the planning of speech movements. *Psychological Review, 105,* 611–633.

Guenther, F. H., & Perkell, J. S. (2004). A neural model of speech production and its application to studies of the role of auditory feedback in speech. In B. Maassen, R. Kent, H. Peters, P. Van Lieshout, & W. Hulstijn (Eds.), *Speech motor control in normal and disordered speech* (pp. 29–50). Oxford: Oxford University Press.

Guitar, B. (1998). *Stuttering: An integrated approach to its nature and treatment* (2nd ed.). Baltimore: Lippincott Williams & Wilkins.

Guralnick, M. J. (1997). *The effectiveness of early intervention.* Baltimore: Paul H. Brookes.

Gutiérrez-Clellen, V. F., & Peña, E. (2001). Dynamic assessment of diverse children: A tutorial. *Language, Speech, and Hearing Services in Schools, 32,* 212–224.

Haelsig, P. C., & Madison, C. L. (1986). A study of phonological processes exhibited by 3-, 4-, and 5-year-old children. *Language, Speech, and Hearing Services in Schools, 17,* 107–114.

Hagen, C. (1981). Language disorders secondary to closed head injury. *Topics in Language Disorders, 1,* 73–87.

Hall, J. W., & Mueller, H. G. (1997). *Audiologists' desk reference: Volume I.* San Diego, CA: Singular.

Hall, K. D., Amir, O., & Yairi, E. (1999). A longitudinal investigation of speaking rate in preschool children who stutter. *Journal of Speech, Language, and Hearing Research, 42,* 1367–1377.

Hall, P. K., Jordan, L. S., & Robin, D. A. (1993). *Developmental apraxia of speech. Theory and clinical practice.* Austin, TX: Pro-Ed.

Halliday, M. A. K. (1975). *Learning how to mean: Explorations in the development of language.* New York: Edward Arnold.

Halliday, M. A. K. (1977). *Exploration in the functions of language.* New York: Elsevier North-Holland.

Halliday, M. A. K. (1978). *Language as a social semiotic: The social interpretation of language and meaning.* Baltimore, MD: University Park Press.

Halper, A., Cherney, L. R., & Burn, M. S. (1996). *Clinical management of right hemisphere dysfunction* (2nd ed.). Rockville, MD: Aspen.

Hanks, R. A., Wood, D. L., Millis, S., Harrison-Felix, C., Pierce, C. A., Rosenthal, M., et al. (2003). Violent traumatic brain injury: Occurrence, patient characteristics, and risk factors from the Traumatic Brain Injury Model Systems Project. *Archives of Physical Medicine and Rehabilitation, 84,* 249–254.

Hardy, J. C. (1983). *Cerebral palsy.* Upper Saddle River, NJ: Prentice Hall.

Harrison, M. (1999, June). *Auditory-verbal therapy for children with hearing loss presented at Listening to Learn: Partnering Families and Professionals to Teach Children with Hearing Loss.* Celebrate the Power! Conference. Ypsilanti, MI: Eastern Michigan University.

Harrison, P., Kaufman, A., Kaufman, N., Bruinicks, R., Rynders, J., Ilmer, S., Sparrow, C., & Cicchetti, D. (1990). *Early screening profiles.* Circle Pines, MN: American Guidance Service.

Hart, B., & Risley, T. R. (1995). *Meaningful differences in the everyday experience of young American children.* Baltimore: Paul H. Brookes.

Hartman-Maeir, A., Soroker, N., Oman, S. D., Katz, N. (2003). Awareness of disabilities in stroke rehabilitation: A clinical trial. *Disability and Rehabilitation, 25*(1), 35–44.

Harvey, P. L. (1996). *Behavioral management of the performing voice.* In M. P. Fried (Ed.), *The larynx: A multidisciplinary approach* (2nd ed., pp. 253–269). Baltimore: Mosby.

Hawking, S. (2003). *My experience with ALS.* Retrieved from http://www.hawking.org.u/disable/disable.html

Hecker, D. E. (2001). Occupational employment projections to 2010. *Monthly Labor Review Online, 124*(11), 57–84

Heflin, L. J., & Simpson, R. L. (1998). Interventions for children and youth with autism: Prudent choices in a world of exaggerated claims and empty promises: Part 1. Intervention and treatment option review. *Focus on Autism and Other Developmental Disabilities, 13,* 194–211.

Heilman, K. M. (2004). Intentional neglect. *Frontiers in Bioscience, 9,* 694–705.

Helm-Estabrooks, N., & Albert, M. L. (1991). *Manual of aphasia therapy.* Austin, TX: Pro-Ed.

Helm-Estabrooks, N., & Hotz, G. (1991). *Brief test of head injury.* Chicago: Riverside.

Herrington-Hall, B., Lee, L., Stemple, J., Niemi, K., & McHone, M. (1988). Description of laryngeal pathologies by age, sex, and occupation in a treatment-seeking sample. *Journal of Speech and Hearing Disorders, 53,* 57–65.

Heward, W. L. (2003). *Exceptional children: An introduction to special education* (7th ed.). Upper Saddle River, NJ: Merrill/Prentice Hall.

Hillenbrand, J., Cleveland, R. A., & Erickson, R. L. (1994). Acoustic correlates of breathy vocal quality. *Journal of Speech and Hearing Research, 37,* 769–778.

Hirano, M. (1990). Surgical and medical management of voice disorders. In R. H. Colton & J. K. Casper (Eds.), *Understanding voice problems.* Baltimore: Williams & Wilkins.

Hirsh-Pasek, K., & Golinkoff, R. M. (Eds.). (1996). *The origins of grammar: Evidence from early language comprehension* (pp. 123–158). Cambridge, MA: MIT Press.

Hodson, B. (1997). Disordered phonologies: What have we learned about assessment and treatment? In B. W. Hodson & M. L. Edwards (Eds.),

Perspectives in applied phonology (pp. 197–224). Gaithersburg, MD: Aspen Publishers.

Hodson, B. W., & Paden, E. P. (1991). *Targeting intelligible speech* (2nd ed.). Austin, TX: Pro-Ed.

Hoff, E. (2003). The specificity of environmental influence: Socioeconomic status affects early vocabulary development via maternal speech. *Child Development, 74,* 1368–1378.

Hoff-Ginsberg, E. (1997). *Language development.* Pacific Grove, CA: Brooks Cole.

Holland, A. L., Frattali, C. M., & Fromm, D. (1999). *Communication activities of daily living* (2nd ed.). Austin, TX: Pro-Ed.

Horner, J., Alberts, M. J., Dawson, D. V., & Cook, G. M. (1994). Swallowing in Alzheimer's disease. *Alzheimer Disease and Associated Disorders, 8,* 177–189.

Huckabee, M. (2004). *New Zealand Index for Multidisciplinary Evaluation of Swallowing.* Christchurch, NZ: University of Canterbury.

Hughes, D., McGillivray, L., & Schmidek, M. (1997). *Guide to narrative language: Procedures for assessment.* Eau Claire, WI: Thinking Publications.

Hymes, D. H. (1972). On communicative competence. In J. B. Pride & J. Holmes (Eds.), *Sociolinguistics.* Baltimore: Penguin Books.

Individuals with Disabilities Education Act Data. (2003). Retrieved from *Annual report tables.* http://www.ideadata.org/AnnualTables.asp

Ingham, J. C. (2003). Evidence-based treatment of stuttering. I. Definition and application. *Journal of Fluency Disorders, 28,* 197–207.

International Phonetic Association (1996). *International Phonetic Alphabet.* London: Author.

Iverson, J. M., & Thal, D. J. (1998). Communicative transitions: There's more to the hand than meets the eye. In A. M. Wetherby, S. F. Warren, & J. Reichle (Eds.), *Transitions to prelinguistic communication* (pp. 59–86). Baltimore: Paul H. Brookes.

Jakielski, K. J., & Davis, B. L. (1995, April). *Differentiating developmental apraxia of speech from other disorders of speech and language.* Short course presented at the annual meeting of the Texas Speech-Language-Hearing Association, Houston, TX.

James, J. M., & Burks, A. W. (1999). Adverse reactions to foods. In D. B. Kessler & P. Dawson (Eds.), *Failure to thrive and pediatric undernutrition: A transdisciplinary approach* (pp. 261–268). Baltimore: Paul H. Brookes.

Johnson, C. J., Beitchman, J. H., Young, A., Escobar, M., Atkinson, L., Wilson, B., Brownlie, E. B., Douglas, L., Taback, N., Lam, I., & Wang, M. (1999). Fourteen-year follow-up of children with and without speech/language impairments: Speech/language stability and outcomes. *Journal of Speech, Language, and Hearing Research, 42,* 744–760.

Johnson, R., & Harris, G. (2004). A preliminary study of the predictors of feeding problems in late infancy. *Journal of Reproductive and Infant Psychology, 22,* 183–188.

Joint Committee on Infant Hearing. (1991). Joint Committee on Infant Hearing 1990 position statement. *ASHA, 3* (Supplement 5), 3–6.

Joint Committee on Infant Hearing. (1995). 1994 position statement. *Pediatrics, 95,* 315.

Joint Committee on Infant Hearing. (2000). Year 2000 position statement: Principles and guidelines for early hearing detection and intervention programs. *Pediatrics, 106*(4), 798–817.

Jones, M., Onslow, M., Harrison, E., & Packman, A. (2000). Treating stuttering in young children: Predicting treatment time in the Lidcombe Program. *Journal of Speech, Language, and Hearing Research, 43,* 1440–1450.

Jusczyk, P. (2003). Chunking language input to find patterns. In D. H. Rakison & L. M. Oakes (Eds.), *Early category and concept development.* New York: Oxford University Press.

Justice, L. M., & Ezell, H. K. (1999). Vygotskian theory and its application to language assessment: An overview for speech-language pathologists. *Contemporary Issues in Communication Science and Disorders, 26,* 111–118.

Justice, L. M., & Ezell, H. K. (2001). Descriptive analysis of written language awareness in children from low income households. *Communication Disorders Quarterly, 22,* 123–134.

Justice, L. M., & Ezell, H. K. (2001). Written language awareness in preschool children from low-income households: A descriptive analysis. *Communication Disorders Quarterly, 22,* 123–134.

Justice, L. M., & Ezell, H. K. (2002). *The syntax handbook.* Eau Claire, WI: Thinking Publications.

Justice, L. M., & Ezell, H. K. (2004). Print referencing: An emergent literacy enhancement technique and its clinical applications. *Language, Speech, and Hearing Services in Schools, 35,* 185–193.

Justice, L. M., & Fey, M. (2004). Evidence-based practices in schools: Integrating craft and theory with science and data. *ASHA Leader, 4–5,* 30–32.

Justice, L. M., & Kaderavek, J. (2004). Embedded-explicit emergent literacy: I. Background and description of approach. *Language, Speech, and Hearing Services in Schools, 35,* 201–211.

Justice, L. M., & Pullen, P. (2003). Promising interventions for promoting emergent literacy skills: Three evidence-based approaches. *Topics in Early Childhood Special Education, 23,* 99–113.

Justice, L. M., & Schuele, C. M. (2004). Phonological awareness: Description, assessment, and intervention. In J. Bernthal & N. Bankson, *Articulation and phonological disorders* (5th ed., pp. 376–406). New York: Allyn & Bacon.

Kaderavek, J., & Justice, L. M. (2002). Shared storybook reading as an intervention context: Practices and potential pitfalls. *American Journal of Speech-Language Pathology, 11,* 395–406.

Kaderavek, J., & Justice, L. M. (2004). Embedded-explicit emergent literacy: II. Goal selection and implementation in the early childhood classroom. *Language, Speech, and Hearing Services in Schools, 25,* 212–228.

Kalia, M. (2003). Dysphagia and aspiration pneumonia in patients with Alzheimer's disease. *Metabolism, 52,* 36–38.

Kalinowski, J., Stuart, A., & Armson, J. (1996). Perceptions of stutterers and nonstutterers during speaking and nonspeaking situations. *American Journal of Speech-Language Pathology, 5,* 61–66.

Kalmanson, B., & Seligman, S. (1992). Family-provider relationships: The basis of all interventions. *Infants and Young Children, 4,* 46–52.

Kandel, E. R., Schwartz, J. H., & Jessell, T. M. (2001). *Principles of neural science.* (4th ed.). New York: McGraw-Hill.

Karmody, C. S. (1996). The history of laryngology. In M. P. Fried (Ed.), *The larynx: A multidisciplinary approach* (2nd ed., pp. 3–14). Baltimore: Mosby.

Kart, C. S., & Kinney, J. M. (2001). *The realities of aging: An introduction to gerontology* (6th ed.). Boston: Allyn & Bacon.

Katz, J. (Ed.) (1994). *Handbook of clinical audiology* (4th ed.). Baltimore: Williams & Wilkins.

Kaufman, A. S., & Kaufman, N. L. (1990). *Kaufman Brief Intelligence Test.* Circle Pines, MN: American Guidance Service.

Kaut, K. P., DePompei, R., Kerr, J., & Congeni, J. (2003). Reports of head injury and symptom knowledge among college athletes: Implications for assessment and intervention. *Clinical Journal of Sport Medicine, 13*(4), 213–221.

Kedesdy, J. H., & Budd, K. S. (1998). *Childhood feeding disorders: Biobehavioral asessment and intervention.* Baltimore: Paul H. Brookes.

Keenan, J. S., & Brassell, E. G. (1975). *Aphasia language performance scales.* Murfreesboro, TN: Pinnacle Press.

Keller, H. (1933). *Helen Keller in Scotland: A personal record by herself* (J. Love, Ed.). London: Methuen.

Kelso, J. A. S., Tuller, B., Bateson, E. V., & Fowler, C. A. (1984). Functionally specific articulatory cooperation following jaw perturbations during speech: Evidence for coordinative structures. *Journal of Experimental Psychology: Human Perception and Performance, 10,* 812–832.

Kenneally, S. M., Bruck, G. E., Frank, E. M., & Nalty, L. (1998). Language intervention after three years of isolation: A case study of a feral child. *Education and Training in Mental Retardation and Developmental Disabilities, 33,* 13–23.

Kent, R. D. (1994). *Reference manual for communicative sciences and disorders: Speech and language.* Austin, TX: Pro-Ed.

Kent, R. D. (1997). *The speech sciences.* San Diego, CA: Singular.

Kent, R. D., Adams, S. G., & Turner, G. S. (1996). Models of speech production. In N. J. Lass (Ed.), *Principles of experimental phonetics* (pp. 3–45). St. Louis, MO: Mosby.

Kent, R. D., & Rosenbek, J. C. (1983). Acoustic patterns of apraxia of speech. *Journal of Speech and Hearing Research, 26,* 231–249.

Kertesz, A. (1982). *Western aphasia battery.* New York: Grune & Stratton.

Kesey, K. (1973). *One flew over the cuckoo's nest.* New York: Viking Press.

Kessler, D. B. (1999). Failure to thrive and pediatric undernutrition: Historical and theoretical context. In D. B. Kessler & P. Dawson (Eds.), *Failure to thrive and pediatric undernutrition: A transdisciplinary approach* (pp. 3–18). Baltimore: Paul H. Brookes.

Kessler, D. B., & Dawson, B. (Eds.). (1999). *Failure to thrive and pediatric undernutrition: A transdisciplinary approach.* Baltimore: Paul H. Brookes.

Kessler, J. W. (1966). *Psychopathology of childhood.* Upper Saddle River, NJ: Prentice Hall.

Khan, L. M. (2002). The sixth view: Assessing preschoolers' articulation and phonology from the trenches. *American Journal of Speech-Language Pathology, 11,* 250–254.

Killion, M. C., & Christensen, L. (1998). The case of the missing dots: AI and SNR loss. *The Hearing Journal, 51*(5), 32–47.

Killion, M. C., & Niquette, P. A. (2000). What can the pure-tone audiogram tell us about a patient's SNR loss? *Hearing Journal, 53,* 46–53.

Kiran, S., & Thompson, C. K. (2003). The role of semantic complexity in treatment of naming deficits: Training semantic categories in fluent aphasia by controlling exemplar typicality. *Journal of Speech, Language, and Hearing Research, 46*(3), 608–622.

Kirkwood, D. (1999). Major survey documents negative impact of untreated hearing loss on quality of life. *Hearing Journal, 52,* 32–40.

Klapp, S. T. (1995). Motor response programming during simple and choice reaction time: The role of practice. *Journal of Experimental Psychology: Human Perception and Performance, 21*(5), 1015–1027.

Klein, E. S. (1996). Phonological/traditional approaches to articulation therapy: A retrospective group comparison. *Language, Speech, and Hearing Services in Schools, 27,* 314–323.

Klein, H. B., & Moses, N. (1999). *Intervention planning for children with communication disorders.* Boston: Allyn & Bacon.

Kleinow, J., & Smith, A. (2000). Influences of length and syntactic complexity on the speech motor stability of the fluent speech of adults who stutter. *Journal of Speech, Language, and Hearing Research, 43,* 548–559.

Knock, T., Ballard, K. J., Robin, D. A., & Schmidt, R. A. (2000). Influence of order of stimulus presentation on speech motor learning: A principled approach to treatment for apraxia of speech. *Aphasiology, 14*(5/6), 653–668.

Kochkin, S. (1993). MarkTrak III: Why 20 million in U.S. don't use hearing aids for their hearing loss. *Hearing Journal, 46,* 20–27.

Kochkin, S. (1999). "Baby boomers" spur growth in potential market, but penetration rate declines. *Hearing Journal, 52,* 1.

Kochkin, S. (2002). MarkTrak V: Why my hearing aids are in the drawer: The consumer perspective. *Hearing Journal, 53,* 34–42.

Kopun, J., & Stelmachowicz, P. (1998). Perceived communication difficulties of children with hearing loss. *American Journal of Audiology, 7,* 30–38.

Kravitz, T. R., Kamps, D. M., Kemmerer, K., & Potucek, J. (2002). Brief report: Increasing communication skills for an elementary-aged student with autism using the Picture Exchange Communication System. *Journal of Autism and Developmental Disorders, 32,* 225–230.

Krebs, N. F. (1999). Gastrointestinal problems and disorders. In D. B. Kessler & P. Dawson (Eds.), *Failure to thrive and pediatric undernutrition: A transdisciplinary approach* (pp. 215–226). Baltimore: Paul H. Brookes.

Kuban, K. C., & Leviton, A. (1994). Cerebral palsy. *New England Journal of Medicine, 330*(3), 188–195.

Kuder, S. (1997). *Teaching students with language and communication disabilities.* Boston: Allyn & Bacon.

Kwiatkowski, J., & Shriberg, L. D. (1993). Speech normalization in developmental phonological disorders: A retrospective study of capability-focus theory. *Language, Speech, and Hearing Services in Schools, 24,* 10–18.

Ladefoged, P. (2001). *A course in phonetics* (4th ed.). Fort Worth: Harcourt Brace Jovanovich.

Lahey, M. (1988). *Language disorders and language development.* New York: Macmillan.

Laing, S. P., & Kamhi, A. (2003). Alternative assessment of language and literacy in culturally and linguistically diverse populations. *Language, Speech, and Hearing Services in Schools, 34,* 44–55.

Landry, S. H., Miller-Loncar, C. L., Smith, K. E., & Swank, P. R. (1997). Predicting cognitive-language and social growth curves from early maternal behaviors in children at varying degrees of biological risk. *Developmental Psychology, 33,* 1040–1053.

Laws, G., & Bishop, D. V. M. (2003). A comparison of language abilities in adolescents with Down syndrome and children with specific language impairment. *Journal of Speech, Language, and Hearing Research, 46,* 1324–1339.

Lazarus, C., & Logemann, J. A. (1987). Swallowing disorders in closed head trauma patients. *Archives of Physical Medicine and Rehabilitation, 68,* 79–84.

Lee, L., Stemple, J. C., & Glaze, L. (2003). *Your child's voice.* Gainesville, FL: Communicare.

Lemons, J. A., Bauer, C. R., Oh, W., et al. (2001). Very low birth weight outcomes of the National Institute of Child Health and Human Development neonatal research network, January 1995 through December 1996. *Pediatrics, 107*(1), E1.

Leonard, L. B. (2000). *Children with specific language impairment.* Cambridge, MA: MIT Press.

Levelt, W. J. M., Roelofs, A., & Meyer, A. S. (1999). A theory of lexical access in speech production. *Behavioral and Brain Sciences, 22,* 1–75.

Lewis, M. S., Crandell, C. C., Valente, M., Enrietto, J., Kreisman, N. V., Kreisman, B. M., & Bancroft, L. (2003). Study measures impact of hearing aids plus FM on the quality of life in older adults. *Hearing Journal, 56,* 30–33.

Liberman, A. M. (1998). When theories of speech meet the real world. *Journal of Psycholinguistic Research, 27,* 111–122.

Light, J. (1988). Interaction involving individuals using augmentative and alternative communication systems: State of the art and future directions. *Augmentative and Alternative Communication, 4,* 66–82.

Light, J. (1997). "Communication is the essence of human life": Reflections on communicative competence. *Augmentative and Alternative Communication, 13,* 61–70.

Light, J. C. (2003). Shattering the silence: Development of communicative competence by individuals who use AAC. In J. C. Light, D. R. Beukelman, & J. Reichle (Eds.), *Communicative competence for individuals who use AAC: From research to effective practice* (pp. 3–38). Baltimore: Paul H. Brookes.

Lincoln, M., Onslow, M., Lewis, C., & Wilson, L. (1996). A clinical trial of an operant treatment for school-age children who stutter. *American Journal of Speech-Language Pathology, 5,* 73–85.

Lincoln, M. A., & Onslow, M. (1997). Long-term outcome of early intervention for stuttering. *American Journal of Speech-Language Pathology, 6*(1), 51–58.

Ling, D. (2001). Speech development for children who are hearing impaired. In R. H. Hull (Ed.), *Aural rehabilitation: Serving children and adults* (pp. 145–167). San Diego, CA: Singular.

Linscheid, T. R. (1992). Eating problems in children. In C. E. Walker & M. C. Roberts (Eds.), *Handbook of clinical child psychology* (2nd ed., pp. 451–473). New York: John Wiley & Sons.

Locke, J. L. (1983). *Phonological acquisition and change.* New York: Academic Press.

Lof, G. L. (2004). What does the research report about non-speech oral motor exercises and the treatment of speech sound disorders? Retrieved March 10, 2004, from www.apraxia-kids.org/faqs/responsefromlof.html

Logemann, J. (1998). *Evaluation and treatment of swallowing disorders* (2nd ed.). Austin, TX: Pro-Ed.

Logemann, J. A. (1995). Dysphagia: Evaluation and treatment. *Folia Phoniatrica et Logopedica, 47,* 140–164.

Lord, C., & Risi, S. (2000). Diagnosis of autism spectrum disorders in young children. In A. M. Wetherby & B. M. Prizant (Eds.), *Autism spectrum disorders: A transactional developmental perspective* (pp. 11–30). Baltimore: Paul H. Brookes.

Love, R. J. (1992). *Childhood motor speech disability.* New York: Macmillan.

Love, R. J. (1994). *Phonology: Assessment and intervention applications in speech pathology.* Baltimore, MD: Williams & Wilkins.

Luetke-Stahlman, B., & Nielsen, D. (2003). The contribution of phonological awareness and receptive and expressive English to the reading ability of deaf students with varying degrees of exposure to accurate English. *Journal of Deaf Studies & Deaf Education* (8), 464–484.

Luiselli, J. K. (1989). Behavioral assessment and treatment of pediatric feeding disorders in developmental disabilities. In M. Hersen, R. K. Eisler, & P. M. Miller (Eds.), *Progress in behavior modification* (vol. 24, pp. 91–131). Beverly Hills, CA: Sage.

Maas, E., Barlow, J. A., Robin, D. A., & Shapiro, L. P. (2002). Treatment of sound production errors in aphasia and apraxia of speech: Effects of phonological complexity. *Aphasiology, 16,* 609–622.

MacDorman, M. F., Minino, A. M., Strobino, D. M., & Guyer, B. (2002). Annual summary of vital statistics—2001. *Pediatrics, 112,* 1037–1052.

Mackey, L. E., Morgan, A. S., & Bernstein, B. A. (1999). Swallowing disorders in severe brain injury: Risk factors affecting return to oral intake. *Archives of Physical Medicine and Rehabilitation, 80,* 365–371.

Maclean, L. K., & Cripe, J. J. (1997). The effectiveness of early intervention for children with communication disorders. In M. Guralnick (Ed.), *The effectiveness of early intervention.* Baltimore: Paul H. Brookes.

Madsen, K. M., Hviid, A., Vestergaard, M., Schendel, D., Wohlfahrt, J., Thorsen, P., Olsen, J., & Melbye, M. (2002). A population-based study of measles, mumps, and rubella vaccination and autism. *New England Journal of Medicine, 347*(19), 1477–1482.

Magnusson, E., & Naucler, K. (1993). The development of linguistic awareness in language-disordered children. *First Language, 13,* 93–111.

Malkus, D., Booth, B., & Kodimer, C. (1980). *Rehabilitation of the head-injured adult: Comprehensive cognitive management.* Downey, CA: Professional Staff Association of Rancho Los Amigos Hospital.

Maner, K. J., Smith, A., & Grayson, L. (2000). Influences of utterance length and complexity on speech motor performance in children and adults. *Journal of Speech, Language, and Hearing Research, 43,* 560–573.

Manjula, R. & Patil, G. S. (2004). Declination of F0 in the speech of Broca's aphasics: Reflection into speech planning? Poster presented at the Clinical Aphasiology Conference, Park City, Utah.

Mann, G., Hankey, G. J., & Cameron, D. (1999). Swallowing function after stroke: Prognosis and prognostic factors at six months. *Stroke, 30,* 744–748.

Martin, F. (1994). *Introduction to audiology* (5th ed.). Upper Saddle River, NJ: Prentice Hall.

Martin, F., & Greer Clark, J. (2002). *Introduction to audiology* (8th ed.). Boston: Allyn & Bacon.

Martino, R., Pron, G., & Diamant, N. (2000). Screening for oropharyngeal dysphagia in stroke: Insufficient evidence for guidelines. *Dysphagia, 15,* 19–30.

Marx, J., Osguthorpe, D., & Parsons, G. (1995). Day care and the incidence of otitis media in young children. *Otolaryngology—Head and Neck Surgery, 112,* 695–699.

Mashima, P. A., Birkmire-Peters, D. P., Syms, M. J., Holtel, M. R., Burgess, L. P., & Peters, L. J. (2003). Telehealth: Voice therapy using telecommunications technology. *American Journal of Speech-Language Pathology, 12,* 432–439.

Maternal and Child Health Bureau. (2002). *Child Health U.S.A.* Washington, DC: U. S. Department of Health and Human Services.

Mathy, P., Yorkston, K. M., & Gutmann, M. L. (2000). AAC for individuals with amyotrophic lateral sclerosis. In D. R. Beukelman, K. M. Yorkston, & J. Reichle (Eds.), *Augmentative and alternative communication for adults with acquired neurologic disorders* (pp. 183–231). Baltimore: Paul H. Brookes.

May, P. A., & Gossage, J. P. (2001). Estimating the prevalence of fetal alcohol syndrome: A summary. *Alcohol Research & Health, 25,* 159–167.

McCauley, R. J., & Swisher, L. (1984). Psychometric review of language and articulation tests for preschool children. *Journal of Speech and Hearing Disorders, 49,* 34–42.

McClean, M. D., & Runyan, C. M. (2000). Variations in the relative speeds of orofacial structures with stuttering severity. *Journal of Speech, Language, and Hearing Research, 43,* 1524–1531.

McConnel, F. M., Cerenko, D., Jackson, R. T., & Guffin, T. N. (1988). Timing of major events of pharyngeal swallowing. *Archives of Otolaryngology—Head and Neck Surgery, 21,* 625–635.

McDonald, E. T. (1987). *Treating cerebral palsy: For clinicians by clinicians.* Austin, TX: Pro-Ed.

McFarlane, S. C., & Watterson, T. L. (1990). Vocal nodules: Endoscopic study of their variations and treatment. In S. C. McFarlane (Ed.), *Seminars in Speech and Language, 11*(1). New York: Thieme Medical.

McGregor, K. K. (1997). The nature of word-finding errors of preschoolers with and without word-finding deficits. *Journal of Speech, Language, and Hearing Research, 40,* 1232–1244.

McGregor, K. K., Friedman, R. M., Reilly, R. M., & Newman, R. M. (2002). Semantic representations and naming in young children. *Journal of Speech, Language, and Hearing Research, 45,* 332–346.

McGregor, K. K., & Leonard, L. B. (1995). Intervention for word-finding deficits in children. In M. Fey, J. Windsor, & S. Warren (Eds.), *Language intervention: Preschool through the elementary years* (pp. 85–105). Baltimore: Paul H. Brookes.

McKevitt, C., Redfern, J., LaPlaca, V., & Wolfe, C. D. (2003). Defining and using quality of life: A survey of health care professionals. *Clinical Rehabilitation, 17,* 865–870.

McNeil, M. R., Doyle, P. J., & Wambaugh, J. (2000). Apraxia of speech: A treatable disorder of motor planning and programming. In S. E. Nadeau, L. J. Gonzalez-Rothi, & B. Crosson (Eds.), *Aphasia and language: Theory to practice* (pp. 221–266) New York: Guilford Press.

McNeil, M. R., Robin, D. A., & Schmidt, R. A. (1997). Apraxia of speech: Definition, differentiation, and treatment. In M. R. McNeil (Ed.), *Clinical management of sensorimotor speech disorders* (pp. 311–344). New York: Thieme.

Mehr, A. S. (2005). *Understanding your audiogram.* Reston, VA: American Academy of Audiology. Retrieved January 10, 2005, from http://www.audiology.org/consumer/guides/uya.php

Menyuk, P., Chesnick, M., Liebergott, J. W., Korngold, B., D'Agostino, R., & Belander, A. (1991). Predicting reading problems in at-risk children. *Journal of Speech and Hearing Research, 34,* 893–903.

Mercer, C. (1997), *Students with learning disabilities* (5th ed). Upper Saddle River, NJ: Merrill/Prentice Hall.

Merritt, D. B., Barton, J., & Culatta, B. (1998). Instructional discourse: A framework for learning. In D. D. Merritt & B. Culatta (Eds.), *Language intervention in the classroom* (pp. 143– 174). San Diego, CA: Singular.

Merritt, D. B., Culatta, B., & Trostle, S. (1998). Narratives: Implementing a discourse framework. In D. D. Merritt & B. Culatta (Eds.), *Language intervention in the classroom* (pp. 277–330). San Diego, CA: Singular.

Merzenic, M. M., Jenkins, W. M., Johnston, P., Schreiner, C., Miller, S. L., & Tallal, P. (1996). Temporal processing deficits of language-learning impaired children ameliorated by training. *Science, 271,* 77–81.

Meyer, J. (1997). Models of service delivery. In P. F. O'Connell (Ed.), *Speech, language, and hearing programs in schools: A guide for students and practitioners* (pp. 241–277). Gaithersburg, MD: Aspect Publications.

Meyerhoff, W. L., & Rice, D. H. (1992). *Otolaryngology—Head and neck surgery*. Philadelphia: W. B. Saunders.

Miccio, A. W. (2002). Clinical problem solving: Assessment of phonological disorders. *American Journal of Speech-Language Pathology, 11,* 221–229.

Miccio, A. W., Yont, K. M., Clemons, H. L., & Vernon-Feagans, L. (2002). Otitis media and the acquisition of consonants. In F. Windsor, M. L. Kelly, & N. Hewlett (Eds.), *Investigations in clinical phonetics and linguistics* (pp. 429–436). Mahwah, NJ: Lawrence Erlbaum.

Miles, S., & Bernstein Ratner, N. (2001). Parental language input to children at stuttering onset. *Journal of Speech, Language, and Hearing Research, 44,* 1116–1130.

Miller, E. K. (2000). The prefrontal cortex and cognitive control. *Nature reviews: Neuroscience, 1,* 59–65.

Miller, J. F., & Chapman, R. (1981). The relation between age and mean length of utterance in morphemes. *Journal of Speech and Hearing Research, 24,* 154–161.

Mohr, P. E., Feldman, J. J., Dunbar, J. L., McConkey-Robbins, A., Niparko, J. K., Rittenhouse, R. K., & Skinner, M. W. (2000). The societal costs of severe to profound hearing loss in the United States. *International Journal of Technology Assessment in Health Care, 16,* 1120–1135.

Montgomery, A. A., & Houston, T. (2000). The hearing-impaired adult: Management of communication deficits and tinnitus. In J. G. Alpiner & P. A. McCarthy (Eds.), *Rehabilitative audiology: Children and adults* (pp. 337–401). Baltimore: Lippincott Williams & Wilkins.

Moore, C. A., & Ruark, J. L. (1996). Does speech emerge from earlier appearing oral motor behaviors? *Journal of Speech & Hearing Research, 39*(5), 1034–1047.

Moore, D. R. (1993). Plasticity of binaural hearing and some possible mechanisms following late-onset deprivation. *Journal of the American Academy of Audiology, 4,* 277–283.

Morgan, A. S., & Mackey, L. E. (1999). Causes and complications associated with swallowing disorders in traumatic brain injury. *Journal of Head Trauma Rehabilitation, 14,* 454–461.

Mori, K. (1999). Vocal fold nodules in children: Preferable therapy. *International Journal of Pediatric Otorhinolaryngology, 49,* S303–S306.

Morris, R. J., Brown, W. S., Hicks, D. M., & Howell, E. (1995). Phonational profiles of male trained singers and nonsingers. *Journal of Voice, 9*(2), 142–148.

Moskovsky, C. (2001). *The critical period hypothesis revisited.* Paper presented at the 2001 Conference of the Australian Linguistic Society. Abstract retrieved November 12, 2003, from http://linguistics.anu.edu.au/ALS2001/proceedings.html

Münte, T. F., Altenmüller, E., & Jäncke, L. (2002). The musician's brain as a model of neuroplasticity. *Nature reviews: Neuroscience, 3,* 473–478.

Murdoch, B. E., Thompson, E. C., & Theodoros, D. G. (1997). Spastic dysarthria. In M. R. McNeil (Ed.), *Clinical management of sensorimotor speech disorders* (pp. 287–310). New York: Thieme.

Murry, T., & Carrau, R. L. (2001). *Clinical manual for swallowing disorders.* San Diego, CA: Singular.

Mysak, E. D. (1989). *Pathology of the speech system: A system approach to organic speech disorders* (2nd ed.). Springfield, IL: Charles C. Thomas.

National Academy of Sciences. (1989). *Recommended dietary allowances* (9th ed.). Washington, DC: National Research Council, Food and Nutrition Board.

National Center for Education Statistics. (2003). *State profiles.* Retrieved from http://nces.ed.gov/nationsreportcard/states/

National Center for Voice and Speech. (2004). *Voice production tutorial.* Available at http://www.ncvs.org/ncvs/tutorials/voiceprod/tutorial/quality.html

National Health Interview Survey. (2002). Summary health statistics for U. S. adults. *Vital and Health Statistics, 10*(222). Hyattsville, MD: U. S. Department of Health and Human Services.

National Institute of Dental and Craniofacial Research. (2003). *Oral-systemic health connection.* Retrieved from http://www.nidr.nih.gov/spectrum/NIDCR2/2menu.htm

National Institute on Deafness and Other Communication Disorders. (1995). *National strategic research plan for language and language disorders, balance and balance disorders, and voice and voice disorders* (NIH Publication No. 97-3217). Bethesda, MD: Author.

National Institute on Deafness and Other Communication Disorders. (2003). *Auditory processing disorder in children: What does it mean?* NIH Publication No. 01-4949. Retrieved September 14, 2003, from http://www.nidcd.nih.gov/health/voice/auditory.asp

National Institute on Deafness and Other Communication Disorders (2003). *Traumatic brain injury: Cognitive and communication disorders.* Retrieved from http://www.nidcd.nih.gov/health/voice/tbrain.asp

National Institute on Deafness and Other Communication Disorders (2005). *Statistics about hearing disorders, ear infections, and deafness*. Retrieved January 20, 2005, from http://www.nidcd.nih.gov/health/statistics/hearing.asp

National Institutes of Health. (1995). Cochlear implants in adults and children. *NIH Consensus Statement 1995, 13*(2), 1–30.

National Institutes of Health. (2000, October). Phenylketonuria: Screening and management. *NIH Consensus Statement Online, 17*(3), 1–27.

National Institutes of Health. (2002). *Stuttering* (NIH Pub. No. 97-4232). Bethesda, MD: Author.

National Joint Committee for the Communication Needs of Persons with Severe Disabilities. (1992). Guidelines for meeting the communication needs of persons with severe disabilities. *ASHA, 34,* (March, Suppl. 7), 1–8.

National Stroke Association. *What is a stroke?* Retrieved September 22, 2003, from http://www.stroke.org/TemplateSingleHTMLTextArea.aspx?P=1233987865564

Nelson, L. (1985). Language formulation related to dysfluency and stuttering. In *Stuttering therapy: Prevention and intervention with children.* Memphis, TN: Stuttering Foundation of America.

Nelson, N. W. (1998). *Childhood language disorders in context: Infancy through adolescence* (2nd ed.). Boston: Allyn & Bacon.

Newman, C. W., Hug, G. A., Jacobson, G. P., & Sandridge, S. A. (1997). Perceived hearing handicap of patients with unilateral or mild hearing loss. *Annals of Otolaryngology, Rhinology, and Laryngology, 106,* 210–214.

Newman, C. W., & Sandridge, S. A. (2004). Hearing loss is often undiscovered, but screening is easy. *Cleveland Clinic Journal of Medicine, 71,* 225–232.

Nicely, P., Tamis-LeMonda, C. S., & Bornstein, M. H. (1999). Mothers' attuned responses to infant affect expressivity promote earlier achievement of language milestones. *Infant Behavior and Development, 22,* 557–568.

Niemeier, J. P., Burnett, D. M., & Whitaker, D. A. (2003). Cultural competence in the multidisciplinary rehabilitation setting: Are we falling short of meeting needs? *Archives of Physical Medicine and Rehabilitation, 84*(8), 1240–1245.

Nilsson, H., Ekberg, O., Olsson, R., & Hindfelt, B. (1996). Quantitative assessment of oral and pharyngeal function in Parkinson's disease. *Dysphagia, 11,* 274–275.

Nippold, M. A. (1998). *Later language development: The school age and adolescent years.* Austin, TX; Pro-Ed.

Nippold, M. A. (2000). Language development during the adolescent years: Aspects of pragmatics, syntax, and semantics. *Topics in Language Disorders, 20,* 15–28.

Nittrouer, S. (1996). The relation between speech perception and phonemic awareness: Evidence from low-SES children and children with chronic OM. *Journal of Speech and Hearing Research, 39,* 1059–1070.

Nittrouer, S. (1999). Do temporal processing deficits cause phonological processing problems? *Journal of Speech, Language, and Hearing Research, 42,* 925–942.

Northern, J., & Downs, M. (1991). *Hearing in children* (4th ed.). Baltimore: Williams & Wilkins.

Nuss, R. C., Hillman, R. E., & Eavey, R. D. (1996). Office and operative diagnostic techniques: The pediatric patient and the use of videolaryngoscopy. In M. P. Fried (Ed.), *The larynx: A multidisciplinary approach* (2nd ed., pp. 65–74). Baltimore: Mosby.

O'Brien, S., Repp, A. D., Williams, G. E., & Christopherson, E. R. (1991). Pediatric feeding disorders. *Behavioral Modification, 15,* 394–418.

Occupational Safety and Health Administration (OSHA) (1992). *Occupational noise exposure—1926.52 standards.* Retrieved February 22, 2004, from http://www.osha.gov/pls/oshaweb/owadisp.show_document?p_table=STANDARDS&p_id=10625

Odderson, M. D., Keaton, J. C., & McKenna, B. S. (1995). Swallow management in patients on an acute stroke pathway: Quality is cost effective. *Archives of Physical Medicine and Rehabilitation, 76,* 1130–1133.

Oetting, J., Rice, M., & Swank, L. (1995). Quick incidental learning (QUIL) of words by school-age children with and without SLI. *Journal of Speech and Hearing Research, 38,* 434–445.

Oller, D. K. (1980). The emergence of speech sounds in infancy. In G. Yeni-Komshian, J. A. Kavanagh, & C. A. Ferguson (Eds.), *Child phonology: Vol. 1. Production* (pp. 93–112). New York: Academic Press.

Onslow, M., Andrews, C., & Lincoln, M. (1994). A control/experimental trial of an operant treatment for early stuttering. *Journal of Speech and Hearing Research, 37,* 1244–1259.

Orenstein, S. R. (1994). Gastroesophageal reflux disease. *Seminars in Gastrointestinal Disease, 5,* 2–14.

Owens, R. E., Jr. (2001). *Language development: An introduction* (5th ed.). Needham Heights, MA: Allyn & Bacon.

Pakulski, L. A., & Hinkle, A. (2003). Patient perception of aural rehabilitation. Poster presented at the Ohio Speech-Language-Hearing Association, Columbus, OH.

Palmer, E. P. (1979). Language dysfunction in cerebrovascular disease. *Primary Care,* 6(4), 827–842.

Paradise, J. L., Rockette, H. E., Colborn, D. K., Bernard, B. S., Smith, C. G., Kurs-Lasky, M., & Janosky, J. E. (1999). Otitis media in 2253 Pittsburgh-area infants: Prevalence and risk factors during the first two years of life. *Pediatrics, 103* (3), 670–672.

Paul, R. (1995). *Language disorders from infancy through adolescence: Assessment and intervention.* St. Louis, MO: Mosby-Year Book, Inc.

Paul, R. (1996). Clinical implications of the natural history of slow expressive language development. *American Journal of Speech-Language Pathology, 5,* 5–21.

Paul, R. (1998). *Literacy and deafness: The development of reading, writing, and literate thought.* Needham Heights, MA: Allyn & Bacon.

Paul, R. (2001). *Language disorders from infancy through adolescence: Assessment and intervention* (2nd ed.). St. Louis, MO: Mosby.

Paul, R., & Smith, R. L. (1993). Narrative skills in 4-year-olds with normal, impaired, and late developing language. *Journal of Speech and Hearing Research, 36,* 592–598.

Pauloski, B. R., Rademaker, A. W., Logemann, J. A., Stein, D., Beery, Q., Newman, L., et al. (2000). Pretreatment swallowing function in patients with head and neck cancer. *Head and Neck, 22,* 474–482.

Payne, V. G., & Isaacs, L. D. (1995). *Human motor development: A lifespan approach* (3rd ed.). Mountain View, CA: Mayfield Publishing Company.

Peck, K. (1997). Decibel (loudness) comparison chart. Retrieved from http://www.Hearnet.com/at_risk/risk_trivia.shtml

Pellowski, M. W., & Conture, E. G. (2002). Characteristics of speech disfluency and stuttering behaviors in 3- and 4-year-old children. *Journal of Speech, Language, and Hearing Research, 45,* 20–34.

Peña, E., Iglesias, A., & Lidz, C. S. (2001). Reducing test bias through dynamic assessment of children's word learning ability. *American Journal of Speech-Language Pathology, 10,* 138–154.

Perkell, J. S., Guenther, F. H., Lane, H., Matthies, M. L., Perrier, P., Vick, J., Wilhelms-Tricarico, R., & Zandipour, M. (2000). A theory of speech motor control and supporting data from speakers with normal hearing and with profound hearing loss. *Journal of Phonetics, 28,* 233–272.

Perlman, A. L., & Christensen, J. (1997). Topography and functional anatomy of the swallowing structures. In A. L. Perlman & K. S. Schulze-Delrieu (Eds.), *Deglutition and its disorders: Anatomy, physiology, clinical diagnosis, and management* (pp. 15–42). San Diego, CA: Singular.

Peters, T. J., & Guitar, B. (1991). *Stuttering: An integrated approach to its nature and treatment.* Baltimore: Williams & Wilkins.

Peterson, C., Jesso, B., & McCabe, A. (1999). Encouraging narratives in preschoolers: An intervention study. *Journal of Child Language, 26,* 49–67.

Petitto, L. A., Holowka, S., Sergio, L. E., & Ostry, S. (2001). Language rhythms in baby hand movements. *Nature, 413,* 35–36.

Philips, B. J., & Ruscello, D. (1998). *Differential diagnosis in speech-language pathology.* Boston: Butterworth-Heinemann.

Pimental, P. A., & Kinsbury, N. A. (1989). *Mini inventory of right brain injury.* Austin, TX: Pro-Ed.

Pinker, S. (1994). *The language instinct.* New York: HarperCollins.

Pinker, S. (1999). *Words and rules.* New York: Basic Books.

Poole, I. (1934). Genetic development of articulation of consonant sounds in speech. *Elementary English Review, 11,* 159–161.

Pore, S. G., & Reed, K. L. (1999). *Quick reference to speech-language pathology.* Gaithersburg, MD: Aspen.

Powell, M., Filter, M., & Williams, B. (1989). A longitudinal study of the prevalence of voice disorders in children from a rural school division. *Journal of Communication Disorders, 22,* 375–382.

Prather, E. M., Hedrick, D., & Kern, C. (1975). Articulation development in children aged two to four years. *Journal of Speech and Hearing Disorders, 40,* 179–191.

Prendergast, S., & Kelley, L. (2002). Aural rehabilitation services: Survey reports who offers which ones and how often. *Hearing Journal, 55,* 30–35.

Pulverman, R., Sootsman, J. L., Golinkoff, R. M., & Hirsh-Pasek, K. (2002). Infants' nonlinguistic processing of motion events: One-year-old English speakers are interested in manner and path. *Proceedings of the 31st Stanford Child Language Research Forum,* Stanford, CT.

Purdy, S. C., Farrington, D. R., Moran, C. A., Chard, L. L., & Hodgson, S. (2002). A parent questionnaire to evaluate children's auditory behavior in everyday life (ABEL), *American Journal of Audiology, 11,* 72–82.

Purdy, S. C., Moran, C. A., Chard, L., & Hodgson, S. A. (2002). Auditory behavior in everyday life. *American Journal of Audiology, 11,* 82.

Radcliffe, D. (1998). The high cost of hearing lost: What our public needs to know. *Hearing Journal, 51,* 21–30.

Ramig, L. O., Countryman, S., Thompson, L. L., & Horii, Y. (1995). Comparison of two forms of intensive speech treatment for Parkinson disease. *Journal of Speech and Hearing Research, 38,* 1232–1251.

Ramig, L. O., & Dromey, C. (1996). Aerodynamic mechanisms underlying treatment-related changes in vocal intensity in patients with Parkinson disease. *Journal of Speech and Hearing Research, 39,* 798–807.

Ramig, L. O., Pawlas, A. A., & Countryman, C. (1995). *The Lee Silverman voice treatment (LSVT): A practical guide for treating the voice and speech disorders in Parkinson disease.* Iowa City, IA: National Center for Voice and Speech.

Ramig, L. O., & Verdolini, K. (1998). Treatment efficacy: Voice disorders. *Journal of Speech, Language, and Hearing Research, 41,* S101–S116.

Ramig, P. R., & Bennett, E. M. (1995). Working with 7- to 12-year-old children who stutter: Ideas for intervention in the public schools. *Language, Speech, and Hearing Services in Schools, 26,* 138–150.

Ramsay, M. (1995). Feeding disorder and failure to thrive. *Child and Adolescent Psychiatric Clinics of North America, 4,* 605–616.

Ramsay, M., Gisel, E. G., & Boutry, M. (1993). Non-organic failure to thrive: Growth failure secondary to feeding-skills disorder. *Developmental Medicine and Child Neurology, 35,* 285–297.

Rao, P. R. (1994). The aphasia syndromes: Localization and classification. *Topics in Stroke Rehabilitation, 1*(2), 1–13.

Ratner, V. L., & Harris, L. R. (1994). *Understanding language disorders: The impact on learning.* Eau Claire, WS: Thinking Publications.

Raymer, A. M. (2001). Acquired language disorders. *Topics in Language Disorders, 21*(3), 42–59.

Reau, N. R., Senturia, Y. D., Lebailly, S. A., & Christoffel, K. K. (1996). Infant and toddler feeding patterns and problems: Normative data and a new direction. *Journal of Developmental and Behavioral Pediatrics, 17,* 149–153.

Redmond, S., & Rice, M. L. (1998). The socioemotional behaviors of children with SLI: Social adaptation or social deviance? *Journal of Speech, Language, and Hearing Research, 41,* 688–700.

Reilly, S., Skuse, D. H., & Poblete, X. (1996) The prevalence of feeding problems in pre-school children with cerebral palsy. *Journal of Pediatrics, 129,* 877–882.

Renout, K. A., Leeper, H. A., Bandur, D. L., & Hudson, A. J. (1995). Vocal fold diadochokinetic function of individuals with amyotrophic lateral sclerosis. *American Journal of Speech-Language Pathology, 4,* 73–79.

Rescorla, L. (1980). Overextension in early language development. *Journal of Child Language, 7,* 321–335.

Rescorla, L., Hadicke-Wiley, M., & Escarce, E. (1993). Epidemiological investigation of expressive language delay at age two. *First Language, 13,* 5–22.

Rescorla, L., Roberts, J., & Dahlsgaard, K. (1997). Late talkers at 2: Outcome at age 3. *Journal of Speech, Language, and Hearing Research, 40,* 556–566.

Rescorla, L., & Schwartz, E. (1990). Outcome of toddlers with specific expressive language delay. *Applied Psycholinguistics, 11,* 393–407.

Restrepo, M. A., & Silverman, S. W. (2001). Validity of the Spanish Preschool Language Scale-3 for use with bilingual children. *American Journal of Speech-Language Pathology, 10,* 382–393.

Rice, M. L. (1996). *Toward a genetics of language.* Mahwah, NJ: Lawrence Erlbaum.

Rice, M. L., Haney, K. R., & Wexler, K. (1998). Family histories of children with SLI who show extended optional infinitives. *Journal of Speech, Language, and Hearing Research, 41,* 419–432.

Rickett, D. (1998). *Review: Sandler should have punted "Waterboy."* Retrieved June 15, 2004 from http://www.cnn.com/SHOWBIZ/Movies/9811/13/review.waterboy/

Rider, E. A., & Bithoney, W. G. (1999). *Medical assessment and management and the organization of medical services.* In D. B. Kessler & P. Dawson (Eds.), *Failure to thrive and pediatric nutrition: A transdisciplinary approach* (pp. 173–193). Baltimore: Paul H. Brookes.

Riley, G. (1972). A stuttering severity instrument for children and adults. *Journal of Speech and Hearing Disorders, 37,* 314–322.

Riley, G., Maguire, G., Franklin, D., & Ortiz, T. (2001). Medical perspectives in the treatment of stuttering. *Contemporary Issues in Communication Science and Disorders, 28,* 104–110.

Robb, M. P., & Smith, A. B. (2002). Fundamental frequency onset and offset behavior: A comparative study of children and adults. *Journal of Speech, Language, and Hearing Research, 45,* 446–456.

Roberts, J. E., Burchinal, M. R., & Zeisel, S. A. (2002). Otitis media in early childhood in relation to children's school-age language and academic skills. *Pediatrics, 110*(4), 1–11.

Roberts, J. E., Wallace, I. F., & Henderson, F. W. (1997). *Otitis media in young children. Medical, developmental, and educational considerations.* Baltimore: Paul H. Brookes.

Roberts, P. (2001). Aphasia assessment and treatment for bilingual and culturally diverse patients. In R. Chapey (Ed.), *Language intervention strategies in aphasia and related communication disorders* (pp. 208–232). Philadelphia: Lippincott Williams & Wilkins.

Robertson, C., & Salter, W. (1995). *Phonological Awareness Test.* East Moline, IL: LinguiSystems.

Robertson, L. (2000). *Literacy learning for children who are deaf or hard of hearing.* Washington, DC: Alexander Graham Bell Association for the Deaf and Hard of Hearing.

Robertson, L., & Flexer, C. (1993). Reading development: A survey of children with hearing loss who developed speech and language through the auditory-verbal method. *The Volta Review, 95,* 253–261.

Robey, R. R. (1998a). The effectiveness of group treatments for aphasia: A meta-analysis. *Hearsay, 12*(1), 5–9.

Robey, R. R. (1998b). A meta-analysis of clinical outcomes in the treatment of aphasia. *Journal of Speech, Language, and Hearing Research, 41,* 172–187.

Robin, D. A., Klouda, G. V., & Hug, L. N. (1991). Neurogenic disorders of prosody. In J. Vogel & M. P. Cannito (Eds.), *Treating disordered speech motor control* (pp. 241–274). Austin, TX: Pro-Ed.

Robin, D. A., Solomon, N. P., Moon, J. B., & Folkins, J. W. (1997). Nonspeech assessment of the speech production mechanism. In M. R. McNeil (Ed.), *Clinical management of sensorimotor speech disorders* (pp. 49–62). New York: Thieme.

Robinson, T. L., & Crowe, T. A. (1998). Culture-based considerations in programming for stuttering intervention with African American clients and their families. *Language, Speech, and Hearing Services in Schools, 29,* 172–179.

Rodriguez, B. L., & Olswang, L. B. (2003). Mexican-American and Anglo-American mothers' beliefs and values about child rearing, education, and language impairment. *American Journal of Speech-Language Pathology, 12,* 452–462.

Rogers, M. A., King, J. M., & Alarcon, N. B. (2000). Proactive management of primary progressive aphasia. In D. R. Beukelman, K. M. Yorkston, & J. Reichle (Eds.), *Augmentative and alternative communication for adults with acquired neurologic disorders* (pp. 305–337). Baltimore: Paul H. Brookes.

Rood, D. S., & Taylor, A. R. (1996). *Handbook of North American Indians: Vol. 17, languages.* Washington, DC: The Smithsonian Institution.

Rosen, D. C., & Sataloff, R. T. (1997). *Psychology of voice disorders.* San Diego, CA: Singular.

Rosenbek, J. C., LaPointe, L. L., & Wertz, R. T. (1989). *Aphasia: A clinical approach.* Austin, TX: Pro-Ed.

Rosenbek, J. C., Robbins, J. A., Roecker, E. B., Coyle, J. L., & Wood, J. L. (1996). A penetration-aspiration scale. *Dysphagia, 11,* 93–98.

Rosenberg, S., & Abbeduto, L. (1993). *Language and communication in mental retardation.* Hillsdale, NJ: Lawrence Erlbaum.

Ross, D. G. (1996). *Ross information processing assessment* (2nd ed.). Austin, TX: Pro-Ed.

Rossetti, L. M. (2001). *Communication intervention: Birth to three* (3rd ed.). Albany, NY: Delmar.

Roth, C., Aronson, A., & Davis, L. (1989). Clinical studies in psychogenic stuttering of adult onset. *Journal of Speech and Hearing Disorders, 54,* 634–646.

Roy, N., Merrill, R. M., Thibeault, S., Parsa, R. A., Gray, S. D., & Smith, E. M. (2004). Prevalence of voice disorders in teachers and the general population. *Journal of Speech, Language, and Hearing Research, 47,* 281–293.

Russell, A., Penny, L., & Pemberton, C. (1995). Speaking fundamental frequency changes over time in women: A longitudinal study. *Journal of Speech and Hearing Research, 38,* 101–109.

Russell, N. K. (1993). Educational considerations in traumatic brain injury: The role of the speech-language pathologist. *Language, Speech, and Hearing Services in Schools, 24,* 67–75.

Rustin, L., & Cook, F. (1995). Parental involvement in the treatment of stuttering. *Language, Speech, and Hearing Services in Schools, 26,* 127–137.

Rvachew, S., Rafaat, S., & Martin, M. (1999). Stimulability, speech perception skills, and the treatment of phonological disorders. *American Journal of Speech-Language Pathology, 8,* 33–43.

Sala, E., Laine, A., Simberg, S., Pentti, J., & Suonpaa, J. (2001). The prevalence of voice disorders among day care center teachers compared with nurses: A questionnaire and clinical study. *Journal of Voice, 15,* 413–423.

Salend, S. J., & Salinas, A. (2003). Language differences or learning difficulties: The work of the multidisciplinary team. *Teaching Exceptional Children, 35*(4), 36–43.

Sambunaris, A., & Hyde, T. M. (1994). Stroke-related aphasia mistaken for psychotic speech: Two case reports. *Journal of Geriatric Psychiatry and Neurology, 7*(3), 144–147.

Sander, E. K. (1972). When are speech sounds learned? *Journal of Speech and Hearing Disorders, 37,* 55–63.

Sapienza, C. M., Ruddy, B. H., & Baker, S. (2004). Laryngeal structure and function in the pediatric larynx: Clinical applications. *Language, Speech, and Hearing Services in Schools, 35,* 299–307.

Satter, E. M. (1986). The feeding relationship. *Journal of American Dietetic Association, 86,* 352–356.

Satter, E. M. (1996). *Feeding with love and good sense: Training manual for the VISIONS workshop* (pp. 49–51) Madison, WI: Ellen Satter Institute.

Satter, E. M. (1999). *Secrets of feeding a healthy family*. Madison, WI: Ellen Satter Institute.

Scarborough, H. S. (2000). Connecting early language and literacy to later reading (dis)abilities: Evidence, theory, and practice. In S. B. Neuman & D. K. Dickinson (Eds.), *Handbook of early literacy research* (pp. 97–110). New York: Guilford Press.

Schauster, H., & Dwyer, J. (1996). Transition from tube feedings to feedings by mouth in children: Preventing eating dysfunction. *Journal of the American Dietetic Association, 96,* 277–281.

Scheetz, N. A. (2001). *Orientation to deafness* (2nd ed.). Nordham Heights, MA: Allyn & Bacon.

Schmidt, R. A. (1976). The schema as a solution to some persistent problems in motor learning theory. In G. L. Stelmach (Ed.), *Motor control: Issues and trends* (pp. 41–65). New York: Academic

Schmidt, R. A. (2003). Motor schema theory after 27 years: Reflections and implications for a new theory. *Research Quarterly for Exercise and Sport, 74*(4), 366–375.

Schmidt, R. A., & Bjork, R. A. (1992). New conceptualizations of practice: common principles in three paradigms suggest new concepts for training. *Psychological Science, 3*(4), 207–217.

Schmidt, R. A., & Lee, T. D. (1999). *Motor control and learning: A behavioral emphasis* (3rd ed.). Champaign, IL: Human Kinetics.

Schow, R., Balsara, N., Smedley, T., & Whitcomb, C. (1993). Aural rehabilitation by ASHA audiologists: 1980–1990. *American Journal of Audiology, 2,* 28–37.

Schow, R. L. (2001). A standardized AR battery for dispensers is proposed, *Hearing Journal, 54,* 10–20.

Schow, R. L., & Nerbonne, M. (1982). Communication screening profile uses with elderly clients. *Ear and Hearing, 3,* 133–147.

Schow, R. L., Seikel, J. A., Chermak, G. D., & Berent, M. (2000). Central auditory processes and test measures: ASHA 1996 revisited. *American Journal of Audiology, 9,* 63–68.

Schuele, C. M., & Hadley, P. A. (1999). Potential advantages of introducing specific language impairment to families. *American Journal of Speech-Language Pathology, 8,* 11–22.

Schulze-Delrieu, K. S., & Miller, R. M. (1997). Clinical assessment of dysphagia. In A. L. Perlman & K. S. Schulze-Delrieu (Eds.), *Deglutition and its disorders: Anatomy, physiology, clinical diagnosis, and management* (pp. 125–152). San Diego, CA: Singular.

Schurr, M. J., Ebner, K. A., Maser, A. L., Sperling, K. B., Helgerson, R. B., & Harms, B. (1999). Formal swallowing evaluation and therapy after traumatic brain injury improves dysphagia outcomes. *Journal of Trauma, 46,* 817–821.

Sears, H. (2003). *Average brain weights*. Retrieved November 2003, from http://www.sc.edu/union/Sears/brain.htm

Secord, W. A., & Wiig, E. H. (2003). *Practical performance assessment.* Sedona, AZ: Red Rock Educational Publications.

Seddoh, S. A. K., & Robin, D. A. (2001). Neurogenic disorders of prosody. In D. Vogel & M. Cannito (Eds.), *Treating disordered speech motor control: For clinicians by clinicians* (2nd ed., pp. 277–320). Austin, TX: Pro-Ed.

Shapiro, L., Swinney, D., & Borsky, S. (1998). Online examination of language performance in normal and neurologically impaired adults. *American Journal of Speech-Language Pathology, 7,* 49–60.

Shea, C. H., Lai, Q., Wright, D. L., Immink, M., & Black, C. (2001). Consistent and variable practice conditions: Effects on relative and absolute timing. *Journal of Motor Behavior, 33*(2), 139–152.

Shipley, K. G., & McAfee, J. G. (1998). *Assessment in speech-language pathology: A resource manual* (2nd ed.). San Diego, CA: Singular.

Shiro, M. (2003). Genre and evaluation in narrative development. *Journal of Child Language, 30,* 165–195.

Shriberg, L. (1997). Developmental phonological disorders: One or many? In B. W. Hodson & M. L. Edwards (Eds.), *Perspectives in applied phonology* (pp. 105–131). Gaithersburg, MD: Aspen Publishers.

Shriberg, L. D., Austin, D., Lewis, B. A., McSweeney, J. L., & Wilson, D. L. (1997a). The percentage of consonants correct (PCC) metric: Extensions and reliability data. *Journal of Speech-Languge-Hearing Research, 40,* 708–722.

Shriberg, L. D., Austin, D., Lewis, B. A., McSweeney, J. L., & Wilson, D. L. (1997b). The Speech Disorders Classification System (SDCS): Extensions and lifespan reference data. *Journal of Speech-Language-Hearing Research, 40,* 723–740.

Shriberg, L. D., Flipsen, P., Kwiatkowski, J., & McSweeney, J. L. (2003). A diagnostic marker for speech delay associated with otitis media with effusion: The intelligibility-speech gap. *Clinical Linguistics and Phonetics, 17,* 507–528.

Shriberg, L. D., Gruber, F. A., & Kwiatkowski, J. (1994). Developmental phonological disorders: III. Long-term speech-sound normalization. *Journal of Speech and Hearing Research, 37,* 1151–1177.

Shriberg, L. D., Kent, R. D., Karlsson, H. B., McSweeney, J. L., Nadler, C. J., & Brown, R. L. (2003). A diagnostic marker for speech delay associated with otitis media with effusion: Backing of obstruents. *Clinical Linguistics and Phonetics, 17,* 529–547.

Shriberg, L. D., & Kwiatkowski, J. (1994). Developmental phonological disorders: I. A clinical profile. *Journal of Speech and Hearing Research, 37,* 1100–1126.

Shriberg, L. D., Kwiatkowski, J., & Gruber, F. A. (1994). Developmental phonological disorders: II. Short-term speech-sound normalization. *Journal of Speech and Hearing Research, 37,* 1127–1150.

Shriberg, L. D., Tomblin, J. B., & McSweeney, J. L. (1999). Prevalence of speech delay in 6-year-old children with comorbidity with language impairment. *Journal of Speech, Language, and Hearing Research, 42,* 1461–1481.

Shuster, L. I., & Wambaugh, J. L. (2003). Consistency of speech sound errors in apraxia of speech accompanied by aphasia. Poster presented at the Clinical Aphasiology Conference, Orca's Island, WA.

Sicher, H., & DuBrul, E. L. (1975). *Oral anatomy* (6th ed.). St. Louis, MO: Mosby.

Simon, C. S. (1991). Functional flexibility: Developing communicative competence in the speaker and listener roles. In C. S. Simon (Ed.), *Communication skills and classroom success.* Eau Claire, WI: Thinking Publications.

Simser, J. (1995, October). *Assessment and goal setting.* Paper presented at the Natural Communications—Auditory Verbal International Conference. Cuyahoga Falls, OH.

Siren, K. (2004). Cleft lip and palate. In L. Schoenbrodt (Ed.), *Childhood communication disorders: Organic bases* (pp. 187–228). Clifton Park, NY: Delmar Learning.

Smith, A., Denny, M., Shaffer, L. A., Kelly, E. M., & Hirano, M. (1996). Activity of intrinsic laryngeal muscles in fluent and disfluent speech. *Journal of Speech and Hearing Research, 39,* 329–348.

Smith, A., & Goffman, L. (1998). Stability and patterning of speech movement sequences in children and adults. *Journal of Speech, Language, and Hearing Research, 41,* 18–31.

Smith, B. C., & Pederson, A. L. (1990, September/October). Nutrition focus: Tube feeding update. *Nutrition for Children with Special Health Care Needs, 5*(5), 1–5.

Society for Neuroscience. (2004). *Hearing loss: Making a difference today.* Washington, DC: Author.

Solomon, N. P., McKee, A. S., & Garcia-Barry, S. (2001). Intensive voice treatment and respiration treatment for hypokinetic-spastic dysarthria after traumatic brain injury. *American Journal of Speech-Language Pathology, 10,* 51–64.

Soto, G., Blake Huer, M., & Taylor O. (1997). Multicultural issues. In L. L. Lloyd, D. R. Fuller, & H. H. Arvidson (Eds.), *Augmentative and alternative communication: A handbook of principles and practices* (pp. 406–413). Needham Heights, MA: Allyn & Bacon.

St. Louis, K. O., & Myers, F. L. (1995). Clinical management of cluttering. *Language, Speech, and Hearing Services in Schools, 26,* 187–195.

Stager, C. L., & Werker, J. F. (1997). Infants listen for more phonetic detail in speech perception than in word-learning tasks. *Nature, 388,* 381–382.

Stanovich, K. E. (2000). *Progress in understanding reading: Scientific foundations and new frontiers.* New York: Guilford Press.

Stemple, J. C., Glaze, L. E., & Gerdeman, B. K. (1995). *Clinical voice pathology: Theory and management* (2nd ed.). San Diego, CA: Singular.

Stevenson, R. D., & Allaire, J. H. (1991). The development of normal feeding and swallowing. *Pediatric Clinics of North America, 38,* 1439–1453.

Stika, C. J., Ross, M., & Cuevas, C. (2002). Hearing aid services and satisfaction: The consumer viewpoint. *Hearing Loss, 23*(3), 25–31.

Stoel-Gammon, C., & Dunn, C. (1985). *Normal and disordered phonology in children.* Austin, TX: Pro-Ed.

Storkel, H. L., & Morrisette, M. L. (2002). The lexicon and phonology: Interactions in language acquisition. *Language, Speech, and Hearing Services in Schools, 33,* 24–37.

Stothard, S. E., Snowling, M. J., Bishop, D. V. M., Chipchase, B. B., & Kaplan, C. A. (1998). Language-impaired preschoolers: A follow-up into adolescence. *Journal of Speech, Language, and Hearing Research, 41,* 407–418.

Strand, E. A., Buder, E. H., Yorkston, K. M., & Ramig, L. O. (1994). Differential phonatory characteristics of four women with amyotrophic lateral sclerosis. *Journal of Voice, 8,* 327–339.

Strom, K. E. (2001). The HR 2000 dispenser survey. *The Hearing Review, 8*(6), 20–42.

Stroudley, J., & Walsh, M. (1991). Radiological assessment of dysphagia in Parkinson's disease. *The British Journal of Radiology, 64,* 890–893.

Sturm, L., & Dawson, P. (1999). Working with families: An overview for providers. In D. B. Kessler & P. Dawson (Eds.), *Failure to thrive and pediatric undernutrition: A transdisciplinary approach* (pp. 65–76). Baltimore: Paul H. Brookes.

Stuttering Foundation of America (2004). *Famous people who stutter.* Retrieved June 10, 2004, from http://www.stutteringhelp.org/celebrit.htm

Surveillance, Epidemiology, and End Results (SEER) Program: SEER*Stat Database (Incidence–SEER 9 Regs Public-Use, Nov. 2003 Sub [1973–2001]). National Cancer Institute, DCCPS, Surveillance Research Program, Cancer Statistics Branch. Released April 2004, based on the November 2003 submission. Retrieved from http://www.seer.cancer.gov

Tamis-LeMonda, C. S., Bornstein, M., & Baumwell, L. (2001). Maternal responsiveness and children's achievement of language milestones. *Child Development, 72,* 748–767.

Taylor, G. R. (2001). *Educational interventions and services for children with exceptionalities.* Springfield, IL: Charles C Thomas.

Taylor, K., & Jurma, W. (1999). Study suggests that group rehabilitation increases benefit of hearing aid fittings. *Hearing Journal, 52,* 48–54.

Taylor, O. (1986). *Nature of communication disorders in culturally and linguistically diverse populations.* San Diego, CA: College-Hill Press.

Teasdale, G., & Jennett, B. (1974). Assessment of coma and impaired consciousness. *Lancet,* 2, 81–84.

Templin, M. (1957). *Certain language skills in children: Their development and interrelationships* (Institute of Child Welfare Monograph No. 26). Minneapolis, MN: University of Minnesota Press.

Thal, D., & Tobias, S. (1992). Communicative gestures in children with delayed onset of oral expressive vocabulary. *Journal of Speech and Hearing Research, 35,* 1281–1289.

Thompson, C. K., Ballard, K. J., & Shapiro, L. P. (1998). Role of syntactic complexity in training Wh-movement structures in agrammatic aphasia: Optimal order for promoting generalization. *Journal of the International Neuropsychological Society, 4,* 661–674.

Thompson, C. K., & Robin, D. A. (1993). Developmental dysarthria. In G. Blanken, J. Dittmann, H. Grimm, J. C. Marshall, & C. W. Wallesch (Eds.), *Linguistic disorders and pathologies: An international handbook* (pp. 834–858). Berlin: Walter de Gruyter.

Thurman, D. J., Alverson, C., Dunn, K. A., Guerrero, J., & Sniezek, J. E. (1999). Traumatic brain injury in the United States: A public health perspective. *Journal of Head Trauma Rehabilitation, 14,* 602–615.

Titze, I. R. (1994). *Principles of voice production.* Upper Saddle River, NJ: Prentice Hall.

Tomasello, M., & Todd, J. (1983). Joint attention and lexical acquisition style. *First Language, 4,* 197–212.

Tomblin, J. B. (1989). Familial concentration of developmental language impairment. *Journal of Speech and Hearing Disorders, 54,* 287–295.

Tomblin, J. B., Records, N. L., Buckwalter, P., Zhang, X., Smith, E., & O'Brien, M. (1997). Prevalence of specific language impairment in kindergarten children. *Journal of Speech, Language, and Hearing Research, 40,* 1245–1260.

Tomoeda, C., & Bayles, K. (2002, April 2). Cultivating cultural competence in the workplace, classroom, and clinic. *ASHA Leader, 7*(6), 4.

Torgesen, J. (1993). Variations of theory in learning disabilities. In G. R. Lyon, D. B. Gray, J. F. Kavanagh, & N. A. Krasnegor (Eds.), *Better understanding learning disabilities* (pp. 153–170). Baltimore: Paul H. Brookes.

Torgesen, J., Wagner, R., & Rashotte, C. (1994). Longitudinal studies of phonological processing and reading. *Journal of Learning Disabilities, 27,* 276–286.

Torres, L. Y., & Sirbegovic, D. J. (2004). Clinical benefits of the Passy-Muir tracheostomy and ventilator speaking valves in the NICU. *Neonatal Intensive Care, 17*(4), 20–23.

Tremblay, K. (2003). Central auditory plasticity: Implications for audiologic rehabilitation. *Hearing Journal, 56,* 10–15.

Tremblay, K., & Cunningham, L. (2002). Is there a genetic link between noise-induced and age-related hearing loss? *Audiology Today 14,* 21.

Trychin, S. (2002). *Living with hearing loss workbook,* Erie, PA: Author. Obtained November, 2004, from the American Speech-Language-Hearing Association annual conference, Chigago.

Turkstra, L. S. (1999). Language testing in adolescents with brain injury: A consideration of the CELF-3. *Language, Speech, and Hearing Services in Schools, 30,* 132–140.

Tye-Murray, N. (1998). *Foundations of audiological rehabilitation: Children, adults, and their family members.* San Diego, CA: Singular.

Tye-Murray, N. (2000). The child who has severe or profound hearing loss. In J. B. Tomblin, H. L. Morris, & D. C. Spriestersbach (Eds.), *Diagnosis in speech-language pathology* (2nd ed.). San Diego, CA: Singular.

Tyler, A. A., Lewis, K. E., Haskill, A., & Tolbert, L. C. (2002). Efficacy and cross-domain effects of a morphosyntax and a phonology intervention. *Language, Speech, and Hearing Services in Schools, 33,* 52–66.

Tyler, A. A., Lewis, K. E., Haskill, A., & Tolbert, L. C. (2003). Outcomes of different speech and language goal attack strategies. *Journal of Speech, Language, and Hearing Research, 46,* 1077–1094.

U. S. Congress. (1997). *Individuals with Disabilities Education Act Amendments of 1997.* Washington, DC: Government Printing Office.

U. S. Department of Education. (1999). Assistance to states for the education of children with disabilities and the early intervention program for infants and toddlers with disabilities: Final regulations. *Federal Register, 64*(48), CFR Parts 300 and 303.

U. S. Department of Education. (2001). *Twenty-third annual report to Congress on the implementation of the Individuals with Disabilities Education Act.* Washington, DC: Author.

U. S. Department of Education. (2002). *Digest of education statistics, 2003.* Washington, DC: U. S. Department of Education, National Center for Education Statistics.

U. S. Department of Education. (2002). *Twenty-fourth annual report to Congress on the implementation of the Individuals with Disabilities Education Act.* Washington, DC: Author.

U. S. Department of Health and Human Services. (1999). *Traumatic brain injury in the United States: A report to Congress.* Washington, DC: Author.

U. S. Department of Health and Human Services. (2000). *Healthy People 2010: Vol. II* (2nd ed.). *Objective for improving health* (Part B: Focus areas 15–28). Washington, DC: Author.

Van Bergeijk, W. A., Pierce, J. R., & David, E. E. (1960). *Waves and the ear.* New York: Doubleday.

Vanderheiden, G. C., & Yoder, D. E. (1986). Overview. In S. W. Blackstone (Ed.), *Augmentative communication: An introduction.* Rockville, MD: American Speech-Language-Hearing Association.

Van Der Lely, H. K. J., & Stollwerck, L. (1996). A grammatical specific language impairment in children: An autosomal dominant inheritance? *Brain and Language, 52,* 484–504.

Van der Merwe, A. (1997). A theoretical framework for the characterization of pathological speech sensorimotor control. In M. R. McNeil (Ed.), *Clinical management of sensorimotor speech disorders* (pp. 1–25). New York: Thieme.

Van de Sandt-Koenderman, W. M. E., Wielaert, S., & Wiegers, J. (2003). *Back in control: The benefits of a palmtop computer with a personalized vocabulary.* Paper presented at the Clinical Aphasiology Conference, Orca's Island, WA.

van Lieshout, P. H. H., Hulstijn, W., & Peters, H. F. M. (1996). From planning to articulation in speech production: What differentiates a person who stutters from a person who does not stutter? *Journal of Speech and Hearing Research, 39,* 546–564.

Van Riper, C. (1963). *Speech correction: Principles and methods* (4th ed.). Upper Saddle River, NJ: Prentice Hall.

Van Riper, C. (1973). *The treatment of stuttering.* Upper Saddle River, NJ: Prentice Hall.

Van Riper, C. (1982). *The nature of stuttering* (2nd ed.). Upper Saddle River, NJ: Prentice Hall.

Vanryckeghem, M., & Brutten, G. J. (1997). The speech-associated attitude of children who do and do not stutter and the differential effect of age. *American Journal of Speech-Language Pathology, 6,* 67–73.

Ventry, I., & Weinstein, B. (1982). The hearing handicap inventory for the elderly, a new tool. *Ear and Hearing, 3,* 128–134.

Verdolini, K. (2000). Voice disorders. In J. B. Tomblin, H. L. Morris, & D. C. Spriestersbach (Eds.), *Diagnosis in speech-language pathology* (2nd ed., pp. 233–280). San Diego, CA: Singular.

Vihman, M. M. (1998). Early phonological development. In J. E. Bernthal & N. W. Bankson (Eds.), *Articulation and phonological disorders* (4th ed.). Boston: Allyn & Bacon.

Vihman, M. M., & Greenlee, M. (1987). Individual differences in phonological development: Ages one and three years. *Journal of Speech and Hearing Research, 30,* 503–521.

von Leden, H. (1985). Vocal nodules in children. *Ear Nose Throat Journal, 64*(10), 473–480.

Vygotsky, L. (1978). *Mind in society: The development of higher psychological processes.* Cambridge, MA: Harvard University Press.

Wada, H., Nakajoh, K., Satoh-Nakagawa, T., Suzuki, T., Ohrui, T, Arai, H., et al. (2001). Risk factors of aspiration pneumonia in Alzheimer's disease patients. *Gerontology, 47,* 271–276.

Wagner, C. W. (1996). Speech rehabilitation following total laryngectomy. In M. P. Fried (Ed.), *The larynx: A multidisciplinary approach* (2nd ed., pp. 611–629). Baltimore: Mosby.

Wagner, R. K., Torgesen, J. K., & Rashotte, C. A. (1999). *Comprehensive test of phonological processing.* Austin, TX: Pro-Ed.

Wambaugh, J. L., Kalinyak-Fliszar, M., West, J. E., & Doyle, P. J. (1998). Effects of treatment for sound errors in apraxia of speech and aphasia. *Journal of Speech Language and Hearing Research, 41,* 725–743.

Wambaugh, J. L., Martinez, A. L., McNeil, M. R., & Rogers, M. A. (1999). Sound production treatment for apraxia of speech: Overgeneralization and maintenance effects. *Aphasiology, 13*(9–11), 821–837.

Wambaugh, J. L., West, J. E., & Doyle, P. J. (1998). Treatment for apraxia of speech: Effects of targeting sound groups. *Aphasiology, 12*(7/8), 731–743.

Watkins, R., & Rice, M. L. (Eds.). (1994). *Specific language impairments in children.* Baltimore: Paul H. Brookes.

Watkins, R., Rice, M., & Molz, C. (1993). Verb use by language-impaired and normally developing children. *First Language, 37,* 133–143.

Watterson, T., Hansen-Magorian, H. J., & McFarlane, S. C. (1990). A demographic description of laryngeal contact ulcer patients. *Journal of Voice, 4,* 71–75.

Wehler, C. A., Scott, R. A., & Anderson, J. J. (1991). A survey of childhood hunger in the United States. Washington, DC: Food Research and Action Center.

Weinstein, B. E. (2000). *Geriatric audiology.* New York: Thieme.

Weintraub, S., Rubin, N. P., & Mesulam, M. M. (1990). Primary progressive aphasia: Longitudinal course, neuropsychological profile, and language features. *Archives of Neurology, 47,* 1329–1335.

Weismer, S. E., Evans, J., & Hesketh, L. J. (1999). An examination of verbal working memory capacity in children with specific language impairment. *Journal of Speech, Language, and Hearing Research, 42,* 1249–1260.

Wellman, B. L., Case, I. M., Mengert, I. G., & Bradbury, D. E. (1931). Speech sounds of young children. *University of Iowa Studies in Child Welfare, 5,* Iowa City: University of Iowa Press.

Wertz, R. T., LaPointe, L. L., & Rosenbek, J. C. (1984). *Apraxia of speech in adults: The disorder and its management*. Orlando, FL: Grune & Stratton.

Westby, C. (1980). Assessment of cognitive and language abilities through play. *Language, Speech, and Hearing Services in Schools, 11,* 155–168.

Westby, C. (2000). Multicultural issues in speech and language assessment. In J. B. Tomblin, H. L. Morris, & D. C. Spriestersbach (Eds.), *Diagnosis in speech-language pathology* (2nd ed., pp. 35–61). San Diego, CA: Singular.

Westby, C. E. (1985). Learning to talk—Talking to learn: Oral-literate language differences. In C. S. Simon (Ed.), *Communication skills and classroom success: Assessment and therapy methodologies for language-learning disabled students* (pp. 181–213). San Diego, CA: College-Hill Press.

Westby, C. E. (1991). Learning to talk—Talking to learn: Oral-literate language differences. In C. S. Simon (Ed.), *Communication skills and classroom success: Assessment and therapy methodologies for language and learning disabled students.* Eau Claire, WI: Thinking Publications.

Whorf, B. (1956). *Language, thought, and reality.* New York: Wiley.

Wilbarger, P., & Wilbarger, J. (1991). *Sensory defensiveness in children: An intervention guide for parents and other caretakers.* Santa Barbara, CA: Avanti Educational Programs.

Wilkins, D. P. (2003). *Psycholinguistic considerations in representation selection for communicative interaction: Why it is that interactions are impaired, not individuals.* Paper presented at the meeting of the Department of Special Education and Communicative Disorders, San Francisco State University, San Francisco, CA.

Williams, A. L. (1993). Phonological reorganization: A qualitative measure of phonological improvement. *American Journal of Speech-Language Pathology, 2,* 44–51.

Williams, A. L. (2000). Multiple oppositions: Theoretical foundations for an alternative contrastive intervention approach. *American Journal of Speech-Language Pathology, 9,* 282–288.

Williams, A. L. (2002). Epilogue: Perspectives in the assessment of children's speech. *American Journal of Speech-Language Pathology, 11,* 259–263.

Wilson, W. J., & Herbstein, N. (2003). The role of music intensity in aerobics: Implications for hearing conservation. *Journal of the American Academy of Audiology, 14,* 29–38.

Wingate, M. (1976). *Stuttering theory and treatment.* New York: Irvington Publishers.

Wingate, M. E. (2001). SLD is not stuttering [Letter to the editor]. *Journal of Speech, Language, and Hearing Research, 44,* 381–383.

Winkworth, A. L., Davis, P. J., Adams, R. D., & Ellis, E. (1995). Breathing patterns during spontaneous speech. *Journal of Speech and Hearing Research, 38,* 124–144.

Wohlert, A. B., & Smith, A. (2002). Developmental change in variability of lip muscle activity during speech. *Journal of Speech, Language, and Hearing Research, 45,* 1077–1087.

World Health Organization. (2001). *International classification of diseases, disabilities, and handicaps.* Geneva: Author.

Yairi, E., & Ambrose, N. (1992). A longitudinal study of stuttering in children: A preliminary report. *Journal of Speech and Hearing Research, 35,* 755–760.

Yairi, E., & Ambrose, N. (1999). Early childhood stuttering: I. Persistency and recovery rates. *Journal of Speech, Language, and Hearing Research, 42,* 1097–1112.

Yairi, E., Ambrose, N., & Cox, N. (1996). Genetics of stuttering: A critical review. *Journal of Speech and Hearing Research, 39,* 771–784.

Yamamoto, L., & Magamonk, E. (2003). Outcome measures in stroke. *Critical Care Nursing Quarterly, 26*(4), 283–293.

Yaruss, J. S. (1997). Clinical measurement of stuttering behaviors. *Contemporary Issues in Communication Science and Disorders, 24,* 33–44.

Yaruss, J. S., LaSalle, L. R., & Conture, E. G. (1998). Evaluating stuttering in young children: Diagnostic data. *American Journal of Speech-Language Pathology, 7*(4), 62–76.

Yoos, H. L., Kitzman, H., & Cole, R. (1999). Family routines and the feeding process. In D. B. Kessler & P. Dawson (Eds.), *Failure to thrive and pediatric undernutrition: A transdisciplinary approach* (pp. 375–384). Baltimore: Paul H. Brookes.

Yorkston, K. M., Beukelman, D. R., Strand, E., & Bell, K. R. (1999). *Clinical management of motor speech disorders in children and adults.* Boston, MA: Little Brown.

Yorkston, K. M., Beukelman, D. R., & Tice, R. (1996). *Sentence intelligibility test.* Lincoln, NE: Tice Technology Services.

Yorkston, K. M., Miller, R. M., & Strand, E. A. (1995). *Management of speech and swallowing in degenerative diseases.* Tucson, AZ: Communication Skill Builders.

Yoshinaga-Itano, C. (2003). From screening to early identification and intervention: Discovering predictors to successful outcomes for children with significant hearing loss. *Journal of Deaf Studies and Deaf Education, 8,* 11–30.

Yoshinaga-Itano, C., Sedey, A., Coulter, D., & Mehl, A. (1998). Language of early- and later-identified children with hearing loss. *Pediatrics, 100,* 135–164.

Young, B., & Drewett, R. (2000). Eating behavior and its variability in 1-year-old children. *Appetite, 35,* 171–177.

Yueh, B., Shapiro, N., MacLean, C. H., & Shekelle, P. G. (2003). Screening and management of adult hearing loss in primary care. *Journal of the American Medical Association, 289,* 1976–1985.

Zebrowski, P. M. (1994). Duration of sound prolongation and sound/syllable repetition in children who stutter: Preliminary observations. *Journal of Speech and Hearing Research, 37,* 254–263.

Zebrowski, P. M. (1997). Assisting young children who stutter and their families: Defining the role of the speech-language pathologist. *American*

Journal of Speech-Language Pathology, 6(2), 19–28.

Zebrowski, P. M. (2000). Stuttering. In J. B. Tomblin, H. L. Morris, & D. C. Spriestersbach (Eds.), *Diagnosis in speech-language pathology* (2nd ed., pp. 199–232). San Diego, CA: Singular.

Zemlin, W. R. (1988). *Speech and hearing science: Anatomy and physiology* (3rd ed.). Upper Saddle River, NJ: Prentice Hall.

Zhang, C., & Bennett, T. (2004). Embracing cultural and linguistic diversity during the IFSP and IEP process: Implications from DEC recommended practice. In *Serving the underserved: A review of the research and practice in child find, assessment, and the IFSP/IEP process for culturally and linguistically diverse young children.* Washington, DC: ERIC Clearinghouse on Disabilities and Gifted Education.

Name Index

Subject Index